Dearborn High Athletic Dept.
19501 Outer Drive
Dearborn, MI 48124

ATHLETIC TRAINING AND SPORTS MEDICINE

FIRST EDITION

Published by

 AMERICAN ACADEMY OF ORTHOPAEDIC SURGEONS

444 North Michigan Avenue, Suite 1500, Chicago, Illinois 60611

CREDITS

Book design and production: The Book Department, Inc.
Medical illustration: Susan Banta, Laurel Cook, and Sharon Ellis
Technical illustration: Paul S. Foti, Boston Graphics, Inc.
Photography: Dr. Edgardo Gonzalez-Ramirez and Katie Zernhelt
Cover design: Wilken / Reich / Wilder

EDITORIAL BOARD

FIRST EDITION

Copyright © 1984 by American Academy of Orthopaedic Surgeons.

Library of Congress Cataloging in Publication Data

American Academy of Orthopaedic Surgeons
Athletic Training and Sports Medicine
ISBN 0–89203–002–X

Published by The American Academy of Orthopaedic Surgeons
444 North Michigan Avenue, Suite 1500
Chicago, Illinois 60611-3981
November 15, 1984

Table of Contents

Preface		*v*
Acknowledgements		*vi*
PART 1	INTRODUCTION	1
Chapter 1	Pioneers in Sports Medicine	3
Chapter 2	The Sports Medicine Team	7
Chapter 3	Organization of a Sports Medicine Program	12
PART 2	ANATOMY AND DIAGNOSTIC SIGNS	21
Chapter 4	General and Topographic Anatomy	23
Chapter 5	Diagnostic Signs and Triage	36
PART 3	TAPING AND BANDAGING	45
Chapter 6	Introduction to Taping and Bandaging	47
Chapter 7	Upper Extremity Taping	51
Chapter 8	Lower Extremity Taping	66
Chapter 9	Elastic Bandaging Procedures	81
PART 4	PROTECTIVE DEVICES	93
Chapter 10	Principles of Protective Devices	95
Chapter 11	Upper and Lower Extremities	97
Chapter 12	Other Protective Devices	101
PART 5	CONDITIONING, REHABILITATION AND USE OF MODALITIES	109
Chapter 13	Psychological Considerations in Working with Athletes	111
Chapter 14	Athletic Training, Conditioning and Reconditioning	115
Chapter 15	Modalities in Athletic Training	133
PART 6	MUSCULOSKELETAL SYSTEM	145
Chapter 16	Injuries to the Musculoskeletal System	147
Chapter 17	Introduction to Biomechanics	178
Chapter 18	The Shoulder and Upper Extremity	189
Chapter 19	The Pelvis	229
Chapter 20	The Hip and Thigh	230
Chapter 21	The Knee	236
Chapter 22	The Lower Leg	306

Chapter 23	The Ankle	314
Chapter 24	The Foot	321
PART 7	CARDIORESPIRATORY SYSTEM	329
Chapter 25	The Respiratory System	331
Chapter 26	Injuries to the Chest	340
Chapter 27	The Hematologic System	350
Chapter 28	The Cardiovascular System	353
Chapter 29	Control of Bleeding	361
Chapter 30	Shock	365
Chapter 31	Basic Life Support	374
PART 8	NERVOUS SYSTEM	391
Chapter 32	Injuries of the Head and Spine	393
Chapter 33	Facial Injuries	412
PART 9	GASTROINTESTINAL AND GENITOURINARY SYSTEMS	415
Chapter 34	The Abdomen and Digestive System	417
Chapter 35	The Acute Abdomen	425
Chapter 36	Injuries of the Abdomen	429
Chapter 37	The Genitourinary System	432
Chapter 38	Common Gastrointestinal and Genitourinary Complaints	438
PART 10	MEDICAL EMERGENCIES	445
Chapter 39	Acute Chest Pain	447
Chapter 40	Shortness of Breath	452
Chapter 41	Sudden Loss of Consciousness	456
PART 11	SPECIAL MEDICAL CONSIDERATIONS	463
Chapter 42	Women Athletes	465
Chapter 43	The Diabetic Athlete	473
Chapter 44	The Asthmatic Athlete	476
Chapter 45	The Physically Impaired Athlete	478
Chapter 46	Communicable Diseases	481
Chapter 47	Common Dermatological Problems	486
Chapter 48	Nutrition	496
Chapter 49	Alcohol and Drugs	516
Chapter 50	Environmental Problems	526
Chapter 51	Poisons, Stings and Bites	540
	GLOSSARY	549
	INDEX	581

Preface

An inevitable byproduct of the physical nature of athletic activities is injury. Thus, the prevention and care of athletic injuries must be given top priority in sports. Injuries often determine individual and team accomplishments, an important factor often overlooked, particularly by those managing youth sport programs. Adequate provision for the prevention and care of athletic injuries is crucial, especially at the high school level. Unfortunately, high school and other youth sports have lagged behind the college and professional teams in attention given to prevention and treatment of athletic injuries.

This manual is designed for individuals concerned with the health and safety of the athlete, particularly those interested in upgrading sport programs in their schools. The athlete wants to compete, even when injured. Unfortunately, competitive desires are often compounded by the external pressures of coaches, fans and media. Whereas the athletic trainer and team physician are primarily responsible for the athlete's health, they must control the athlete's environment to the point that he is able to compete to the best of his ability without jeopardizing his health. They must maintain the fine balance between the desired competition and the external forces that influence competition. We hope this volume assists trainers and team physicians to make their valuable contributions to the physical well-being of athletes central to participation in any sport.

The reader is encouraged to consider this text to be in less than ultimate form. Sports medicine is dynamic and will continue to evolve, and content cannot be all-inclusive. It is the nature of Academy publications to grow and improve through revisions and subsequent editions. We hope this volume will be no exception, and that it will continue to evolve to better serve all of those who are concerned with and care for the athlete.

As the text is not intended for the exclusive use of physicians or experienced athletic trainers, a word of caution is in order. Readers who do not possess the training and experience of the contributors should exercise care in attempting treatments and procedures recommended herein with which they are unfamiliar. Whenever there is doubt, particularly in serious cases, expert help should be sought.

Thoughtful use of this book may prove of great benefit to the student or practitioner who is reminded that the opinions expressed herein are those of the contributors, not of the Academy, and do not represent the only way to manage athletic injuries.

Acknowledgements

Over the past decade there has been a dramatic increase in the body of scientific knowledge and in the professionalism required by the athletic trainer and physician involved in sports medicine. The absence of a single volume containing the in-depth scientific information needed to fulfill these increasingly sophisticated demands has been of great concern to the leadership of the athletic training and sports medicine fields.

In 1974, a workshop composed of representatives from the National Athletic Trainers Association (N.A.T.A.), led by President Frank George, as well as members of the American Academy of Orthopaedic Surgeons (A.A.O.S.), met at Mount Hope Farm, a conference center in Williamstown, Massachusetts. The purpose of the workshop was to devise programs to improve the health care of the athlete. Two major accomplishments resulted from this effort. The first, designed to increase the availability of skilled athletic trainers, was a proposed ''alternative route'' that would permit interested faculty members to complete an approved training curriculum. Ultimately, these potential trainers would then be eligible to sit for the comprehensive certification exam. This alternative process was greatly aided by the contributions of Frank George, Lindsay McLean and the late Sayers ''Bud'' Miller.

The second accomplishment was the development of a curriculum that would constitute an educational core. This achievement received its major thrust from Phillip B. Donley and William E. ''Pinky'' Newell. It was the strong recommendation of Phil Donley that a text be created for this educational program, and through his impetus, this volume began to take shape.

Under the N.A.T.A. presidential administrations of Bill Chambers and, more recently, Bobby Barton, there have been major alterations leading to improvements in the certification process. Such change has, hopefully, been reflected in the content of this volume, and may be attributed to the tireless work of Paul Grace and the Board of Certification.

The role of the Sports Medicine Committee of the American Academy of Orthopaedic Surgeons has also been critically important. Virtually the entire text originated through the efforts of this Committee. The final manuscript was shaped by editorial subgroups of N.A.T.A. and the Academy's Sports Medicine Committee members. The enormous efforts of these combined editorial groups greatly facilitated the preparation of the final manuscript.

The magnitude of the assistance provided by Academy staff, particularly, Fred V. Featherstone, M.D., Andrea Korogi and Patricia Becker; that of The Book Department, Inc. and the editorial assistance of Susan Berman; and my office staff, including Mary Bennett, Edgardo Gonzalez-Ramirez, M.D. and, most emphatically, Heather Calehuff, P.A.-C., can only be ''duty above and beyond the call.'' In truth, without them, there would be no volume.

Arthur E. Ellison, M.D.
Williamstown, Massachusetts

Contributors

Margaret Alford, R.D.

William C. Allen, M.D.

B. A. Baker, M.D.

Dave Barringer, A.T.,C.

Bobby Barton, A.T.,C.

Frank H. Bassett, III, M.D.

R. W. Beart, Jr., M.D.

Harold Bennett, Jr., A.T.,C.

Wilma Bergfeld, M.D.

John Bernfield, A.T.,C.

Arthur L. Boland, Jr., M.D.

John Bruno, M.D.

William J. Bryan, M.D.

Robert E. Burdge, M.D.

Heather Calehuff, A.T.,C., P.A.-C.

O. Donald Chrisman, M.D.

William G. Clancy, Jr., M.D.

H. Royer Collins, M.D.

Rod Compton, A.T.,C.

James G. Cotanche, M.D.

Kenneth E. DeHaven, M.D.

David J. Drez, Jr., M.D.

Arthur E. Ellison, M.D.

John E. Feagin, M.D.

Frank Frangione, Ph.D.

Victor H. Frankel, M.D.

Keith Frary, A.T.,C.

F. James Funk, Jr., M.D.

Joseph Gieck, A.T.,C.

Joseph D. Godfrey, M.D.

Edgardo Gonzalez-Ramirez, M.D.

Paul Grace, A.T.,C.

William A. Grana, M.D.

Perry W. Greene, Jr., M.D.

Kathy Heck, A.T.,C.

George F. Hewson, M.D.

James Hill, M.D.

H. C. Hoagland, M.D.

William Hopfinger, B.S., R.P.T.

Timothy M. Hosea, M.D.

Letha Y. Hunter, M.D.

Wiley C. Hutchins, M.D.

Douglas W. Jackson, M.D.

Edward M. Jewusiak, M.D.

Frank W. Jobe, M.D.

Rollin M. Johnson, M.D.

Carl Krein, A.T.,C.

Bernie LaReau, A.T.,C.

John Leard, A.T.,C.

Clarence L. Livingood, M.D.

Don Lowe, A.T.,C.

George B. McManama

Robert P. Mack, M.D.

Robert Mathias, A.T.,C.

J. A. Meadows, III, M.D.

Duane G. Messner, M.D.

B. F. Morrey, M.D.

Kurt W. M. Niemann, M.D.

Frank R. Noyes, M.D.

Robert R. Oden, M.D.

Phillip L. Parr, M.D.

Bobby Patton, Ph.D.

Thomas R. Peterson, M.D.

Robert R. Protzman, M.D.

James R. Ralph, M.D.

J. Rand, M.D.

John Repsher, A.T.,C.

David Schultz, A.T.,C.

Arthur J. Siegel, M.D.

Franklin Sim, M.D.

George A. Snook, M.D.

Spanky Stephens, A.T.,C.

Timothy N. Taft, M.D.

Robert A. Teitge, M.D.

James E. Tibone, M.D.

Hugh S. Tullos, M.D.

Harold J. VanderZwaag, Ph.D.

D. Wiebers, M.D.

Thomas C. Wilson, M.D.

Michael Yager, P.A.-C.

George Young, A.T.,C.

Katie Zernhelt

National Athletic Trainers Association, Inc.

1001 EAST FOURTH STREET • P.O. DRAWER 1865 • GREENVILLE, NC 27835-1865 • TELEPHONE (919) 752-1725

Gentlemen:

It is indeed an honor to introduce this outstanding contribution to the literature of both professional organizations. Since the **National Athletic Trainers' Association** began in 1950 the relationship between the athletic trainer and the orthopaedic physician has been extremely close and congenial. This publication is the first joint venture available to the athletic training and medical world, which is indicative of our unique and special relationship.

The growth of our professions has many parallels. However, the trainer/team physician relationship has improved to the point that it is unsurpassed in the sports medicine profession.

Unquestionably we have laid the foundation for improved health care for the future generations of the athlete. This text will surely become a corner stone for future educational programs in athletic training.

Your continued support and encouragement is sincerely appreciated.

Sincerely,

National Athletic Trainers' Association, Inc.

Bobby Barton
President

Part 1

INTRODUCTION

Pioneers in Sports Medicine

Throughout human history, man's ability to survive has depended upon his physical capabilities. The speed, skill and strength early man needed for survival were transformed into games of skill during times of peace and as civilization progressed. As contests became more organized, more highly trained and skilled athletes competed in teams. Maintaining fitness and recovering from injuries became more important as the sophistication and popularity of athletic events grew. The need for physicians, trainers and therapists knowledgeable in the care and rehabilitation of athletes grew simultaneously.

The use of therapeutic exercises (medical gymnastics) was recorded as early as 800 to 100 B.C. in the Atharva-Veda, a medical manuscript from India. The first sports physician was Herodicus, who during the Fifth Century B.C. treated the athletes and other injured patients in Athens with therapeutic exercises and diet. His colleagues considered his approach harsh and radical. Yet, his fame spread, and other physicians came to observe and evaluate his techniques. His most famous pupil was Hippocrates, who later wrote of the value of exercise in treating many illnesses.

In the Second Century A.D., Galen was appointed physician to the gladiators and thus became the first physician known to occupy a position analogous to the team physician of today. Although he recognized the brutality and danger of some of the sporting events of his day, he taught and did an enormous amount of research in anatomy, physiology and sports injuries. While he did not believe in excessive exercise, he did recommend exercise in moderation for health and to help cure many diseases.

In the Fourth Century A.D., Oribasius of Pergamum believed that the body's organs functioned better when physically stressed. He therefore endorsed an intensified form of exercise.

In the Fifth Century A.D., the physician Aurelianus first recommended exercise during convalescence from surgery, prescribing hydrotherapy and the use of weights and pulleys.

During the first five centuries of the Christian era, the combination of invasions by Barbarians and the medieval church's zealous destruction of Greek and, to some extent, Roman knowledge led to the loss of much of the early medical texts. We are indebted to the Muslim culture for preserving this Greek and early Roman heritage. The great Islamic center of Baghdad under the caliphate of al-Mansur and Harun al-Rashid encouraged science and education. The earlier Greek, Roman and Hebrew medical documents were copied into Arabic and subsequently returned to the West in this form.

Hakim Avicenna (ibn-e-Sina), who lived from 980 to 1037 A.D., was probably the most famous Muslim writer. His standing in Islam was certainly equal to that of Galen in Rome. Included among the approximately 100 books he wrote was the Canon (Al-Qanun), his most famous medical book, which not only describes prophylactic medical gymnastics but also proposes rest, heat, massage and exercise to aid recovery from illness and injury.

In the Fifteenth Century, Vittorino de Feltre and Maffeus Veginus reintroduced the Greek tradition of obligatory exercise and sport into the educational curriculum. This concept has influenced Western education ever since.

A Sixteenth Century landmark was the publication of the "Six Books on the Art of Gymnastics" by Gerolamo Mercuriale. He classified exercises into preventative and therapeutic. His concepts were presented in a popular pictorial style that appealed to the general public, and his work was still being published 150 years later.

Marsillus Cagnatus first recognized the need for sports physicians who were knowledgeable and interested in the care of athletes. Laurent Joubert, professor of medicine at Montpelier University, first introduced therapeutic exercises (medical gymnastics) into the medical school curriculum. Cristobal Mendez was the first physician to write a book on exercise, while Ambrose Pare was the first to recommend rehabilitative exercises following the treatment of fractures.

In 1743, Nicholas Andry published *Orthopaedia*, in which he prescribed exercises for prevention and treatment of diseases in children. He also recommended exercises and sports for weight reduction as well as to help cure many diseases.

In the Nineteenth Century, physical education, separate from therapeutic exercise and unassociated with medicine, had its inception due to contributions by such men as Ling, Zander and Bernard. Ling introduced a system of exercise, based on his method of active, assisted and resistive techniques. Because of the shortage of therapists and the enthusiasm for his system, Zander developed machines using levers, wheels and weights for performing these exercises. Claude Bernard laid the foundations for modern physiology with his experimental work in nutrition and the nervous system.

Physical education in the United States received its start at Amherst College in Amherst, Massachusetts, with the appointment in 1854 of Edward Hitchcock, Jr., as professor of physical education and hygiene. He developed a system of coordinated physical education for the college, incorporating not only the Swedish and German systems of gymnastics and running but also the American style games of football, basketball, baseball and track. Dr. Hitchcock was also the school physician for Amherst College and instituted the study of anthropomorphic measurements of Amherst College students and also kept systematic records of the incidence of disease and injury at Amherst College, including athletic injuries. His writings covered a broad range of subjects such as "Athletics in American Colleges," "Basketball for Women" and "The Gymnastic Era and Athletic Era of Our Country." He is correctly identified as the founder of physical education in America, but he was also the first team physician in America.

In 1873, Dr. John Morgan, a former oarsman in England, published a paper comparing the longevity of 299 former oarsmen with that of the general population. The first text in English on medical treatment was written by two other Englishmen, J. B. Byles and Samuel Osbin, who wrote a section on first aid for athletics and a book called the *Encyclopedia of Sport*, published in 1898. They not only described the emergency treatment of various maladies, but also described injuries sustained in angling, boxing, cricket, football, hunting, lawn tennis, mountaineering, rowing and shooting and how to manage them.

In 1899, E. A. Darling, a physician at Harvard University, undertook a study of the Harvard University crews called "The Effects of Training," which was published in the *Boston Medical and Surgical Journal* the same year. In 1905, Edward H. Nichols published the first of two articles on football injuries at a time when the government was seriously considering banning the game because of its injury and fatality rate. Following the rule changes brought about by Walter Camp and his committee, a second article by Dr. Nichols in 1909 analyzed the injury situation of the Harvard football team.

The Twentieth Century has seen great development and expansion in the field of sports medicine. Weissbein published the first book dealing comprehensively with sports medicine. Outstanding and major publications by McKenzie, Hill, Bock, Dill, Schneider and

Dawson were influential in establishing the modern concepts of physiology and rehabilitative exercises.

In 1931 Walter Meanwell collaborated with Knute Rockne to produce the first American work in sports medicine which discussed the role of the athletic trainer and team physician in caring for the athlete. Augustus Thorndike published the first book on athletic injuries in the United States in 1938, emphasizing not only the diagnosis and treatment but also prevention of injuries.

Outstanding contributions all over the world have been and are still being made that continue to expand the knowledge of sports medicine. To mention some would be an injustice to others.

Many organizations now bring together individuals and groups interested in sports medicine. Among the first was the Federation of Sports Medicine (FIMS), established at the Olympic Winter Games at St. Moritz in 1928. The American Medical Association appointed an ad hoc committee on Injuries in Sports in 1951, which later became a standing committee. One of the largest and most productive organizations, the American College of Sports Medicine, was founded in 1954. Many disciplines interested in sports medicine form the membership of this organization. The American Orthopaedic Society for Sports Medicine was established in 1971 and is actively involved in research and education in sports medicine.

The National Athletic Trainers Association is an active organization devoted to education of athletic trainers, research in sports medicine, and establishment of a certificate of standards for athletic trainers. This organization began in the spring of 1938, when a group of trainers met at the Drake Relays in Des Moines, Iowa. The association first published a monthly bulletin, *NATA Bulletin,* and now *Athletic Training,* the journal of the National Athletic Trainers Association, is published quarterly.

Growth of this organization paralleled the growth of organized sports in the United States. It was not until 1950, however, that the present national organization for athletic trainers was organized. In Kansas City, Missouri, on June 24-25, 1950, the National Athletic Trainers Association was officially formed. The continued growth of this organization has worked to raise the standards of its members by exchanging and disseminating information valuable to every phase of athletic training.

This review is not meant to be a comprehensive analysis of the entire field of sports medicine but to recall some of the major developments. Even though sports medicine is often seen as a new discipline, its roots and traditions are ancient.

*SPORTS MEDICINE ORGANIZATIONS

1. Physician Organizations

A. The American Academy of Orthopaedic Surgeons, Sports Medicine Committee. Suite 1500, 444 North Michigan Avenue, Chicago, IL 60611. (312) 822-0970

B. American Orthopaedic Society for Sports Medicine. Suite 202, 70 West Hubbard, Chicago, IL 60610. (312) 644-2623

C. American College of Sports Medicine. 1440 Monroe Street, Madison, WI 53706. (608) 262-3632

D. American Academy of Pediatrics, Sports Committee. 1801 Hinman Avenue, Evanston, IL 60204. (312) 869-4255

E. American Medical Association. 535 North Dearborn Street, Chicago, IL 60610

---

*Many of the national organizations on this list have regional, state or local chapters, with committees that deal with aspects of sports medicine.

F. American Academy of Family Physicians, Sports Committee. 1740 West 92nd Street, Kansas City, MO 64114. (816) 531-0377

2. Athletic Trainers Associations

A. National Athletic Trainers Association. 112 S. Pitt Street, Greenville, NC 27834. (919) 752-1725

3. High School Organizations

A. The National Federation of State High School Athletic Associations. 11724 Plaza Circle, P.O. Box 20626, Kansas City, MO 64195

4. College Organizations

A. National Collegiate Athletic Association, Competitive Safeguards and Medical Aspects of Sports Committee. P.O. Box 1906, Mission, KS 66201

B. American Football Coaches Association, Committee on Injuries and Fatalities. Box 8705, Durham, NC 27702. (919) 489-8160

C. National Association for Intercollegiate Athletics. 1221 Baltimore, Kansas City, MO 64105. (816) 842-5050

5. Athletic Injury Data Sources

A. National Athletic Injury Reporting Services. 131 White Bldg., Penn State, University Park, PA 16812. (814) 865-9593

B. National Head and Neck Injury Registry. 235 South 33rd Street, Weightman Hall, Philadelphia, PA 19104. (215) 662-4090

C. National Safety Council. 444 North Michigan Avenue, Chicago, IL 60611

D. New York State Public High School Athletic Association. Executive Park South, Stuyvesant Plaza, Albany, NY 12203

E. Risks Associated with Certain Sports Activities, U.S. Department of Commerce, Performance and Safety Analysis Section, Product Systems Division, Center for Consumer Product Technology, Institute for Applied Technology, 1974

The Sports Medicine Team

This volume focuses on the athlete participating in organized athletics, particularly at the professional, collegiate, high school and junior high school levels. Yet, its scope encompasses organized industrial, community, intramural, physical education and youth programs. Beyond organized athletics, numerous recreational athletes who are playing various racquet sports, jogging, skiing, swimming, cycling, skating and participating in many other recreational sports activities are at risk of sustaining sports-related injuries.

In some ways athletes are no different from nonathletic patients who sustain the same injuries and illnesses. However, athletes are different from the general population in that they impose higher functional demands on their cardiovascular, respiratory and musculoskeletal systems. As otherwise healthy, highly motivated people, athletes want to recover maximum function. The primary goals of sports medicine are both to prevent as many injuries and illnesses as possible, and to treat injuries and illnesses that do occur with prompt, complete rehabilitation so that the athletes have the opportunity to return to their sports.

The special needs of today's athletes can be best provided for through a team approach. Historically, the health care of athletes was left to the coach or trainer. The modern approach calls for a highly organized and qualified team to provide comprehensive medical care for today's athlete. Although the specific setting may affect its magnitude, the team approach is appropriate for all levels of operation, i.e., high school, college or professional competition.

THE TEAM APPROACH

The team should, in actuality, be two teams: an active team and an assistive team. The active team consists of:

1. Team physician
2. Certified athletic trainer
3. Coaches
4. Student athletic trainers
5. Resident physicians
6. Athletic administrators

Each member of the active team plays a vital role in the health, safety and welfare of the athlete.

The assistive team is comprised of individuals who play important but secondary roles in the care of athletes.

1. Medical consultant specialists
2. Allied medical personnel
3. General consultants

Several medical specialists should be readily available for consultation to the team.

1. Allergist
2. Cardiologist
3. Dermatologist
4. Dentist/oral surgeon
5. Gynecologist
6. Internist
7. Neurological surgeon
8. Ophthalmologist
9. Orthopedist (unless the team physician is same)
10. Otolaryngologist
11. General surgeon
12. Urologist
13. Radiologist

2

7

Allied medical personnel who may be needed include:

1. Emergency medical technician
2. Podiatrist
3. Laboratory technicians
4. Nurse
5. Optometrist
6. Optician
7. Pharmacist
8. Physical therapist
9. Psychologist/mental health specialist

The general consultants whose involvement is advantageous to the team approach for the care of athletes are:

1. Administrators
2. Brace maker
3. Coaches
4. Equipment manager
5. Exercise physiologist
6. Health educator
7. Kinesiologist
8. Lawyer
9. Nutritionist
10. Substance abuse personnel
11. Strength coach

The interaction of the active medical team with these consulting groups enhances the success of the medical team's efforts to care for today's athletes adequately and properly.

COMMUNICATIONS

The active medical team members are responsible for providing medical care for the athlete. The success of the entire operation depends on their qualifications, interest and abilities. Certainly, the knowledge, skills and experience of the physician and trainer are key factors in developing a successful team, but also vital are organization, development of policies, procedures and a clear line of authority. Communications and preplanning are necessary for an efficient operation.

The chain of command and lines of communication should be well established and followed. In a well organized program, the team trainer is the liaison between all parties.

The physician should communicate directly with parents regarding special or serious problems, particularly in a high school setting. The physician–trainer relationship is most important for the smooth, efficient operation of the sports medicine program. These two individuals should be compatible, with mutual respect and confidence in each other's abilities.

They must be willing and able to communicate regarding procedures and policies on the care, treatment and follow-up of all injuries and illnesses. Possibly the key ingredient in the physician–trainer relationship is the understanding of the other's roles, which usually results in a cooperative and successful effort (Fig. 2:1).

The ability to compromise on methodology without compromising oneself can be important as well. The ability to plan ahead for problems and emergencies and then to act in tandem to detect common and unique problems and devise appropriate care results in efficient medical care.

Within the realm of the athlete–coach–trainer–physician interaction, it is paramount that all involved have complete understanding of *who* makes medical decisions regarding who plays or practices. The final decision on availability rests solely with the team physician. Vital input from the trainer, however, who has more day-to-day contact with the athlete, is necessary for this decision.

For this approach to be effective, the athlete must have respect and confidence in the medical team's capabilities and techniques. The physician and trainer must keep the athlete's best interests in mind at all times, and not yield to outside pressure.

When a coach acts intelligently and maturely, has trust and confidence in the trainer and medical team, the necessary environment for cooperation and proper care can be realized. Policies must assure that everyone understands the process of deciding availability. An administrator must be aware of these policies and ready to control situations in which con-

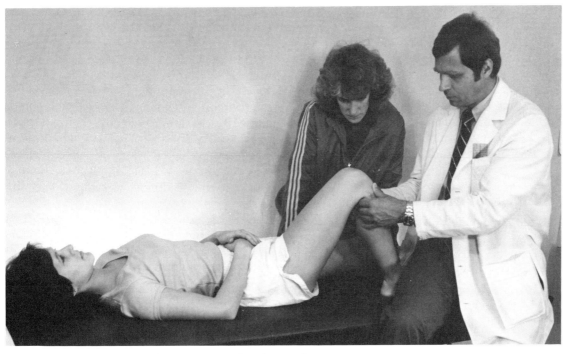

FIGURE 2:1. Physicians and trainers: mutual understanding

flict might develop. Strong administrative support is a must for the medical team's control of availability of athletes for practice or competition.

Triage

Triage, although important, usually is much simpler in an athletic training room or on the playing field than in the hospital emergency department. Simultaneous multiple injuries are uncommon in sports. However, when they do occur, the team physician or trainer can rapidly assess the injuries and relegate care for the less severe injuries to graduate trainers or student trainers.

RESPONSIBILITIES OF TEAM MEMBERS

Family Physician or Pediatrician

The family physician provides important continuity of care and general counseling for the athlete. The family physician is often the primary source of preparticipation medical history and growth and development data. This physician may also perform the preparticipation physical evaluation.

Team Physician

The team physician directly supervises the athletic trainer, and advises on the overall conditioning program. He is responsible for performing or collecting and reviewing the preparticipation physical evaluation, and making the final determination of fitness for participation.

The team physician provides medical coverage for competitive events, especially contact sports, supplying emergency evaluation, treatment, and triage of athletic injuries and illnesses. He also will provide primary care of athletic injuries or arrange referrals to the family physician or specialist consultants as indicated. Additionally, he oversees or establishes the guidelines and procedures for trainer personnel to respond to emergencies and can suggest emergency equipment needed.

Following injury or illness, the team physician is responsible for insuring that rehabilitation has been adequate. He should assess the athlete for readiness to return to activity.

Finally, the team physician should educate coaches, trainers, administrators, athletes and parents regarding the medical aspects of sports.

Athletic Director

The athletic director is responsible for organizing athletic activities and taking steps to insure that athletes are adequately protected and informed of potential risks. The athletic director should project the school's concern for injury prevention and care. This concern could be demonstrated to coaches by setting minimum standards of proficiency in cardiopulmonary resuscitation and first aid, and by providing numerous opportunities for in-service training in injury prevention and care.

The athletic director should reflect the school's concern for the care of the athlete by providing adequate medical coverage. This should include a medical insurance program, an athletic training program with adequate training room equipment and facilities and, ideally, a certified athletic trainer to administer the program.

The athletic director should provide supervision of the practice and playing environment as well as insure that all athletic equipment is adequate and suitably maintained. In addition, he should provide the best possible officiating for competitive events and arrange for emergency transport of injured athletes as well as insure the security of athletes and spectators.

Coach

The coach is responsible for teaching playing skills. As a member of the sports medicine team, he should impart a proper game philosophy and an overall safety awareness. Coaches can establish the credibility of their concern for injuries and injury prevention by communicating with athletes and parents. One means of doing this is to have a meeting with team members and perhaps parents to inform them of potential injuries, outlining means of prevention. The "win at all cost" syndrome can be dangerous and shows little regard for the safety of the athlete.

Football coaches in particular should specifically warn athletes of the potential for head and neck injuries, insisting on techniques of blocking and tackling that reduce the chance of injury. All coaches should recognize areas of physical hazards in their sports, inform athletes of injuries that might occur, and insist on skill techniques that minimize risk.

Teams should follow effective and safe conditioning programs, including off-season, preseason and in-season programs with endurance, strength, flexibility and agility components. The conditioning program and practice schedules should be structured to prevent excessive fatigue and heat injuries.

The coach must also provide, or delegate to a competent aid, emergency care of athletic injuries and application of first aid in the absence of the trainer or team physician. At least one member of any coaching staff should have training in cardiopulmonary resuscitation and basic first aid. The coach should also communicate freely with the trainer and team physician regarding health and safety matters. When the coach is called upon to carry out athletic training functions, there is a potential conflict of interest. The safety and well-being of the athlete must always have the highest priority.

Athletic Trainer

The basic role of the athletic trainer is to stand at the "crossroads" between the athlete and coach, the athlete and physician and the physician and coach. The trainer has important record-keeping responsibilities, including preparticipation evaluations and a daily injury log. These records document types of injuries and illnesses, treatments given, and time lost from participation. The trainer also insures that communication with the school nurse, physician and parents is adequate.

The athletic trainer should advise with regard to basic conditioning programs and purchase and use of various types of exercise equipment. In addition, the trainer is responsible for administering and maintaining the training room. In the absence of an equipment manager, the trainer may be called upon to supervise equipment purchase and fitting.

The athletic trainer's primary responsibility is to prevent injury and also assure that when injuries do occur, proper medical care is given. He must be knowledgeable in the techniques of taping, bracing and use of special padding and other protective equipment. The athletic trainer must evaluate injuries, provide warranted first aid and make appropriate follow-up referrals in addition to providing care for the numerous injuries that do not require physician referrals.

While working closely with the team or school physician, the athletic trainer's duties should include supervising the rehabilitation of the injured athlete and assessing readiness for return to activity.

Finally, the athletic trainer should assist the physician in educating the coach, athlete, parents and administration as to injury trends, injury potential, and prevention and care of injuries.

Student Trainers

The student trainers act as extensions of the head athletic trainer. They provide the all important work force for routine duties in practices and games. They should be aware of their limitations and work within them, yet be encouraged to expand their knowledge and experience.

At first, observing the program should be the student trainers' main activity. As they become familiar and comfortable with the procedures and skills, they should start with easy duties and progress to more involved duties.

The head trainer and team physician should supervise the student trainers, advising and counseling as necessary and requested. An in-service educational program should provide student trainers with information and skills to make them more proficient.

Athletes

Athletes must play an active role in their own physical conditioning, and understand the importance of getting adequate rest and nutrition and refraining from alcoholic beverages and ingestion of drugs. Athletes should promptly report illnesses and injuries to the coach, trainer or a team physician and not attempt to hide medical problems, which may become more severe and create more disability and time lost. Athletes should become knowledgeable about injury and illness risks involved with their sports, and about safety and preventive measures that minimize those risks. Athletes are also responsible for the proper care and fit of their own equipment.

Parents

Parents should provide and encourage proper nutrition and rest for the athlete in the home, and encourage athletic participation without forcing an unwilling child into athletics. They should help the athlete strike the important balance between educational needs and sports.

The parents should also become aware of the hazards of athletic participation and take an active role in insuring that the proper coaching, equipment and playing environment are provided. They should also be actively involved in booster organizations to help finance and support safe athletic programs.

School Nurse

In some situations, the school nurse may be an active participant in the athletic program. The nurse's functions can include keeping records of injuries sustained and time lost, processing insurance forms, helping to organize and carry out the preparticipation physical evaluations, coordinating the schedule of special diagnostic tests, and assisting in first aid for athletic injuries and illnesses.

Organization of a
Sports Medicine Program*

3

The size and scope of a sports medicine program depends on the locale, the facilities available, the funding available and the age and number of athletes to be cared for. Whether the athletes are junior high school students in a small community cared for by a family physician and a faculty athletic trainer or students in a large university with consultants available in each area of expertise and a large budget, the purpose of a sports medicine program is to provide the most efficient medical care and protection to the athlete. Proper care is best provided by adhering to certain guidelines.

1. Prevention of illness and injury
   A. Preseason physical examination
   B. Careful evaluation of playing fields and equipment
   C. Preseason conditioning programs
   D. Daily environmental testing for heat, cold and humidity
2. Prompt evaluation of illness or injury
3. Initial treatment of illness or injury
4. Referral of the injured or sick athlete through proper referral channels to a physician or consultant
5. Rehabilitation following injury to maximize functional recovery and minimize risk of reinjury
6. Record keeping

PREVENTION OF ILLNESS AND INJURY

Preseason Physical Examination

A preseason or preparticipation medical evaluation is required before any athlete can participate in an organized sport. This evaluation not only fulfills legal and insurance requirements, but also yields a base line of the athlete's fitness for participation. The examination may reveal disqualifying abnormalities and correctable or treatable physical conditions, and produces a base line record for later comparison should illness or injury occur during the course of the season. The exam should include:

1. History of prior medical problems or injury
2. Childhood immunization record
3. Orthopedic examination
4. Complete general physical
5. Urinalysis
6. Eye examination

The preseason examination should be conducted in an area large enough to permit easy traffic flow and multiple simultaneous examinations. The number of examiners varies according to the number of athletes to be examined at one time and the skill of the examiners. The athletes should present in gym shorts or gym suits with past history and immunization records filled out. If any athletes give positive answers to past medical illnesses, the team physician should take an individual history. For efficiency and thoroughness, the athletes should rotate through a series of stations, the number depending on the number

---

*This chapter is taken from *The Law of Sports*, John C. Weistart and Lowell Smith. The Bobbs-Merrill Co., Inc., 1976.

of examiners and available space. Basically the examination should be conducted as follows.

Station I. *Blood pressure:* can be done by student trainer or trainer.

II. *Urinalysis:* athlete should be provided with paper cup. A student trainer can test urine with Clini-stix or Lab-stix.

III. *Mouthpiece:* fitted individually; ideally done by dentist, or can be done by a trainer or student trainer.

IV. *Snellen Vision Chart:* student trainer or manager.

V. *Skin, mouth, eyes:* physician.

VI. *Chest:* physician.

VII. *Lymphatics, genitalia, abdomen:* physician.

VIII. *Orthopedic:* physician, preferably an orthopedic surgeon, or a physical therapist.

IX. *Review:* team physician.

Decisions to permit participation should be made at this preparticipation physical. If additional testing is recommended, clearance to participate is withheld until the problem is proved of no consequence. Examples of these problems are diastolic blood pressure above 90 mm Hg, protein or sugar in the urine, acute or chronic infection, skin rash, inguinal hernia, undescended testicle or scoliosis. Limited participation may be permitted with certain disqualifying abnormalities, noted on the history or physical examination, until the abnormality is corrected. Specific sports in which the athlete may participate should be listed. Copies of the examination should be kept on file, sent to the family or personal physician and, ideally, be sent to the athlete's parents. The disqualifying conditions listed in the *Medical Evaluation of the Athlete—A Guide* (Revised, American Medical Association, Chicago, 1976) should be consulted.

Preseason Conditioning Programs

A preseason conditioning program can help prevent injury. As part of their overall pre-season evaluation, athletes should be tested for cardiovascular fitness, flexibility and muscle strength. Those who have particular injury potential due to weakness or tightness should be put on a special exercise program.

Evaluation of Playing Fields and Equipment

Playing fields and surfaces should be examined regularly for obstacles that might cause injury. All hard obstacles that cannot be removed should be padded to reduce impact forces. Field equipment should also be inspected periodically to determine wear and impending failure that could cause injury. In addition, the athletes should personally inspect all their protective gear routinely and report any defects to the coach or athletic trainer.

Daily Environmental Testing

Environmental factors directly affect the safety of athletes. Athletes should be allowed unlimited access to drinking water during practices and games. In hot, humid weather, practice plans should be adjusted to protect athletes from heat illness. (See Chapter 51.)

Athletes practicing in cold weather should be adequately protected. Extremities in particular should be kept warm. If the wind chill index is extremely low, practice should be held indoors.

PROMPT EVALUATION AND INITIAL TREATMENT OF ILLNESS OR INJURY

Although ideally a physician is readily available to evaluate injuries during games and practices, in reality, this is not economically feasible. Therefore, in the absence of a physician, the athletic trainer evaluates injuries. Many injuries do not require referral to a physician and can be adequately treated and followed by the athletic trainer. Each injury should be reported to the team physician.

In the absence of the physician or trainer, the coach usually must make an initial evaluation and provide first aid. The athlete can then be referred to the trainer or an emergency facility as appropriate.

REFERRAL OF THE ATHLETE

Those responsible for administering the athletic medicine program should have a written policy statement listing proper channels for referring more extensive injuries for further evaluation and x-ray films. When the coach is responsible for this referral, a written guideline is especially helpful. This written policy should include procedures for ambulance transport and a list of emergency equipment as well as emergency telephone numbers.

REHABILITATION

When an athlete must discontinue activity due to injury, a comprehensive plan of rehabilitation and reconditioning should be instituted. The athletic trainer, after consultation with the physician, is responsible for this program. Written guidelines for return to activity help avoid confusion and misunderstanding. These guidelines should cover general strength and flexibility requirements as well as functional requirements, such as running figure-of-eights and jumping.

RECORD KEEPING

As in all instances when medical care is provided, record keeping is very important. This is usually the responsibility of the athletic trainer.

The athletic trainer should fill out a referral form when referring an athlete to the team physician. This form should indicate whether the player was hurt in practice or in a game, in what sport the player was participating, the body part injured and a brief sentence of how the injury happened. At the conclusion of the examination, the physician should have enough space to add the diagnosis, the recommended treatment, when the patient can resume athletic participation and at what level.

The form should state whether the trainer is to provide treatment. Referral to another physician should be written in the space provided. If a third party such as a physical therapist is to provide treatment, instructions for therapy should be outlined on the form. Specific return appointments should be noted. A copy of the form should be kept in the trainer's office.

The trainer should keep a daily report and daily log on each sport and for each sick or injured athlete. This gives an accurate record of days lost from practice and the response to treatment. The coaches should be informed daily of the medical status of the sick or injured athlete and the anticipated date of return to full practice.

Figure 3:1 is an example of a form used to report all injuries that occur in a college athletic department, whether intramural, recreational or intercollegiate. The person who evaluates and cares for the injury fills out the form and then submits it to the head athletic trainer. This form is then filed in an intramural or recreational injury file or, in the case of athletes, filed with the daily medical report form (Fig. 3:2) in that athlete's individual file.

The Athletic Injury Report and the Daily Medical Report can be kept in a three-ring binder until the athlete is ready to return to full activity. At this time, totals are filled in at the bottom, the injury is recorded on a master log and the form is then filed.

Insurance

It is impossible to recommend a complete program of insurance coverage for the athlete, but there are three basic methods of insurance coverage.

1. The school provides the insurance policy and pays for it.
2. The school provides the insurance policy, but it is paid for by the athlete.
3. Athletes carry their own insurance coverage and pay for it.

Any policy carried by an athlete should be carefully examined to be sure that the policy covers interscholastic or intercollegiate athletic injuries.

Department of Sports and Recreation
ATHLETIC INJURY REPORT FORM

Name of Injured _____ SS# _____ Age _____

Date of Injury _____ Sport/Activity _____

Describe how injury occurred (include time and place) _____

_____

Describe injury (pain, swelling, probable injury) _____

_____

Describe immediate care and treatment _____

_____

Referrals (emergency, UHS, training room) _____

Specific follow up instructions _____

Witnesses (serious injury)

   1. Name _____ Address_____

   2. Name _____ Address_____

   3. Name _____ Address_____

Name of person reporting _____

Signature _____ Date _____

Additional comments

FIGURE 3:1. Injury Report Form

Department of Sports and Recreation

ATHLETIC TRAINING AND INJURY CARE

DAILY MEDICAL REPORT

NAME _____ AGE _____ SPORT/POSITION _____

INJURY _____ Trauma _____ Stress _____ Reinjury _____

Practice Game	Date	Actvity or Rehabilitation	Treatment	Comments

TOTALS: Days Injured _____ Practices Missed _____ Modified _____

Physician Referrals_____ Diagnostic Tests _____

FIGURE 3:2. Daily Medical Report Form

LEGAL RESPONSIBILITIES

General Principles of Negligence Liability

The athlete and parents should be aware of their responsibilities and that they can be held legally responsible for their actions in athletics. Negligence refers to conduct that falls below the standard established by law for the protection of others against unreasonable risks of harm. Under most circumstances, this considers what an ordinary, reasonable person would do under like circumstances.

Legal doctrines can modify legal considerations regarding injuries suffered because of the injured party's conduct. The first is the doctrine of "contributory negligence." In contributory negligence, conduct by the injured party falls below the standard necessary for his or her own protection, and is a legally contributing cause in bringing about the injury. The second doctrine is the "assumption of risk," stating that a party who voluntarily assumes a risk of harm arising from the conduct of another cannot recover if harm is caused to him or her.

Recent court decisions have substantially modified the doctrine of assumption of risk. These court decisions have served notice that assumption of risk no longer applies if the injured party was unaware of the risks and if techniques that can contribute to injury were not discouraged. Not only should any dangerous technique be discouraged, but the coach is obligated to inform the athlete of the specific potential outcome of employing that technique.

In general, the sponsoring institution should do everything possible to prevent injury, project a general atmosphere of concern for injuries and inform the athlete and parents of injury potential. In addition, signed information sheets should document attempts to inform athletes of injury potential.

Athletic Trainer Personal Liability

The law requires that in regard to injury, an individual or an institution must act or behave toward others in a certain definable way (standard of care). These standards of care are established in many different ways, including local custom, statutes, ordinances, case law, administrative law, or professional standards. In a law suit, a judge and jury decide the performance of the defendant as compared to those standards.

While the athletic trainer's professional competence and credibility have greatly improved through national certification and state licensure and certification, the trainer's personal liability has increased in direct proportion to the strength of the credentials. When the position of the athletic director was not as clearly defined as it is now, the court-defined standard of care was similar to the population. However, as expertise and credibility improve, the expected standard of care increases. Athletic trainers working in states with licensure or certification are expected to conform to standards of other trainers in that state. In the absence of state-regulated credentials, the national certification will probably be the expected standard of care. An uncertified individual who performs the duties of an athletic trainer will probably still be expected to meet the standards of certified athletic trainers.

Team Physician Legal Responsibilities

Principles of Medical Malpractice Liability

The physician must practice with the level of reasonable skill and knowledge common for members of the medical profession in good standing. The physician is not in a position to guarantee all treatment and procedures, and is not held liable for honest mistakes of judgment where proper treatment is open to reasonable doubt. The general standard of care is not altered by the fact that the physician may be acting gratuitously.

As applied to sports medicine, a physician in general practice who treats a sports injury is expected to perform with the degree of reasonable skill and knowledge that would be used by members of the profession in good standing. However, if the physician is practicing as a specialist in sports medicine, the standard of care is slightly altered. The specialist will be held to a standard of care measured in terms of the specialty itself rather than the standard of the medical profession in general; i.e., the sports medicine practitioner would be required to perform with the degree of reasonable skill and knowledge that would be used by sports medicine experts.

If the physician is unable to determine what "good medical practice" requires, then it is appropriate to contact other members of the profession for aid in making that determination. Where uncertainty continues to exist in spite of such consultations, there may be an important legal responsibility issue, and preliminary legal analysis could help avoid serious legal problems.

Physician–Athlete Relationship

When the athlete is accepted as a patient by the treating physician, there then exists a physician–patient relationship, and the physician is obligated to treat the athlete in accordance with recognized standards of care. These duties will not be affected by the fact that the physician may be acting gratuitously.

Consent for Treatment

Under normal circumstances, the physician must obtain the consent of an adult patient before administering medical care. The general rule for treatment of minors is that consent must be obtained from the parent or guardian, since the minor is deemed incapable of giving valid consent. Exceptions exist where minors can give valid consent in emergency situations when the parent or guardian is inaccessible, or when the minor is near adulthood and able to give informed consent.

Informed consent indicates that the physician has "imparted some quantum of medical information relative to a proposed treatment which is sufficient to enable the patient to make an intelligent choice as to whether he should undergo such treatment." This typical-

ly includes a reasonable disclosure of alternatives, the danger of each, and their relative advantages and disadvantages. If informed consent cannot be obtained from the patient, it may be implied from the circumstances, such as in emergency situations.

Disclosure of Information

There is potential liability for disclosure of medical information without consent from the patient, and sports medicine physicians or athletic trainers should give no information to outside individuals or teams without the specific written consent of the athlete. Legitimate requests for information regarding prior injury should normally be restricted to disclosure of the nature of the injury and the method of treatment, leaving the requesting party the burden of determining the current fitness of the athlete.

Physician–School Relationship

A formal physician–patient relationship exists whenever a physician treats a student pursuant to a contract with the athlete's school. The school has a duty to provide reasonable medical care to athletes who are injured in school-related athletic programs.

If a team physician is acting as an employee of the school rather than an independent contractor, vicarious liability exists and the school is responsible for the conduct of the physician, since he is acting under the school's authority. The basis for distinction is whether the school exerts control over the physical conduct of the physician and, if so, vicarious liability can exist. But, if the physician is considered an independent contractor, the school would not be subjected to vicarious liability.

Examination of Athletes

The standard guidelines apply for preparticipation physical evaluations, in that a sports medicine physician must act with the skill and knowledge that other members of the profession would use acting in similar circumstances.

Important considerations are the purpose of the evaluation; the nature of the conditions under which it was performed; procedures generally used by other members of the profession in conducting such examinations; and the requirements of good medical practice in responding to the results of the examination.

Prescription Drugs

Sports medicine physicians can be considered negligent in prescribing drugs that could cause injury or worsen an existing injury, especially if the athlete has not given informed consent based upon a disclosure of the potential damages that the drugs might pose. A physician's duty in prescribing drugs to athletes is to use the level of responsible skill and knowledge that is common for members of the medical profession or physicians practicing a given specialty. The principal issue is whether good medical practice allows prescription of the drug in question to a given athlete in the manner and dosage used. The necessity of obtaining informed consent is one aspect of good medical practice. If informed consent was not obtained prior to prescribing the drug, that might itself constitute physician negligence.

Part 2

ANATOMY AND DIAGNOSTIC SIGNS

General and Topographic Anatomy

4

The surface of the body has many definite features. These landmarks are guides to structures that lie beneath them, giving clues to the anatomy of the body through its external features, its topography. A knowledge of the superficial landmarks of the body, or the topographic anatomy, allows the well-trained examiner to evaluate the seriousness of an injury quickly and to anticipate complications. Inspection is the simplest component of the primary and secondary survey of injured persons. It requires no special dexterity or strength on the part of the examiner. It causes the patient no pain or risk of further injury. Thorough inspection yields much information regarding the extent of injury. The importance of this inspection cannot be overemphasized; more facts are missed by not looking at a patient thoroughly than by not knowing a specific anatomic relation.

All medical personnel should be familiar with the language of topographic anatomy so they can pass on specific information with the least possible confusion. Picture the body in the standard position, which is always standing erect, facing the examiner, with the arms at the sides, palms forward. When the terms right and left are used, they refer to the patient's right and left. The principal regions of the body are the head, neck, thorax (chest), abdomen and the extremities (arms and legs).

The surface of the front of the body, facing the examiner, is the anterior surface. An imaginary vertical line drawn from midforehead through the nose and the umbilicus (navel) to the floor is termed the midline. Areas lying away from this line are termed lateral, and areas lying toward it are termed medial; we speak, for example, of the medial and lateral surfaces of the knee, elbow or ankle. Toward the head is the superior or cephalad end; toward the feet is the inferior or caudad end. The nose is superior to the mouth, while the umbilicus is inferior to the chest.

Proximal refers to a location on an extremity that is nearer to the trunk, and to any location on the trunk nearer to the midline or to the point of reference named. Distal is the opposite of proximal and refers to a location on an extremity nearer to the free end—the end not attached to the trunk. Similarly, it refers to any location on the trunk that is farther from the midline or from the point of reference named. For example, the elbow is distal to the shoulder, yet proximal to the wrist and hand (Fig. 4:1).

In general, arms and legs are taken to mean the upper and lower extremities. Specifically, the upper portion of the lower extremity from the hip joint to the knee is the thigh. The lower portion from the knee to the ankle is the leg. The upper part of the upper extremity from the shoulder to the elbow is the arm. The lower portion from the elbow to the wrist is the forearm.

By using these terms and recalling the description of the standard anatomic position, one examiner can describe the location of an injury so that another examiner will know immediately where to look and what to expect. The examiner can choose how to inspect the patient, but it should be systematic, thorough

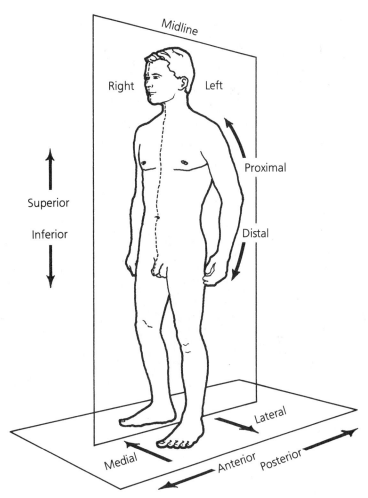

FIGURE 4:1. The general terms of topographic anatomy are routinely used to describe wounds and injuries.

across the top of the ears and eyes separates the superior (top) and inferior (bottom) portions of the head. The area above this imaginary plane is the cranium. It contains the brain that connects with the spinal cord through a large opening at the base of the skull and in the center of the upper neck. The most posterior portion of the cranium is the occiput. On each side, the lateral and most anterior portions of the cranium are called the temples or temporal regions; more posteriorly are the parietal regions. One can feel the pulse of the temporal artery just anterior to the ear (Fig. 4:2).

Just below the horizontal plane lie the ears, eyes, nose, mouth, cheeks and jowls, which make up the face. The orbital rim of the maxilla is prominent below the eye, while the mandible (jawbone) is also obvious. The most apparent landmarks of the face are, of course, the eyes, ears, nose and mouth. Gross injuries of these structures are not difficult to recognize.

Viewing the face from the side, the eyeball is recessed (Fig. 4:3). It is protected superiorly and inferiorly by bony ridges and medially by the bridge of the nose. These ridges protect the eye but obviously receive the greatest force of any impact. A bruise, laceration or abrasion in these locations must always be viewed, therefore, as a possible sign of a major underlying fracture. Frequently, a fracture of the maxilla will trap one or more of the muscles that control motion of the eye. In this situation, the affected eye will often look down and its motion in other directions will be limited. This type of fracture is called a "blowout" fracture of the floor of the orbit.

Only the proximal third of the nose, the bridge, is formed by bone. The remainder is a cartilaginous framework. Any injury of the proximal third is therefore cause to suspect an underlying fracture, while an abrasion on the tip of the nose usually is a minor lesion. Bleeding or discharge from the nose after an injury of the head should always be investigated further. A nasal discharge of clear cerebrospinal fluid is an indication of a fracture of the

and performed in exactly the same sequence for all patients. Developing a routine will help the examiner avoid overlooking a critical but perhaps subtle sign. Examination should begin at the head and proceed through the neck, thorax, abdomen, pelvis and the extremities. It is especially crucial to compare a given injured region with the corresponding uninjured region on the opposite side.

HEAD

The head is divided into the cranium and the face. An imaginary horizontal plane passing

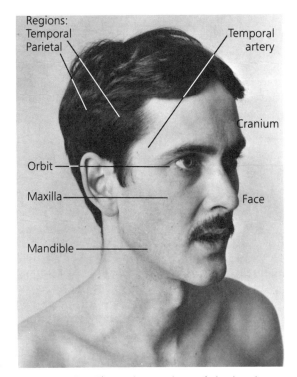

FIGURE 4:2. The major portions of the head

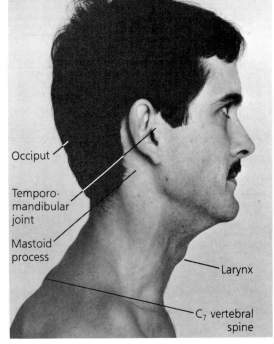

FIGURE 4:3. Lateral view of the head and neck

anterior portion of the skull. A bloody discharge or leaking of clear fluid from the ear suggests a fracture of the skull involving its base.

Unlike the nose, the exposed portion of the ear is composed entirely of cartilage covered by skin and injuries are usually obvious. Immediately anterior to the notch at the middle of the anterior border of the exposed ear is the easily palpable temporal artery. If you hold a finger gently on the temporal artery at this site and then open your mouth, you will immediately appreciate that the articulation of the mandible with the undersurface of the skull, the temporomandibular joint, lies at this location. The tragus, or small, rounded, fleshy protuberance immediately at the front of the ear canal, lies just over the area where the temporal artery may be palpated. The pinna is the name given to the ear itself. The lobes are the dependent fleshy portions at the bottom of each ear.

The prominent, hard, bony mass at the base of the skull 1 cm posterior to the tip of the lobe of the ear is called the mastoid process. In patients who have suffered a serious skull fracture involving the base, an ecchymosis or purplish-blue discoloration (bruise) may appear in this region some hours after the injury. This finding is subtle and is often overlooked or misdiagnosed as a simple bruise.

NECK

The neck contains many structures, including the cervical or upper esophagus and the trachea (windpipe). The first seven vertebrae form the cervical spine, lying in the neck. The carotid arteries may be found at either side of the trachea, together with the jugular veins and several nerves (Fig. 4:4).

Several useful landmarks are present in the neck. Most obvious is the firm, prominent thyroid cartilage in the center of the anterior

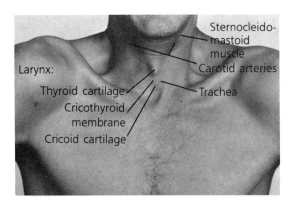

FIGURE 4:4. Anterior view of the neck

surface known as the "Adam's apple," more prominent in men than women. Approximately ¾ inch inferior to the upper border of this prominence is a marked soft tissue depression about ¼ inch wide that separates the thyroid cartilage from a second, somewhat less noticeable, cartilage—the cricoid cartilage. This cricoid cartilage is palpable as a firm ridge 1/8 to ¼ inch thick. The thyroid and cricoid cartilages together form the framework of the larynx (voice box). The soft tissue depression represents the area of the cricothyroid membrane, which is a substantial sheet of fascia (connective tissue) connecting the two cartilages. The cricothyroid membrane is covered at this point only by skin.

Inferiorly from the larynx, several additional firm ridges are palpable in the trachea. These ridges are the cartilages of the trachea. The trachea connects the larynx with the main bronchi (airways) of the lungs.

On either side of the lower larynx and the upper trachea lies the thyroid gland. Unless it is enlarged, this gland is usually not palpable.

Pulsations of the carotid arteries are easily palpable 1 to 2 cm lateral to the larynx. Lying immediately adjacent to these arteries are the internal jugular veins and important nerves. Obviously, injuries that involve these areas of the neck may cause rapid, fatal bleeding.

Posteriorly, the spines of the cervical vertebrae are palpable prominences in the midline of the neck and become more obvious as they progress down the spine. They are most easily palpable when the neck is in extreme flexion. At the base of the neck posteriorly the spine of the seventh cervical vertebra is usually the most prominent (see Fig. 4:4). Ordinarily, the larynx lies just anterior to the fifth and sixth cervical vertebrae.

THORAX

The thorax (chest) is the cavity that contains the heart, lungs, esophagus and the great vessels (the aorta and the two venae cavae). It is formed by the 12 thoracic vertebrae and 12 pairs of ribs. The clavicle (collarbone) overlies its upper boundaries in front and articulates with the scapula (shoulder blade), which lies in the muscular tissue of the thoracic wall posteriorly. Pleura lines the chest cavity, arches high in a dome behind each clavicle superiorly, and inferiorly covers the upper surface of the diaphragm, the lower boundary of the thorax (Figs. 4:5A, B).

The dimensions of the thorax are defined by the bony rib cage and its attachments. Anteriorly, in the midline of the chest, is the sternum (breastbone). The superior border of the sternum forms the easily palpable jugular notch. The inferior end of the sternum forms a narrow cartilaginous tip called the xiphoid process.

In the midline of the upper back, the spines of the 12 thoracic vertebrae can be palpated. Ten of these vertebrae are connected anteriorly to the sternum or to the costal arch by the first through the tenth ribs. The eleventh and twelfth ribs do not connect to the sternum or the arch and are therefore called floating ribs. An interposed costal cartilage forms the articulation between the ribs and the sternum or the arch. Inferiorly, the cartilages themselves become longer and form the palpable costal arch, which is the definite boundary of the lower border of the thorax and the upper border of the abdomen. The arch itself is made up of the fused costal cartilages of the sixth through the tenth ribs. The jugular notch of

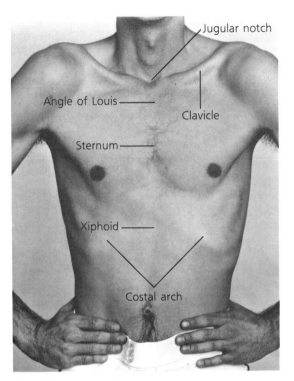

FIGURE 4:5A. Anterior aspect of the chest wall

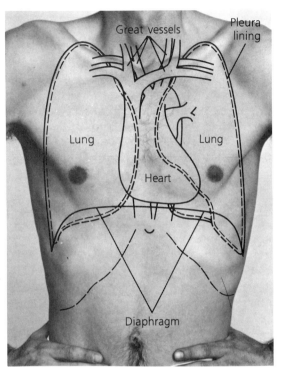

FIGURE 4:5B. Anterior aspect of the chest with the positions of the important chest organs.

the sternum lies at the level of the second thoracic vertebra. The xiphoid tip lies approximately at the level of the ninth thoracic vertebra.

On the male chest the nipples lie at the level of the interspace between the fourth and fifth ribs. In the female, breasts obviously vary in size, and consequently nipple position may vary. The center of the breast, however, still lies at the interspace between the fourth and fifth ribs.

Posteriorly, the scapula overlies the thoracic wall and is contained within heavy muscles. When the patient is erect, the two scapulae should lie at approximately the same level, with their inferior tips at about the seventh thoracic vertebra. If one scapula lies noticeably higher, it may be an indication of neuromuscular or bony injury.

The diaphragm is a muscular dome forming the undersurface of the thorax, separating the chest and abdominal cavities. Anteriorly, it is attached to the costal arch. Posteriorly, it is attached to the lumbar vertebrae. It moves up and down with normal breathing for a distance of one or two intercostal spaces. Injuries of the lower portion of the lung and the diaphram from penetrating wounds obviously depend on the position of the diaphragm at the time of injury. Similarly, injuries of the lower chest may easily involve the abdomen.

Within the thoracic cage, the most prominent structures are the heart and lungs. The heart lies within the pericardial sac immediately under the sternum and immediately above the midportion of the diaphragm. It extends from the second to the sixth ribs anteriorly and from the fifth to the eighth thoracic vertebrae posteriorly. Ordinarily it lies from the midline to the left midclavicular line in the fifth intercostal space. Diseased hearts may be larger or smaller.

The major palpable landmarks in the chest are obviously the ribs, most of which can be easily felt. The first rib is not palpable on either side, since it is hidden under and behind the clavicle, which joins the sternum. Both clavicle and sternum are easily felt. Just inferior to the junction of the clavicle and sternum is a prominence on the breastbone, the angle of Louis. This prominence always lies opposite the space between the second and third ribs (second intercostal space). Orientation for counting ribs can be from this prominence and the palpable interspace opposite it.

The major blood vessels traveling to and from the heart lie deep within the chest. On the right side of the spinal column the superior and inferior venae cavae carry blood to the heart. Just beneath the upper third of the sternum, the arch of the aorta and the pulmonary artery rise to distribute blood to the body and to the lungs, respectively. The arch of the aorta passes to the left and lies alongside the left side of the spinal column as it descends deep within the chest and into the abdomen. The esophagus lies behind the trachea and directly on the spinal column as it passes through the chest into the abdomen.

All the space within the chest not occupied by the heart, the great vessels and the esophagus is occupied by the lungs. Anteriorly, the lungs extend down to the surface of the diaphragm at the level of the xiphoid process. Posteriorly, the lungs continue in contact with the surface of the diaphragm down to the level of the twelfth thoracic vertebra.

ABDOMEN

The abdomen is the second major body cavity. It is bounded superiorly by the diaphragm, inferiorly by a plane extending from the pubic symphysis through the sacrum, anteriorly by the anterior abdominal wall and posteriorly by the posterior abdominal wall. It contains the major organs of digestion and excretion.

Although there are several methods of referring to the various portions of the abdomen, the simplest and most common uses abdomi-

nal quadrants. In this system, the abdomen is divided into four equal parts by two lines that intersect at right angles at the umbilicus. The quadrants thus formed are right upper, right lower, left upper and left lower (Fig. 4:6), where right and left are the patient's right and left, not the observer's. Pain or injury in a given quadrant usually arises from or involves the organs in that quadrant. This specification of that quadrant allows the organs that are injured or diseased or that may require emergency attention to be identified quickly and clearly.

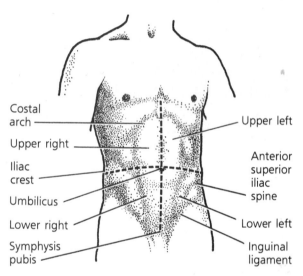

FIGURE 4:6. In the abdomen, quadrants are the easiest system for identifying areas. Major bony landmarks are also shown.

In the upper right quadrant, the major organs are the liver, gallbladder, and a portion of the colon (Fig. 4:7). The greater portion of the liver lies in this quadrant almost entirely under the protection of the eighth to twelfth ribs. It extends through the entire anteroposterior depth of the abdomen. Injuries in this area are frequently associated with injuries of the liver. Tenderness without injury in the right upper quadrant is usually due to gallbladder disease.

In the left upper quadrant, the principal organs are the stomach, the spleen, a portion

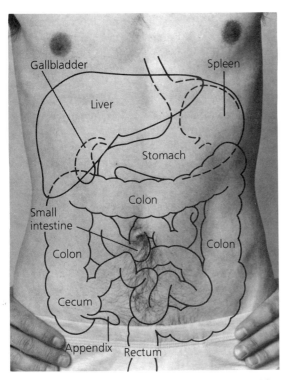

FIGURE 4:7.   Anterior view of the abdomen with the position of the major abdominal organs outlined

quadrants. The large bowel arises laterally in the right lower quadrant and completely encircles the abdomen in one sweep, coming to lie in all four quadrants also. The urinary bladder lies just behind the junction of the pubic bones at the middle of the abdomen; therefore, it lies in both lower quadrants. The pancreas lies transversely on the posterior body wall behind the abdominal cavity and therefore is in both upper quadrants. The kidneys lie in the same plane as the pancreas, behind the abdominal cavity. They lie completely above the level of the umbilicus, extending from the eleventh thoracic vertebra to the third lumbar vertebra. They are approximately 4 to 6 inches long and lie in an angle formed by the spinal column and the lower ribs, the costovertebral angle. They are each attached to the bladder by tubular structures called ureters, which lie in the same plane behind the abdominal cavity. These tubes pass on either side of the spinal column along the posterior wall of the abdomen into the pelvis to enter the bladder (Fig. 4:8).

of the transverse and descending colon and a small portion of the liver. The stomach and the spleen are almost entirely protected by the left rib cage. The spleen lies lateral and posterior in this quadrant, under the diaphragm and immediately beneath the ninth to eleventh ribs. This organ is frequently injured, especially in association with fracture of these ribs. Tenderness or pain in the left upper quadrant often indicates a ruptured spleen.

In the right lower quadrant, the principal organs are the cecum and the ascending colon. The appendix is a small tubular structure attached to the lower border of the cecum. Appendicitis is the most frequent cause of tenderness and pain in this region. In the left lower quadrant the principal organs are the descending colon and the rectosigmoid colon.

Many organs lie in one or more quadrants. The small bowel, for instance, encircles the umbilicus, and parts of it occupy all four

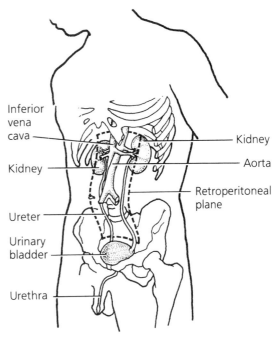

FIGURE 4:8.   Several organs lie in more than one quadrant.

Posteriorly, one does not usually refer to quadrants. The posterior portions of the iliac crest and the midline spines of the five lumbar vertebrae are the predominant landmarks of reference.

Properly speaking, organs that lie in the lowest portions of the abdominal cavity are in the pelvic cavity. This cavity is bounded by the sacrum behind and the pubis in front. It lies between the most inferior portions of the pelvic bone. The female reproductive organs (the uterus, ovaries and fallopian tubes) and the rectum and urinary bladder are situated in this cavity, which is continuous with the abdominal cavity above.

In the abdomen the chief topographic landmarks are the costal arch, the umbilicus, the anterior superior iliac spines, the iliac crests and the pubic symphysis. The costal arch is the fused cartilages of the sixth through the tenth ribs. It forms the superior arching boundary of the abdomen. The umbilicus, a constant structure, is in the same horizontal plane as the fourth lumbar vertebra and the superior edge of the iliac crests. It overlies the division of the aorta into the two common iliac arteries. The anterior superior iliac spines are the hard bony prominences at the front on each side of the lower abdomen just below the plane of the umbilicus. At the center of the lowermost portion of the abdomen, another hard bony prominence, the pubic symphysis, can be felt. The bladder lies just behind this bone. Injuries of the bladder frequently accompany fractures of the pelvis. Between the pubic symphysis and the anterior superior iliac spine on each side, one can palpate the tough inguinal ligament, a useful soft tissue landmark which directly overlies the femoral vessels.

PELVIS

The pelvis is a closed bony ring consisting of the sacrum in the midline posteriorly, two iliac bones laterally, two ischial bones inferiorly and two pubic bones anteriorly. The latter three bones, ilium, ischium and pubis, are fused to form a single bone, commonly called the innominate bone (Fig. 4:9). On each side of the pelvis are deep sockets. They receive each femoral head and form the hip joints. Gentle pressure on each anterior superior iliac spine or on the iliac crests in a patient with a pelvic fracture usually causes pain at the fracture site.

Located between the pubic symphysis and the anterior superior iliac spine on each side of the lower abdomen is a palpable, tough band of tissue, the inguinal ligament. Deep to this ligament pass the femoral nerve, artery, vein and muscles to the lower extremity. The femoral artery is easily palpable just distal to the midpoint of the ligament. The femoral nerve lies immediately lateral to the artery, and the femoral vein lies just medial to it.

Posteriorly, the pelvis presents a flattened appearance, mainly because of the configuration of the sacrum. In the sitting position, a bony prominence is easily felt in the middle of each buttock. These prominences are the ischial tuberositas. The sciatic nerve carrying major motor and sensory innervation to the foot and leg passes lateral to the tuberosity as it enters the thigh. With fractures of the pelvis in this region or a posterior hip dislocation, pressure on this nerve results in pain or paralysis.

LOWER EXTREMITY

The lower extremity consists of the hip, thigh, knee, leg, ankle and foot. Strictly speaking, the hip is a joint articulating the femur with the innominate bone. Just distal and posterolateral to this joint is a bony prominence present on each femur called the greater trochanter (Fig. 4:10). In examination, the position of this prominence should always be compared with that on the opposite side. Changes in the relative positions of these prominences may indicate underlying hip fractures or dislocations. The hip joint itself is superior and medial to the greater trochanter and about 1 inch lateral and 1 inch inferior to the pulsations of the femoral artery at the inguinal ligament (Fig. 4:11).

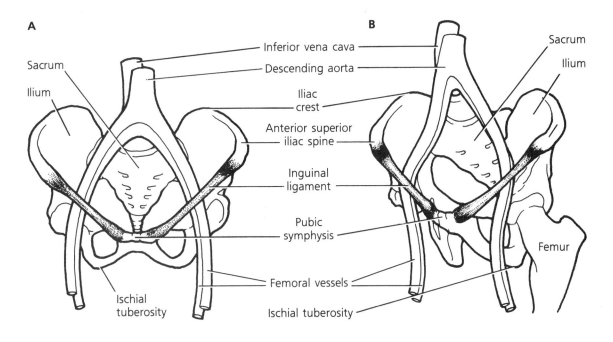

FIGURE 4:9. The pelvis is composed of several separate elements and bears the sockets for the hip joints. The inguinal ligament lies just above the femoral vessels and helps protect them.

The thigh extends from the hip joint to the knee. The underlying femur has few landmarks, except the greater trochanter and the distal femoral condyles, but fractures of this large bone, when displaced or angulated, can be localized without great difficulty. The powerful muscles which attach to the femur can drive fractured segments of bone through the skin after an injury. The examination of a suspected femoral fracture must be done carefully to avoid converting a closed fracture into an open one.

The patella lies anteriorly to the knee joint, within the quadriceps tendon, and thus is an important part of the extensor mechanism of the knee. A fracture of the patella will frequently interrupt this tendon, and the patient will be unable to extend the leg at the knee. A gap in the patella itself may also be palpated in these cases. Normally the patella rides smoothly in a groove on the anterior surface of the distal femur. This groove lies between the rounded condyles that make up the distal end of the femur and the articular surface of the knee joint. When the patella is dislocated, it is usually displaced laterally from the groove beyond the lateral condyle. In such instances the leg is fixed in flexion at the knee, and the pain is extreme. The actual joint line of the knee is usually 1 inch inferior to the lower margin of the patella and it can be easily felt by palpating on either side of the patella tendon with the knee flexed at 90°.

The leg is the portion of the lower extremity extending from the knee joint to the ankle joint. The bones of the leg are the tibia and the fibula. The broad tibial plateau forms the lower surface of the knee joint. The entire extent of the tibia, the familiar shinbone, can be palpated just under the skin on the medial surface.

At the posterolateral corner of the knee lies the head of the fibula, and this bone is most easily palpated with the knee flexed at 90°.

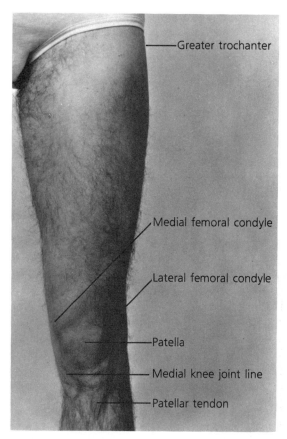

FIGURE 4:10. Anterior view of the thigh and knee

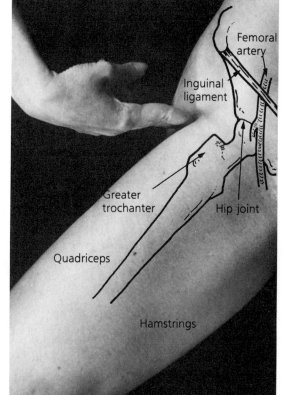

FIGURE 4:11. Anatomy of the hip

Passing immediately distally around this bony prominence is the peroneal nerve, which controls movement at the ankle and sensation over the top of the foot. Injury of the fibula in this region should always prompt comparison of the function of the nerve with that on the opposite side of the patient's body.

The ankle is easily located by identifying the prominent distal ends of both tibia and fibula (Fig. 4:12). Usually visible even in patients with large or fat legs, these knobs are called, respectively, the medial malleolus and lateral malleolus, and form the socket of the ankle joint. Within the socket sits the talus (anklebone), which in turn articulates with the calcaneus (heelbone or os calcis) inferiorly.

The calcaneus is palpable through the skin of the heel. The extremity is completed by the tarsal bones, five metatarsal bones, which form the substance of the foot, and the five toes formed of 14 phalanges.

Inspection of the lower extremity can give many clues to an injury, particularly fractures and dislocations. Noting the relative position of bilateral structures helps diagnose other injuries from the hip joint to more distal areas in the extremity. In assessing injuries in the lower extremity, if the patellae are at the same level on either side, the injury is probably below the knee. If they are not, the injury may be above the knee. Most patients with hip fractures have a shortened, externally rotated leg. In these patients, the patella may be above the patella on the opposite side, facing outward. A dislocated hip may cause the extremity to shorten, flex and internally rotate, in which

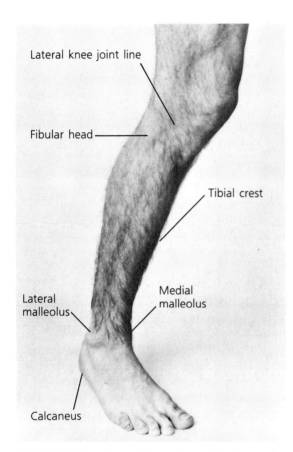

FIGURE 4:12. Anterolateral view of the leg and foot, showing the bony prominences

The scapula is a broad, flat bone overlying the posterior wall of the thorax and articulating with the clavicle and humerus. Injury of this bone is rare because of its protected situation. It ordinarily is palpable, especially the transverse ridge or spine running across the upper portion of each scapula.

The external appearance of the shoulder as a unit is that of a gently rounded area without major noticeable prominences. The very top of the shoulder corresponds to the acromioclavicular joint. This joint lies 3 cm from the lateral surface of the arm. The most lateral structure of the shoulder is the rounded head of the humerus, the bone of the arm, which accounts for the rounded appearance of the shoulder in general. If the humeral head is dislocated from its articulation with the scapula, it is no longer laterally located and the configuration of the shoulder may change from a rounded to a more angular appearance. Injuries that do not involve the joint itself fail to produce this change.

case the patella may face its neighbor. Careful inspection allows the examiner to make all these observations.

SHOULDER GIRDLE

The shoulder girdle (Fig. 4:13) is composed of the clavicle anteriorly, scapula posteriorly and the humeral head laterally. Injury of these structures may present as "pain in the shoulder." The clavicle is attached medially to the sternum at the sternoclavicular joint. It is palpable throughout its entire length, from the sternum to its attachment to the scapula at the acromioclavicular joint. Acromioclavicular dislocations or separations can be easily palpated. Fractures of the clavicle are not only easily palpable but also usually visible.

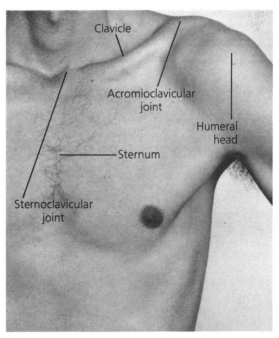

FIGURE 4:13. The rounded prominence of the shoulder girdle laterally is created by the humeral head, covered by muscle.

UPPER EXTREMITY

The upper extremity extends from the shoulder to the fingertips. It is composed of the arm, elbow, forearm, wrist, hand and fingers. The arm extends from the shoulder to the elbow, and the supporting bone is the humerus. The arm offers few specific landmarks. Displaced or angulated fractures of the humerus are generally easy to diagnose. The radial nerve, carrying sensation to the greater portion of the back of the hand and motor function that controls extension of the hand at the wrist, wraps very closely around the shaft of the humerus in its midportion. Fractures in this region demand careful testing of the function of this nerve.

The elbow presents several bony landmarks (Fig. 4:14). The medial and lateral condyles of the humerus form the medial and lateral borders of the upper surface of the elbow joint.

They are easy to palpate at the distal end of the elbow joint and at the distal end of the humerus with the elbow flexed. A third prominence is the most posterior portion of the elbow at its apex, called the olecranon process of the ulna. Fractures about the elbow usually result in distortion of the normal alignment of these three prominences.

Immediately posterior to the medial condyle of the humerus is a groove in which the ulnar nerve passes. This groove can be easily felt by extending the elbow fully. The ulnar nerve is extremely important, controlling sensation over the fourth and fifth fingers and most of the muscular function of the hand. The ulnar nerve is easily damaged in elbow injuries. Contusions to this nerve at the elbow produce tingling in the fourth and fifth fingers, an event referred to as injuring the "funny bone."

The median nerve may also be injured about the elbow. This nerve lies near the anterior surface of the elbow, approximately in the midline. It is more protected in this area by adjacent muscles than is the ulnar nerve.

At the wrist (Fig. 4:15), a bony prominence is easily felt at the distal end of the ulna, the ulnar styloid. A similar, less obvious, bony process is present on the lateral (thumb or radial) side of the wrist. This is the radial styloid process and represents the distal end of the radius. Simultaneous palpation of these distal tips shows that the radial styloid process usually lies about 1 cm distal to that of the ulna. With displaced wrist fractures, this rela-

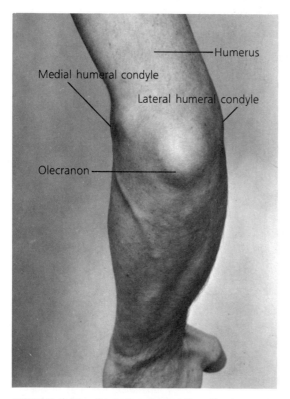

FIGURE 4:14. Posterior view of the elbow, showing the three bony prominences

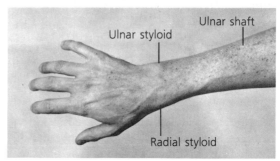

FIGURE 4:15. Dorsal view of the forearm and wrist

tionship may be reversed, or the processes may lie at the same level.

The hand articulates with the forearm through the eight carpal bones. The palm of the hand is formed by five metacarpal bones and the thumb and fingers by the 14 phalanges.

ARTERIAL PULSE POINTS

At any point where an artery passes over a bony prominence or lies close to the skin, it can be palpated and the arterial pulse taken. These points were called arterial pressure points because it was felt that compression at one of these points would help control hemorrhage distal to it. Although this principle is sound and applies to any artery in the body, pressure over any single artery rarely completely stops circulation distal to that point because more than one artery is always supplying blood to an injury site. Therefore, local pressure on the wound remains the best method to control hemorrhage.

At major arterial pulse points (Fig. 4:16) it is usually easy to find the arterial pulse and to ascertain correctly the presence of cardiac activity or the absence of a proximal arterial injury.

Anterior to the upper portion of the ear, just over the temporomandibular joints, lie the superficial temporal arteries that supply the scalp. Anterior to the angle of the mandible, on the inner surface of the lower jaw on either side, one may palpate the external maxillary arteries, which contribute much of the blood supply to the face. The carotid arteries may be compressed anteriorly against the transverse processes of the sixth cervical vertebra just behind the artery. At the inner surface of the arm, the brachial artery may be palpated approximately 4 cm above the elbow. Arterial

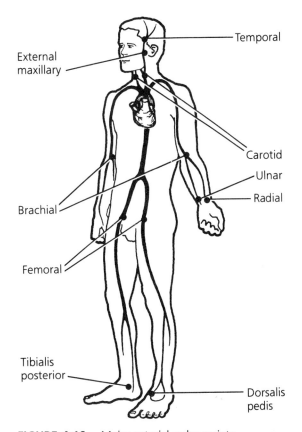

FIGURE 4:16. Major arterial pulse points

pulsation may be felt in both the radial and ulnar arteries at the wrist, at the bases of the thumb and little finger, respectively.

The femoral artery may be palpated as it issues from beneath the inguinal ligament in the groin. Just posterior to the medial malleolus is the posterior tibial artery. On the anterior surface of the foot just lateral to the major extensor tendon of the great toe is the dorsalis pedis artery. This artery is not as constantly present as the posterior tibial artery, but when present, its pulsations may be felt easily.

Diagnostic Signs and Triage

5

A rapid but accurate examination of an injured or critically ill patient is essential for adequate emergency medical care. This examination includes observing diagnostic signs and evaluating symptoms. Signs are manifestations of changes in body function apparent to the trainer, while symptoms are evidence of changes in body function apparent to the patient and expressed to the trainer as subjective complaints. The nine essential diagnostic signs—pulse, respiration, blood pressure, body temperature, condition of the skin, status of pupils, state of consciousness, ability to move and reaction to pain—can be observed rapidly during examination. Together with questioning about symptoms and examination, they form the basis for diagnosis.

THE NINE DIAGNOSTIC SIGNS

1. Pulse

The pulse is the pressure wave, traveling along the arteries, caused by the contraction of the heart. The usual pulse rate in adults is 60 to 100 beats per minute; in children it is 80 to 100 beats per minute. The pulse can be palpated (felt by touch) at any area where an artery passes over a bony prominence or is close to the skin.

Commonly, the place to palpate the pulse is at the base of the thumb over the palmar surface of the wrist (Fig. 5:1A), where the radial artery is fairly superficial. However, palpation of the radial pulse may be difficult in an emergency and not always accurate. Instead, the carotid artery in the neck is the preferred site to palpate the pulse, although it can be felt in other major arteries. One must palpate gently

under the anterior border of the sternocleidomastoid muscle (Fig. 5:1B). The patient must always be lying down or sitting. If no pulse is detected, the unconscious patient should be considered pulseless.

Changes in the rate and volume of the pulse are important findings in emergency medical care. The pulse rate is easily checked and reflects the rapidity of the heart contractions. The pulse volume describes the sensation the contraction itself gives to the palpating finger.

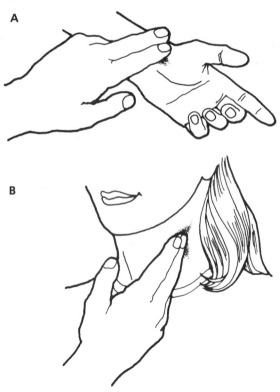

FIGURE 5:1. **A** Radial and **B** carotid pulses are usually easily palpated.

Normally the pulse is a strong, easily felt impulse reflecting a full blood volume. A rapid, weak pulse can be the result of shock from loss of blood; a rapid, bounding pulse is present in fright or hypertension. The absence of a pulse means that the specific artery is blocked or injured, that the heart has stopped functioning (cardiac arrest), or that death has occurred. Changes in the pulse directly reflect changes in heart rate in response to injury or alarm, changes in circulating blood volume, or changes in the vascular bed. The pulse should be taken immediately and then periodically during emergency treatment to note any changes. The pulse rates must be written down as they are taken and the character of the pulse described (weak or strong).

2. Respiration

Normal breathing is easy, without pain or effort. The rate can vary widely. Usually it is between 12 and 20 breaths per minute, but well-trained athletes may breathe only six to eight times a minute. Rarely does the resting rate exceed 20 breaths per minute. A record should be made of the initial rate and character of respiration when the patient is first seen, and any change should be observed.

Rapid, shallow respirations are seen in shock. Deep, gasping, labored breathing may indicate partial airway obstruction or pulmonary disease. In respiratory depression or respiratory arrest, there is little or no movement of the chest and abdomen with respiration and little air flow at the nose and mouth. Severe metabolic disturbances, such as acidosis or alkalosis, may produce characteristic breathing patterns.

Frothy sputum with blood at the nose and mouth accompanied by coughing following an injury indicates lung damage. Fractured ribs can tear the lung. In each instance, bleeding within the lung may appear as coughed-up pink froth. Frothy pink or bloody sputum is also an indication of pulmonary edema, which can accompany acute cardiac failure or severe lung contusion.

Occasionally one can learn much from the smell of the athlete's breath. Obviously, the intoxicated patient may smell of alcohol. The breath of patients in severe diabetic acidosis frequently has a sweet or fruity odor. Any particularly obvious odor should be noted and recorded.

3. Blood Pressure

Blood pressure is the pressure of the circulating blood against the walls of the arteries. Since in the normal person the arterial system is a closed system attached to a pump and completely filled with blood, changes in the pressure indicate changes in the volume of the blood, in the capacity of the vessels or in the ability of the heart to pump. Changes in blood pressure, like those in the pulse, can be rapid. They are not as rapid as pulse changes, however, because normal protective mechanisms maintain blood pressure in spite of injury or disease.

Blood pressure can fall markedly in states of shock, after severe bleeding or after a heart attack. Lowered blood pressure means that there is insufficient pressure in the arterial system to supply blood to all of the organs of the body. Some of these organs may thus be severely damaged. The causes of low blood pressure must be rapidly ascertained and treated.

If blood pressure is abnormally high, the vessels in the arterial circuit may be damaged or ruptured. It is equally important that the cause of this state be ascertained and treated. The treatment of elevated blood pressure may require hospitalization. This therapy is complex and is not a function of the trainer. On the other hand, the treatment of low blood pressure from bleeding requires emergency control of such bleeding by direct pressure on the source if accessible.

Blood pressure can change rapidly during transport of a patient to the hospital. Emergency department personnel must know the status of the blood pressure as early as possible, and any changes before arrival at the hospital. Therefore, during emergency medical care of the patient, the trainer should check and record the pressure at intervals as necessary, together with the time taken.

Blood pressure is recorded at systolic and diastolic levels. Systolic pressure is the level present during contraction of the heart. Diastolic pressure is the level present during relaxation of the heart. Systolic pressure is the maximum pressure to which the arteries are subjected, while diastolic pressure is the minimum pressure constantly present in the arteries. Usually these pressures change in a parallel fashion, both rising or falling. Brain damage in a patient with a head injury at times causes a rise in the systolic pressure with a stable or falling diastolic pressure. Systolic and diastolic pressures that approach each other, as the former falls and the latter rises, occur in cardiac tamponade.

Blood pressure is determined with a sphygmomanometer and a stethoscope (Fig. 5:2). The cuff of the sphygmomanometer is fastened about either arm above the elbow and is inflated with a rubber bulb until the mercury column or the needle of the dial stops moving with the pulse. This point is usually between 150 and 200 mm on the scale. The stethoscope diaphragm or bell is placed over the brachial artery at the front of the elbow. Air is slowly released from the bulb as the gauge returns to zero. The point at which the first sounds of the pulse are heard through the stethoscope is the systolic pressure. The point at which the sounds disappear is the diastolic pressure. The pressure reading is in millimeters of mercury (mm Hg) and is recorded in the form systolic/diastolic.

Blood pressure levels vary with age and sex. A useful rule of thumb for normal systolic pressure in the male is 100 plus the age of the athlete, up to a level of 140 to 150 mm Hg. Normal diastolic pressure in the male is 65 to 90 mm Hg. Both pressures are about 10 mm Hg lower in the female. Sounds at the elbow are at times impossible to hear, so the trainer must rely on the movement in the gauge at the moment of systolic pressure and the stopping of such movement at the diastolic level.

Alternatively, the systolic pressure can only be obtained by the palpation method. With this technique, the patient's radial pulse is palpated and then the sphygmomanometer cuff is inflated. The pulse will disappear when the cuff pressure exceeds the systolic blood pressure. The cuff pressure is increased approximately 50 mm Hg above the point at which the pulse disappears. The cuff is then deflated gradually. When the palpating finger first feels a return of the radial pulse, the pressure recording on the gauge equals the systolic blood pressure.

One of the most useful diagnostic instruments the trainer has is the stethoscope. It is used to determine blood pressure and to detect heart, breath and bowel sounds. Heart sounds are detected by listening over the heart, detection of breath sounds by listening in the interspaces between the ribs on each side of the chest, and bowel sounds are detected by listening in all four quadrants of the abdomen.

When the stethoscope is used correctly, the

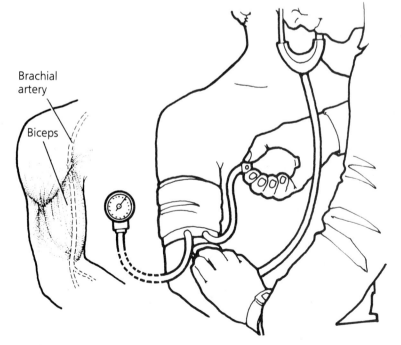

Brachial artery

Biceps

FIGURE 5:2. The proper location for and application of the sphygmomanometer and stethoscope

earpieces fit into the ears comfortably and exclude outside sounds. The stethoscope should be worn with the earpieces pointing forward. The principal mistakes made in using a stethoscope are selecting one that is too small or too tight, or putting it into the ears backward. Before applying it to the patient, always make sure the stethoscope is picking up sounds by tapping the diaphragm or bell lightly with the finger.

4. Temperature

Normal body temperature is 37 Centigrade (98.6 Fahrenheit). The skin is largely responsible for regulating this temperature by radiation of heat from skin blood vessels and the evaporation of water as sweat.

Illness or injury produces changes in temperature. A cool, clammy (damp) skin indicates a general response of the sympathetic nervous system to body insult, i.e., blood loss (shock) or heat exhaustion. As a result of nervous stimulation, sweat glands are hyperactive and skin blood vessels are contracted, resulting in cold, pale, wet or clammy skin. These signs are often the first indication of shock, and they must be recognized as such. Exposure to cold will produce a cool, dry skin. A dry, hot skin may be caused by fever or by exposure to excessive heat, as in heatstroke (Chapter 51).

Temperature is usually taken by mouth, with the bulb of the thermometer placed beneath the tongue. The thermometer should be left in place with the athlete's mouth closed for three minutes. In a child or uncooperative adult, the thermometer can be placed in the axilla (armpit), and the arm kept at the side. Axillary temperatures are notoriously inaccurate, take a long time to register accurately (10 minutes) and should be used only as a last resort. Rectal temperature is very accurate and usually taken, if necessary, in the emergency department. It is routinely one-half to one degree above oral temperature and is taken with a special thermometer left in place for one minute.

5. Skin Color

In lightly pigmented people, skin color depends primarily on the presence of circulating blood in the subcutaneous blood vessels. In deeply pigmented people, skin color depends primarily on the pigment. Pigment may hide skin color changes resulting from illness or injury. In patients with deeply pigmented skin, color changes may be apparent in the fingernail beds, in the sclera, or under the tongue. In lightly pigmented patients where changes may be seen more easily, colors of medical importance are red, white and blue.

A red color may accompany high blood pressure, certain stages of carbon monoxide poisoning and heatstroke. The patient who has severe high blood pressure may sometimes be plethoric (dark, reddish-purple skin color, and all visible blood vessels full). The patient with carbon monoxide poisoning is usually cherry red, as is the heatstroke patient.

A pale, white, ashen or grayish skin indicates insufficient circulation and is seen in shock, acute heart attack, or certain stages of fright. Here there is literally not enough blood circulating in the skin.

A bluish skin color, cyanosis, results from poor oxygenation of the circulating blood. As a result, blood is very dark, and the overlying tissue appears blue. Cyanosis is caused by respiratory insufficiency due to airway obstruction or inadequate lung function. It is usually first seen in the fingertips and around the mouth. Cyanosis always indicates a significant lack of oxygen and demands rapid correction of the underlying respiratory problems.

Chronic illness may also produce color changes, such as the yellow color, jaundice, in liver disease. In such cases bilirubin, a reddish-yellow pigment normally present in the liver and the gastrointestinal tract, is deposited in the patient's skin.

Assessment of the patient's color can lead to a decision about the immediate treatment. Oxygen, control of bleeding or resuscitation may be needed. Sometimes only a glance at the patient is needed to decide on priority treatment.

6. Pupils

The pupils, when normal, are regular in outline and usually the same size. In examining the pupils, always consider the presence of contact lenses or prostheses (glass eyes).

Changes and variation in size of one or both pupils are important signs in emergency medical care. Constricted pupils (Fig. 5:3) are often present in a drug addict or an athlete with a central nervous system disease. Dilated pupils indicate a relaxed or unconscious state. Such dilation usually occurs rapidly, within 30 seconds after cardiac arrest. Head injury or prior drug use, however, may cause the pupils to remain constricted even in patients with cardiac arrest.

Variation in the size of the pupils is seen in patients with head injuries or strokes. A small percentage of normal persons have anisocoria (unequal pupil size). The incidence of this is so small, however, that in the injured athlete pupil variation is a reliable sign of brain damage. Pupils ordinarily constrict promptly when light shines into the eye. This is the eye's normal protective reaction. The pupils fail to constrict when a light shines into the eye in disease, poisoning, drug overdose and injury. In death, the pupils are widely dilated and fail to respond to light.

Constricted pupil

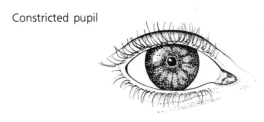

Dilated pupil

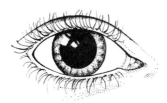

FIGURE 5:3. Normal pupillary diameter is 2 to 3 mm.

Progressive changes in the pupils rapidly reflect central nervous system dysfunction. Any such changes should be noted early in the examination of patients, reported and written down.

7. State of Consciousness

Normally a person is alert, oriented (knows time, place and what day it is), and responsive to vocal or physical stimuli (Fig. 5:4). Any change from that state is indicative of illness or injury. Recording such a change is extremely important in emergency medical care. Such changes may vary from mild confusion in an alcoholic or mental patient to deep coma as a result of a head injury or poisoning. The patient's state of consciousness is probably the single most reliable sign in assessing the status of the nervous system.

It is extremely important to note immediately the state of consciousness of a patient and all subsequent changes. Progressive development of coma or increasing difficulty in rousing a patient means that the patient urgently needs prompt attention at the hospital. This is especially true in the patient who is unconscious following an injury, rouses and seems normal for a period of time (lucid interval), and then suddenly becomes unconscious and collapses. Such a patient may have intracranial bleeding and need immediate surgery.

8. Ability to Move

The inability of a conscious patient to move voluntarily is known as paralysis. It results from illness or injury. Paralysis of one side of the body (hemiplegia) may be caused by bleeding within the brain or a clot in a vessel (stroke). Some drugs, if used over long periods of time, may also cause paralysis.

Inability to move the legs or arms after an accident indicates injury to the spinal cord until proven otherwise. Inability to move the legs while the arms remain normal indicates a spinal injury below the neck. Paralysis is a particularly important sign, and its presence and onset with regard to an injury must be recorded. The patient who has a completely severed spinal cord is paralyzed below the level of the injury, immediately and permanently. The patient who has a spinal injury in which the cord is gradually compressed experiences progressive onset of paralysis.

9. Reaction to Pain

Reaction by vocal response or body movement to painful physical stimulation is a normal function of the body. Loss of sensation following an injury or illness may change this reaction.

The loss of voluntary movement of the extremities after an injury is usually accompanied by loss of sensation in these extremities. Occasionally, however, movement is retained and the patient complains of numbness or tingling in the extremities. This fact must be recognized as a sign of probable spinal cord injury so that mishandling does not aggravate the condition.

Severe pain in an extremity with loss of skin sensation may be the result of occlusion of the extremity's main artery. In such a case the pulse in the extremity is absent. The patient can usually move the extremity, although often holds it immobile because of pain.

Frequently, patients suffering from hysteria, violent shock or excessive drug or alcohol use may feel no pain from an injury for several hours. This is not accompanied by paralysis, and usually other signs will support a diagnosis of hysteria or other such reaction.

PATIENT ASSESSMENT

A good general survey usually results in appropriate judgment and action. In the case of the injured athlete, this includes observation of the mechanism of injury. The trainer should observe the position in which the player lies on the field or floor. If the trainer has seen the injury occur, such as an athlete being struck against the lateral side of his knee by an opposing player, he should immediately suspect certain injuries.

NEUROLOGICAL CHECKLIST				
Time				
Talks	yes / no	yes / no	yes / no	yes / no
Follows commands	yes / no	yes / no	yes / no	yes / no
Pupil diameter	L R mm mm	L R mm mm	L R mm mm	L R mm mm

FIGURE 5:4. The neurological checklist used to record periodic observations of the patient's level of consciousness

Primary Survey

This primary survey (Fig. 5:5) is designed to discover and correct any immediate life-threatening problems. An initial survey begins as soon as the trainer reaches the injured player. During the primary survey, the trainer needs only to talk, feel and observe. No diagnostic equipment is needed. Inquiries should be brief and pertinent, with no detailed questioning at this time. Five diagnostic signs—position, state of consciousness, respiration, skin color and pulse—should be evaluated.

During the primary survey, a definitive step-by-step outline of action must be followed. A disorganized or unplanned approach will result in lost time and inhibit emergency care, creating confusion at the scene. The trainer must remain calm no matter what the situation. This attitude instills confidence in the athlete and others as to the trainer's knowledge and ability to handle the situation. A record of initial observations can be started.

Secondary Survey

Upon completing the primary survey and controlling of any immediate life-threatening problem, the trainer should examine the athlete more thoroughly to prepare for transport from the field and to decide whether hospital-

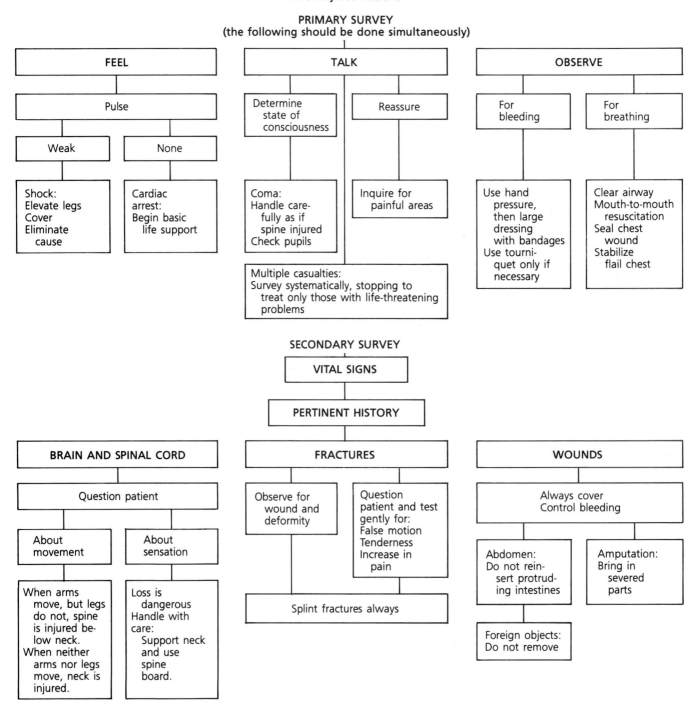

FIGURE 5:5. Primary and secondary surveys for patient assessment

ization is necessary (see Fig. 5:5). A working diagnosis should be established as soon as possible. The conscious athlete should be questioned to determine symptoms. All of the athlete's complaints should be noted and recorded. This is the best guide to the identification of an underlying disease or injury process. The trainer should be familiar with any important medical history and, if not, should ask the athlete whether any previous, similar episodes have occurred. Allowing the athlete to talk is very helpful but, at times, the trainer must direct the history. Once as much pertinent medical information as possible has been obtained, the trainer should thoroughly examine the area of injury. The examination should be conducted in a standard fashion. The effective survey requires inspection, palpation, listening and even, occasionally, the sense of smell to identify all abnormalities. The trainer should become proficient enough to complete this examination within a few minutes. With the exception of life-threatening emergencies, this secondary survey should be completed before beginning stabilization.

In the case of the unconscious athlete, life-threatening situations should first be attended to, followed by evaluation of the diagnostic signs. Immediate observers, such as other players, officials or coaches may provide important information and should be consulted. If there is no immediate improvement in the athlete's condition, the athlete should be transported from the field on a stretcher with back board to prevent further injury.

Triage

Athletes with certain conditions or injuries have a priority for treatment and transportation, as outlined below.

1. Highest priority (must be treated first at the scene and transported immediately)
   A. Airway and breathing difficulties
   B. Cardiac arrest
   C. Uncontrolled or suspected severe hidden bleeding
   D. Open chest or abdominal wounds

   E. Severe head injuries with evidence of brain damage, however slight
   F. Several medical problems: diabetes with complications, cardiac disease with failure
   G. Dislocations associated with lost pulses
2. Second priority
   A. Major or multiple fractures
   B. Back injuries with or without spinal damage
3. Lowest priority
   A. Minor fractures or other minor injuries

Leadership is paramount during triage. Someone must be in command to guide the player's management and to use any help as it arrives. This is the duty of the most highly skilled trainer or of the accompanying physician.

Injury Site Duties

The following actions are routine duties at the site of injury.

1. Obtain assistance, where necessary, with cardiopulmonary resuscitation on the field, in placing the injured athlete on a back board and stretcher and in carrying him from the field. Even with less severe injuries, help is necessary to remove the injured player from the field for further evaluation on the sideline or in the locker room.
2. Reassure relatives and inform them of the patient's condition.
3. Assess the ability of the athlete to go back into the contest. With minor injuries, the trainer can frequently make that judgment but, if the injury is major, a team physician must be consulted. Minor injuries may be evaluated on the field but the patient may have to be brought to the locker room or the physician's office or hospital.

The telephone numbers of the rescue squad, hospital emergency department, team physicians and consultants (home and office) should always be attached to the training room phones. In the case of the severely injured player, emergency medical care continues during loading for transportation.

Accurate assessment of the patient at the scene of the injury along with immobilization of injured parts and clear communication to the physician and hospital personnel aids later care.

By adopting a standardized approach the trainer does not overlook important details and has a plan for any situation that arises.

Part 3

TAPING
AND
BANDAGING

Introduction to Taping and Bandaging

6

The athletic trainer is responsible for the prevention, immediate care and rehabilitation of athletic injuries. Prevention of athletic injury is concerned with the preparticipation screening for muscular strength, muscular imbalances, stress testing, joint range of motion measurements and the application of adhesive tape strapping and support bandages. In addition, the trainer should serve as an advisor for the basic athletic conditioning program. The athletic trainer's response to athletic injuries includes early recognition of injuries, immediate care, arranging for transportation and referral to the team physician when necessary.

The athletic trainer's role includes all procedures that enable the athlete to return to participation with maximal efficiency and minimal risk of reinjury. These procedures include application of hot and cold to injured body parts, use of therapeutic modalities (ultrasound, galvanic stimulation, etc.), specific range of motion and strengthening exercises, adhesive and elastic bandaging techniques, fabrication and fitting of special pads and other protective devices, and monitoring and coordinating the gradual resumption of full activity.

ADHESIVE TAPING

Adhesive taping, commonly used in athletic training, has two functions: injury management and injury protection. In injury management adhesive tape is applied to stabilize the body part to prevent injury or reinjury. Taping procedures are designed to limit range of motion of specific joints and to support in-jured body parts to reduce the possibility of further injury. Taping will not totally prevent an injury recurrence, but may reduce the severity of injury.

Recent studies of the effects of adhesive strapping techniques on reducing the incidence of specific injuries have shown that adhesive techniques do contribute to a lower rate of injury and reinjury. One particular study conducted by Garrick and Requa during two intramural basketball seasons at the University of Washington concluded that basketball players who played with their ankles taped had a significantly lower incidence of injury and reinjury.

The application of adhesive tape helps prevent injury by providing specific ligaments with external support. A joint can never receive the stability from adhesive tape that it does from its own normal ligamentous structure, but in cases where these structures have been repeatedly injured, adhesive tape can provide sufficient stability to permit the athlete to participate without disability.

The application of adhesive taping varies from athletic trainer to athletic trainer, but all procedures must follow these essential rules:

1. The injured site must be properly stabilized.
2. The anatomy of the injured part must be considered with regard to the type and severity of the injury.
3. The adhesive taping cannot compromise the sport skill of the athlete.
4. Always support the ligament in a shortened state. For example, when taping an ankle

to support the lateral ligamentous structure, tape from the medial side to the lateral side of the ankle.

Certain guidelines should be followed when applying adhesive tape to the skin:

1. The area to be taped must be dry and free of body hair (Fig. 6:1), though not always shaved when prewrap is used.
2. Some form of skin adherent must be used to assure bonding of the tape to the skin. If foam underwrap is used, one layer should be applied over the skin adherent. Underwrap helps protect the skin but decreases the efficiency of the tape.
3. In areas with potential for friction blisters or burns, a lubricated pad (grease pad) can be applied. A pad is made by spreading a nonwater soluble lubricant over a cotton sponge or Telfa pad that is placed between the skin and the tape.
4. Continuous circular strapping should be applied cautiously, especially with acute or recent injuries, because of the possibility of circulatory embarrassment.
5. Each strip of adhesive tape should overlap the previous strip of tape by half. Spaces between tape segments must be avoided. This space can cause blisters at the tape site.

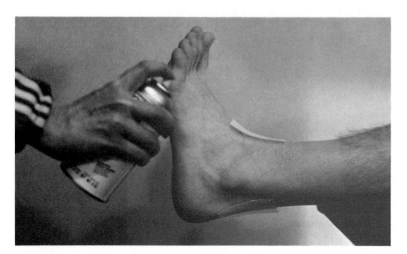

FIGURE 6:1. Skin adherent assures bonding of tape to skin while heel and lace pads prevent blister formation.

ELASTIC BANDAGING

While each athletic trainer has a particular technique for applying adhesive tape, elastic bandage techniques are less variable. Elastic bandages provide compression to help control internal and external hemorrhaging from injuries such as sprains, strains and contusions. They also help limit stressed or strained soft tissues by adding support.

In initial injury management, a compression wrap can help control internal hemorrhaging associated with sprains, strains and muscle tissue injury.

Guidelines in applying compression wraps include:

1. Wet the wrap so that it can enhance the conductivity of various cold application agents.
2. Half-inch household sponges dipped in ice water and placed over the injured area can greatly enhance the wrap's ability to provide compression.
3. Start the wrap distal to the injury site. For example, if an athlete suffers an ankle sprain, start the wrap at the base of the toes.
4. The wrap should be tighter distal than proximal to the injury site to minimize venous congestion.
5. After the wet elastic wrap is in place, ice packs can be applied to assist in controlling the bleeding and swelling (Fig. 6:2A).
6. A dry elastic wrap can then be placed over the ice packs to secure them in place and assist in compression (Fig. 6:2B).

SOFT TISSUE SUPPORT

An elastic bandage for soft tissue support is used primarily to reduce stresses on muscle tissue. Guidelines for applying include:

1. Spray the area to be bandaged with a skin adherent to reduce the chance of slipping.
2. A pad made of felt or foam rubber approximately 1 inch larger than the injured area may provide additional support.

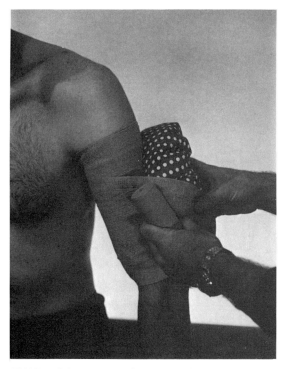

FIGURE 6:2A. Ice pack to control bleeding and swelling

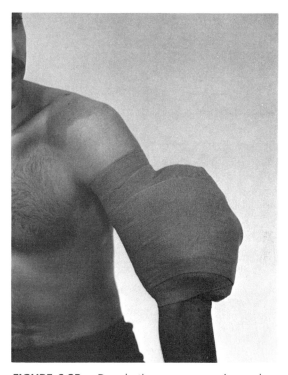

FIGURE 6:2B. Dry elastic wrap secures ice pack.

3. If the wrap is applied where friction with the skin or clothing may be excessive, a skin lubricant pad should be used.
4. Wrapping should allow for contraction and relaxation of major muscle groups.
5. Begin distal to the injury and wrap toward and beyond the injury site applying constant, even support.
6. Check for vascular compromise after the athlete has had sufficient time to warm up.

COTTON WRAPS

Cotton wrap is used for ankle support. The most common ankle wrap is a piece of cotton material 92 to 102 inches long, depending upon the size of the athlete. Ankle wraps are becoming popular to prevent ankle injuries because they combine adequate protection with ease of application and durability and are cost efficient compared to tape.

Most ankle wrap procedures involve a series of figure-of-eight turns in combination with heel locks. The purpose of the heel lock is to limit rotational movement in the ankle. This technique does not limit ankle extension or flexion. The Louisiana ankle wrap, universally used by athletic trainers, is illustrated in Figure 6:3.

Guidelines for applying cotton ankle wraps include:

1. Make sure the sock over which the wrap is applied is snugly fitted.
2. In areas where friction blisters may develop, apply grease pads between the sock and the wrap.
3. Avoid wrinkling the wrap when applying.
4. Secure the completed wrap with strips of adhesive tape.
5. For additional support, two additional heel locks with adhesive tape may be applied over the standard ankle wrap.

50

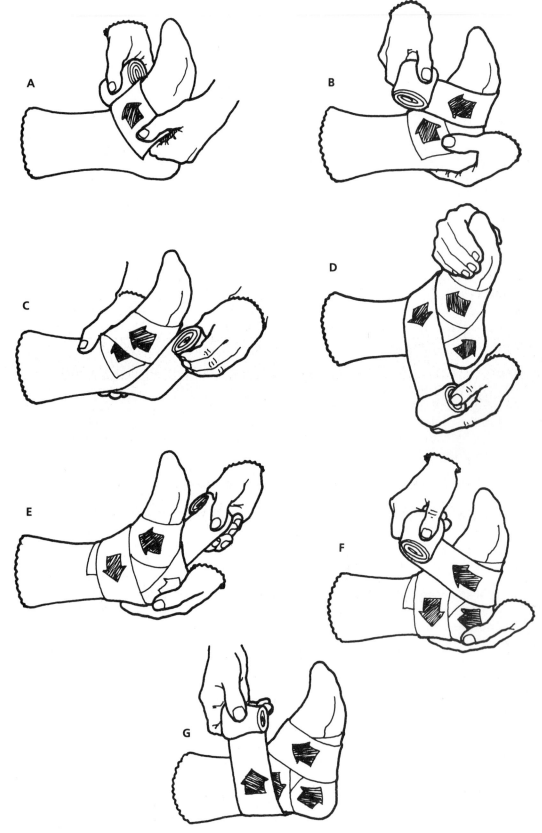

FIGURE 6:3. The Louisiana ankle wrap. Apply additional support with adhesive tape in the same manner.

Upper Extremity Taping

Often athletes with upper extremity injuries can participate in their sports if their injuries are protected. Certain types of taping procedures, if used appropriately, may allow athletes to safely return to their sports.

SHOULDER STRAPPINGS

Protective acromioclavicular joint taping is designed to stabilize the acromioclavicular articulation but allow movement of the shoulder.

Material

- one ¼ inch thick felt pad
- 2 inch adhesive tape
- 2 × 2 inch gauze pad
- 3 inch elastic bandage

Position

The athlete sits in a chair with the affected arm resting, slightly abducted (Fig. 7:1). The operator stands facing the athlete's abducted arm.

Procedure

1. Apply three anchor strips, the first in a three-quarter circle just below the deltoid insertion, the second just below the nipple encircling half the chest and the third over the trapezius near the neck and then attaching to the second anchor in front and back. Cover the nipple with the 2 × 2 gauze pad and the acromioclavicular joint with the ¼ inch felt pad to achieve greater compression at this area (Fig. 7:1A).
2. Apply the next two strips of tape from the front and back of the first anchor, crossing each other at the acromio-clavicular articulation and attaching to the third anchor strip (Figs. 7:1B, C).
3. Place the third support strip over the ends of the first and second pieces, following the line of the third anchor strip.
4. Lay the fourth support strip over the second anchor strip.
5. Continue this basketweave pattern until the entire shoulder complex is covered (Figs. 7:1D, E). Then apply a shoulder spica with an elastic bandage.

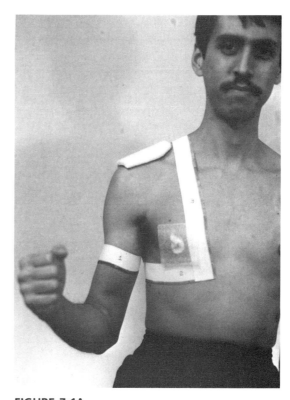

FIGURE 7:1A.

51

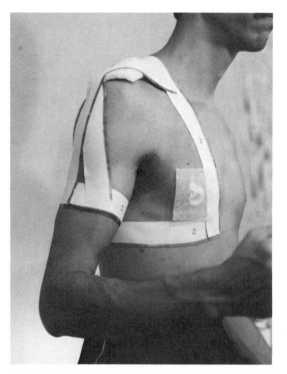

FIGURE 7:1B.

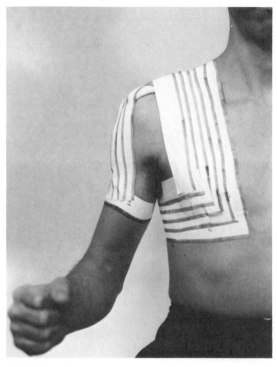

FIGURE 7:1D.

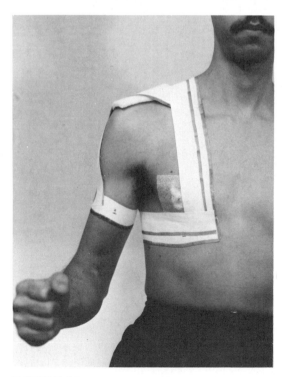

FIGURE 7:1C.

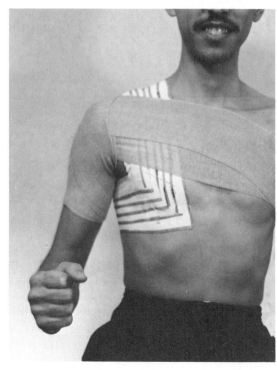

FIGURE 7:1E.

Taping for shoulder support and restraint is designed to support the soft tissues of the shoulder complexes and to restrain the arm from abducting more than 90°.

Material

- one ½ inch thick felt pad
- 2 inch adhesive tape
- tape adherent
- 2 × 2 inch gauze pad
- 3 inch elastic bandage

Position

The athlete sits in a chair with the affected arm resting, slightly abducted. The operator stands facing the abducted arm.

Procedure

1. The first phase is designed to support the capsule of the shoulder joint. After placing a cotton pad in the axilla, apply a series of three loops around the shoulder joint. Start the first loop at the top of the scapula, pulling it anteriorly across the acromion process and around the anterior aspect of the glenohumeral joint, posteriorly under the axilla, over the posterior glenohumeral joint, crossing the acromioclavicular joint again and terminating at the clavicle.
2. Next run strips of tape upward from a point just below the insertion of the deltoid muscle and crossing over the acromion process, completely covering the outer surface of the shoulder joint.
3. Before applying the final basketweave shoulder taping place a gauze pad over the nipple area. Lay a strip of tape over the shoulder near the neck and carry it to the nipple line in front and to the scapular line in back.
4. Take a second strip from the end of the first strip, around the middle of the humerus, ending at the back end of the first strip.
5. Continue the above alternating pattern, overlapping each preceding strip by at least one half of its width, until the shoulder is completely capped.

6. Apply a shoulder spica to keep the taping in place.

Shoulder Dislocation Taping

The purpose of this taping is to support the structures around the glenohumeral joint after dislocation. It can often successfully support the glenohumeral joint for activity.

Shave the chest area if body hair is dense. Place a gauze pad with skin lubricant over the nipple on the breast nearest the affected arm. To correctly position the athlete's body, the athlete places the hand of the affected side behind his body, on the buttocks area (Fig. 7:2A). This movement internally rotates the arm and yet allows for some degree of abduction.

Apply two figure-of-eights (shoulder spicas) around the affected upper arm using 3 inch elastic tape. Begin on the vertebral border of the scapula, cross over the affected deltoid and

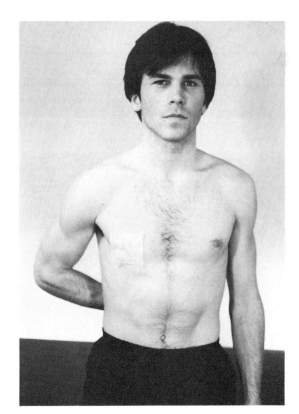

FIGURE 7:2A.

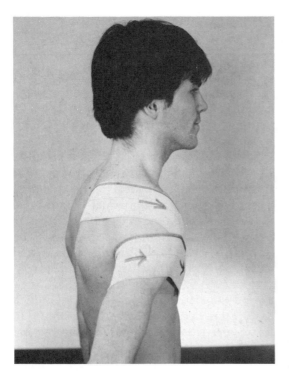

FIGURE 7:2B.

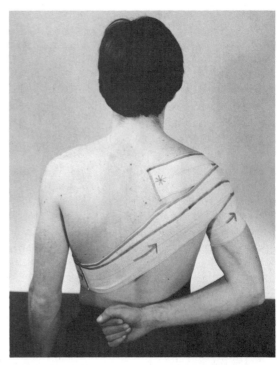

FIGURE 7:2D.

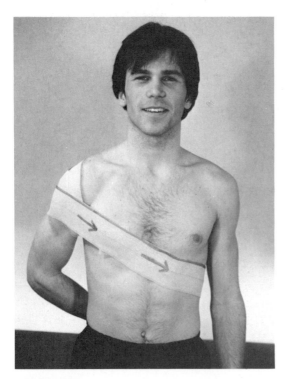

FIGURE 7:2C.

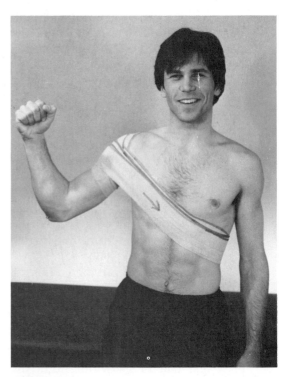

FIGURE 7:2E.

encircle the upper arm from posterior to anterior, cross the chest below the nipple line, go around the upper body and continue on around the upper arm. Overlap the tape just one half the width of the first strip of tape and encircle the body a second time (Figs. 7:2B, C, D). Continue applying elastic tape until the entire roll is used. Assure that the tape encircling the upper arm is not too constricting. In addition, the tape must come down far enough onto the upper arm to obtain an appropriate angle of pull to prevent external rotation and abduction (Fig. 7:2E). Numerous types of shoulder harnesses have been used with varied degrees of success in preventing a recurrence of glenohumeral dislocation.

ELBOW HYPEREXTENSION TAPING

Method #1

Material

- 1½ inch adhesive tape
- tape adherent
- 2 inch elastic bandage

Position

The athlete stands with the affected elbow flexed 90° and the forearm in a neutral position. The operator stands facing the side of the affected arm.

Procedure

1. Apply two anchor strips loosely around the arm, approximately 2 inches above and below the elbow joint (antecubital fossa) (Fig. 7:3A).
2. Construct a checkrein by cutting a 10 inch and a 4 inch strip of tape and laying the 4 inch strip against the center of the 10 inch strip, blanking out that portion. Next, place the checkrein so that it spans the two anchor strips, with the blanked-out side facing downward (Fig. 7:3B).
3. Place five additional 10 inch strips of tape over the basic checkrein (Fig. 7:3C). (A leather strap or a rubber bandage [AT6843, minimum length 14 feet,

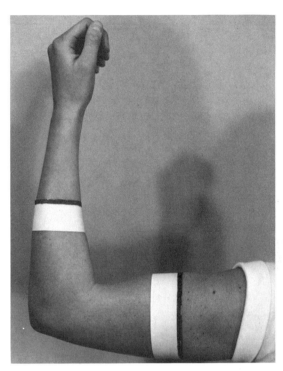

FIGURE 7:3A.

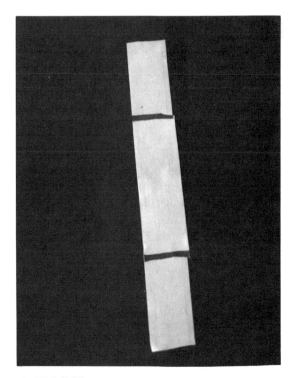

FIGURE 7:3B.

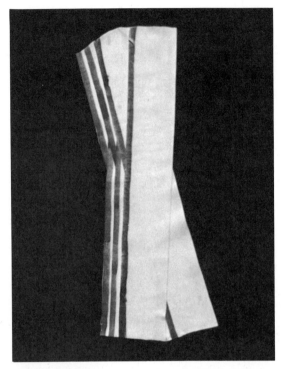

FIGURE 7:3C.

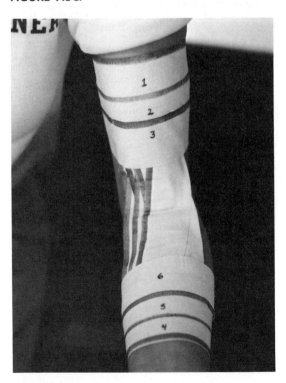

FIGURE 7:3D.

Fulflex, Inc., Bristol, RI 02809] can serve as the checkrein.)
4. Finish the procedure by securing the checkrein with three lock strips on each end (Fig. 7:3D).
5. Apply a figure-of-eight elastic wrap over the taping to close the strapping.

Method #2

Material
- tape adherent
- 1½ inch adhesive tape
- 2 inch elastic tape
- underwrap (optional)

Position
The athlete stands with the elbow flexed at 90° and the forearm in a neutral position. The operator stands facing the side of the athlete's affected arm.

Procedure
1. Apply two anchor strips loosely around the arm, approximately 3 inches above and below the elbow joint (antecubital fossa).
2. Begin on the medial side of the forearm on the anchor strip with 1½ inch tape, bringing it obliquely upward and crossing the antecubital fossa to the superior anchor strip.
3. Repeat this lateral to medial creating a criss-cross effect over the antecubital area.
4. Each set of oblique strappings should move laterally and overlap the previous pair by one half width.
5. Place lock strips to secure oblique taping in place.
6. Close loosely with a 2 inch elastic tape.

WRIST TAPING

Wrist bands are designed for mild wrist injuries where slight limitation of motion in all directions is necessary. Wrist taping can also be used for compression or to support the retinaculum of the wrist.

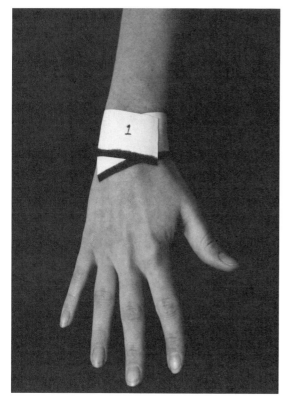

FIGURE 7:4A.

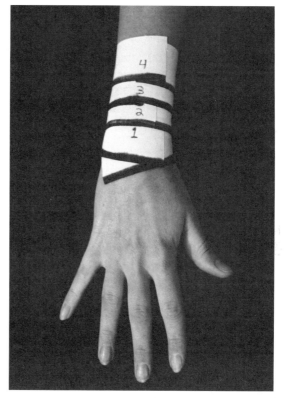

FIGURE 7:4B.

Material

- tape adherent
- 1 or 1½ inch adhesive tape (depending on the athlete's size)
- underwrap (optional)

Position

The athlete stands with the affected wrist in a neutral position, fingers moderately abducted, elbow flexed to 90°, forearm in neutral position. The operator stands facing the athlete's affected wrist.

Procedure

1. Starting at the base of the wrist, bring a strip of tape from the palmar side upward and encircle the wrist (Fig. 7:4A).
2. In the same pattern, lay in place three additional strips with each strip overlapping the preceding one by at least one half its width (Fig. 7:4B).

Wrist hyperextension/flexion taping prohibits movement of wrist flexion or extension and hence protects and stabilizes the injured wrist.

Material

- tape adherent
- 1 inch adhesive tape
- 1½ inch adhesive tape
- underwrap (optional)

Position

The athlete stands with elbow flexed at 90°, forearm in neutral position, fingers abducted, wrist placed toward injured side (either flexion or extension). The operator stands facing the athlete's affected wrist.

Procedure

1. Place anchor strips 3 inches proximal to the styloid process, with another around

the spread hand proximal to the base of the metacarpal heads (Fig. 7:5A).

2. With the wrist flexed, or extended, toward the injured side, take a strip of tape from the anchor strip near the little finger and carry it obliquely across the wrist joint to the wrist anchor strip. Take another strip from the anchor strip on the index finger side and carry it obliquely across the wrist joint to the wrist anchor. This forms a criss-cross over the wrist joint (Fig. 7:5B). A series of four or five criss-crosses may be applied (Fig. 7:5C). A checkrein may be used instead of the criss-cross, formed in a manner similar to the elbow hyperextension strapping.

3. Apply two or three series of figure-of-eight tapings over the criss-cross taping.

Figure-of-eight wrist hyperflexion taping is another technique used to prevent excessive wrist flexion.

Material
- tape adherent
- 1 inch adhesive tape
- 1½ inch adhesive tape
- underwrap (optional)

Position

The athlete stands with the elbow at the side, flexed to 90°, wrist extended and fingers abducted. The forearm is in neutral position. The operator stands facing the athlete's affected wrist.

Procedure

1. Start a strip of 1 inch tape on the palmar aspect of the hand and bring it radially through the web space.
2. Continuing with the tape, move obliquely toward the ulnar styloid process.
3. Wrap around the wrist once and continue for one half turn, until the tape can then obliquely cross the dorsal surface of the hand to the original anchor.

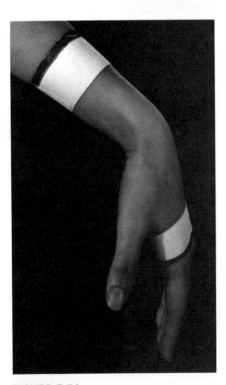

FIGURE 7:5A.

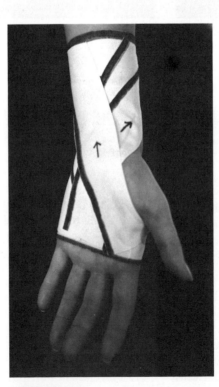

FIGURE 7:5B.

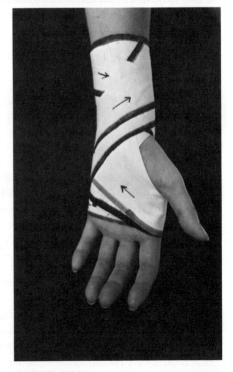

FIGURE 7:5C.

4. Cut tape and repeat.
5. Close with 1½ inch tape around anchors to lock tape in place.

Figure-of-eight wrist hyperextension taping is a mirror image of the figure-of-eight wrist hyperflexion taping, since its purpose is to prevent wrist extension. The oblique strapping will be on the palmar surface of the hand. The wrist is held in flexion while tape is applied.

Ulnar deviation assist taping is designed to support the wrist in ulnar deviation while allowing radial deviation.

Material

• tape adherent
• 1½ inch adhesive tape
• 2 inch elastic tape
• one pair of scissors
• underwrap (optional)

Position

The athlete sits with the arm supported by a table and the elbow flexed to 90°. Forearm is in neutral position with wrist in ulnar deviation and fingers abducted. The operator stands facing the athlete's affected wrist.

Procedure

1. Place two anchor strips loosely—one two thirds of the way down the forearm and the other around the metacarpals.
2. Measure and split elastic tape at both ends and wrap it around the anchor strip. It should pull the wrist into ulnar deviation. This can be repeated.
3. Secure the elastic tape with 1½ inch tape all the way up the ulnar surface. Repeat if necessary.
4. Lock in place with 1½ inch tape.
5. Close in the taping with elastic tape using figure-of-eights around the wrist and loose spiral strapping on the forearm.

Radial deviation assist taping is the same as ulnar deviation assist taping using radial deviation rather than ulnar deviation. Place elastic tape on the radial side of the forearm and close in the tape as in steps 3, 4, and 5

above. Notice that these assistive taping techniques can be used for flexion or extension and/or combinations of these movements.

THUMB TAPING

Thumb spica taping is designed to protect the musculature and joint of the thumb.

Method 1

Material

• tape adherent
• 1 inch adhesive tape
• underwrap (optional)

Position

The athlete should hold the thumb in a relaxed, neutral position—usually the functional position, as if holding a can, is the instruction to the athlete. The operator stands in front of the athlete's injured thumb.

Procedure

1. Place an anchor loosely around the wrist with another around the distal phalanx of the thumb (Fig. 7:6A).
2. From the anchor at the tip of the thumb to the anchor around the wrist, apply four splint strips in a series on the side, either dorsal or palmar, and hold them in place by one lock strip around the wrist and the distal phalanx (Fig. 7:6B).
3. Now add a series of three thumb strips in a "spica" fashion. Start the first strip, which goes around the metacarpophalangeal (MCP) joint, on the radial side at the base of the thumb and carry it under the thumb, completely encircling it, and then cross to the starting point (Fig. 7:6C). Each of the following spica strips should overlap the preceding strip by at least ⅔ inch and move downward on the thumb.

Method 2

Material

Same as Method 1

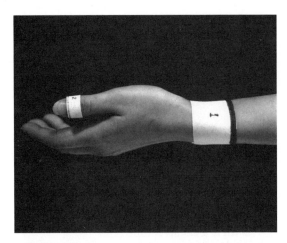

FIGURE 7:6A.

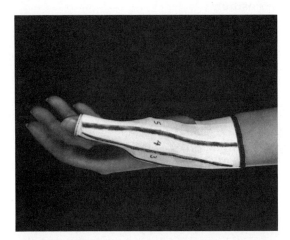

FIGURE 7:6B.

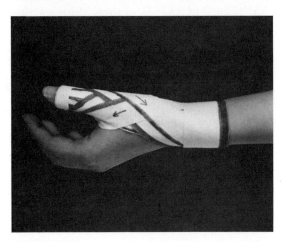

FIGURE 7:6C.

Position

Same as Method 1

Procedure

1. Place one anchor around the wrist over the styloid process.
2. Place one thumb spica strip over the MCP joint as in step 3, above.
3. Start at the anchor on the ulnar side. Place a strip that will cross the palmar surface and wrap around the base of the thumb, beginning radially, and return to the starting point, forming a horse shoe.
4. Start a strip on the dorsal ulnar side of the anchor and place it through the web space. Then wrap it around the thumb and return to the starting point (horse shoe).
5. Place another thumb spica around the MCP joint to hold the horse shoes in place.
6. Place 1 inch lateral horizontal support strips from the base of the first metacarpal distally to the base of the proximal phalanx. These strips should be long enough to reach the third metacarpal (hoods).
7. Place one strip through the web space to lock the hood strips in place. The first distal interphalangeal (DIP) and second through fifth MCP joints should not be covered by tape.

Thumb checkreins can be a reinforcing strapping for the previous two thumb tapings. This taping provides additional protection to an injured MCP joint of the thumb by preventing any extreme range of motion. It can also be used as a strapping by itself.

Material

• 1 inch tape

Position

The athlete spreads his injured fingers widely but within a pain-free range of motion. The operator faces the athlete's injured thumb.

Procedure

1. After encircling the middle phalanx of the injured thumb, bring a strip of 1 inch tape around the hand just proximal to the metatarsal heads and return to the middle phalanx of the thumb. Leave enough slack between the thumb and second phalanx to protect the joint but still allow some function.
2. Encircle the center of the checkrein for additional strength.

Pancake thumb strapping is designed to protect the thumb from reinjury but does not allow the thumb to be used functionally for grasping.

Material

- tape adherent
- 2 inch elastic tape
- 1½ inch adhesive tape
- underwrap (optional)

Position

The athlete should stand with elbow flexed 90°, wrist and forearm in neutral position, thumb and fingers abducted. The operator faces the athlete's injured thumb.

Procedure

1. Begin a spiral wrap of elastic tape at the MCP joints of the fingers, holding the thumb abducted to the second metacarpal.
2. Continue to loosely wrap the hand, overlapping the strips by one half until the ulnar and radial styloid processes are covered.
3. Close the strapping with 1½ inch tape around the wrist, covering the end of the elastic tape.

HAND STRAPPING

Gymnast hand taping is designed to protect the upper palm of the hand where there has been a partial or complete tear in the skin.

Material

- tape adherent
- 1½ inch adhesive tape
- 1 inch gauze roll (optional)

Position

The athlete should be seated with arm resting on a table, elbow flexed at 90°, forearm and wrist in neutral position, fingers and thumb abducted. The operator faces the injured hand.

Procedure

1. Apply tape adherent to hand and wrist, making sure that none is on the fingers (Fig. 7:7A).
2. Apply one layer of 1½ inch tape around the palm and wrist for anchors (Fig. 7:7B).
3. Tear thin strips of tape and place them between the fingers without rolling the edges (Fig. 7:7C), anchoring them on the wrist. (Optional: place 1 inch gauze between fingers so it covers the palm and dorsum of the hand.)
4. Place lock strips around the wrist, and possibly the palm, to hold the thin strips in place (Fig. 7:7D).

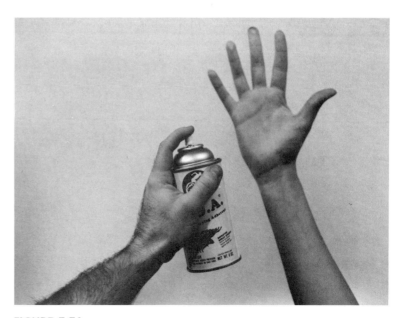

FIGURE 7:7A.

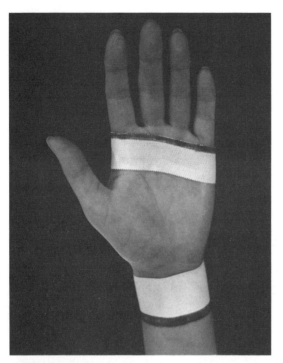

FIGURE 7:7B.

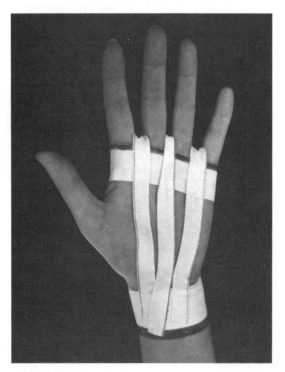

FIGURE 7:7C.

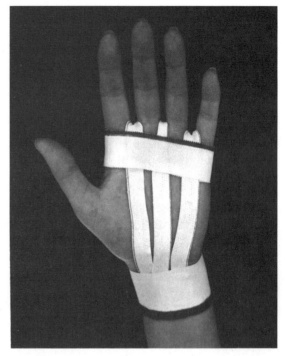

FIGURE 7:7D.

5. For the gymnast, apply chalk over the tape as normally done.

Metacarpal strapping is designed to support the metacarpals and to protect the heads of the metacarpal phalanges from bruising when punching with a fist.

Material
- tape adherent
- 1 inch adhesive tape
- 1½ inch adhesive tape
- 2 inch rolled gauze
- ½ inch thick soft sponge rubber pad

Position
The athlete should stand, elbow flexed 90°, forearm in neutral position, fingers abducted. The operator faces the athlete's hand.

Procedure
1. Lay the pad over the dorsum of the hand.

2. Wrap 2 inch rolled gauze around the styloid process of the wrist twice. Then continue the gauze distally to the web space between the fourth and fifth digits. Loop it around the fifth digit and back around the wrist for a complete turn. Repeat for the second, third and fourth digits.
3. Using 1 inch tape, apply thumb horse shoes, followed by a spica.
4. Apply a figure-of-eight using 1 inch tape to hold the wrist in slight extension.
5. With 1½ inch tape, lock the strapping into place around the wrist and the palm, covering the metacarpal phalanges.

FINGER TAPING

Buddy taping is designed to support the joint of an injured finger with the longer of the neighboring fingers without impeding functional range of motion.

Material
• 1 inch adhesive tape

Position
The athlete should stand, with elbow at 90° flexion, wrist and forearm in neutral position, with the fingers that are to be taped together. The operator stands in front of the athlete's injured finger.

Procedure
1. Place a 1 or ½ inch tape strip around the injured finger and the adjoining proximal phalanx and distal phalanx to hold them together.
2. Place tape above and below the proximal interphalangeal (PIP) joint to allow fullest mobility possible (Fig. 7:8).

Circular finger strapping is designed to give compression and support while limiting motion of the DIP and PIP joints.

Material
• 1 inch adhesive tape

Position
The athlete stands, elbow at 90° flexion, wrist and forearm in neutral position, extending the injured finger as much as possible. Operator stands in front of the athlete's injured finger.

Procedure
1. Place a 1 inch or a ½ inch strip of tape around the finger distal to the injured joint.
2. Repeat this with individual strips moving proximally, overlapping slightly, until the joint is completely covered.
3. Be careful not to impede circulation.

Finger joint hyperextension/flexion stop strapping is designed to eliminate as much motion as possible at the PIP joint.

Material
• 1 inch adhesive tape

Position
The athlete stands, elbow flexed to 90°, wrist and forearm in neutral position, and the injured finger in the position to be fixed. The operator stands in front of the athlete's injured finger.

Procedure
1. Wrap a 1 inch or ½ inch strip of tape around the proximal phalanx.
2. As the turn is completed, pull the tape obliquely across the dorsal surface (to prevent flexion) or the palmar surface (to prevent extension). Then wrap the middle phalanx twice.
3. As the second turn is completed, pull the tape down obliquely across the PIP joint, forming a criss-cross over the joint.
4. Turn the wrap once around the proximal phalanx to lock it in place.

Immobilization of one digit is designed to splint and limit motion of an entire finger in a functional position using only tape.

Material
• tape adherent

- 1 inch adhesive tape
- gauze
- 2 inch elastic tape

Position

The athlete is seated with arm resting on table, elbow flexed to 90°, forearm in neutral, wrist slightly extended, fingers abducted and slightly flexed. The operator stands in front of the athlete's injured finger.

Procedure

1. Place anchor strips around the wrist, the palm of the hand and the phalanx to be immobilized (Fig. 7:9A).
2. Starting at the wrist, place a strip of tape the length of the metacarpal and phalanx to be immobilized from the distal phalanx to the anchor strip at the wrist on the palmar surface (Fig. 7:9B).
3. Place a piece of gauze on the tip of the finger and continue the tape down the dorsal side until reaching the wrist.
4. Place lock strips between the DIP and PIP joints, between the PIP and MCP joints, and around the palm and the wrist.
5. Close with a figure-of-eight elastic taping to hold in place (Fig. 7:9C).

Immobilization of multiple digits is designed to allow functional use of some fingers while allowing support and stabilization of others, generally the fourth and fifth digits.

Material

- underwrap
- 1½ inch adhesive tape
- elastic tape
- 1 inch gauze

Position

The athlete sits or stands with elbow flexed, wrist extended, forearm in neutral, and the fourth and fifth digits flexed. The operator is in front of the athlete's injured hand.

Procedure

1. The athlete holds onto 1 inch gauze with fourth and fifth digits while underwrap is applied around digits, palm and wrist.
2. Apply an anchor strip to wrist with 1½ inch tape.
3. Place a longitudinal strip of 1½ inch tape over the top of the fourth and fifth digits and anchor it at the wrist.
4. Place lock strips at the wrist and, loosely, around the palm.
5. Close strapping with elastic tape in a figure-of-eight fashion to hold in place.

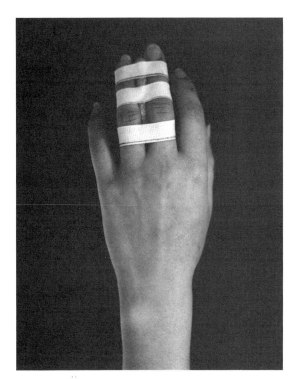

FIGURE 7:8.

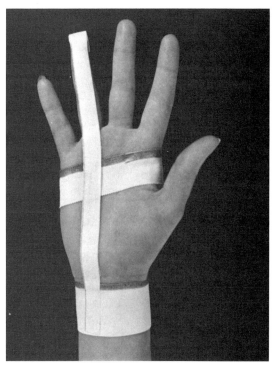

FIGURE 7:9B.

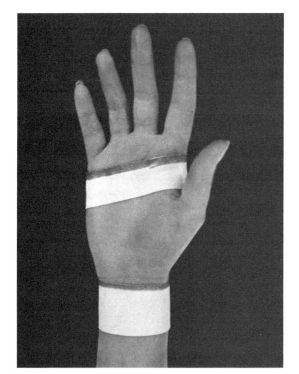

FIGURE 7:9A.

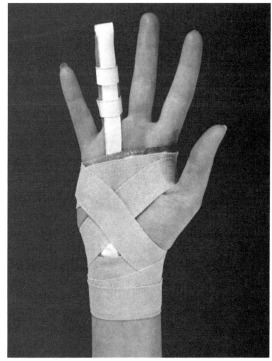

FIGURE 7:9C.

Lower Extremity Taping

8

For the past few decades, athletic trainers, coaches and team physicians have traditionally used adhesive taping to limit the amount of ankle motion (particularly inversion) available to the athlete. A very high incidence of ankle sprains involves the lateral ligament complex, primarily as a result of excessive inversion stress. The ligaments of the knee also sustain numerous types of sprains. These sprains are a result of excessive valgus, varus or hyper-extension of torsion forces. Proper application of adhesive tape can support both the ankle and the knee for activity.

The effectiveness of adhesive taping has been a matter of controversy for many years. Arguments against taping include the following:

1. Tape usually becomes loose with wear.
2. The skin is mobile, thus taping cannot be effective.
3. Taping the ankle weakens the leg muscles.
4. The prophylactic use of ankle taping removes the body's safety valve. The subtalar joint of the ankle is prevented from sprain. Thus, the force is transferred to the knee, resulting in ligament damage.
5. Moisture develops between the skin and tape, thus affecting the adherence of the tape.
6. Tape tears under stress.

However, a review of recent literature concerned with effectiveness of adhesive strapping techniques on reducing the incidence of specific injuries (ankle sprains) concluded that adhesive techniques do contribute to a lower incidence of ankle and knee injury and re-injury.

Possible complications with tape use include:

1. Skin allergies
2. Skin irritations
3. Blisters
4. Lacerations
5. Reactions to tape adherent (benzoin)

Some people have allergies to adhesive tape. Skin irritations commonly develop with prolonged use of taping over a sport season. Usually, these irritations are minor. Proper daily cleaning of the area taped can sometimes prevent irritation. Improper application techniques can result in blisters or small skin lacerations. Finally, certain athletes have skin reactions (allergies) not to the tape itself but to the tape adherents which contain benzoin.

Several general considerations apply to all lower extremity tapings:

1. Select nontear tape of proper width.
2. Tape directly to the skin for maximum protection.
3. Properly prepare the area to be taped. This includes (a) covering all areas of skin irritation, (b) protecting areas of potential irritation, and (c) applying adherent or benzoin as needed.
4. Stretch elastic tape 85% to 90%.
5. Contour all tape strips to tapered body parts to prevent wrinkles.
6. Always tape from high to low, i.e., toward the heart.

KNEE TAPING

Tape application techniques to the knee area to support various types of ligament sprains depends upon the type, area and severity of injury, i.e., medial collateral ligament (MCL) sprain, lateral collateral ligament (LCL) sprain or hyperextension injury. Most athletic trainers prefer a nontear tape of proper width when taping the knee. An elastic, nontear tape provides the ultimate tape strength and, at the same time, retains an adequate amount of mobility. Figure 8:1 illustrates general points in knee taping.

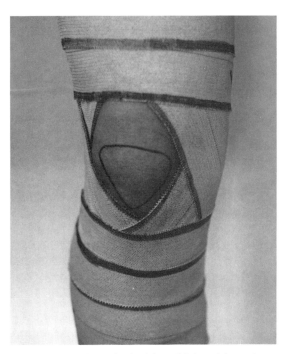

FIGURE 8:1. Tape both sides of injured knee but keep patella free of tape.

When taping an injured knee, do not apply tape simply over the side of the knee injured. Tape both sides of the knee to afford as much support as possible. It is extremely important to keep all tape off the patella to prevent patellofemoral complications.

MCL Injury

Material

- tape adherent
- underwrap (optional)

Basic Knee Taping Formulas

MCL Injury	LCL Injury	Hyperextension Injury
1. 6 strips inside	1. 6 strips outside	1. 3 strips posterior
2. 3 strips outside	2. 3 strips inside	2. anchors
3. anchors	3. anchors	

- 1½ inch adhesive tape
- 3 inch elastic tape

Position

The athlete stands with the heel of his foot elevated on a 2 inch object. The affected knee should be in 15° to 20° flexion. The operator stands facing the athlete.

Procedure

1. Apply anchor strips at midthigh and midcalf (Fig. 8:2A).
2. Using elastic tape, apply six strips to the medial aspect of the knee (Fig. 8:2B). Begin at the lower midlateral aspect of

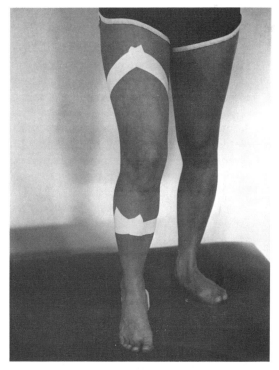

FIGURE 8:2A.

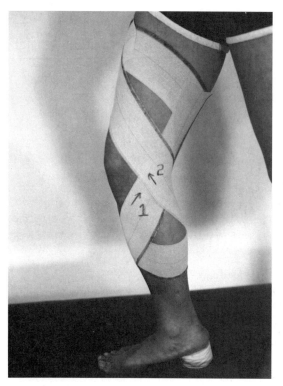

FIGURE 8:2B.

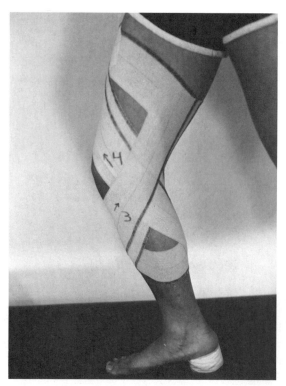

FIGURE 8:2C.

the calf, cross the medial joint line to the midmedial aspect of the thigh. A second strip starts at the midmedial aspect of the calf, crossing the previous strip at the joint line and progressing to the midlateral aspect of the thigh. Care should be taken to assure the patella is free of tape. Apply a second set of crossing strips in the previously described manner, overlapping the previous strips by three fourths (Fig. 8:2C). Apply two vertical strips from midmedial calf to midmedial thigh (Fig. 8:2D).

3. Apply three strips of elastic tape to the lateral aspect of the knee. Begin at the midlateral calf, cross the lateral joint line and progress to the midmedial thigh (Fig. 8:2E). A second strip starts at the midlateral calf, crosses the previous strip at the joint line, and progresses to the midmedial thigh. Apply a vertical strip

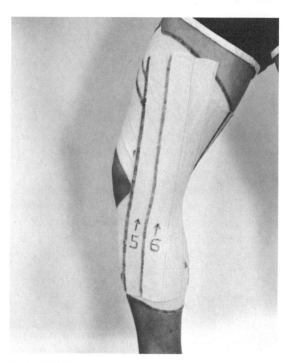

FIGURE 8:2D.

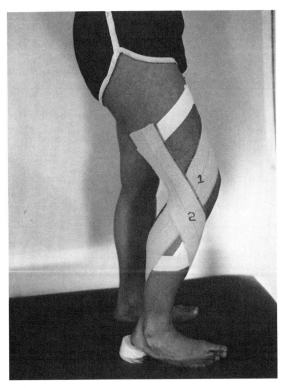

FIGURE 8:2E.

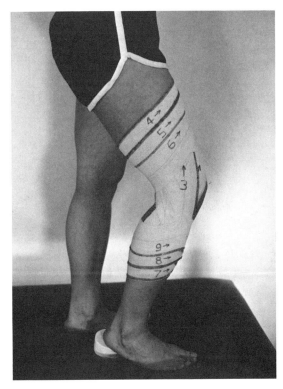

FIGURE 8:2G.

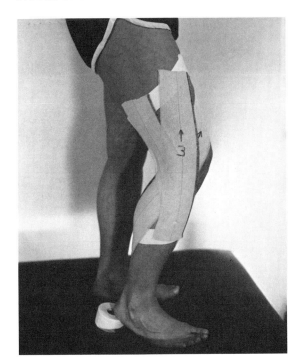

FIGURE 8:2F.

from midlateral calf to the midlateral thigh (Fig. 8:2F).

4. Apply anchor strips to the calf and thigh to hold previous strips in place (Fig. 8:2G). The number may vary with the size of the athlete.

Knee Hyperextension

Material

- tape adherent
- 4 × 4 gauze or felt pad
- 1½ inch adhesive tape
- 6 inch elastic tape (optional)

Position

The athlete stands with the heel of his foot elevated on a 2 inch object, with knee in full extension.

Procedure

1. Apply anchor strips at midthigh and midcalf (Fig. 8:3A).

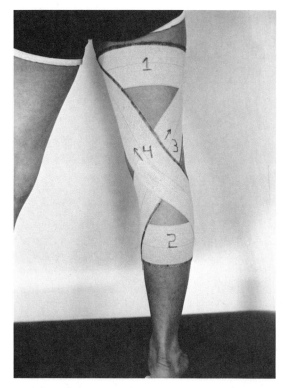

FIGURE 8:3A.

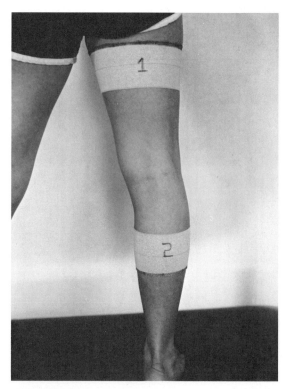

FIGURE 8:3B.

2. Place a 4 × 4 gauze or felt pad in the popliteal space.

3. Cross two strips in the popliteal area to form an **X** and run the third strip up and down the posterior aspect of the leg (Fig. 8:3B). Begin the first strip in the midmedial calf and pass it through the popliteal area, ending on the midlateral upper thigh. Begin the second strip on the midlateral calf and pass it through the popliteal area to end on the midmedial upper thigh. These two strips form an **X** behind the knee. The third strip begins on the posterior calf and ends on the midposterior thigh (Fig. 8:3C).

4. Repeat this procedure as necessary, depending upon the amount of restriction desired.

5. Apply anchors around the calf, thigh and knee area to secure longitudinal strips (Fig. 8:3D).

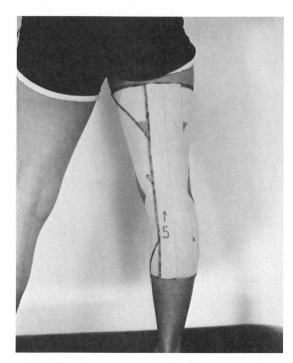

FIGURE 8:3C.

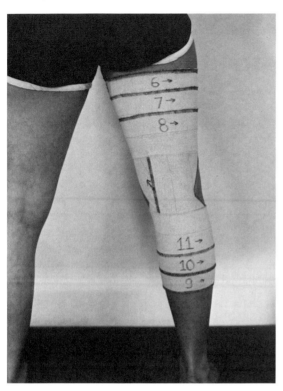

FIGURE 8:3D.

When placing anchor strips encircling the thigh and calf, have the athlete contract the thigh and calf musculature in turn as you encircle each area very cautiously with elastic tape. Often, trainers apply anchor strips too tightly, resulting in discomfort or muscle cramping. A little caution prevents this. Some people elect to close knee taping procedures with 6 inch elastic wraps to hold the basic support strips in place. This alternative method might be used to reduce tape costs.

ANKLE TAPING

The method for applying tape to support the ankle joint depends upon the purpose for the taping. The purposes usually are (1) preventive taping; (2) lateral (inversion) sprain (talofibular or calcaneofibular ligament); (3) medial (eversion) sprain (deltoid ligament). Tape ap-

plication for both the lateral sprain of the ankle and for injury prevention is basically the same, and usually only the amount of tape applied varies.

Lateral Inversion Sprains

Material
- heel and lace pads with lubrication, i.e., Vaseline
- tape adherent
- 1½ inch adhesive tape
- underwrap (optional)

Position

The athlete sits on a table with knee extended and lower third of calf extended past the edge of the table. Athlete's foot is in dorsification. Trainer faces plantar aspect of the athlete's foot.

Procedure

1. Apply heel and lace pads appropriately.
2. Apply two anchor strips. Place one at the base of the gastrocnemius heads and the second at the distal third of the longitudinal arch (Fig. 8:4A). Assure that the fifth metatarsal head is not constricted.

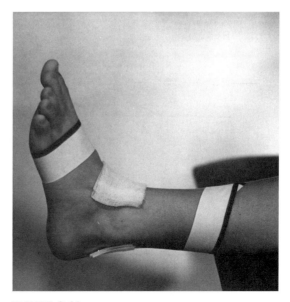

FIGURE 8:4A.

3. Apply stirrup strips, beginning on the medial calf. Pass under the foot (heel) and pull up on the lateral aspect of the leg with moderate tension (Figs. 8:4B, C). This direction of application results in slight eversion of the foot, thus counteracting the inversion sprain. Apply between three and ten stirrups, depending on the amount of support desired.

4. Apply heel locks using one of several methods. One simple method is to begin the tape on the lateral lower leg, cross the tibia at a 45° angle just above the medial malleolus, pass directly over the Achilles tendon and down onto the lateral calcaneus, under the foot and up onto the top of the forefoot. Reverse this process for the medial lock. Begin the heel lock strip on the top of the forefoot. Cross in front of the lateral malleolus at a 45° angle. Going downward, under the calcaneus and up behind the medial malleolus, cross the Achilles tendon and continue to the top of the forefoot (Fig. 8:4D). Usually two or three heel locks in each direction are adequate.

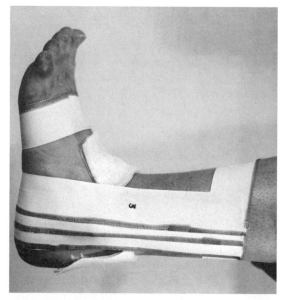

FIGURE 8:4C. Additional stirrups (3-10) are added depending upon the amount of support needed. A wide band of moleskin is sometimes used in place of these stirrups.

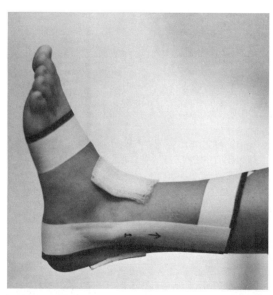

FIGURE 8:4B. A stirrup is applied with tension pulling up on the lateral side.

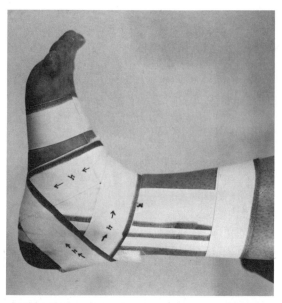

FIGURE 8:4D. Heel locks are applied next. Care should be taken to avoid wrinkles along the achilles, as they are a frequent cause of blisters.

5. Apply figure-of-eight strips with force to cause slight foot eversion. Start the tape strip just in front of the medial malleolus, passing the tape under the foot and up the outside of the foot. As the tape passes under the foot, use your free hand to evert the foot while applying the tape firmly. The foot should be flattened as well as everted to prevent the tape from encircling the foot too tightly. The ''8's'' continue on up and around the foot and around the lower leg (Fig. 8:4E). (The ''8's'' acquire their name from encircling both the foot and the lower leg in the figure-of-eight fashion.) Usually, two, three or four ''8's'' produce adequate foot eversion. Encircling the foot too tightly distal to the head of the fifth metatarsal can result in foot discomfort. Applying the tape properly in conjunction with pressure to the foot, causing the foot to spread to a greater width, decreases the chances of this.

6. Apply fill-in strips to hold other tape components (stirrups, heel locks, figure-

of-eights) in place. The fill-in strips encircle the lower leg, ankle area and foot with overlapping strips that encase the entire area with tape (Fig. 8:4F). They should begin at the bottom of the stirrups and encase the entire area upward to the proximal anchor.

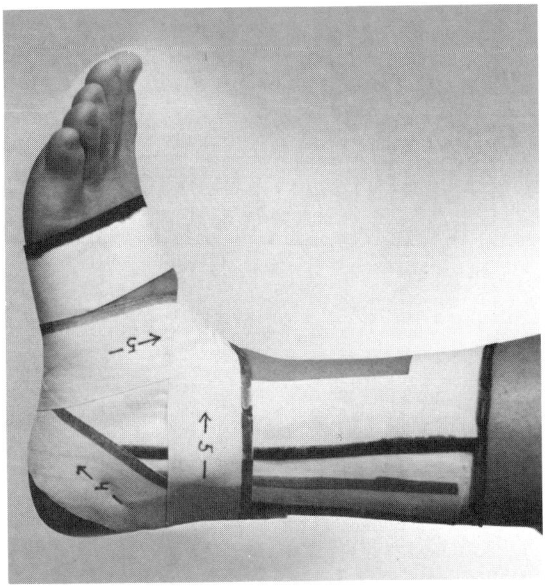

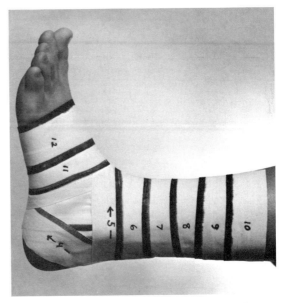

FIGURE 8:4F. Circular fill-in strips start distally and move proximally, overlapping by half the previous strip.

As stated earlier, the primary difference for postinjury taping compared with preventive taping is the amount of tape applied. The more support required, the more tape required, i.e., more stirrups, more heel locks and more figures-of-eight.

When taping for the medial (deltoid/eversion) sprain, follow the previously described routine except apply the stirrups and figures-of-eight outside to inside to effect an inversion of the foot. Only 5% to 10% of ankle sprains are medial or eversion sprains, so this application is the exception. It is, however, recommended with a deltoid ligament (eversion) sprain.

FIGURE 8:4E. Figure-of-eights also evert the foot with lateral pull upward.

Special Note on an Alternate Technique

When the maximum support or protection is required for a severe ankle sprain, some trainers use 3 inch strips of mole skin for the stirrups and elastic tape for figure-of-eight strips, followed with regular adhesive tape to complete the taping. This taping technique greatly limits motion and thus function.

ACHILLES TENDON TAPING

Achilles tendon taping is designed to prevent extreme dorsiflexion of the ankle when Achilles tendonitis or a mild Achilles tendon strain is present.

Material
- tape adherent
- heel pad with lubricant, i.e., Vaseline
- 2 and 3 inch elastic tape
- 1½ inch adhesive tape

Position
The athlete lies prone on the table, with his lower leg extending over the edge and the foot in relaxed plantar flexion.

Procedure
1. Apply anchors below the metatarsal heads and at midcalf with 1½ inch tape (Fig. 8:5A).
2. Using 2 or 3 inch elastic tape, apply a longitudinal strip starting at the plantar surface of the first metatarsal head and ending at the lateral aspect of the gastrocnemius muscle (Fig. 8:5B).
3. Using the same material, apply a second longitudinal strip starting at the plantar surface of the fifth metatarsal head and ending at the medial aspect of the gastrocnemius muscle (Fig. 8:5C).
4. Center a third longitudinal strip between the two prior strips, beginning at the center of the metatarsal arch and ending at the posterior aspect of the calf (Fig. 8:5D).

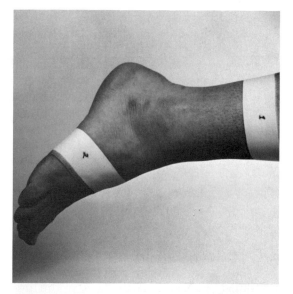

FIGURE 8:5A.

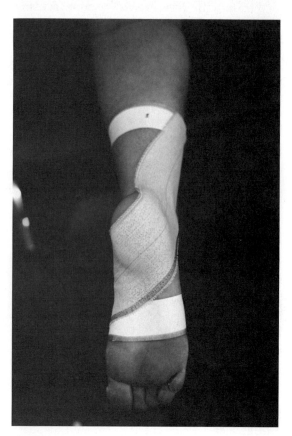

FIGURE 8:5B.

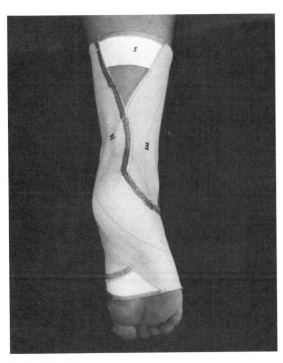

FIGURE 8:5C.

5. Use circular strips of 3 inch elastic tape to close off the forefoot and lower calf (Fig. 8:5E). Be sure these closing strips do not cause binding of the midfoot or calf.

LONGITUDINAL ARCH TAPING

The purpose of longitudinal arch taping is to give support to the structures of the longitudinal arch. It has been successfully used to treat posterior tibial tendonitis, plantar fasciitis and other midfoot dysfunctions.

Material
- tape adherent
- 1 inch elastic tape
- 1½ inch adhesive tape
- underwrap (optional)

Position
The athlete sits on a table with the ankle in a slightly dorsiflexed and neutral position throughout the taping procedure.

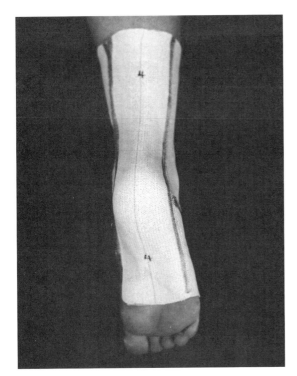

FIGURE 8:5D.

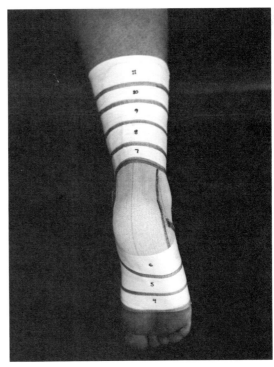

FIGURE 8:5E.

Procedure

1. Prepare the area to be taped. The sole of the foot must be clean and dry before applying tape adherent. Sometimes underwrap is applied to protect the hair on the dorsum of the foot, but should not extend beyond the anchor strip.

2. Apply anchor strips to the skin at the heads of the metatarsals, encircling the forefoot. The tape must be wrinkle free to avoid skin irritation and not too tight.

3. Apply supportive strips to the longitudinal arch (Figs. 8:6A, B, C), usually beginning at the fifth metatarsal head, wrapping around the heel not too tightly, and returning either to the head of the fifth or the first metatarsal head. Repeat this procedure until the entire sole of the foot is covered.

4. Apply fill-ins with strips of tape that encircle the forefoot, overlapping one third to one half to prevent spacing between layers of tape (Fig. 8:6D). These strips are usually placed from a lateral to medial direction to give added support to the medial plantar surface of the foot. Be sure strips encircling the midfoot do not cause binding.

GREAT TOE TAPING

The purpose of great toe taping is to decrease the range of motion at the first metacarpophalangeal (MCP) joint to support injured structures and prevent further damage. Depending on the application, the taping can restrict abduction, flexion or extension.

Material
- tape adherent
- 1 inch adhesive tape

Position
Athlete sits on a table with knee in full extension and foot off edge of table.

Procedure
1. Begin the taping by applying tape adherent to the dorsum and plantar aspects

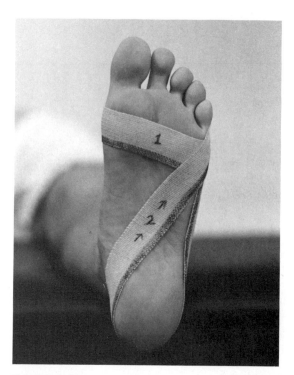

FIGURE 8:6A.

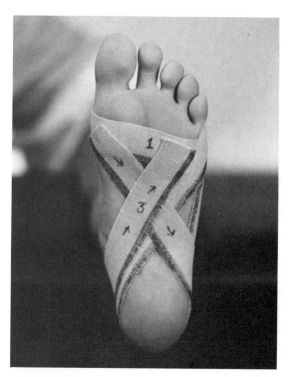

FIGURE 8:6B.

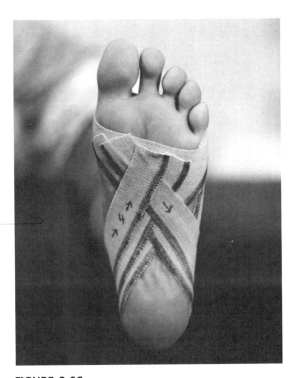

FIGURE 8:6C.

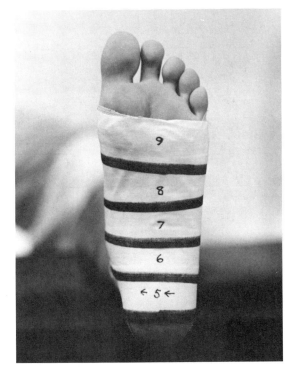

FIGURE 8:6D.

of the forefoot and great toe. Tape directly to the skin for maximum protection.

2. Place an anchor around the forefoot, encircling the metatarsals (Fig. 8:7A). Allow the tape to conform to the contours of the body part to prevent wrinkles and binding.

3. Apply half figure-of-eight taping by starting at the superior medial aspect of the first MCP and encircle the great toe, ending on the superior aspect of the second MCP joint (Figs. 8:7B, C). This prevents flexion/abduction. To prevent extension, begin on the inferior medial aspect of the first MCP and encircle the great toe (Fig. 8:7D).

4. Close in the toe and forefoot with overlapping strips applied distal to proximal (Fig. 8:7E).

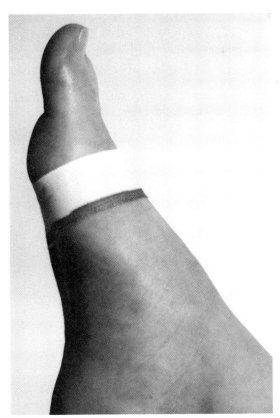

FIGURE 8:7A.

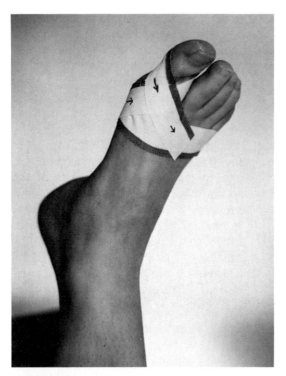

FIGURE 8:7B.

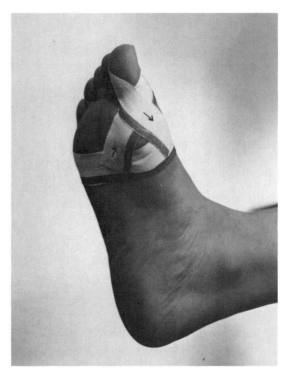

FIGURE 8:7D.

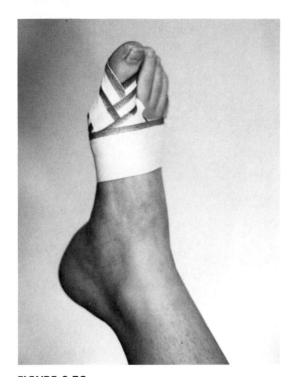

FIGURE 8:7C.

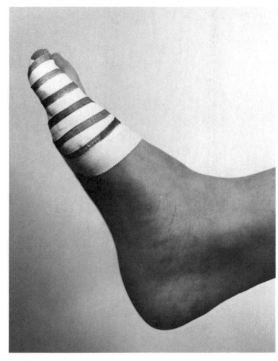

FIGURE 8:7E.

SUPPORTIVE PADS

Frequently, pads rather than tape can be used for support, especially for the lower extremity. Pads can be made from felt, foam rubber or similar material. Felt has an advantage over foam in that it is less compressible. Sorbethane is another popular padding material because of its cushioning qualities. In addition, it is fairly noncompressible but is far more expensive than felt.

To make supportive pads:

1. Draw an outline of the area to be supported, i.e., longitudinal arch, on the bottom of the athlete's foot with magic marker or liquid adherent (Fig. 8:8A).
2. Immediately place the foam, felt or Sorbethane on the outlined area. The imprint of the drawing will remain.
3. Cut along the imprinted line and bevel the edges. This gives the padding a gradual, rather than sharp, drop-off in line with the foot's normal contour (Fig. 8:8B).
4. Covering the felt or foam pad with moleskin helps give it longevity.
5. Hold the pad in place with circular strips of tape (Fig. 8:8C).

A longitudinal arch pad supports the arch in cases of foot pronation (Fig. 8:9A). It is therefore useful in treating shin splints, plantar fasciitis, etc.

Metatarsal cookies can take the pressure off metatarsal heads, and therefore can be used to treat metatarsalgia (Fig. 8:9B).

Heel pads may be used to elevate the heel, thereby decreasing the tension placed on the Achilles tendon when treating Achilles tendonitis (Fig. 8:9C).

Heel pads may also be used to take the pressure off a particularly painful area on the heel, such as with heel spurs or bone bruises (Fig. 8:9D).

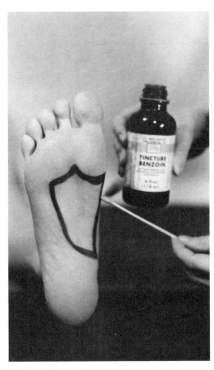

FIGURE 8:8A.

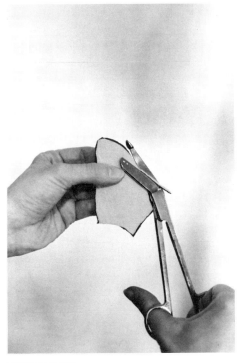

FIGURE 8:8B.

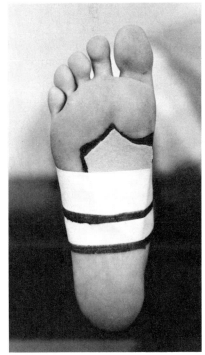

FIGURE 8:8C.

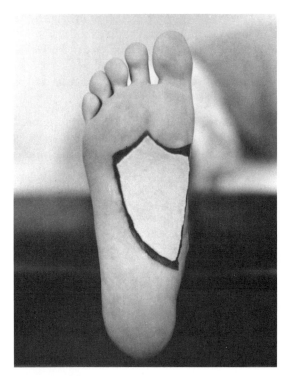

FIGURE 8:9A.

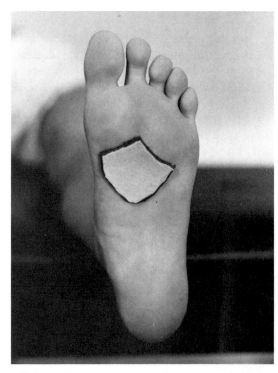

FIGURE 8:9C.

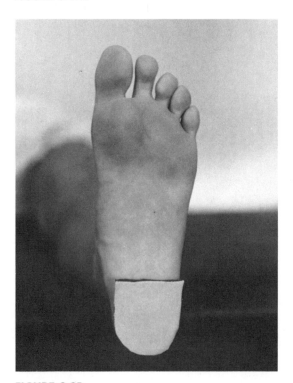

FIGURE 8:9B.

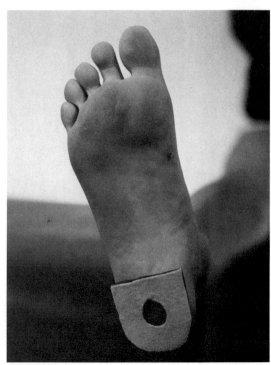

FIGURE 8:9D.

Elastic Bandaging Procedures

Properly applied elastic bandages serve many needs in sports medicine.

1. Pressure (first aid compression)
2. Secure ice packs, dressings, splints and protective pads
3. Mild support of joints
4. Support of large muscle groups
5. Retard and/or reduce swelling and hemorrhaging
6. Restrict movement

The wraps are available in 2, 3, 4, 5 and 6 inch widths. Select the proper size wrap for the area, such as a 2 inch wrap for the hand and wrist or 3 to 4 inch for the ankle and forearm. The 6 inch bandage is probably the most frequently used, since it can cover large areas of the body as well as ice packs, pads, etc. The 6 inch wrap is used for the knee, thigh, shoulder, groin, etc.

Elastic bandages are manufactured with several grades of tension, depending upon the amount of rubber in the fabric and the type of weave. Mild tension is usually used for first aid applications. Stronger tension is used to support large muscle groups and the trunk. Some elastic bandages are free of rubber but stretch because of the type of weave. These are not often used in athletics since they do not hold up with heavy use.

APPLICATION/REMOVAL GUIDELINES

Some basic guidelines should be followed when using elastic bandages.

1. Tape adherent may be sprayed onto the skin to prevent slippage.

2. Anchor at the distal end of the body segment (covering the end with the first turn).
3. In most cases, apply the bandage in a distal to proximal direction.
4. Overlap turns by one half width on each turn.
5. Do not leave skin exposed between strips.
6. Make the bandage contour to the part with equal tension on both the upper and lower edges.
7. For the greatest support and compression, take most of the stretch in the wrap as it is applied. If less support is needed, apply with less stretch.
8. Fasten the wrap with clips if the athlete is not going to participate (Fig. 9:1). Use tape

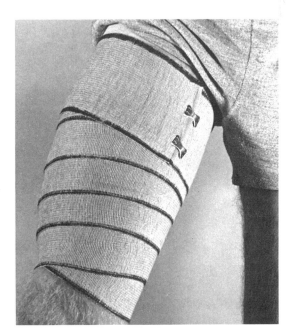

FIGURE 9:1. Spiral wrap of thigh with end secured by clips

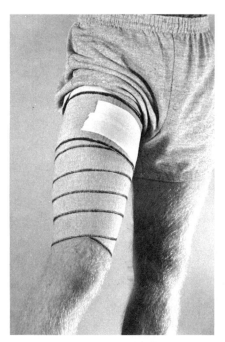

FIGURE 9:2A. Secure end of spiral wrap with adhesive tape applied halfway around the thigh.

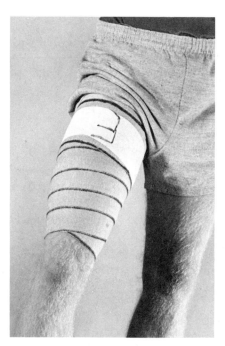

FIGURE 9:2B. Apply more adhesive tape in opposite direction to completely secure spiral wrap for activity.

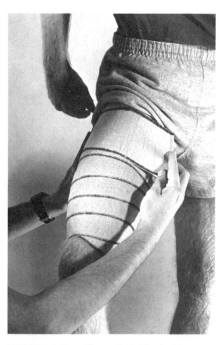

FIGURE 9:3. The spiral 4″ elastic wrap on the thigh begins at the distal thigh and is covered by the completed wrap.

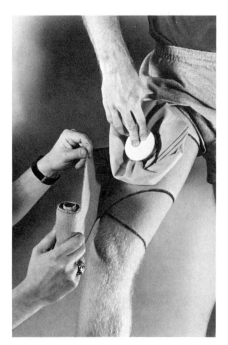

FIGURE 9:4A. Spiral wrap applied to secure an ice bag to the thigh

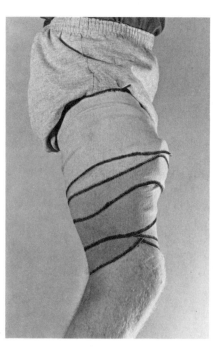

FIGURE 9:4B. Completed spiral wrap securing ice bag over thigh

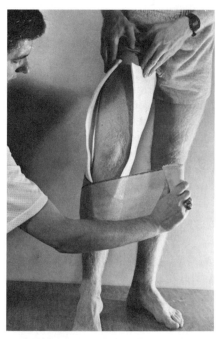

FIGURE 9:5A. Spiral wrap applied over felt strips as a splint for the knee

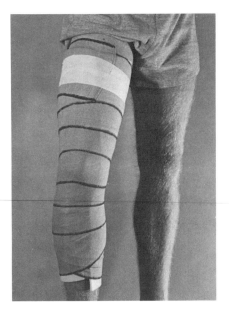

FIGURE 9:5B. Completed spiral wrap securing felt strips over the knee

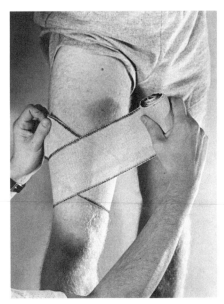

FIGURE 9:6A. To anchor the figure-of-eight wrap of the thigh, position the beginning of the wrap so the completed wrap will cover it.

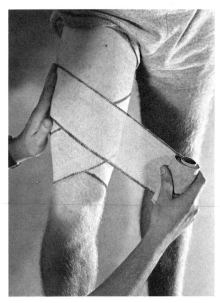

FIGURE 9:6B. The end of the first turn in the figure-of-eight wrap for the thigh

if the athlete intends to participate (Figs. 9:2A, B).

9. The wrap should be comfortable to wear. A wrap that is too tight may cause the extremity to swell.
10. In removing tape or clips, be careful not to damage the bandage.
11. The soiled bandage may be laundered in mild soap and warm water. It can be dried in mild heat in the dryer or in the open air. Both hot water and hot air drying tend to reduce the effectiveness of the rubber and shorten the life of the bandage.

COMMON APPLICATION METHODS

The most common types of bandages are the spiral, figure-of-eight, spica, and combinations of the above. Each bandage type has advantages for certain situations.

The spiral wrap is simply anchored and spiraled around the area, overlapping each turn by one half the width of the wrap (Fig. 9:3). It is quick and easy to apply and can cover a large area. As a first aid measure with an ice pack, the anchor and first layer may be moistened with water and applied under the ice pack (Figs. 9:4A, B). This provides compression directly to the skin and makes the cold pack more comfortable. The major disadvantage is that the spiral wrap tends to slip easily when the athlete is very active.

The spiral wrap is effective over felt strip splints as a first aid measure on the field for care of injuries such as knee sprains (Figs. 9:5A, B). Also, the spiral may be used over tape jobs to help "set" and protect the taping.

The figure-of-eight wrap is a very good bandage for many areas of the body, especially over large muscle groups such as the thigh, knee and calf. With some practice, it is easy to apply and does not slip as easily as the spiral wrap.

The wrap is anchored, and the first turn is taken at a sharp angle (Fig. 9:6A). The returning turn is taken at a downward angle (Fig. 9:6B). The additional loops in the pattern overlap the previous loops by half the width of the

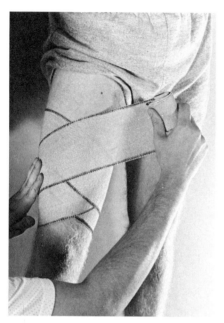

FIGURE 9:6C. The beginning of the second turn of the thigh figure-of-eight wrap

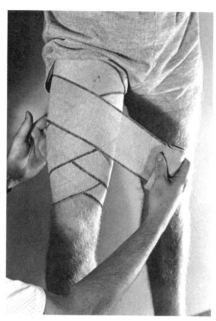

FIGURE 9:6D. Completion of the second turn of the thigh figure-of-eight wrap

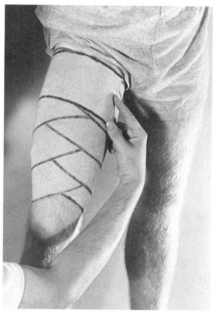

FIGURE 9:6E. Continue the figure-of-eight pattern up the thigh and end it at the top. Secure it by tape or clips.

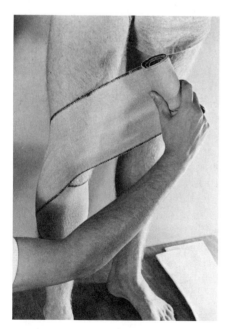

FIGURE 9:7A. To start the figure-of-eight wrap for the knee, anchor it below the knee and carry it up over the kneecap at a sharp angle.

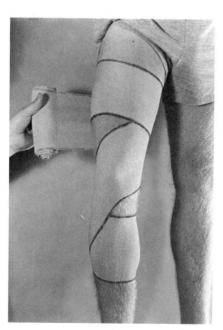

FIGURE 9:7B. Anchor the knee figure-of-eight around the thigh, thus providing anchors above and below the knee.

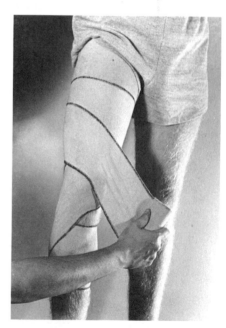

FIGURE 9:7C. Start the figure-of-eight pattern back down the leg by pulling the beginning of the first turn down at a sharp angle.

wrap (Fig. 9:6C). This pattern is continued, normally from the distal to the proximal portion of the body segment (Fig. 9:6D). The wrap should be secured with nonelastic tape at the top and bottom. The top tape may be carried partially onto the skin to prevent slippage (Fig. 9:6E). The securing tapes are applied in two pieces, each going only half the way around the extremity, front to back and back to front, thus preventing a circulation problem when the muscles are contracted.

The figure-of-eight is especially effective for the knee, thigh and calf, forearm, elbow and upper arm. When applying the wrap to the knee or elbow, it is better to anchor low, carry the first turn over the joint (Figs. 9:7A–H), anchor at the top and work the pattern down to the original anchor. Starting at the bottom and ending at the bottom usually prevents slippage with participation in these very active joints.

The figure-of-eight wrap provides excellent compression. If adherent is not available, or if the athlete has a sensitivity to the adherent, a piece of white tape, folded lengthwise with the adhesive side out, can be used under the wrap (Figs. 9:8A, B).

The spica wrap is basically a figure-of-eight in which one loop is substantially larger than the other loop. This wrap is especially effective for the foot/ankle, shoulder and groin areas (Figs. 9:9A–D).

The wrap is anchored on the extremity and carried over the joint and around the body. Normally, at least two sets of loops are used, with more if additional support is desired.

Care must be taken not to apply the wrap too tightly. Also, the direction in which the spica is applied should support the injured structures. For example, with an adductor strain (groin), the first loop, after the anchor,

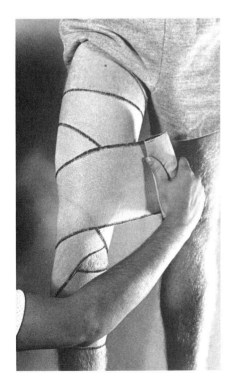

FIGURE 9:7D. Pull the end of the first turn of the knee figure-of-eight up at a sharp angle.

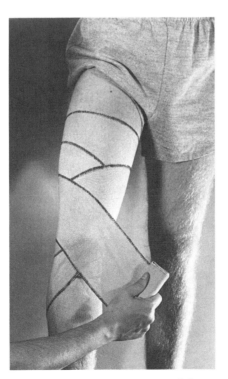

FIGURE 9:7E. The beginning of the second turn follows the first turn, overlapping by at least one half width at the same angle.

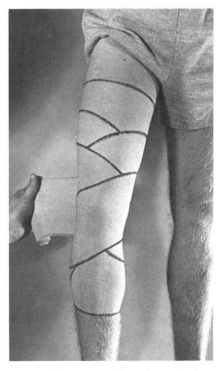

FIGURE 9:7F. Complete the end of the second turn by following the upward angle of the first turn and overlapping by at least one half width.

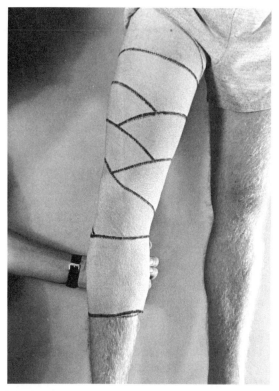

FIGURE 9:7G. Continue the knee figure-of-eight pattern down to the bottom anchor and complete it below the knee.

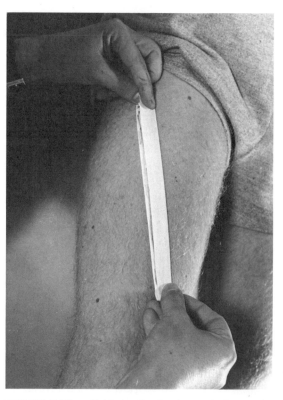

FIGURE 9:8A. Folded adhesive tape can be used in place of spray adhesive.

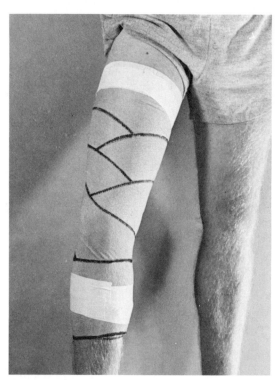

FIGURE 9:7H. Secure the knee figure-of-eight with adhesive tape over the top and bottom. The top tape can override onto the skin (shaved) to prevent slippage.

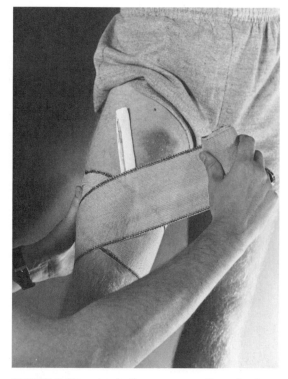

FIGURE 9:8B. Apply the wrap over the adhesive tape. The folded tape helps to prevent slippage of the wrap.

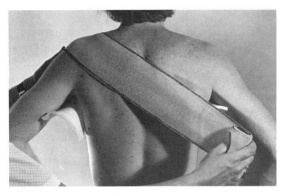

FIGURE 9:9A. The clavicle figure-of-eight wrap is used for emergency care of clavicle fractures. The athlete places his hands on his hips and throws his shoulders back. Start the wrap on one shoulder and carry it down and across the back.

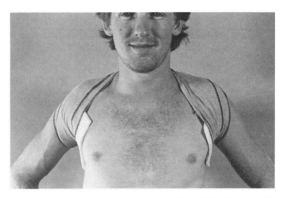

FIGURE 9:9D. In the completed clavicle figure-of-eight wrap, note the padding under the arms to prevent discomfort.

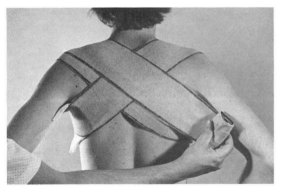

FIGURE 9:9B. Pull the wrap under the opposite shoulder, around and across the back, following this pattern at least twice.

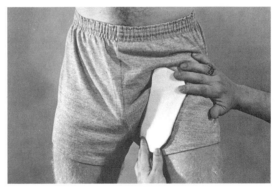

FIGURE 9:10A. A felt pad fitted for the area can provide additional support for a groin (adductor) strain. This is held in place by a hip spica wrap.

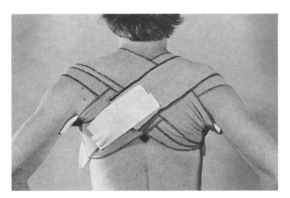

FIGURE 9:9C. Secure the completed clavicle figure-of-eight with tape.

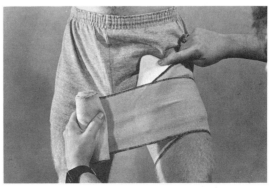

FIGURE 9:10B. To apply the hip spica wrap, pull it from the lateral aspect to the medial, pulling the leg into the groin.

should be pulled around the outside of the leg, across, up and over the front of the abdomen to the opposite hip (Figs. 9:10A–F), pulling the leg into the groin, not away from it.

The opposite is true in supporting the muscles of the buttocks. The initial large loop is pulled from the leg across, up, and over the back of the buttocks (Figs. 9:11A–D). This pulls the buttocks into the midline of the body. In a shoulder spica, a soft pad may be applied under the armpit to avoid chafing. In a hip spica, additional support for a groin strain may be given by incorporating a felt pad fitted into the groin.

Combinations of the above wraps are sometimes used for special situations. The 4 **S** wrap is such a combination, used as a first aid measure for many shoulder injuries. This wrap requires a double-length 4 inch or 6 inch wrap, or two or three regular length wraps. This ban-

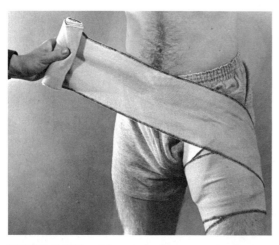

FIGURE 9:10C. After anchoring, carry the first large loop of the hip spica up and over the groin, onto the opposite hip. Again, note the pull is from lateral to medial.

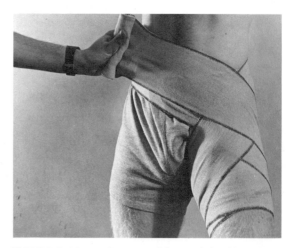

FIGURE 9:10E. The second loop of the hip spica wrap follows the pattern of the first, overlapping by at least one half width (usually more).

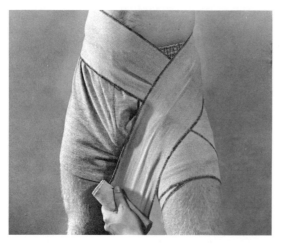

FIGURE 9:10D. Complete the first large loop of the hip spica by pulling the wrap around, behind the waist and down firmly into the groin.

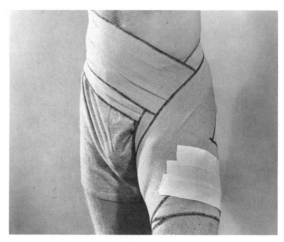

FIGURE 9:10F. The completed hip spica wrap for an adductor strain

dage incorporates the spica bandage, the sling, the swathe and stabilizing acromioclavicular joint straps (Figs. 9:12A–I). An ice bag may be incorporated where necessary. The wrap supports the entire shoulder area and is especially useful when a sling is not available.

The foot/ankle pressure wrap is a combination of wrapping techniques used to retard and/or prevent swelling and hemorrhage in injuries such as an ankle sprain. A pressure gradient is created by applying more pressure at the toe of the bandage, gradually decreasing the pressure going up the foot, with almost no pressure at the top of the ankle (Figs. 9:13A–H). This greater pressure discourages the accumulation of swelling in the foot and toes. The swelling tends to gather in the area with the least resistance (pressure). The better circulation of the lower leg can more efficiently absorb the swelling.

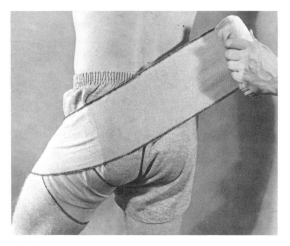

FIGURE 9:11A. To anchor the hip spica for a buttocks strain, pull the wrap from lateral to medial, pulling the muscle group into the midline of the body.

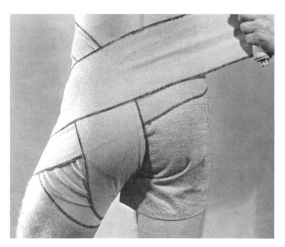

FIGURE 9:11C. The second large loop of the hip spica overlaps the first by at least one half width.

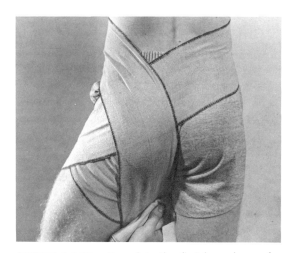

FIGURE 9:11B. Complete the first large loop of the hip spica around the waist, over and into the buttocks.

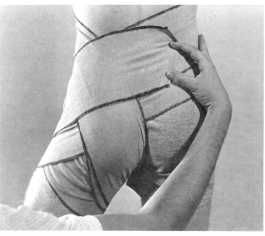

FIGURE 9:11D. The completed hip spica, supporting the buttocks. This wrap can be used to hold dressings over abrasions, common in sliding injuries.

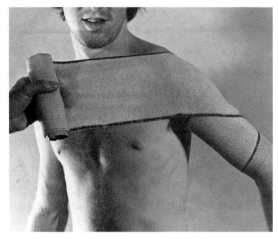

FIGURE 9:12A. The 4 S wrap starts with a shoulder spica, normally pulled from the lateral to the medial aspects.

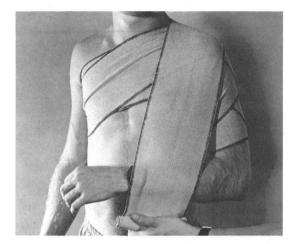

FIGURE 9:12D. After completing the second large loop of the shoulder spica, pull the wrap over the acromioclavicular (AC) joint and down under the bent forearm. This supports the AC joint and a sling.

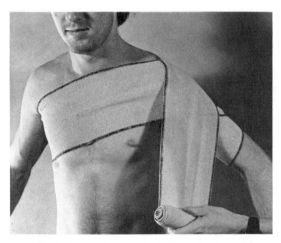

FIGURE 9:12B. Completion of the first shoulder spica in the 4 S wrap.

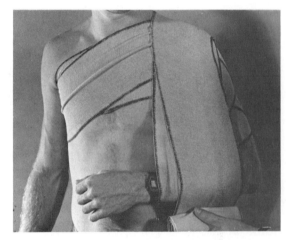

FIGURE 9:12E. Apply a second sling loop.

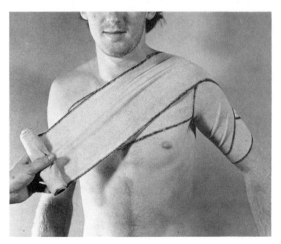

FIGURE 9:12C. Beginning of second shoulder spica in the 4 S wrap.

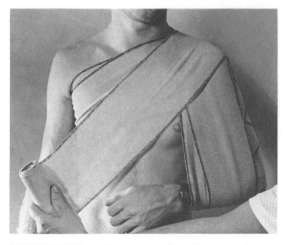

FIGURE 9:12F. After completing the second sling loop, pull the wrap down across the chest to start the swathe portion of the wrap.

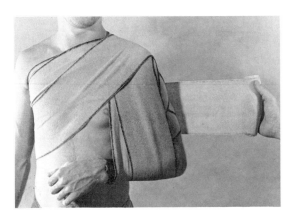

FIGURE 9:12G. Start the swathe portion by pulling the wrap around the back.

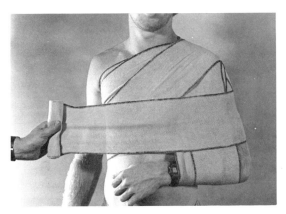

FIGURE 9:12H. Complete the swathe portion of the wrap by going around the injured arm and around the chest (usually twice).

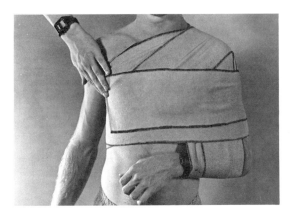

FIGURE 9:12I. The completed 4 S shoulder wrap. It can include an ice bag and be secured with tape. It provides a shoulder spica, a sling, a swathe, and a stabilizing strap for the AC joint.

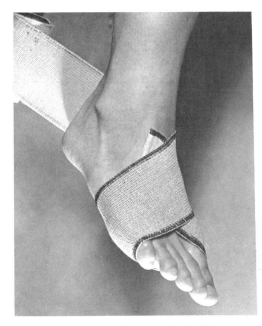

FIGURE 9:13A. Anchor the foot/ankle pressure wrap just behind the toes. Start the spica by pulling the wrap low across the medial aspect of the foot and behind the heel.

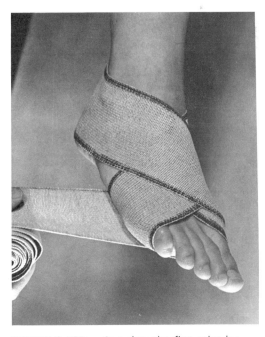

FIGURE 9:13B. Complete the first spica by covering the low, lateral aspect of the foot and pulling the wrap up over the foot, then repeat.

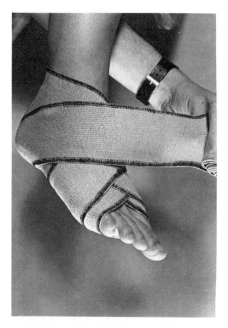

FIGURE 9:13C. After covering the point of the heel, bring the wrap up over the front of the ankle.

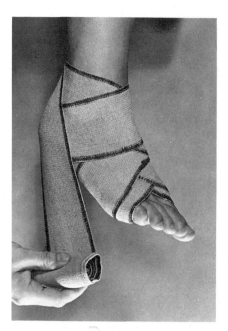

FIGURE 9:13D. Then pull the wrap behind the ankle diagonally down over the lateral aspect of the heel. This is similar to a heel lock in ankle taping.

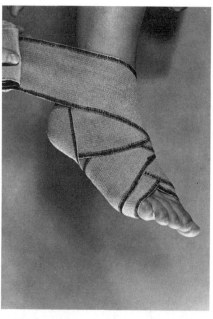

FIGURE 9:13E. Pull the wrap under the heel, over the high front of the ankle to start the inside heel lock.

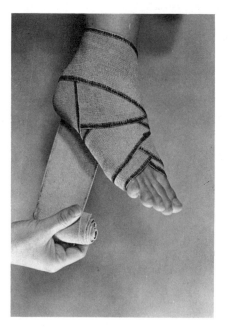

FIGURE 9:13F. Pull the second heel lock behind the heel diagonally down across the medial aspect of the ankle.

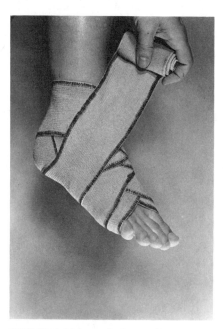

FIGURE 9:13G. After completing the heel locks, bring the wrap up over the lateral aspect of the foot and over the high front of the ankle.

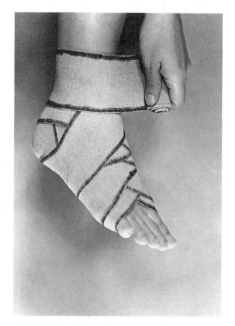

FIGURE 9:13H. Complete the wrap by loosely spiraling the end of the wrap just above the ankle.

Part 4

PROTECTIVE DEVICES

Principles of Protective Devices

10

OBJECTIVES

Protective devices in sports should be designed to:

1. Protect body parts against injury
2. Protect injured parts against further aggravation
3. Prevent recurrent injury to areas that are healed or susceptible

Ideal protective equipment causes minimal functional interference and is not harmful to other participants. Practicality dictates that such equipment be simple to fit and maintain, be durable and reliable and not prohibitively expensive.

Injury Prevention

The need for specific types of protection is dictated by the hazard demonstrated in each individual sport. New sports, e.g., racquetball, present new problems and require changing techniques, and some sports require reanalysis of injury problems. In contact sports such as football and hockey, exposed and vulnerable areas must be protected. Players must be protected from the sticks in lacrosse and field hockey. Vulnerable and vital areas such as the head, eyes, neck, kidneys and genitalia must have priority for protection. High-velocity, low-mass hazards are seen in baseball, lacrosse, hockey and racquet sports, and protection is by means of helmets, face masks, and various types of eye protection for athletes with and without glasses. The primary contact points such as the shoulder, arms and the anterior leg regions must be protected with appropriate pads. Dental protection by mouth-guards is mandatory in football and recommended in other sports because of proven protective value. The injurious effects of rigid protective equipment such as the football helmet are still a problem.

The prophylactic value of bracing or taping at susceptible joints such as the knee and ankle is well established but not practical for routine use at all levels. This is an individual matter and is still treated as such. The relationship of footwear to turf fixation has been recognized, and the type of shoe surface has to be tailored according to the playing surface. The condition of the playing surface also affects the choice of footwear and ankle taping. The wear factors on artificial surfaces, the decreased impact absorption and interface friction have to be monitored because of the changing hazard.

Protection of Injured Parts

When medical supervision indicates the athlete can return to sporting activity with appropriate protection, the protective devices are often individually chosen by training personnel. In football, improved impact absorption helmet linings provide protection subsequent to concussion. Commercial or individualized cervical collars or straps can prevent recurrent neck strain but must be properly fitted to be safe and of value. Contused areas on the body can be protected with customized resilient padding around the contused area using semi-rigid or firm materials to disperse the impact. All materials must be sufficiently padded on the exterior to prevent injury to other participants. Joint mobility is best limited with adequate taping procedures. Common examples

95

are protection against hyperextension of the knee, attempted control of rotational stresses on the knee, and limitation of either flexion or extension of the elbow. Shoulder pad extensions as well as various types of hip padding are available for injured areas on the rib cage and the pelvic bones.

Protection Against Reinjury

When joint injuries are considered stable enough to allow return to participation, the joint should have protective restriction, usually supplied by appropriate tape protection. Tape protection is directed at restricting stress on the affected area while still permitting functional movement of the joint. Some braces are effective, particularly in combination with tape protection. Again, any brace used to protect a joint must be noninjurious to opponents. Ankle instability can usually be protected with good tape support for athletic participation, remembering that tape support tends to lose its effectiveness with time, perspiration and use.

PROTECTIVE EQUIPMENT REGULATIONS

Increasing effort toward regulation and mandatory use of protective equipment including mouthguards, head, eye and facial protection has made great strides in preventing injury. The quality of protective equipment has improved greatly with attempts at standardization and improved methods of testing

materials. Sports regulatory bodies have established National Operating Committee on Standards for Athletic Equipment (NOCSAE) certification standards for protective devices such as football helmets. The Sports Equipment and Facilities Committee of American Society for Testing Material has established testing standards for skiing equipment and is involved in establishing standards in other protective areas. These movements focus upon eliminating protective devices that are inadequate. Biomechanical principles increasingly employed in developing protective devices allow material with maximal impact resistance, shock attenuation and durability under various conditions to be identified. Protective equipment will continue to improve because the materials available and understanding of the mechanical forces that affect the body in sports continue to improve.

The characteristics of playing surfaces of all kinds and their relationship to traction and various types of footwear are being further evaluated. Again, standardizing testing methods will be focused upon increasingly. The variety of footwear available designed for different sports and different playing surfaces is evidence of growing understanding of shoe and surface interface problems. Equipment that is standardized and regulated must not be altered. Any modification of such devices must be done by certified reconditioners. Protective devices must be continually updated and matched to the needs of changing athletic activities.

Upper and Lower Extremities

UPPER EXTREMITY

The shoulder girdle is generally protected against forceful contact with opponents and hard surfaces and objects. Commercial shoulder pads used in football, ice hockey and lacrosse are generally adequate to protect this region (Fig. 11:1). Additional customized padding can be readily fashioned to further protect local areas of susceptibility, such as the acromioclavicular joint (Fig. 11:2). Standard shoulder protective devices do not substantially restrict or protect the glenohumeral joint. Tape restraints or commercial devices that limit abduction movements can provide protective restriction of motion at this point (Fig. 11:3).

Football Shoulder Pad Fitting

Although different styles and types of shoulder pads are used in football today, the principles used in fitting have remained the same over the years. The width of the shoulder is measured to determine what size pad is needed. When fitted correctly, the shoulder pad should meet the following criteria:

1. The inner padding should cover the tip of the shoulders.
2. The neck opening should not be constrictive yet should minimize the areas exposed to injury.
3. The epaulets and cups should cover the deltoid and allow those movements required by the athlete's specific position.
4. Straps and lacings should be as snug as possible without constricting breathing.
5. If a split clavicle shoulder pad is used, the channel for the acromioclavicular joint should be in proper position. Collars and drop down pads can be added as adjuncts to shoulder pad protection.

11

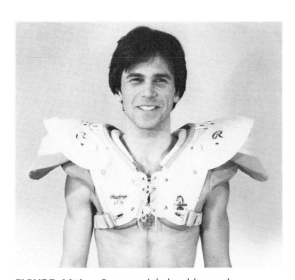

FIGURE 11:1. Commercial shoulder pads

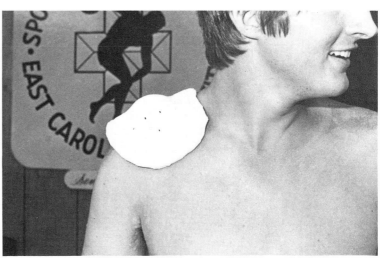

FIGURE 11:2. Pad over the acromioclavicular joint

97

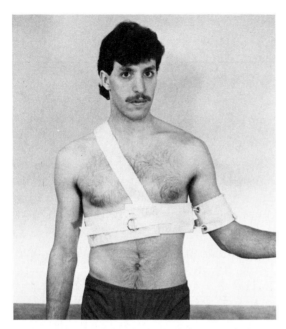

FIGURE 11:3. Device to limit abduction of gleno-humeral joint

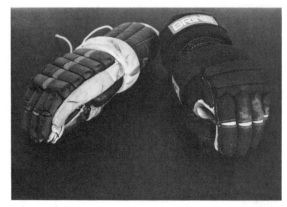

FIGURE 11:4. Padding in the form of gloves to protect hands

Silicone rubber has been used extensively to mold protective padding for joints such as the wrist and hand, particularly in enabling injured athletes to participate in contact activities. Innovative coaches and trainers can salvage external firm and padding materials from old sports equipment to provide inexpensive, custom-made materials (Figs. 11:5, 11:6).

The ribs and thorax may be protected primarily, or following injury shielded from further trauma, by commercially available ''flak jackets.'' Running backs who are exposed to repeated thoracic contusion or quarterbacks with prior rib cage injury may derive significant benefit from this padding.

The humeral or arm region can be protected in any sport by commercial padding similar to types available for the elbow. Additionally, protective padding can be modified to cover broader or more specific areas and attached with elastic bandages and tape. The motion of the elbow can be limited by appropriate tape methods. Similarly, forearm musculature and bone structures can be adequately protected with commercial cushion pads.

Commercial pads in the form of gloves to protect the hands are traditional and well developed in ice hockey, lacrosse and, for goal-keepers, field hockey. In the sport of boxing, the gloves serve a twofold purpose: protection of the boxer's hands and protection of the impact site of the opponent (Fig. 11:4).

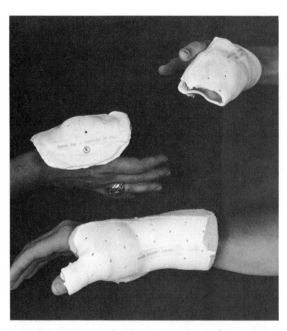

FIGURE 11:5. Orthoplast uses. Top to bottom: sandwich splint for fingers; bubble pad for thumb; thumb/wrist splint

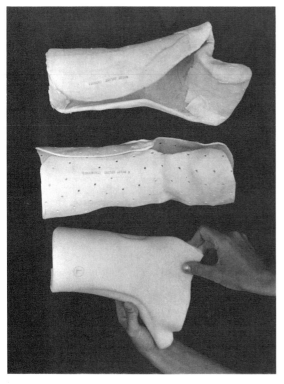

FIGURE 11:6. Splints for the hand and wrist. Top and middle: Orthoplast; bottom: softer Plastazote

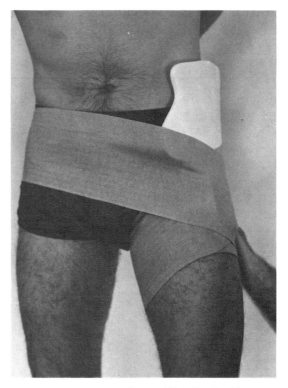

FIGURE 11:7. Protective padding for the hip to protect injured areas

LOWER EXTREMITY

Standard protective padding for the hip and pelvic area is adequate for contact sports when varied in structure, weight and application according to the sport for which it is used. As in other areas, commercial and custom pads can be used to protect injured areas such as contusions of the iliac crest and muscular attachments thereon (Fig. 11:7). Likewise, commercially available soft and rigid protection for the genital region is adequate in most instances for contact sports. In the thigh region, the standard padding available in uniforms, particularly for football, is effective, although coverage is limited to the most susceptible anterior region. Larger or adequate pads for this region can be easily made from materials readily available. Padding and strapping can minimize, by tension, the sensitivity to use in some muscular injuries.

Knee Protection

The knee is well protected against direct blows by padding in hockey uniforms as well as in the leg guards used in sports such as baseball and field hockey. Commercially available supplementary padding as well as custom pads are available for additional protection from external blows to the knee region. All wrestlers should wear standard knee pads to protect the prepatellar and infrapatellar bursae from excessive friction.

The prophylactic taping of the knee joints is usually not considered practical, although it may be potentially useful. Currently, some feel that single upright knee braces may protect the collateral knee structures in the interior linemen in football (Fig. 11:8). Whether this type of protection can be translated into more standard use in all sports and other positions is uncertain.

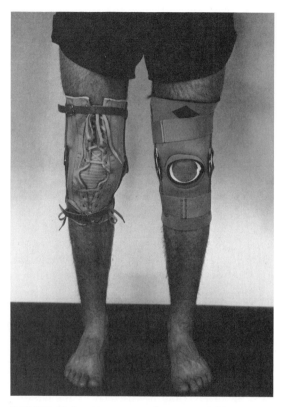

FIGURE 11:8. Two types of commercial knee braces to protect collateral knee structures

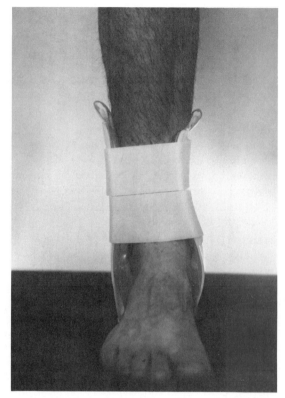

FIGURE 11:9. Commercial ankle brace for prophylactic or protective use

Lower Leg, Foot and Ankle

External padding for the tibial region is available for baseball catchers, ice hockey, field hockey, soccer, and several other sports. These shields are designed to protect against the blow of the high velocity missile used in these sports as well as the stick devices in the hands of players. Again, supplementary customized padding is easily devised with semirigid ex-ternal surfaces and dispersion type resilient materials beneath.

The ankle region can be effectively protected with taping as described in other sections. Numerous commercial and customized ankle braces can be used prophylactically and for protection following injury (Fig. 11:9). External padding is similarly simple to devise for contused areas in the ankle region.

Other Protective Devices

The effectiveness of protection for the brain and skull has greatly increased in recent years. Head protection is desirable in many sports including football, ice hockey, lacrosse, boxing, baseball, cycling, automobile and motorcycle racing. The most complete development of head protection is presently seen in the evolution of the football helmet. Mandatory head protection in sports such as football and ice hockey has reduced the number and severity of injuries.

In several sports the combination of face masks and helmets provides essential protection to the face and head. The wide variety of facial protection reflects the nature of the dangerous contacts. Obviously, the face mask in ice hockey, lacrosse and baseball has to limit the entry of the puck, ball and stick. A moveable pad to protect the throat is desirable. Ear protection is afforded in wrestling and boxing by standard head gear.

Eye protection has become extremely important in recent years due to the many eye injuries that can occur from paddles, racquets and the high-velocity small balls. The football face mask is of great benefit in protecting the facial bones, nose and eyes. The fencing mask should be of strong, fine metal mesh with an extra shell over the top of head and ears for saber. It must be adjustable to head size and have a thick bib to protect the throat from thrusting weapons. The glove must be heavier for saber and epee, and women fencers need extra protection in their jackets for the breasts.

Mouth guards are mandatory in football and are extremely effective. They are increasingly used in sports such as basketball and hockey. Development of mouth protection has followed its long, proven use in boxing. The effectiveness of intraoral mouth guards in reducing impact to the brain is documented. Mouthpieces are manufactured to provide intraoral, extraoral, or combination protection. They can be obtained in three styles: the preformed, or stock, mouthpiece; the form-fitted or moldable mouthpiece, which is placed in boiling water and molded to the athlete's mouth; and the custom-fitted variety, which is made from a mold taken of the athlete's teeth.

SELECTION AND FITTING

Protective equipment serves a twofold function in treating and preventing athletic injuries. It helps to reduce forces that would otherwise cause injury and prevents further insult to areas that have already been injured.

The correct use of protective equipment can substantially minimize the athlete's risk of being injured or reinjured. In selecting and fitting protective equipment, knowledge and expertise in the following areas are vital:

- Fit
- Maintenance
- Rules and regulations specific to the sport
- Design
- Fabrication
- Physical properties of materials used in pad construction
- Types, styles and brand names
- Special equipment
- Safety
- Athlete education
- Cost

12

Clinicians who master the use of protective equipment have an invaluable tool in their efforts to prevent and treat athletic injuries.

Fitting Equipment

Fitting equipment should be a combined effort by the equipment manager, trainer, physician, coach and parents. Correctly fitting equipment is of the utmost importance for injury prevention and protection. Incorrectly fitting equipment can be hazardous. Standards of correct fit should be set and adhered to. Many times, athletes will want to wear smaller, less restrictive equipment because it makes them look better or feel faster. This practice should be discouraged.

To fit athletic equipment correctly, the following factors should be considered.

Size of Athlete

The athlete's size is very important in selecting athletic equipment. Just as a pair of shoes should not be too large or too small, protective equipment should be the proper size.

Equipment that is too small for the athlete does not offer adequate protection (Fig. 12:1).

Correctly fitted equipment protects without inhibiting performance. In fitting equipment in relation to size, measure the area to be protected and then visualize the athlete with the pad in place.

The football helmet must fit correctly to function properly. Football helmets should be able to absorb force levels high enough to fracture the skull. With an improper fitting helmet, a fracture or concussion could result. To insure proper fit of a football helmet, hair length and head shape should be noted. Drastic changes in hair length and head shape can affect the fit. The front of the helmet should be about two finger widths above the eyebrow (Fig. 12:2). This may vary slightly with the air-inflated headgears. The back should cover the

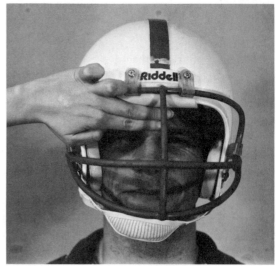

FIGURE 12:2. The front of the helmet should be about two finger-widths above the eyebrow.

base of the skull, but should not dig into the neck on neck extension (Fig. 12:3). Space between the neck band allows the helmet to rotate forward. The side earholes should coincide with the ear canals. The jaw pads should fit snugly to prevent lateral rocking (see Fig. 12:2).

With chin strap buckled, have the athlete hold his head straight forward. Grasp the sides

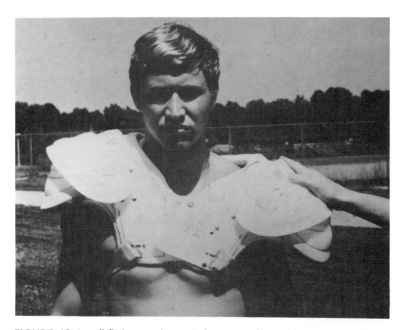

FIGURE 12:1. Ill-fitting equipment does not offer adequate protection.

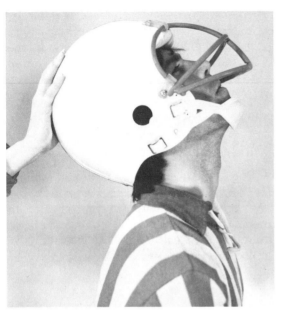

FIGURE 12:3. The back of the helmet should not dig into the neck.

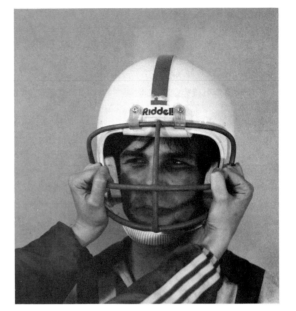

FIGURE 12:4. A properly fitting helmet moves only slightly.

of the helmet and try to turn the helmet on the head, side to side, and then try to rock it front to back. A properly fitting helmet moves only slightly (Fig. 12:4).

Fit of the helmet should be monitored often, as many factors can alter fit:

- Environmental temperature
- Hair length
- Deterioration of internal padding
- Loss of air from cells
- Spread of face mask

The vast number of sports and different types of equipment make it difficult to describe correct fit for each situation, but adhering to the preceding principles increases the likelihood of correctly fitting equipment.

Sport and Sport Position

Sports such as ice hockey, football and baseball have equipment designed for the demands of a specific position—goalie, midfielder, quarterback and catcher. Performance protection should be evaluated closely in selecting equipment for a specific sport position.

Strength

Evaluating the strength of athletes further determines what size equipment is used. If the equipment is too small and restrictive, the strong athlete could be compromised; the inverse could be true of large and bulky equipment used by the weaker athlete.

Age and Physical Development

A tremendous array of equipment is manufactured for different ages and developmental stages. This equipment can be adapted for use by athletes at all levels of competition.

Skill Levels

Some equipment is manufactured to adapt to different skill levels. Equipment such as this is generally not suitable for the amateur athlete.

Maintenance

One of the few standards for protective equipment is the NOCSAE certification for football helmets. Yearly inspection provides some safeguards, but daily monitoring of helmets and all protective equipment most effectively prevents injuries due to faulty equipment. Schedules for equipment inspection, repair and disposal are advisable.

Responsibilities for maintaining equipment should be defined and adhered to for each sport. Daily inspections, cleaning, drying, storage and repair are some maintenance procedures for which athletes can be made responsible, especially where trained maintenance people are not always available.

Although the athlete greatly assists in equipment maintenance, a trained person should be designated to monitor this area. The maintenance person, along with the rest of the sports staff, should constantly watch for ill-fitting or damaged equipment and should establish a weekly schedule for inspection and repair of all equipment.

Basic steps should be followed in maintaining the specific equipment.

Football Helmets: Weekly Maintenance

1. Visually inspect and stress shells to locate defects.
2. Check padding for wear and deterioration.
3. Check air cells for leaks and proper inflation levels.
4. Check face masks for bends or cracks. Also inspect screws and grommets that secure the mask to the helmet for deterioration and looseness.
5. Check chin straps and buckles for wear and looseness.
6. Send helmets to a reconditioner for inspection certification (if required) and overall repair annually.

Football Shoulder Pads: Weekly Maintenance

1. Inspect shell for cracks and loose rivets.
2. Inspect straps, laces and buckles for wear and deterioration.
3. Inspect padding for defects in the padding and its covering. Test the shock absorption capacity of the padding.

4. Inspect cantilevers to make sure they are functioning.
5. Send shoulder pads to a reconditioner for inspection, certification (if required) and overall repair annually.

These same principles can be used for all other protective equipment.

Rules and Regulations

Sports medicine clinicians should familiarize themselves with each sport's specific rules and regulations dealing with protective equipment. The trainer's knowledge of both required and illegal equipment will allow the athlete maximum protection from injury.

Design

The clinician's knowledge of design plays an important part in both selecting manufactured equipment and fabricating equipment in the clinical situation. There are four basic principles used in pad design.

1. *Channeling:* forces are channeled away from anatomical structures.
2. *Dispersive:* forces are dispersed over a large area.
3. *Mechanical:* through the use of a mechanical structure, forces are reduced.
4. *Restriction:* anatomical ranges of motion are reduced to prevent forces that cause injury.

Most manufactured equipment combines these design principles. By knowing design principles, the clinician understands how protective equipment works and can design equipment necessary.

Fabrication

In constructing protective equipment, knowledge and mastery of fabrication techniques are essential. While experience, imagination and practice are the best teachers, a good construction plan for each pad helps the clinician. Factors to consider when developing a plan for pad construction follow.

Injury Protection During Fabrication

While using the athlete as a model to fabricate a pad, great care must be taken not to aggravate the injury. The injury should be protected from undue pressure, temperature, constriction, movement and contact with an unyielding surface. Stockinet, prewrap or positive cast molds are just a few means for protecting the athlete during fabrication.

Materials

Select materials that best serve the design principles selected. Make sure the materials are compatible in terms of physical properties: flexible vs. inflexible, soft vs. hard, etc. (Fig. 12:5).

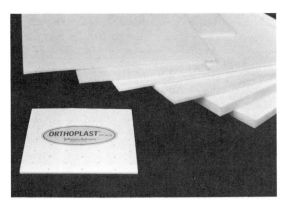

FIGURE 12:5. A perforated piece of Orthoplast, also available in solid sheets, plus various thicknesses and densities of Plastazote (above)

Cutting and Trimming Excess Material

Plan how the pad will be trimmed by using the injured area as a guide. Mark the area to be trimmed while the unfinished pad is still in place on the athlete (Figs. 12:6A, B). The proper tools such as cast saws and scissors are a necessity and should be sharp and in good working order.

Gluing

Fabricating some pads requires gluing different materials. Often it is better to bond the materials together before forming the pad. Experience with different injuries and techniques

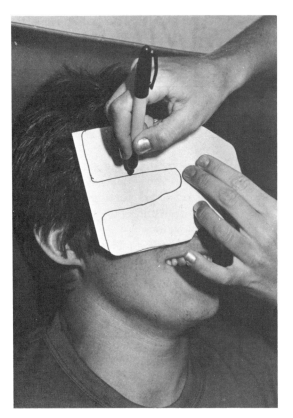

FIGURE 12:6A. A model for a nasal splint can be created with paper.

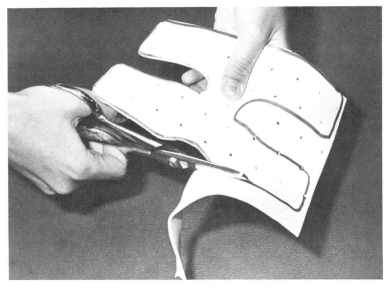

FIGURE 12:6B. After softening Orthoplast slightly in hot water, cut out the nasal splint form.

helps develop this skill. Adhesive materials need to be resistant to water and perspiration to maintain the pad's integrity.

Stabilizing the Pad

This is most important, as an improperly positioned pad can be very detrimental. When constructing the pad, how it will be held in place should be determined. Materials such as velcro, elastic webbing, canvas straps, elastic wraps, elastic sleeves, rubber sleeves and adhesive elastic or nonelastic tape can be used for stabilization. Alteration of the standard uniform (pants, jersey, girdle, etc.) is also an effective technique to stabilize pads located in awkward positions.

Forming Ridges, Channels Bubbles and Donuts

Accentuating or highlighting injured areas during fabrication helps dissipate the force. When a ridge, channel, bubble or donut can be effective, the injured area must be clearly identified. Structural anatomy and kinesiology should also be taken into consideration when forming these structures for force dissipation.

Pad Construction Materials

The clinician needs an understanding of the physical properties of materials used in constructing protective equipment whether for manufactured pads or clinic-made pads. Shock absorption capacity, deflective properties, weight and durability are all factors to be considered when selecting materials for purchase or use.

Foam rubber products on the market provide a wide range of shock absorption and recovery properties. The decision on what type to use is based on injury location, severity, tenderness and other equipment or materials involved in treatment.

Commercial thermoplastics or cast-type materials provide flexibility in the use of deflective, restrictive or hard dispersive materials. The selection of material depends on location, restriction needed, rules that govern

pads and other materials used to protect the injured body part.

Pneumatic (air-filled) devices are currently being used more extensively. Problems with rupture, maintaining inflation levels and stabilization have deterred the use of pneumatic devices.

Types, Styles and Brand Names

Staying abreast of improvements made in protective equipment maintains the quality of care. Clinicians should contact sales representatives and obtain literature to help maintain their knowledge of the latest materials, manufactured equipment and techniques. They can also offer advice on materials and design to help improve the quality of the protective equipment and materials being developed.

Special Equipment

Protective equipment from one sport can often be adapted for use in a different sport. Unique or unusual injuries often require creativity in designing or selecting protective devices.

Safety

Protective equipment should protect both the wearer and fellow athletes. Exposed edges, unyielding surfaces, sharp points and the potential as a weapon should be avoided.

Athlete Education

Athletes should be instructed on the use, maintenance, application and proper limits of all protective equipment worn.

Cost

Protective equipment is so important in preventing and treating athletic injuries that cost should not be a major factor. If the cost of equipment is a major budgetary concern, perhaps the status of the program or the athlete's eligibility should be re-evaluated.

MISCELLANEOUS PROTECTIVE DEVICES

Fabrication, Design and Application

Unusual injuries, the lack of appropriate commercial protective equipment, or the need for custom-fitted protection, at times, requires special protectives devices. Plastics and various padding materials are available for making such devices.

Care should be taken when providing such special equipment. Avoid changing the design or structure of commercially made equipment. Many times such changes can void the manufacturer's warranty and liability and create an additional point of liability. Avoid making guarantees to the athlete as to the protective powers of the device. Educate the athlete as to the device's proper use and the limitations in protection.

Many types of plastics are available to create splints and pads. Two common types are Orthoplast, a rather rigid plastic, and Plastazote, a softer, foam-like material used to pad or softly splint injuries. With considerable practice, the devices can be made to offer the athlete some protection.

The preceding procedures represent only a few special pads and splints that can be made. Of course, all devices are provided with the supervision and approval of the team physician, keeping in mind the types of activities and stresses the athletes will be exposed to during their use.

Part 5

CONDITIONING, REHABILITATION AND USE OF MODALITIES

Psychological Considerations in Working with Athletes

13

An athlete's performance is an integration of physical and psychological factors. Physical factors such as strength, endurance, flexibility and skill obviously influence performance, but the extent to which mental state affects performance has only been recognized recently. Athletic trainers have been primarily concerned with preventing and treating physical injuries. But with increased knowledge of psychological factors, trainers can expand their capability by preventing and treating psychological conditions that impair performance. They can also help insure that athletic participation enhances the athletes' psychological health.

This chapter examines five topics.

1. The relationship between trainers and athletes
2. Improving the athlete's mental state
3. The athletes' perspective on injuries
4. Psychological conditions in the acute treatment of injuries
5. Psychological factors during rehabilitation

DEVELOPING A RELATIONSHIP WITH THE ATHLETE

The relationship that develops between athlete and trainer determines the trainer's ability to promote the athlete's psychological well being. The trainer's expertise, dress, speech, organization, professional membership and training room manner all communicate preparation for and the capability to provide quality care and influence the trust that can develop between trainer and athlete. While occasional humor may be useful, the trainer should listen seriously to the athlete's comments and respond with concern and willingness to assist in improving performance.

One of the complexities in the athletic environment is that several individuals are concerned with the performance of a team or individual. A close, cooperative relationship must be fostered if the organization is to work effectively. When others voice dissatisfactions, the best approach may be to make constructive suggestions or simply listen without comment. On the other hand, trainers should not use players as counselors to help deal with their own complaints. Coaches, athletes and physicians should see the trainer as a team member, willing and eager to fulfill his role and not openly second guessing or criticizing his colleagues.

ENHANCING PSYCHOLOGICAL HEALTH

Athletes can experience psychological difficulties in their personal lives or professional environments. The stress of competition may also aggravate a nonathletic problem. These difficulties make athletes uncomfortable and can detract from performance. Because the coaches decide who plays, athletes may hide problems from them. They are often more willing to discuss their concerns with a trainer.

Athletes may express their psychological discomfort by frequent physical complaints or by showing undue concern over minor injuries. A trainer can help in these situations by assisting the athlete with minor problems or by referring more serious problems to psychiatrists or psychologists with expertise in treating athletes. Referral should be mandatory if psychological stress is intense or persistent and certainly with any suggestion of suicide or loss of contact with reality. The team physician and trainer should together insure that athletes receive professional treatment for serious psychological problems.

If the disturbance is mild but persistent and does not improve with the assistance of trainers and coaches, then it is advisable to seek additional help. Determining the availability of sport psychologists or psychiatrists in the area in advance of any problem is a wise precaution.

When talking with an athlete, some of the conversation will relate to the athlete's personal condition, some will be social, but some of the athlete's communications may express worries, concerns, fears or other psychological states. Be alert for this. In many instances, a good listener is all that is wanted or required.

Effective Listening

Although there is no formula for effective counseling, some frequently helpful methods are suggested.

1. Listen attentively for the message of the athlete. Don't think about what will be said next, thus missing what the athlete is really saying. Keep personal troubles to yourself and do not play down the importance of what the athlete feels is a problem. Exhibit concern for any problem shared and avoid criticism when athletes express fears or discomfort.
2. Many times persons are uncomfortable because they view their feelings as not normal while, in fact, they are typical in such situations. "Normalizing" the behavior by saying that many people feel the same way and considering how others successfully handle the problem often moves an athlete from worrying to problem solving.

3. If the athlete's statements or conclusions do not seem true, suggest that "from your perspective" things look a little different. Athletes often are too self-critical or pessimistic. If they reinterpret the situation more favorably, much of their discomfort diminishes.
4. Athletes may become discouraged when problems seem insurmountable and progress seems too slow. Focusing on goals and progress rather than errors and shortcomings may help. Helping athletes set a series of objectives leading toward a goal and marking progress along the way may enhance performance and satisfaction.

Trainers can usually offer this type of assistance in conjunction with treatments and it need not involve special sessions. While listening to athletes, also provide useful feedback, because they are reassessing their attitudes by the reactions of others. Do not place excess emphasis on past performance and potential failures to the extent of disturbing present performance. Setting realistic goals and expectations makes success more likely, and realistic evaluations of performance and the reaction of others encourages improvements.

The Athlete's Perspective

The treatment of any injury requires attending to both physical and psychological aspects. Athletes depend upon the ability of their bodies to perform at or near optimal levels. Failure to perform optimally is little more than an irritant to the nonathlete or recreational athlete. To the competitive athlete, performance can be the cornerstone of social and economic success and an important determinant of self-esteem. Thus, caring for the psychological needs of the injured athlete is a major challenge.

To an athlete, an injury is any physical problem that interferes with performance. The aches and pains following a contact sport that many nonathletes would consider injuries are usually normal parts of the game to athletes. On the other hand, a sprain that would be merely an inconvenience to a teacher, clerk or plumber could seriously incapacitate an athlete. Thus athletes' psychological reactions depend upon their perceptions of the injury's severity, not as a threat to life or source of unbearable pain, but as an interference with peak performance.

Emotional reactions to injuries are partially caused by pain associated with tissue damage, but also by the meaning placed upon an injury and the amount of attention focused on it. Competitive athletes' self-esteem is frequently tied closely to their capacities to excel physically. Their social roles are often based upon their ability to perform, and they spend a large amount of time attending to their bodies. Athletes are likely to react emotionally if they perceive that an injury will threaten their capacities to perform. The amount and type of reaction varies considerably from athlete to athlete, which complicates the assessment and treatment of injuries.

INTERACTION DURING ACUTE TREATMENT

The focus here is on non-life-threatening injuries and other injuries that do not require immediate hospitalization. With less traumatic injuries, the athlete's psychological needs become particularly important. Trainers should try to be familiar with an athlete's typical reaction to pain. While some athletes frequently overreact to slight injuries, an injury should always be assumed serious until thoroughly evaluated. During and after evaluation, the trainer can help control the athlete's discomfort by reassurance and moving the athlete's attention away from the injury. When the player keeps his eyes open, and talks with the trainer, he is concentrating on something other than the injury. If the athlete has developed confidence in the trainer before the injury, the trainer's presence will reassure him. Indicating to the athlete that he can be helped and the condition treated helps decrease anxiety and control pain. Never lie, but don't make

any unnecessary statements regarding potential complications.

The athlete goes through four psychological phases of injury: (1) denial, (2) anger, (3) depression, and (4) acceptance.

In the denial phase, the athlete says nothing is really wrong, and he will be ready to play on Friday. This can't happen to him, only to others. It is not up to the trainer to convince him otherwise. A physician makes the diagnosis and then advises the necessary treatment. At this point, most athletes leave the denial phase. Others seek second and third opinions, thus prolonging this phase.

After the athlete can no longer deny the injury, he often becomes angry at himself, those around him, and everything in general. Remember that you cannot reason with anger, and back off. To challenge anger only makes matters worse by increasing the anger. Things not meant are often said, thus damaging the player–trainer relationship. Wait until the athlete is more in control of himself before reasoning with him.

Depression is often the longest negative phase. Depression begins after anger subsides and the athlete believes his career, season or game is over. Often his life's goals are related to sport, and now these goals may no longer be achievable. If this is the athlete's first injury, depression may be especially severe. Dealing with this phase takes a great amount of patience. In these first three phases goals must be constantly repeated and exercises and routines reinforced, often daily, as the athlete may not listen very well to what he is being told. The athlete's frustration is often more difficult to deal with than the injury.

In the final, or acceptance, phase maximum effort should be applied to rehabilitation. Hopefully, the athlete will reach this phase in a short time. The skill of the athletic trainer in helping the athlete achieve this phase can determine the length of the rehabilitation.

Some athletes are not only able to blunt or ignore pain signals from injuries but can deny pain or loss of function. They can tolerate high levels of pain and apparently feel that it is to their advantage not to acknowledge discomfort. Trainers should watch athletes during and after competition to try to detect signs of injury, paying particular attention to those who have hidden injuries in the past. Coaches will often see injuries occur or note performance deficits. Their help is important in identifying injuries and convincing athletes that possible injuries require evaluation. The welfare of the athletes and the team is best served by rapid treatment.

Some injured athletes obviously will deny discomfort if it threatens their opportunity to play. But for other athletes, injury is a source of relief rather than a threat. Competition is not only an opportunity to triumph, it holds the chance of a failure. Particularly when others expect the athlete to succeed but circumstances such as more intense competition make the athlete less confident, the threat of failure and the pressure to succeed can produce great psychological discomfort. A small injury may provide a socially acceptable reason to avoid the pressure. If an overreaction to an injury threatens an athlete's ability to compete, and the athlete shows less than expected psychological discomfort, it would be worthwhile to discuss his perception of the situation and reaction to pressure. Trainers can help these athletes perceive the competitive situation as less threat and more opportunity. It is senseless to suggest that an athlete will perform above his potential or succeed without further effort. Urging this type of athlete to focus on possible success, however, and not on possible failure assists him to perceive competition more positively, and feel there is less reason to escape.

REHABILITATION

During treatment, pain and fear are no longer a major psychological factor but depression and impatience may decrease the athlete's contribution to rehabilitation. The athlete's cooperation is essential for successful rehabilitation because he must dedicate the time, exert the effort and endure the pain sometimes involved. The trainer can improve cooperation during rehabilitation with clear explanations. Trainers should outline procedures used in treatment and make a reasonable prediction of the time before returning to competition. Athletes typically want to return to competition more rapidly than possible. Offering an optimistic expectation, measuring progress daily, and breaking programs into small subgoals so that improvement is more visible alleviates some of the emotional discomfort. The ability to return to the previous level of performance or to regain the previous position on the team can be discussed and reasonable and appropriately optimistic estimates used to maintain morale.

To encourage the athlete's participation he can be involved in planning the treatment schedules and setting the goals along the route to complete recovery. If an athlete sees the relationship between a procedure and the eventual return of function and ability to compete, his motivation to follow treatment can increase. Setting goals and measuring improvement also helps convince the athlete that the injury has in fact been repaired and can be trusted when he returns to play. An athlete can lose confidence in his ability to perform at previous levels even when the injury is 100% rehabilitated. Treatment should not only mend the body but teach the athlete to believe in his ability once more.

With prolonged recovery, social status and rewards often dramatically decrease. Friendships based upon team membership become threatened. Efforts should be made to keep players part of the team either with light workouts or suggestions to coaches that a player could assist with coaching or managerial tasks. Maintaining a team association can keep the motivation to return to play from fading.

Athletic Training, Conditioning and Reconditioning

Athletes with superior training and conditioning are stronger, better coordinated and less subject to injury. The improvement in the conditioning of the athlete is the factor most responsible for recent assaults on the record books. Maximum physical and mental fitness requires training of the whole body, including every tissue and cell. This helps the athlete better enjoy the event, prevents injuries and speeds recovery following injuries.

Athletic training and conditioning can be broken down into three basic components: (1) the development of muscle strength, power and endurance; (2) joint flexibility; and (3) cardiovascular endurance. All three components are necessary in a training program to maximize safe athletic performance.

The cornerstone of athletic training is the law of specificity, or the SAID principle, which states that the body makes specific adaptation to imposed demands. The more specific the demands, the more specific the adaptation. Athletic training, therefore, should be as specific as possible to the given sport.

Efficiencies in the lungs, heart and muscles are different in untrained individuals than in highly trained individuals. The difference in VO_2 max (maximal oxygen consumption) of the lungs is near 100%. The difference in Q max (normal cardiac output) of the heart is also near 100%, while the difference in the oxidative efficiency of muscles from untrained to highly trained individuals is near 400%. This is directly related to differences in mitochondrial density of the individual muscle fibers, and supports the concept that athletic train-

ing occurs at the cellular level. It may be inferred that training muscle groups in sport-specific patterns has the greatest carry-over in training, next to the athletic activity itself.

MUSCLE STRENGTH, POWER AND ENDURANCE

The Nature of Muscles

The basic unit of structure and function in skeletal muscle is the sarcomere, which is composed of the contractile proteins actin and myosin. When a muscle contracts (shortens), a series of events result in the interaction of the actin and myosin filaments. The interaction causes the actin filaments to slide over the myosin filaments, shortening the muscle fiber. This shortening process produces the force or tension of muscle contraction. The force of contraction is transmitted to the bones to which the muscles are attached by the muscle tendons (Fig. 14:1).

The immediate source of energy for muscle contraction is ATP–adenosine triphosphate. ATP is synthesized by anaerobic or aerobic metabolic processes (see Fig. 14:1). Anaerobic energy production does not require oxygen, whereas aerobic energy production requires oxygen. Muscle strength training is an anaerobic activity. A brief description of these processes follows.

Anaerobic Systems

ATP-PC System: phosphocreatine (PC) stored in the muscle is broken down into in-

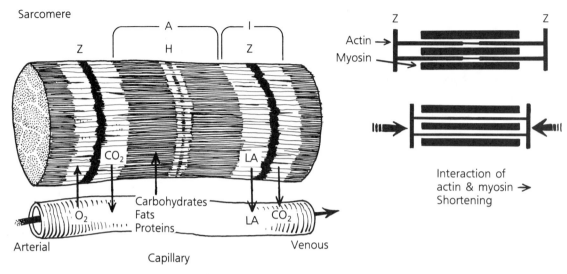

ATP   ADP + Pi + energy for muscle contraction.
Anaerobic processes
    PC   Pi + C + energy to resynthesize ATP
    Glycogen   Lactic Acid + energy to resynthesize ATP
Aerobic process
    Carbohydrates, Fats, Proteins + O_2 CO_2 + H_2O + energy to resynthesize ATP

FIGURE 14:1 A skeletal muscle cell, tissue capillary and the energy systems that supply adenosine triphosphate (ATP) for muscle contraction

organic phosphorus and creatine, releasing energy to synthesize ATP; allows work for up to 10 seconds.

Lactic Acid System: glycogen and glucose are broken down incompletely into lactic acid, releasing energy to synthesize ATP; lactic acid accumulation in the muscle leads to fatigue; allows work for 10 seconds to 3 minutes.

Aerobic System

Oxygen System: carbohydrates, fats and proteins can be completely broken down with oxygen producing carbon dioxide, water and energy to synthesize ATP. This process occurs in the mitochrondria of the muscle cell. Allows work for hours.

Diet and Nutrition

Ultimately, the fuel for the energy systems comes from the food eaten. A balanced diet from the four basic food groups plus water provides the proper nutrition and calories for an athlete involved in strength training. The four basic food groups are:

1. Milk and cheese
2. Meat (veal, pork, beef, lamb), poultry, fish and eggs
3. Bread and cereals
4. Vegetables and fruits

An athlete requires 1 gm of protein per kilogram of body weight. The caloric requirement for an athlete in strength training is between 3,000 and 6,000 calories per day. The recommended percentages of these calories for the three types of foods are protein, 10% to 15%; fats, 25% to 30%; and carbohydrates, 55% to 60%.

Muscle Control

Skeletal muscle is voluntary muscle under the control of the nervous system, and is, therefore, properly termed the neuromuscular system. The basic unit of structure and function in the neuromuscular system is the motor unit. A motor unit is the nerve and all of the muscle fibers it innervates. During different intensities of muscle contraction, the nervous system recruits muscle fibers and fires them at frequencies to perform the desired movement.

Muscle Fiber Types

Of the several muscle fiber types identified, the two major types are type I, fast-twitch fibers, and type II, slow-twitch fibers. (Type I and type II muscle fibers are discussed in more detail in Chapter 16.) The fast-twitch muscle fibers are adapted to function for power/strength activities. Slow-twitch fibers are adapted for endurance activities. Man has mixed muscles; i.e., both fiber types are present in muscles in different proportions as determined genetically. Hence, some individuals are predisposed to be better power athletes, i.e., have more fast-twitch fibers, while others are predisposed to be better endurance athletes, since they have more slow-twitch fibers. Training programs can be designed to develop the slow- or fast-twitch fibers.

Principles of Muscle Training

Thousands of years ago, Milo of Croton began his daily routine of lifting a baby bull until it was full grown and, to the present day, this basic principle of resistance training remains: ''progressive resistance exercise and overload principle.'' This principle is applied in many ways that make up the myriad of today's training programs.

Basic to all of these programs are specificity, intensity, duration and frequency. Specificity refers to developing strength and endurance in the specific muscles exercised. The athlete's movement must be analyzed to identify the muscles involved and to design a muscle training program to specifically develop those muscles. Intensity refers to the degree of resistance offered to the muscles, i.e., 80% of the maximum poundage that can be lifted in the bench press. The closer to maximum, the higher the intensity. The duration is the time necessary to complete the desired exercise. Frequency is the number of workouts carried out per unit of time, i.e., how many workouts per week. The terminology of resistance training is defined below.

1. *Repetition (reps):* performing the particular exercise, e.g., raising and lowering the weight in the bicep curl, is one repetition.
2. *Set:* the grouping of a specific exercise into a number of repetitions; for example ten repetitions of the bicep curl is one set of this exercise, written 1×10.
3. *Resistance:* the opposing force to muscle contraction, offered in many ways—a bag of sand, free-weight barbell or Nautilus machine.
4. *One-repetition maximum (1 RM):* the maximum resistance that can be moved in one time through a full range of motion.
5. *Movement time:* the time it takes to complete one repetition; slower movement is recommended, especially when the muscles are working with gravity.
6. *Relief time:* the time interval between sets and exercises.
7. *Exercise order:* larger muscles should be exercised first (back, legs, chest) and smaller muscles last (bicep, tricep, abdominal).

Muscle Training Prescription

Muscle strength, power and endurance development should begin at least six to eight weeks prior to the competitive season. A maintenance program one day per week throughout the season maintains the gains made preseason.

Strength, power and endurance in muscle groups specific to the sport are developed by using the methods described under reconditioning later in this chapter. The same exercise regime of exercising every other day with one exhaustive workout per week can be adhered to.

Muscle training programs can be designed to develop muscle strength, muscle power and/or muscle endurance, as defined here. Muscle strength is the force or tension that a muscle or muscle group can exert against a resistance, and is usually measured by a 1 RM. Muscle power is the speed of movement or the rate at which a resistance can be moved per unit of time, i.e., the rate of doing work. Muscle endurance refers to repetitive muscle contractions carried out over time without undue fatigue.

In general, strength and power training uses a high resistance and low repetitions. Muscle endurance training programs use low resistance and high repetitions. An example of a strength program for the bench press is:

Exercise: Bench Press
Sets: 3   Resistance: 80%–85% of 1 RM
Reps: 6   Rest Interval: 50–90 seconds

The number of repetitions is based on the percent 1 RM employed.

Percent 1 RM	No. Reps/Set
90–95	1–2
85–90	3–4
80–85	4–6
75–80	6–8
70–75	8–10
65–70	10–12

An example of a program designed for muscle endurance for the bench press is:

Exercise: Bench Press
Sets: 3   Resistance: 65%–70% of 1 RM
Reps: 10–15   Rest Interval: 40–70 seconds

A question often asked is, "When should I add more weight?" In a strength or endurance program, when the prescribed number of repetitions is performed with ease, an increment of weight is added that forces the muscle(s) to fail on the last few reps. When the muscles adapt to the new weight, more weight is added. This is the progressive overload principle.

Rest and recovery time should be included in a muscle training program. Recovery time allows the muscles to build strength. Staleness and retrogression occur when proper recovery time is not allowed. Do not overtrain!

Tables 14.1, 14.2 and 14.3 are muscle conditioning programs designed for free weights, Universal Gym and Nautilus. Note that many strength training experts advocate a free weight program or a combination free weight and machine program.

The free weight program can be combined with the following exercises:

Nautilus	*Universal*
Leg extension	Knee extension
Leg curl	Knee curl
Hip abduction	
Hip adduction	

Periodization of Muscle Training

Periodization of training refers to the different types of muscle training that should be employed during the different phases of the training year.

Muscle Response to Training

Skeletal muscle tissue responds to the stimulus of training by increasing in cross sectional size (hypertrophy) and strength, representing an increase in tension-developing tissue. Hence, the muscle can exert more force. Recent research suggests that the number of muscle cells may also increase (hyperplasia), but this is controversial and must await further research. Muscle tendons and joint ligaments also respond to resistance training by becoming thicker and stronger.

Muscle Training in Youth

Adolescent athletes should not lift heavy weights. The weight to be lifted should be a percentage of body weight, or a percentage of the estimated 1 RM. In either case, 12 to 16 repetitions in three sets should be performed. At the completion of puberty, heavier resistances with a lower number of reps may be used.

TABLE 14:1.   A Free Weight Program for Muscle Strength and Endurance

Exercise	Body Part	Weight, % 1 RM	Sets	Reps
Half squat	Thighs, hips	70	3	10–15
Heel raise	Calf	70	3	10–15
Lunge	Thighs, hips	(10–30 lbs)	3	15–20
Bench press	Chest, upper arm	70	3	10–15
Overhead press	Shoulder, upper arm	70	3	10–15
Good morning	Back	(30–75 lbs)	3	10–15
Bent over row	Upper back	70	3	10–15
Bicep curl	Arm, forearm	70	3	10–15
Tricep extension	Arm, forearm	70	3	10–15
Bent knee sit-ups	Abdominals	(5–25 lbs)	3	10–15
Trunk twists	Trunk	(10–25 lbs)	3	10–15

Note: The exercises should be performed in the order given above. The time interval between sets should be 60 to 70 seconds. Perform all three sets of each exercise before proceeding to the next. The total workout time is approximately 70 minutes. The rest between exercises should be no more than 70 to 80 seconds.

TABLE 14:2.   A Universal Gym Program for Muscle Strength and Endurance

Exercise	Body Part	Weight, % 1 RM	Sets	Reps
Leg press	Thighs, hips	70	3	10–15
Knee extension	Thighs	70	3	10–15
Knee curl	Hamstrings	(10–30 lbs)	3	10–15
Bench press	Chest, arms	70	3	10–15
Overhead press	Shoulder, arms	70	3	10–15
Back hyperextension	Back	(0–15 lbs)	3	10–15
Bicep curl	Arm, forearm	70	3	10–15
Tricep extension	Arm, forearm	70	3	10–15
Lat pull-down	Back, lats	70	3	10–15
Bent knee sit-ups	Abdominals	(5–25 lbs)	3	10–15
Trunk twists	Trunk	(10–15 lbs)	3	10–15

Note: Follow the same instructions as for the free weight program.

Muscle Training in Women

Women are encouraged to participate in resistance training. It will not result in bulky muscles. The lower level of the hormone testosterone in women prevents excessive hypertrophy of muscles.

FLEXIBILITY

Most often a particular sport involves short, intensive movements about the joints within a small part of the full range of motion. If not fully stretched, the muscles involved progressively tighten, limiting active range of motion. Abnormally tight muscles can alter form, thus reducing biomechanical efficiency and creating a climate for athletic injuries, such as muscle strains, chronic muscle fatigue and tendonitis. The population in general falls along a continuum of tightness versus looseness with small segments of the population either loose or tight but the bulk somewhere in between.

TABLE 14:3.   A Nautilus Program for Muscle Strength and Endurance

Exercise	Body Part	Weight	Sets	Reps
Hip and back	Hips, lower back	plates*	3	10–15
Leg extension	Thigh	''	3	10–15
Leg press	Hips, thighs	''	3	10–15
Leg curl	Hamstrings	''	3	10–15
Hip abduction	Gluteus medius	''	3	10–15
Hip adduction	Adductor magnus	''	3	10–15
Lateral raise	Shoulder	''	3	10–15
Seated press	Shoulder, upper arm	''	3	10–15
Decline press	Chest, shoulder	''	3	10–15
Bicep curl	Arm, forearm	''	3	10–15
Tricep curl	Arm, forearm	''	3	10–15
Abdominal curls	Abdominals	''	3	10–15

*The proper plate allows completion of three sets of 10 to 15 repetitions for the first three weeks. The second three weeks, select a plate that allows completion of three sets of six repetitions.

A few simple tests determine where an athlete falls on the spectrum of muscle tightness. The sit and reach test indicates low back and hamstring tightness (Fig. 14:2). The athlete places his feet on the box at right angles and reaches his finger tips over the ruler. The measurement is read in inches either + or −, depending upon the tightness found. Most athletes should strive to achieve either 0 or +

scores. Minus scores indicate muscle tightness, and that particular athlete may have to work harder than average on joint flexibility.

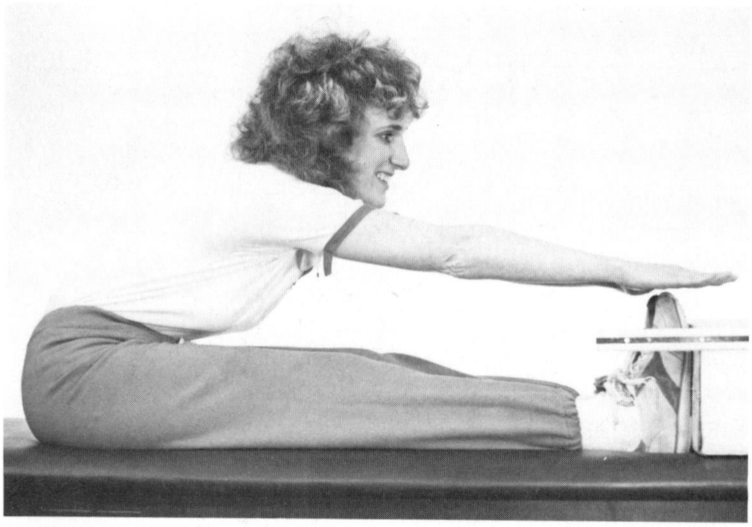

A test of upper extremity flexibility at the shoulder is conducted with the athlete standing with arms flexed at 90°, elbows fully extended (Fig. 14:3). The athlete externally rotates his arms as far as possible. Those who can rotate their palms beyond horizontal, making the hypothenar eminence higher than the thenar eminence, are considered loose.

A simple goniometric test of active dorsiflexion at the ankle can assess tightness and its possible relation to present and future athletic conditions. Athletes should be able to achieve at least +15 of active dorsiflexion to be a guard against athletic injury.

To test hip flexor tightness the athlete lies supine and pulls one knee completely to the chest with both arms while extending the opposite leg onto the floor or table (Fig. 14:4). Athletes should be able to extend the leg fully. The degrees of hip flexion of the extended leg indicate iliopsoas tightness on the same side. The test is reversed for the opposite hip.

All of these tests should be used to determine tightness or looseness for individual athletes. Retesting shows progress after initiating a flexibility program. Stretching exercises

FIGURE 14:2.   The sit and reach test indicates low back and hamstring tightness.

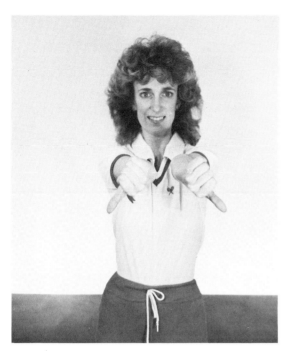

FIGURE 14:3. Test of upper extremity flexibility at the shoulder indicating looseness.

should be conducted after the athlete is warmed to a mild perspiration level. Environmental temperatures determine the amount and intensity of effort required. Stretching exercises are most effective when active muscle contraction is the prime mover into the end point. This aids reflex relaxation of the antagonist muscles. Passive stretching should be done slowly to inhibit the protective stretch response of the muscle. The effectiveness of the stretch depends upon the tension and time of stretch. When in doubt, less tension and more time is best—one to two minutes for each muscle group in 15-second intervals. The flexibility exercises illustrated here are basic to most running sports.

Flexibility Exercises

The objectives of these exercises are to increase the range of the athlete's motion, and to reduce the potential of injuries. This program is designed to increase the range of motion gradually. Each exercise should be taken to the point of tightness and slightly beyond. For safety purposes, work on proper form and *do not* force any motion. All exercises are to be held for three to five seconds and performed only once. The entire program should take no longer than ten minutes, once learned. Count "1,001, 1,002, 1,003, 1,004, 1,005 . . ."

Seat Straddle Lotus Seated position; place soles of feet together and drop knees toward floor. Place forearms on inside of knees and push knees to ground. Lean forward, bringing chin to feet.

Seat Side Straddle Sit with legs spread; place *both* hands on same ankle. Bring chin to knee, keeping leg straight. *Hold.* Perform exercise on opposite leg.

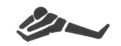

Seat Forward Straddle Sit with legs spread; place *one* hand on *each* ankle. Lean forward, bringing chest to ground. *Hold.*

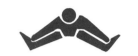

Seat Stretch Sit with legs together, feet flexed, hands on ankles. Bring chin to knees. *Hold.*

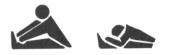

Leg Stretch Seated position; keep legs straight with hands on backs of calves. Lift and pull each leg individually to ear. *Hold.*

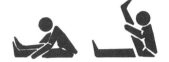

Leg Cross-Over Lie on back, legs spread and arms *out* to the side. Bring R toe to L hand, keeping leg straight. *Hold.* Repeat, with L toe to R hand.

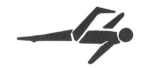

Lying Quad Stretch Lie on back with one leg straight, the other with hip in internal rotation, knee in flexion. Press knee to floor. *Hold.*

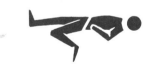

Back Bridge Lie on back; place hands behind head with palms on the ground. Push up, so the back arches and arms and legs are extended. *Hold.* Repeat.

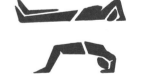

Knees to Chest Lie on back with knees bent. Grasp tops of both knees and bring them out toward the armpits, rocking gently. Repeat.

Forward Lunges Kneel on L leg; R leg forward at a right angle. Lunge forward, keeping the back straight. Stretch should be felt on the L groin. *Hold.* Repeat on opposite leg.

Side Lunges Stand with legs apart; bend the L knee and lean toward the L, keeping the back straight and the R leg straight. Repeat on opposite leg.

Cross-Over Stand with legs crossed; keep feet close together and legs straight. Touch toes. *Hold.* Repeat with opposite leg.

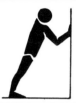

Heel Cord Stretch Stand 3 feet from wall, with feet pointed straight ahead. Drop hips to wall. Heels should not come off floor. *Hold.*

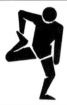

Standing Quad Stretch Stand supported. Pull foot to buttocks as shown. *Hold.*

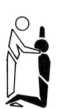

Shoulder Stretch Kneel/sit with arms extended overhead. Partner stands behind and grasps the athlete's arm, between the shoulder with elbow and stretches it backward. The athlete pulls forward, while the partner resists, for three to five seconds. Relax, while partner stretches the arm backward again. Repeat with opposite arm.

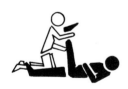

Hamstring Stretch Lie on back. Partner brings leg up *only* to the point of tightness and resists while the athlete pushes downward. Relax while partner pushes leg farther until tightness is felt again. Repeat with opposite leg.

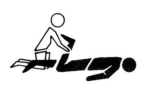

Quad Stretch Lie on stomach. Partner grasps lower leg and bends it until stretch is felt on the front of the thigh. The partner holds the leg while the athlete pushes against the partner for three to five seconds. Relax while the partner bends the leg again until another stretch is felt. Repeat with opposite leg.

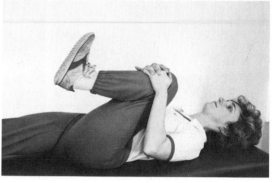

FIGURE 14:4. Test of hip flexor and iliopsoas tightness.

CARDIOVASCULAR ENDURANCE

Cardiovascular endurance determines the ability of the heart to perform work and to maintain efficiency for long periods. Knowing how a person endures a given workload documents physical fitness. This endurance is a measure of fitness. The ability of athletes to reach a high level of performance depends on their maximum oxygen consumption. Strength, power, speed, agility, coordination and body composition are also important. Moreover, physical fitness is specific to a sport. The most important aspect in the truly physically fit, however, is cardiovascular endurance, measured by the difference between the minimum aerobic requirement and the maximum aerobic capacity.

Everyone has the same minimum aerobic requirements, that is, about 3 cc per kilogram per minute. However, maximum aerobic capacity, the index of the ability to work, varies. Since maximum oxygen consumption reflects the capacity of the heart and lungs to take up and deliver oxygen to the tissues and the tissues to process oxygen, consumption also reflects the effectiveness of all the components of the oxygen transport system. Maximum aerobic capacity is a reasonably accurate prediction of performance with exercise. In order to improve the oxygen consumption and develop cardiovascular endurance, aerobic exercises are important. Aerobic exercise implies continuous movement with minimal resistance, that is, dynamically moving the muscle mass to stimulate the heart, lungs and oxygen-carrying capabilities. Cross-country skiing, running, cycling and walking are aerobic exercises because the muscle mass is continuously moved with minimal resistance.

The comparable benefits of the various aerobic activities have been evaluated. Running 1 mile in eight minutes has an aerobic training effect comparable to swimming for 15 minutes, cycling for 5 miles or 20 minutes or playing tennis or racquet ball for 35 minutes. Paddle games take longer because this involves intermittent activity with brief spurts of high intensity. Running is the most efficient way to develop physical fitness, which accounts for its great popularity today.

With the development of physical fitness, the cardiac output increases from 5.8 to 6.6 liters per minute, and the resting stroke volume increases (the amount of blood coming out of the heart with each beat; about 70 cc in the untrained person and about 103 cc in the conditioned aerobic athlete). With the more efficient emptying of the heart, fewer beats are required and the resting heart rate is reduced. This is an index of the cardiac efficiency. Moreover, the blood volume and hemoglobin increases, contributing to the oxygen-carrying capacity of the blood. The maximum cardiac output will increase about 5 liters per minute. With exercise the heart rate of the untrained person increases more than that of the trained athlete, and the recovery period is much longer.

With the development of exercise physiology in the last ten years, scientifically designed exercise prescriptions allow predictable improvement in an individual's oxygen consumption. Prescribed exercise combines the frequency of participation, the intensity and duration of participation and the rate of progression. The individual performs an aerobic activity three to five times a week. The added improvement by training six to seven times a week is not significantly greater than that achieved in five days so is probably not worth the extra effort. This fits into another principle of balancing exercise with rest. Table 14:4 presents a basic aerobic training program.

Duration of the activity is important. In order to get a training effect from aerobic activity, at least 20 to 30 minutes and, if possible, up to 60 minutes of continuous activity is

TABLE 14:4. An Aerobic Program Designed to Improve Cardiovascular Fitness

RUNNING PROGRAM	First Three Weeks*	
	Time (Min)	*Miles*
Tuesday	14–20	2
Thursday	14–20	2
Saturday	14–20	2
	Second Three Weeks	
	Time (Min)	*Miles*
Tuesday	21–30	3
Thursday	21–30	3
Saturday	21–30	3
CYCLING PROGRAM	First Three Weeks*	
	Time (Min)	*Miles*
Tuesday	28–40	7
Thursday	28–40	7
Saturday	28–40	7
	Second Three Weeks	
	Time (Min)	*Miles*
Tuesday	36–54	9
Thursday	36–54	9
Saturday	36–54	9

*Assumes resistance training is performed Monday, Wednesday and Friday.

Note: Conditioning is a progressive program that begins at a low to moderate level and progresses to a higher level. Begin at the beginning! Athletes who start at the end of the program risk injury.

required. Moreover, the intensity of the activity should increase cardiac work to 70% to 85% of the individual's maximum heart rate, which is equivalent to the training heart rate. The formula for calculating maximum heart rate is 220 minus the individual's age, multiplied by 70% to 85%, depending on the percentage of heart rate maximum desired. Thus, a 20-year-old should exercise to a heart rate of 140 three to five times a week for 20 to 30 and preferably 60 minutes, if possible, in a continuous movement. This undoubtedly results in improved oxygen consumption.

Research showed that the untrained Swedish man has an oxygen consumption of about 42 ml per kilogram per minute. However, the cross-country skier demonstrated the highest level of oxygen consumption—about 80 ml per kilogram per minute.

While a number of sophisticated metabolic tests can measure oxygen consumption, several field tests correlate very well with them. For example, maximum oxygen consumption correlates with the 12-minute run test. As applied to the athlete, he should be able to cover about 1.5 miles in 12 minutes—an oxygen consumption of about 42 ml per kilogram per minute. If athletes can run 2 miles in 12 minutes, oxygen consumption is approximately 60 ml per kilogram per minute, and one should have a superbly trained team. On the other hand, a team that can run only 1.2 miles in 12 minutes has an average oxygen consumption of 32, and is in deep trouble from the conditioning standpoint.

Therefore athletes should start an aerobic program two or three months before the opening of the season. Testing athletes on opening day will hopefully show they can cover at least 1¾ miles in 12 minutes and so are in superb condition. Most good college athletes can run 1.5 miles in about 8.15 minutes, where a world class athlete can often cover 1.5 miles in less than 7 minutes.

The aerobic program should be performed three days per week, preferably not on the days of resistance training. A program of running and cycling is recommended (see Table 14:4). Select one activity or use both activities on alternate weeks (cross-training).

In summary, conditioning programs should include a variety of activities—isometric, isotonic (discussed under reconditioning later in this chapter) and aerobic. If nothing is *invested,* nothing will be *gained!* Aerobic conditioning should be a firm base for these other activities. Benefits of endurance are fewer injuries and much less fatigue. As Coach Lombardi said, "Fatigue makes cowards of us all."

RECONDITIONING PROCEDURES

Those involved in the care of the athlete must understand athletics and appreciate the value that today's athlete places upon participation. Keeping this in mind during treatment will pay back dividends many times over by securing the athlete's fullest confidence and cooperation.

The athlete is most often young, highly motivated and in superior physical condition. When injury strikes, this abundance of energy should be channeled into a strict treatment regimen that has the greatest chance of producing a 100% recovery in the shortest time.

Management of Acute Injury

Reconditioning any injury begins with intensive first aid measures to minimize the aftereffects of trauma, which in many cases cause more discomfort than the injury itself. Joint effusion and uncontrolled bleeding into fascial planes are often the rule following second-degree sprains.

The body reacts to all acute injuries in a predictable fashion, with pain, erythema, warmth, swelling and loss of function. These are the means by which the body initiates repair. The severity of the signs directly relates to the severity of injury and the amount of tissue damage. When the insult is severe, the athlete will have a hot, swollen injury with intense pain and total disability. This overreaction or uncontrolled inflammatory response often causes secondary tissue damage that greatly lengthens recovery time. The inflammatory response can be controlled by applying aggressive first aid in the form of cold, compression, elevating the injury above the level of the heart and protecting it with a soft splint, cast or crutches.

Principles of Reconditioning

Reconditioning of athletic injuries means regaining the previous level of training. Specifically, it includes:

1. Regaining former athletic flexibility (which may be greater than normal) of the surrounding joints
2. Regaining muscle strength, power and endurance of the surrounding muscles

3. Regaining prior functional athletic ability including cardiorespiratory endurance

Reconditioning is most accurate when preseason screening exams provide meaningful data with which to judge whether an athlete has achieved his prior level of training. The preseason screening exam also helps to prevent injury or reinjury by identifying muscle weakness, muscle tightness, abnormal joint laxity or prior injury. Exams should be conducted a half to a full season ahead of anticipated sports participation to allow time for rehabilitation if necessary. Rescreening should be scheduled for those athletes involved in rehabilitation just prior to the sport season.

The screening exam may include:

1. Name
2. Date
3. Height
4. Weight
5. Percent fat
6. Complete athletic injury history by interview
7. Grip strength
8. Flexibility across major joints (sit and reach for low back and hamstring)
9. 1.5 mile run time
10. 40 yard dash time
11. Sport-specific agility course time
12. Leg length: proximal tip of anterior superior iliac spine to distal tip of medial malleolus
13. Thigh girth: 3 inches proximal to the patella
14. Posture check
15. Joint laxity check
16. Strength test of right and left quadriceps and hamstrings
    a. Isokinetic dynamometer analysis
    b. 1 and 10 RM using weights attached to iron shoe or table arm (such as Universal Gym or N-K table)
17. Log hoppers in 60 seconds
18. Other sport-specific tests as deemed necessary by coaches and medical personnel

Flexibility in Reconditioning

When an injury or weakness is documented, regaining normal athletic flexibility is the first area of concern during reconditioning. Cryo, contrast and thermotherapy early in the reconditioning program can be used to control the body's sometimes exaggerated response to acute injury. The inflammatory response is not a bad sign, per se, but indicates that the body is in the active process of repair. Immobilization is an important initial first aid measure to control this response and prevent further tissue damage. The greater the extent of injury and the longer the immobilization, the greater the demand upon the mobilization process during recovery. Active assistive exercise performed under cold water is the first step toward regaining full, pain-free strength and motion. The introduction of active exercise is an important milestone for the athlete in the return of joint flexibility and muscle strength. A careful monitoring of reported pain guards against trying to reach this goal too soon, which may cause the inflammatory response to flare up.

Therefore, the athlete should always move within the limits of pain. As assisted exercise increases, the athlete may start to exercise actively out of water and may progress to a heel-toe crutch gait, with partial weight bearing as in, for example, first-degree ankle sprain. The amount of progressive stretching and mobilization techniques is a function of the primary tissue damage and the resulting time needed for tissue repair. Mild injuries often require only active exercise to regain normal range of motion. Daily measurement with a goniometer quickly documents the stubborn knee or shoulder. The ability to regain a full range of motion varies among athletes, and is not solely a result of the time of immobilization and the severity of injury.

Passive exercise is used when the inflammatory response is under control and the athlete is ready to regain the remaining loss of motion. Progressive stretching uses the knowledge of functional anatomy and time vs. tension relationships to elongate the contractile and noncontractile tissue. Pushing to an end point actively under his own control is the safest, most effective means of achieving a normal range of motion. When necessary, passive stretching to the point of discomfort may be necessary to achieve this goal. A rule of thumb is that the discomfort should almost completely subside within five minutes after the stretching exercise. When muscle spasm of the antagonist is responsible for limiting motion of the agonist, the technique of contract-relax can reflexively relax muscle tightness. Traction along the long axis of a limb, dorsal and ventral glide, and rotation may help to increase active motion about joints by increasing passive motion that is normal and necessary in all joints.

Muscle Strength, Power and Endurance

Muscle strength, power and endurance development is the second area of concern in reconditioning athletic injuries. Muscle tissue has the unique ability to produce tension when stimulated. Muscle tissue can produce tension under three sets of circumstances. When a muscle produces tension equal to the external resistance of the musculoskeletal system, the lack of movement is termed isometric contraction. When a muscle produces tension greater than the external resistance of the musculoskeletal system, the shortening movement is termed a concentric contraction (Fig. 14:5). When a muscle produces tension less than the external resistance of the musculoskeletal system, the lengthening movement is termed an eccentric contraction (Fig. 14:6).

The ability of muscle tissue to produce tension or force is termed strength. The tension developed is related to the speed of contraction attempted by the muscle. The greater the speed of contraction, the less muscle tissue is recruited to produce tension. When injury strikes, pain inhibits the ability of muscle tissue to produce tension at all speeds, which is mainly responsible for the early loss of strength and functional movement—the body's own immobilization device. The weakness that follows injury is directly related to the time of immobilization required for tissue repair. Muscle strength continues to decrease until pain and inflammation subside enough to allow the involved muscles to produce a relatively pain-free contraction. Muscle endurance is the product of muscle tension and movement, the ability of muscle tissue to perform work.

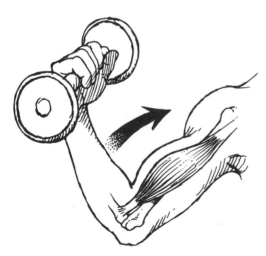

FIGURE 14:5. In concentric contraction muscle shortens against resistance.

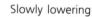

Slowly lowering

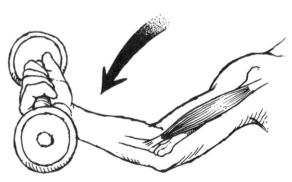

FIGURE 14:6. In eccentric contraction muscle lengthens against resistance.

$$[W = F \times D]$$

Muscle tissue can perform work by a concentric contraction or be worked upon by an external force through an eccentric contraction. Muscle power is the intensity or rate at which muscles are able to perform work.

$$[P = F \times D]$$

Muscle endurance and power both depend upon strength and therefore also decline as a result of injury and immobilization. Too often the parameter that keeps the injured player from attaining full recovery is not the lack of strength or endurance but the lack of power. Power work cannot be attempted until inflammation has almost completely subsided. Reconditioning is concerned with keeping the time from injury to the first tension development at a safe minimum. This muscle ''down time'' may be as short as one day as in the case of isometric contractions being performed in a cylindrical cast following knee injury, or many weeks as in the case of shoulder immobilization following dislocation. Once pain-free active motion is possible throughout most of the range of motion, the athlete is ready for one or more of the active resistive types of exercise, all of which have their advantages and disadvantages.

Resistive Exercises

Table 14:5 lists the similarities and differences among the four basic types of resistive exercise.

Isometric Exercise

An advantage of isometric exercises is that they can be prescribed for conditions requiring immobilization, as in a cylindrical cast applied for certain knee injuries. Substantial strength gains can occur up to $\pm 7°$ from the exercised point on the range of motion with isometric exercise (Fig. 14:7).

Isometric exercise can also be prescribed when points on the range of motion are painful. Tension can be developed at a variety of points, staying clear of the painful ranges. When inflammation is present, this procedure can produce major strength gains, while keeping joint irritation to a minimum. An example is isometric exercise of the knee extensors at 30°, 15° and 0° of extension with chondromalacia patellae.

For maximum safe strength gains, isometric exercise can be performed each day up to 90% tension development, holding six seconds and repeating three to five times per point on the arc of motion. Isometric strength can be subjectively measured by comparing force production of the injured limb to the noninjured limb. Place the athlete's body and limbs in the same position right to left and ask the athlete to produce a maximum, pain-free contraction against the examiner's hand. A cable tension dynamometer as shown in Figure 14:7 can objectively measure strength read in pounds of tension or foot pounds of torque. A disadvantage of isometric exercise is that without movement no external work is performed and therefore little muscular endurance develops.

Isotonic Exercise

Isotonic exercise is the performing of either a concentric or eccentric contraction with a fixed external resistance. An example is lifting and lowering a 10-pound bar bell.

Scientific isotonic regimes date back to the 1940s and Thomas DeLorme. His recommended program of progressive resistance exercise (PRE) is based upon the 10 resistance maximum (10 RM). The 10 RM is the maximum amount of weight a person can successfully lift ten times. His program recommends lifting three sets of ten repetitions, starting with one half the 10 RM, which is one half the 10 RM weight. The individual then progresses to three quarters of the 10 RM and finally to 100% of the 10 RM. This method has been used suc-

TABLE 14:5. Four Types of Resistive Exercise

Exercise	Resistance	Muscle Contraction Possible	Speed Control	Musculoskeletal Loading Possible (%)	Examples	Advantages	Disadvantages
Isotonic	Constant	Concentric Eccentric	No	Less than 100	N.K. table; pulleys; free weights; calisthenics	Inexpensive; easy to exercise most muscle groups	Slow speed only; is likely to cause irritation at inflamed points of range of motion
Variable resistance	Variable, depends upon equipment pattern	Concentric Eccentric	No	Less than 100	Nautilus; Universal; Lifeline Gym, etc. manual resistive exercise	Standardization; excellent for slow speed strength gains	Can be expensive; requires a knowledgeable partner in manual resistance exercise; is likely to cause irritation at inflamed points of range of motion
Isometric	Accommodating to the force applied	None; tension development only	Yes, 0°/sec	100 at one fixed point of exercised range of motion	The application of muscular force to any fixed point	Easily performed; least irritation to inflamed points of range of motion	Little muscular endurance developed
Isokinetic	Accommodating to the force applied	Concentric	Yes, range and accuracy depends upon equipment	100 at all points of exercised range of motion	Cybex II; Orthotron; Mini Gym; Hydra Gym; underwater exercise	Inexpensive when swimming pool is available; wide range of exercise speeds available; 100% musculoskeletal loading; extensive biomechanical information available from read out	Can be expensive; concentric contractions only

cessfully incorporating an infinite number of variations. Research indicates that the more repetitions, the greater the work performed, and the greater endurance development; the more weight lifted, the greater the strength development.

Studies also indicate that, with enough repetitions, there is selective fatiguing of individual motor units, which can cause a substantial increase in muscle strength. This is important when designing strength training programs for muscles around damaged joints. In these cases it may be more effective to use less weight and more repetition to minimize joint irritation. A disadvantage of isotonic exercise is that the musculoskeletal system can be effectively loaded only at slow speeds. When the speed of exercise is increased, the effective load on the muscle is reduced proportionately by acceleration at the end of the range of motion (Fig. 14:8).

For maximum strength gains, isotonic exercise can be performed every other day with only one intensive workout per week. An intensive workout involves increasing the weight and repetitions to full muscle fatigue, and is not recommended early in the rehabilitation program or in the presence of muscle or joint irritation. Isotonic strength can be objectively measured by comparing right-left resistance maximums.

Variable Resistance

Variable resistance exercise is performed on specially designed machines, or with sports medicine personnel providing manual re-

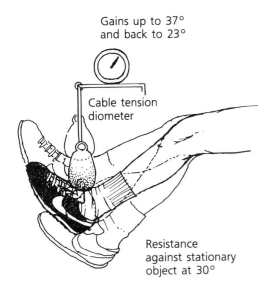

FIGURE 14:7. Isometric exercise can produce strength gains up to ±7° from the exercised point.

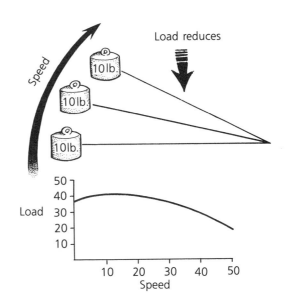

FIGURE 14:8. Effect of increased speed on muscle load with acceleration at end of range of motion

sistance. The machines, such as the Nautilus, produce inherent mechanical changes during an arc of motion to coincide with the skeletal lever changes of human motion. The resistance increases as the mechanical advantage of the body increases. The pattern variation of each machine is constant and does not depend on the length of the skeletal levers of the athletes using them.

Advantages of the Nautilus system are full range of motion exercise; the ability to exercise eccentrically, specific to many sport movement patterns; and standardizing exercise and evaluation of strength gains. A disadvantage of the variable resistance exercise is lack of speed control. Acceleration can occur throughout the range of motion, which reduces the external resistance on the muscles required to complete the range of motion. This is a problem in exercising muscles such as the terminal knee extensors when a full arc of motion is employed. Acceleration can be minimized by exercising at slow speeds and by performing partial arc exercise.

Rehabilitating athletes should regain a full arc of motion before using the full motion variable resistance machines to avoid possible reinjury. Manual resistive exercise by a trained person allows exercise to be performed effectively at slow and medium speeds and at the same time lessens resistance at painful or weak ranges of motion. Maximum strength gains can be achieved by exercising every other day with one exhaustive workout per week.

Isokinetic Exercise

Isokinetic exercise is performed on specially designed machines or underwater. The differences between isokinetic machines and underwater exercise are the accuracy of speed control, the mass of the external resistance arm, the internal drag of the energy-absorbing mechanism and the accuracy of recording torque, work and power scores. Speed control is an advantage of isokinetic exercise.

Certain machines such as the Cybex II and Orthotron can perform reciprocal concentric contractions (Fig. 14:9). Speed control allows exercise to be accurately performed at a wide range of speeds. Concentric contractions of both the agonist and the antagonist during exercise allow for reflex relaxation of the muscles

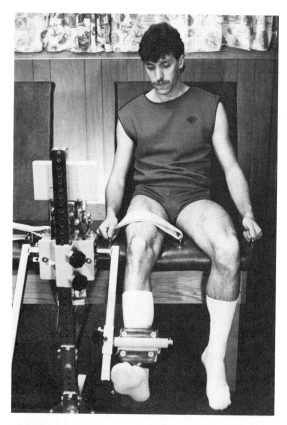

FIGURE 14:9. Lower extremity rehabilitation on Orthotron strengthens quadriceps and hamstrings.

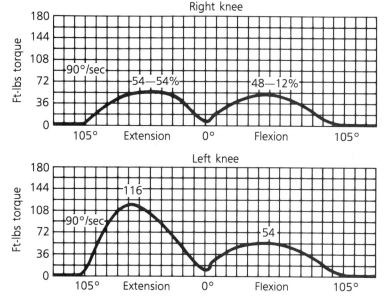

FIGURE 14:10. Cybex printout showing anterior cruciate deficient knee with flat midrange extension pattern

involved, which is especially important in the early phases of an active exercise program since maximum blood flow through the muscles is maintained during exercise. With speed control isokinetic exercise machines accommodate 100% to the tension developed by the muscles. Therefore, 100% loading of the muscles occurs during the entire range of motion, which is especially helpful when there is pain or weakness at one or more points on the range of motion.

An abundance of biomechanical information can be recorded from the Cybex II system, such as torque-motion curves, total work performed and power scores of muscle groups (Fig. 14:10). This information can help detect muscle weakness at specific points in a range of motion. The information can support certain diagnoses, such as flat midrange extension patterns in the anterior cruciate deficient knee, or flat end-range extension patterns in chondromalacia patellae.

Isokinetic exercise equipment is especially helpful in exercising and measuring the power output of muscle groups, the last muscle parameter to be achieved in the rehabilitation process. Isokinetic exercise, however, is not able to perform eccentric contractions, which may be useful in the later stages of training programs for muscle groups required to accept forces eccentrically during the sport activity.

Underwater exercise, although without accurate speed control, tends to dampen acceleration of body parts during the movement pattern, and water absorbs energy. The amount of dampening is related to the surface area of the part moved. Standing in waist deep water and kicking one foot forward and back, rotating at the knee, produces a crude isokinetic movement of approximately 100° per second. When swim fins are attached to the feet, the speed of movement falls according to the surface area of the fins. Underwater exercise can also support injured limbs and the athlete can easily perform partial ranges of motion without stress in weak or painful positions. The temperature of the water can be controlled to either promote circulation or control inflammation of injured tissue. Maximum strength gains can be achieved by exercising every other day with one exhaustive workout per week.

Program of Exercise

When reconditioning an athletic injury, the entire athlete must be reconditioned. The amount of training necessary depends upon the length of down time—the time from injury to return to full competition. Down time need not be equal for all fitness parameters of the body. Whenever possible, the athlete should continue to train and maintain healthy parts of the body while receiving treatment for the injury.

The type of partial training depends upon the site and severity of injury. Underwater exercise in swimming pools is an excellent way to continue cardiorespiratory training while rehabilitating a weight-bearing injury. One-legged stationary bicycle training, flexibility and upper body strength training are also possible with many injuries. Muscles above and below the injury site should be tested for weakness. The muscle strength test, whether it be isotonic, variable resistance, isometric or isokinetic, should be precisely defined and reproducible. Once weakness has been documented, a specific program of exercise can be developed for the weak muscle. During the early stages of active exercise, training can take place every day. As the work load increases to approximately 25% of the noninjured muscle group, the frequency of exercise should be reduced to every other day. The 48 hours between exercise sessions is necessary for cellular adjustments in the muscle tissue, which creates a climate for maximal strength gains. If the injury becomes inflamed again, usually the intensity or frequency of exercise is too great.

Commercially available multistation exercise gyms allow circuit training programs where many athletes can rotate through dif-ferent stations at prescribed intervals (Fig. 14:11). If the intervals are short enough, cardiovascular endurance will also improve.

Functional Activity Progression

In order to insure an orderly and safe return to full competition, a program of functional activities should be developed for each injured athlete. Many of the progressions will be similar, such as those for lower extremity injuries. The progression starts with the initial protection required at injury. The three-point crutch gait is an example as in the case of a sprained ankle. Athletes should realize that early protection of injuries will decrease rehabilitation time. When indicated, the three-point crutch gait, no weight bearing, progresses to three-point crutch gait with soft flat foot and then on to three-point crutch gait with a soft heel-toe strike to promote flexibility and circulation.

Progressions should not continue in the presence of pain. Discomfort should be distinguished from pain. Discomfort with activ-

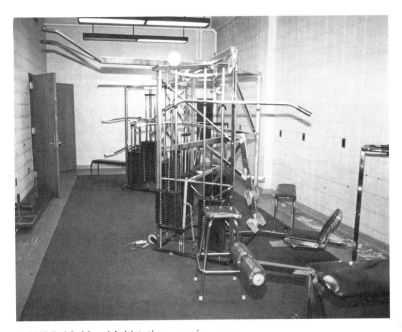

FIGURE 14:11. Multistation exercise gym

ity should not cause facial grimace or gait deviation and should subside within three to five minutes following activity. Although response to injury and pain varies widely, pain is present when the activity is substantially altered from the norm. When able, the athlete progresses to one crutch on the opposite side of injury, then to a cane and finally to walking without a limp.

The athlete performs two-legged and then one-legged heel raisers until he can progress to jumping on two feet and then on one foot. Once the athlete can jump ten times on the injured foot with equal height, no pain or facial grimace and no extra body movements, he is ready for jogging straight. The next progres-

sion is jogging in a figure-of-eight pattern 10 yards long, crossing at 5 yards. When this is accomplished, back pedaling, carioca steps (moving sideways, cross over front, cross over rear), jogging in place with 90° direction changes and sprints are added. Sport-specific activities in a noncompetitive environment are finally added to complete the progression.

Athletes should be aware of the full progression at the beginning of the rehabilitation program to insure their compliance. They should progress only under the direct supervision of the athletic trainer and should be checked each step of the way. There should be a final activity check prior to return to full competition.

Modalities in Athletic Training

15

Minimizing the time lost to injury is a major goal of the athletic training profession. While there is no known way to speed or to aid the body's natural healing process, various modalities or physical agents can create an optimum environment for healing while reducing pain and discomfort. Modalities include forms of heat, cold, light, water, electricity, massage and any mechanical means used in an effort to promote healing or rehabilitation. The selection of specific treatments or combinations of treatments is based upon several factors.

1. Injury site, type and severity
2. Modality indications and contraindications
3. Physician's prescription
4. Athlete's willingness to accept treatment

For legal reasons, treatments must be administered in accordance with local physical therapy regulations by a licensed trainer or therapist. Progress notes and careful documentation of all treatments administered are also essential.

EFFECTS OF INJURY

A knowledge of injury's specific effects upon the body's tissue is a prerequisite to understanding how and why modalities can help create an optimum environment for healing. When tissue is crushed, stretched or torn, inflammation results. Vasodilation of local blood vessels with formation of edema and pain are the major elements of the inflammatory response. Chemically, prostaglandins are synthesized and histamines are released. Both increase local swelling and pain. Subsequent hemorrhage of blood from damaged, dilated vessels adds additional trauma to the injured area. When local circulation is disrupted because of damaged blood vessels, some cells are not damaged by the injury itself but by the ensuing interruption of oxygen supply.

Muscular spasm is induced in the body's effort to splint damaged tissues. Pressure from swelling and from the spasm compresses pain fibers and contributes to the pain-spasm cycle (pain causes spasm which causes pain, etc.).

Limiting swelling and interrupting the pain-spasm cycle minimizes the inflammatory response, which reduces the athlete's time lost to injury. Only the body's natural healing process can repair damaged tissue. But, by limiting the swelling, spasm, pain and bleeding following injury, the time required for healing can be minimized. The athletic trainer's goal, therefore, is to minimize the inflammatory response.

TYPES OF MODALITIES

Four basic types of modalities are used in athletic training.

1. *Cryotherapy/cryokinetics:* cold therapy, contrast therapy, cold therapy combined with exercise
2. *Superficial thermotherapy:* whirlpool, hydrocollator packs, paraffin bath, infrared/ultraviolet light
3. *Penetrating/electrical therapy:* diathermy, ultrasound, phonophoresis, electrical muscle stimulation, iontophoresis, TENS
4. *Mechanical therapy:* massage, manipulation, traction, intermittent compression

Cryotherapy

The physiological effects of cold application, or cold therapy (cryotherapy), are the most effective means of reducing postinjury inflammation. ICE (ice, compression, elevation) is a standard treatment for all acute athletic injuries.

Cryotherapy in the form of ice packs, ice massage, cold water immersion, etc., decreases tissue temperature surrounding the site of the injury. In response to cold, nerve impulses and conduction velocities are diminished and the athlete experiences an anesthetic effect. Cold decreases muscle spindle firing and muscle activity, thus diminishing muscle spasm in the surrounding region. When spasm and pain sensations are decreased, the pain-spasm response also diminishes. The vasoconstriction caused by cryotherapy results in decreased capillary permeability and blood flow into the injured area. Thus, bleeding or hemorrhage into the tissues is lessened. Tissue metabolism is decreased in response to cold, with resultant decrease in the cells' oxygen demand. This decreases the number of cells destroyed because disrupted local circulation was unable to provide their normal supply of oxygen.

The initial constriction of blood vessels following the application of cold is followed by a period of dilation as the body attempts to warm the cooled area. Therefore, cryotherapy to treat acute injuries should be limited to 20 to 30 minutes. The reflex vasodilation caused by the extended application of cold can increase swelling and prevent lowering of skin temperature as the body attempts to protect itself from frostbite.

In acute conditions, cryotherapy is best combined with elevation and compression in the form of an elastic wrap to complete the ICE concept. Elevation of an injured extremity higher than the heart as well as compression of the tissues with an elastic wrap applied distal to proximal can minimize swelling or edema.

Thermotherapy

Thermotherapy, or heat application, is a second major modality of athletic injury care. Heat has the opposite effect of cryotherapy in that it produces an immediate increase in local

TABLE 15:1. Physiological Effects of Cryotherapy and Thermotherapy*

Cold Applications	Short—30 minutes or less	Prolonged—more than 30 minutes
Skin capillaries	Constriction, then dilation	Constriction
Skin color	White, turning red	White
Skeletal muscle	Relaxed after shivering	Rigid voluntary and/or reflex contractions
Cell size	Little change	Slightly decreased
Tissue metabolism	Decreased	Decreased
Pain sensation	Decreased	Decreased
Deep circulation	Little change	Vasodilation

Heat Applications	Short—30 minutes or less	Prolonged—more than 30 minutes
Skin capillaries	Dilation	Continued dilation
Skin color	Pink, then red	Deep red
Skeletal muscle	Relaxed	Irritated
Cell size	Expanded	Less expanded but still larger than normal
Tissue metabolism	Increased	Levels off
Pain sensation	Decreased	Variable

*Donley, P.B. "The Uses of Therapeutic Modalities." Eastern Athletic Trainers Association Convention, Grossinger, NY. January 24, 1977.

circulation. By speeding blood flow and by dilating closed capillary beds, the fluid quantity of the tissue increases. As a result, swelling is also increased. This is the major contraindication for use of thermotherapy in acute inflammatory conditions. Thermotherapy is often advocated 24 to 48 hours following injury. **A safer and more effective guideline is to avoid heat until the active swelling or inflammatory process has ceased.** For this reason, forms of cryotherapy are frequently the exclusive treatment for chronic inflammatory conditions such as tendonitis, fasciitis and tenosynovitis.

Despite its dangers, thermotherapy has the advantage of being a far more comfortable modality than cryotherapy. The increase in local circulation caused by heat speeds cell metabolism. This produces an influx of oxygen and nutrients into the injured area and encourages the removal of waste products. Heat reduces muscle spasm by inhibiting nerve activity, and also produces a sedative effect. Congestion in the injured area is diminished, with resultant diminished pain sensation. Thermotherapy can be very effective in breaking the pain-spasm cycle, particularly in postacute soft tissue injuries (Table 15.1).

Heat or thermotherapy can be introduced to the body by four major methods.

1. *Conduction:* a transfer of heat through direct contact with its source—moist heat packs or paraffin bath
2. *Convection:* a transfer of heat via a medium such as the movement of air or water, i.e., whirlpool bath
3. *Radiation:* a transfer of heat or energy through space by electromagnetic waves, i.e., infrared lamp
4. *Conversion:* heat developed by the passage of sound or electrical current through the tissues, i.e., electrical muscle stimulation, ultrasound or diathermy

The method used to deliver thermotherapy to the body varies with the athlete's specific injury and depends upon each modality's indications and contraindications.

Penetrating/Electrical Therapy

Electrical current to treat injuries relies on three major effects.

1. *Thermal:* the increase in local tissue temperature is a result of resistance offered by the conductor of the current, tissue.
2. *Chemical or Ionic:* When current is passed between two electrodes, ions flow toward their opposite poles. Thus, medication can be introduced into the tissues via the flow of current.
3. *Electromagnetic:* Muscle contraction and nerve conduction are affected by the flow of current through tissues.

Two forms of current are used to treat athletic injuries: direct, or galvanic, current that flows in only one direction, and alternating, or faradic, current that periodically reverses its flow.

Mechanical Therapy

Mechanical therapies used in athletic injury care include massage, mobilization techniques and intermittent compression. For the most part, mechanical therapies are used in conjunction with, or as a supplement to, other methods of treatment.

CRYOTHERAPY MODALITIES

Cryotherapy, or cold therapy, cools tissue by transferring heat energy. Its indications include soft tissue injuries such as sprains, strains, contusions and muscle spasms. Cryotherapy is also indicated for chronic inflammatory conditions such as tendonitis, tenosynovitis and fasciitis. Contraindications include circulatory disturbances, hypersensitivity to cold and prolonged application that can result in skin damage, blisters or frostbite. Techniques for the application of cold include:

1. *Ice massage.* Paper cups filled with water are frozen to form an ice cylinder that can be rubbed or massaged directly onto the skin surface. The ice is rubbed gently over the

site of the injury until the skin becomes bright pink in color, usually seven to ten minutes.

2. *Cold water immersion.* A whirlpool tank, bucket or other similar container is filled with a mixture of water and ice. Immersion lasts for 20 to 30 minutes and is extremely effective in delivering cryotherapy to a large area such as the ankle, shin or lower leg. An elastic wrap applied prior to treatment adds compression to cryotherapy.

3. *Ice packs.* Plastic bags or wet towels filled with cubed or shaved ice can be placed over the site of the injury. A wet elastic wrap can first be applied to provide pressure over the injured site, and the remainder of the wrap can be used to secure the ice pack in place. Treatment is 20 to 30 minutes in length. Elevation can be combined with the ice and compression for injured extremities.

4. *Chemical cold packs.* Commercially manufactured chemical cold packs are expensive but convenient. Mixing the chemical contents produces the cold. Temperatures are not always consistent, nor can the packs be reused. The length of time that the pack stays cold also varies. Chemical burns can result if the pack ruptures.

5. *Flexible gel cold packs.* Refreezable, flexible silicone gel cold packs, encased in plastic, are a convenient means of applying cold therapy. A damp towel must be placed between the skin and the pack to guard against frostbite. Treatment time is 20 to 30 minutes. Compression and elevation can be used in conjunction.

6. *Evaporative cooling.* Cold sprays use rapid evaporation of chemicals sprayed on the surface of the skin. Chemicals commonly contained in commercially prepared cold sprays include ethyl chloride, chloromethane or fluoromethane. The effects of such sprays are temporary and superficial. In addition, cold sprays can damage or burn the skin. Cold sprays are sometimes combined with stretching exercises to help break the pain-spasm cycle of soft tissue injuries, i.e., hamstring or low back strains.

The physiologic effects of cryotherapy are the same despite the method of delivery. The athlete will experience the sensations of cold, burning, aching and, finally, numbness after cold has been applied for a period of time. Care should always be taken to avoid freezing the skin, and to limit ice pack and cold water immersion treatment to 20 to 30 minutes. Cold applications can be repeated several times daily and, in the acute phase of injury, cold can be applied for 20 minutes of every hour.

Contrast Therapy

Contrast therapy alternates cryotherapy and thermotherapy in the postacute phase of injury. By applying cold to constrict circulation followed by heat to increase circulation, circulation and nutrition to the area are stimulated without the dangers of increased swelling. The "pumping" action of alternately speeding and slowing circulation may also help to decrease local swelling, particularly following sprains in the extremities. Contraindications include acute injuries, lesions with active hemorrhaging and peripheral vascular disease.

The most common technique for contrast therapy uses two whirlpools or containers filled with water. One is filled with cold water at 10 to 18.3 C (50 to 65 F), and the second is filled with hot water at 37.8 to 43.3 C (100 to 110 F). The injured extremity is placed in the cold water for one minute, followed by three to five minutes in the hot water. Cold and hot are alternated for four to five cycles, possibly several times daily. Generally all treatments should end with cold to diminish any swelling that the thermotherapy may have produced. Range of motion exercises can be performed while the extremity is in the water. Use cryotherapy exclusively if swelling develops following contrast treatment.

Cryokinetics

Cryokinetics is the use of cold and movement as treatment modalities. Cold therapy decreases pain sensation and allows mobilization or range of motion activities to be incorporated with treatment. Often, pain and spasm result in a decreased range of motion in an injured body part. Increasing joint motion decreases disuse atrophy and prevents adhesions. In cryokinetics standard cold therapy, usually ice massage, is followed by simple pain-free movement. Active motion involving rotary, circular or diagonal patterns versus traditional linear movements can be included. If active motion is painful, isometrics may be substituted. At no time should the athlete force movement or experience pain when performing exercise. Exercises are repeated 10 to 20 times several times daily. Cryokinetics can be easily included in the athlete's home care instructions.

SUPERFICIAL THERMOTHERAPY

Whirlpool Bath

The modality most commonly associated with athletic injury care is the whirlpool bath. Whirlpools can be used in immediate injury care and in cryotherapy when filled with a combination of cold water and ice. Hydrotherapy is most commonly a form of heat treatment in a tank filled with hot water. A turbine circulates the water in the tank, providing a massaging effect in addition to thermotherapy effects of the water. Indications for whirlpool treatment include soft tissue trauma, postimmobilization conditions in need of increasing range of motion, open wounds or abrasions in need of cleansing, and postacute injuries. Perhaps the most effective use of hydrotherapy is in regaining range of motion of the extremities following prolonged immobilization, i.e., after surgery and fracture. Contraindications include active hemorrhaging or swelling, heat stress, acute contusions, and acute sprains and strains.

Whirlpool baths have a sedative and analgesic action, decrease muscle spasm, produce relaxation, stimulate circulation, promote healing and increase superficial tissue temperature. Treatment times and temperatures are:

Treatment	Temperature	Time (min)
Cold whirlpools	4.4–15.5 C (40–60 F)	20–30
Hot whirlpools		
Extremity	37.8–43.3 C (100–110 F)	20
Full body	34.4–37.8 C (94–100 F) maximum	8–12 maximum

Full body whirlpool treatment can produce dizziness and heat stress; therefore, it must be used cautiously. Only those body parts in need of treatment should be in the whirlpool bath. Electrical safety inspections and ground-fault circuit interrupters are essential for the safe operation of whirlpool baths. Athletes receiving treatment should never be left unattended, nor should they turn the unit off or on while in the water. Range of motion activities can be performed in the water during treatment.

Whirlpool water and tanks must be kept clean. Frequent water changes and daily cleaning are essential. Disinfectants may be added to the water when debriding wounds and may also be used regularly to keep whirlpool water clean.

Hydrocollator Packs

Hydrocollator, or moist heat, packs are an efficient and inexpensive means of applying moist heat to an injured body part (Fig. 15:1). Hydrocollator packs are indicated in postacute soft tissue injuries such as contusions, strains and muscle spasms. As with any form of heat, moist heat packs are contraindicated for acute injuries, over areas of impaired thermal sensation, over extremities numb from exposure to cold, over analgesic packs and over the eyes and genitals.

Moist heat packs are fabric packs containing a silicone gel that absorbs and holds heat. Packs are stored in a unit that keeps them at 65.6 to 76.7 C (150 to 170 F). A pack is removed from the unit, wrapped in several layers of

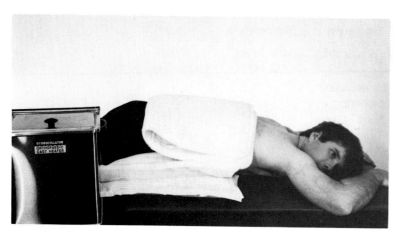

FIGURE 15:1. Hydrocollator, or moist heat, pack

toweling and applied to the body for 20 to 30 minutes. The athlete should be cautioned that hydrocollator packs can burn the skin, and adequate toweling must be placed between the pack and the skin. While receiving treatment, the athlete should be in a comfortable position. If the pack no longer feels hot, layers of toweling can be removed.

Paraffin Bath

Paraffin baths are of particular use in providing superficial heat to angular, bony areas of the body, i.e., hands, feet and wrists. A mixture of paraffin and mineral oil (8:1 ratio) is kept at 51.7 to 57.8 C (125 to 136 F) in a thermostatically controlled unit. With its high melting point and low heat conductivity, paraffin can provide sustained heat, increased circulation and decrease pain in the affected area. The paraffin bath is especially effective in treating sprains and strains to the distal extremities. It is also useful in the hand care of gymnasts since the mineral oil helps to keep callouses soft and pliable. Paraffin should not be used in any conditions where heat is contraindicated or with active hemorrhaging or impairment of local circulation. Techniques for use include:

1. *Dip and soak:* dip the extremity in and out of the paraffin several times to build up a layer of wax; soak in the wax for 15 to 20 minutes.
2. *Dip and wrap:* dip the extremity in the wax for several seconds, 6 to 12 times, and wrap the extremity in toweling for 20 to 30 minutes.
3. *Painting:* paint the extremity with 6 to 12 layers of paraffin; allow it to remain for 20 to 30 minutes.

Infrared and Ultraviolet Light

Infrared and ultraviolet lamps can provide superficial heat to injured areas. Open wounds, lesions resistant to healing and injuries on which the weight of a moist heat pack would be uncomfortable are all conditions that may benefit from infrared and/or ultraviolet light. Individuals on prescription medications causing sensitivity to ultraviolet light, such as tetracycline antibiotics, should not be treated with such devices. Other possible side-effects include erythema production and photochemical reactions. Protective eye goggles should be worn at all times when an ultraviolet light is used. Treatment times and techniques vary with the device used.

PENETRATING/ELECTRICAL THERAPY

Diathermy

Diathermy is the therapeutic application of high frequency electrical current to heat the body's tissues. The effects of local heating by diathermy are the same as for any form of heat therapy: increased blood flow and tissue metabolism, decreased spasm, etc. In addition, internal tissue temperatures can be elevated as much as 9 F. The indications for diathermy are postacute strains and inflammation of musculotendinous units, joints, bursae and tendon sheaths. Contraindications include acute inflammation, nondraining infections, hemorrhage, limited circulation or sensation, peripheral vascular disease, epiphyseal growth plates, casts, dressings and metal implants or screws. There are two forms of diathermy, shortwave and microwave.

Shortwave diathermy uses an oscillating high frequency electrical current of 10 megacycles per second (Fig. 15:2). The dosage is monitored by the athlete's subjective feeling of warmth, and treatment time is 20 to 30 minutes daily. One condensor plate is placed on either side of the area, or an induction coil is wrapped around the area. A double layer of dry toweling should be placed between the skin and the plates or coil.

Microwave diathermy uses current at a rate of 2,450 megacycles per second to heat tissues to 40 C (104 F) at a depth of 2 inches from the surface. Waves travel from the device's reflector head in a beamed or cylinder heating pattern. Microwave diathermy produces a deeper and more localized tissue heating pattern than does short wave diathermy. The reflector head is placed approximately 2 inches above the bare skin, and treatment lasts 15 to 30 minutes. Microwave diathermy treats only one side of a joint at a time, but it is a safer and easier modality.

Ultrasound

Ultrasound therapy involves the conversion of electrical energy into high frequency sound energy (Fig. 15:3). As the sound waves penetrate the tissues, they produce a mechanical vibration, increasing local tissue temperature. Ultrasound is reported to raise tissue temperature 7 to 8 F at 2 inches below the skin's surface, and the ultrasonic waves may also provide a micromassaging action upon the cells. Indications for ultrasound include postacute· soft tissue trauma, bursitis, tendonitis and fasciitis. Contraindications include treatment of acute inflammatory conditions where heat is contraindicated, treatment over areas of limited vascularity or sensation, and treatment over the ears, eyes, heart, reproductive organs, endocrine glands, central nervous system or epiphyses.

Ultrasonic waves can be produced in a pulsed or a continuous manner. Pulsed treat-

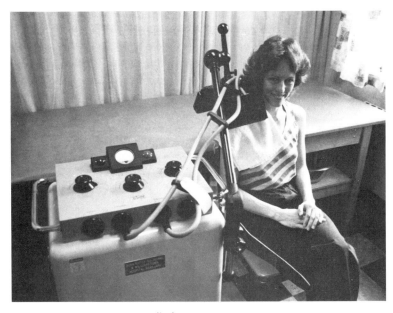

FIGURE 15:2. Shortwave diathermy

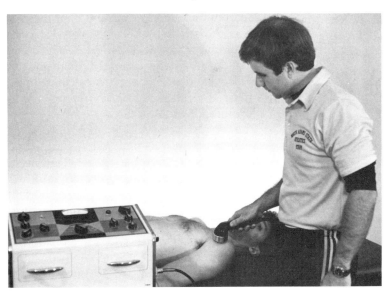

FIGURE 15:3. Ultrasound therapy

ment produces mechanical vibration with only a minimum of heating effect. It is used primarily on bony areas to avoid a heat build-up between the periosteum-bone interface. Continuous treatment provides both heat and mechanical vibration, and is used over smooth, flat surfaces.

A coupling medium such as lotion, mineral oil or water is necessary to transmit sound waves from the transducer to the site of the injury. Treatment can also be given under water with the sound head ½ to 1 inch from the skin surface. For all treatments, the sound head should be kept moving in small circles or longitudinal strokes and kept at a 90° angle to the body. Treatment time is five to eight minutes daily at 1 to 1.5 watts per square centimeter.

Phonophoresis

In phonophoresis whole molecules of a medication are driven through the skin to inflamed structures by ultrasound therapy. The most commonly used medication in phonophoresis is 1% to 10% hydrocortisone cream. Instead of mineral oil, lotion or water, hydrocortisone cream is the coupling medium for standard ultrasound treatment. Other medications such as 10% hydrocortisone with xylocaine ointment (for anesthetic) or a combination of dexamethasone and 2% lidocaine gel can also be used. The purpose of phonophoresis is to place anti-inflammatory medication into affected tissues.

Phonophoresis is indicated in postacute soft tissue trauma such as tendonitis, strains and contusions. And, since it is a noninvasive technique, it is also an alternative to injection therapy. Contraindications for phonophoresis are the same as for any ultrasound treatment. In addition, the contraindications for the medication used must also be considered. Phonophoresis treatment is generally of lower intensity but longer duration than standard ultrasound therapy, i.e., 1 to 1.5 watts per square centimeter for 5 to 15 minutes.

Ultrasound therapy can also combine with electrical muscle stimulation to treat postacute soft tissue trauma, e.g., sprains, muscle spasm, strains and contusions. With combination therapy, the athlete receives both the deep heating effects of ultrasound and the benefits of muscular contractions via electrical muscle stimulation. Treatments generally last 5 to 7 minutes and can be given twice daily.

Electrical Muscle Stimulation

Electricity can be used in a variety of ways to elicit rhythmic muscular contractions in the body (Fig. 15:4). In athletic injury care, the primary purposes of electrical muscle stimulation are to exercise muscle tissue, decrease or prevent atrophy and its accompanying enzymatic and structural changes, encourage circulation, increase tissue temperature, encourage the breakdown of adhesions, reeducate muscles and treat peripheral nerve lesions involving musculotendinous units. Inflammatory conditions, swelling, spasm and sprains can all be treated with electrical muscle stimulation. Contraindications for treatment include acute inflammatory conditions and, in particular, injuries where muscle tissue is torn.

Two types of current are used in electrical muscle stimulation: galvanic, or direct, current and faradic, or alternating, current. Galvanic muscle stimulators use short pulses of 0–500 volts of direct current. Current flow can be reversed between the pads, and a dispersive pad can be used to provide a return path of current flow. Pad placements are determined by the purpose of the treatment. In treating inflammatory conditions, the positive pad is distal to or at the site of the injury, and the negative pad is proximal to the site of the injury. When treating to reduce swelling or effusion, the positive pad is placed proximal to the site of the injury and the negative pad is placed at or distal to the injured area. Effects at the positive and negative poles are:

Positive	*Negative*
Vasoconstriction	Vasodilation
Hardens tissue	Softens tissue
Sedative	Irritation
Local analgesic	Decreases swelling

Galvanic current can also be used in testing isolated muscle responses.

Faradic muscle stimulators involve the use of alternating current and can deliver stimulation to the muscles in a variety of ways, including pulsing, surging and tetanizing contractions. Faradic muscle stimulators are used primarily to exercise muscles through contraction. Treatment times for both galvanic and faradic muscle stimulation are 10 to 30 minutes twice daily.

Iontophoresis

Iontophoresis uses electrical current or ultrasound to drive ionized medications through the skin to injured tissues. Electrical potential causes ions in solution to travel according to their electrical charges. In this fashion, medication can be introduced into the body through the skin. The most commonly used medications for iontophoresis are dexamethasone and hydrocortisone. Postacute soft tissue injuries, contusions, tendonitis, strains, bursitis, etc., can all be treated by iontophoresis. The contraindications for the medications involved and for electrical muscle stimulation or ultrasound apply. Treatment times are 5 to 10 minutes daily for both techniques.

TENS

Transcutaneous electrical nerve stimulation (TENS) devices can be used to treat both acute and chronic pain (Fig. 15:5). The exact effects of TENS are unknown, but its operation is based upon the gate control theory. The stimulation of afferent nerve fibers seems to decrease pain sensations or perceptions. Electrical stimulation is thought to close the gate to the transmission of pain sensations in the dorsal horn level of the spinal cord, thus relieving pain. Other theories center upon the idea that chronic pain is actually a circuit of neuro-reverberating pain that can be broken by the flow of electrical current, or that TENS can cause the body to produce its own pain inhibiting chemicals, i.e., endophins and enkephalins.

While the exact effects of TENS are subject to speculation, it has been shown to diminish pain in many conditions. TENS is contraindicated in pregnant women and in persons with pacemakers, nor should it be used over the

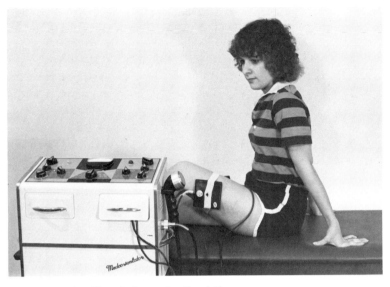

FIGURE 15:4. Electrical muscle stimulation

carotid sinuses. Because TENS can mask pain, participation in physical activity during or after its use must be carefully controlled. TENS units introduce current into the body via two or four electrode pads. Pad placement is subject to trial and error, but, generally, one electrode is placed on the site of pain, and the second is placed proximal to the painful area. TENS units allow adjustment of the current's pulse rate, pulse width and amplitude. The current should be adjusted to a comfortable sensation, but it should not elicit pain or muscular contraction. TENS treatment can be used continuously or intermittently. Treatment generally continues from 1 to 5 days, and electrode pads must be relocated if skin irritation begins to develop.

MECHANICAL THERAPY

Massage

Massage, one of the oldest modalities, is the systematic and scientific manipulation of the body's soft tissue. The therapeutic effects of massage include stimulating cell metabolism, increasing venous flow and lymphatic drainage, increasing circulation and nutrition,

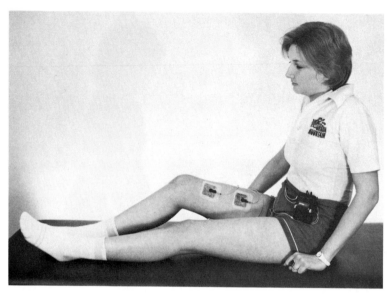

FIGURE 15:5. Transcutaneous electrical nerve stimulation (TENS) to treat acute and chronic pain

stretching superficial scar tissue and relaxing muscle tissues. It is often used as an adjunct in treating postacute soft tissue trauma and strains. Conditions contraindicating the use of massage include acute injuries, hemorrhaging, infection, thromboses, nerve damage, skin disease and the possibility of calcification.

The basic massage techniques include:

1. *Effleurage:* superficial or deep stroking
2. *Pĕtrissage:* kneading
3. *Tapotement:* percussion or tapping
4. *Vibration:* trembling, forward and backward movement
5. *Friction:* pressure across muscles or tendons

The effects of massage are both mechanical and reflexive. Mild stretching of scar and superficial tissue is its major mechanical effect. Reflexive effects include stimulation and relaxation of the tissues. Generally lubricants such as oil, lanolin, lotion or powder should be used during massage therapy. Stroking toward the heart is also recommended to increase and promote venous return and to reduce swelling in the injured areas.

Manipulative Therapy

Manipulative therapy is based on the concepts of joint play and joint dysfunction. Joint play is the normal range of involuntary movement of which a joint is capable. Without normal joint play, pain is experienced. Manipulation restores normal joint play by taking a joint's movement to its limits, thus correcting the joint's dysfunction. Manipulation must be practiced by trained, experienced therapists or physicians. Contraindications for manipulative treatment include bone or joint disease or inflammation, healing ligament sprains or muscle strains, disc injuries and vertebral fractures. The muscle spasm accompanying joint dysfunction can be treated by conventional therapies, but manipulative therapy can often correct the cause of the problem.

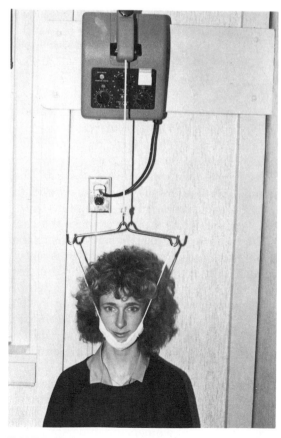

FIGURE 15:6. Cervical traction

Traction

Cervical and lumbar traction is used to treat noninflammatory musculoskeletal conditions, muscle spasm and pain (Fig. 15:6). Its effects are decreased muscle spasm, increased blood flow and length of fibrotic tissue, encouragement of range of motion and relief of nerve pressure. Traction is frequently combined with moist heat packs and can be applied continuously or intermittently. Continuous traction is said to enlarge the intervertebral foramina and to reduce compressive and irritative forces on the nerve routes. Treatment with continuous traction begins with 15 to 20 pounds of pressure for 30 minutes daily. Intermittent traction uses a gradually increasing stretch alternating with periods of relaxation. Intermittent traction is more easily tolerated than continuous traction because it is less likely to cause overstretching and resultant muscle spasm. Treatment may build up to 50 to 75 pounds with 5 to 16 interruptions per minute.

Intermittent Compression

In intermittent compression an air-filled boot or sleeve applies pressure to force edema out of an injured extremity at timed intervals. It should be combined with elevation. Decreased blood flow, limited venous pooling, assistance in venous return and decreased swelling are intermittent compression's effects. It can also be combined with cryotherapy. With the Jobst Cryotemp Unit, the boot or sleeve is filled with refrigerant fluid so that cold, pressure and elevation can be simultaneously applied. By using a flexible gel cold pack, a standard Jobst Compression Boot can also be used to apply ICE. This is an effective initial and postacute therapy for joint sprains or injuries involving swelling.

Part 6

MUSCULOSKELETAL SYSTEM

Injuries to the Musculoskeletal System

16

SOFT TISSUES

The soft tissues of the body, apart from the viscera or specific organs, are the skin and muscles. For the purposes of this chapter, only the muscles of the skeleton are considered, although muscle forms a considerable portion of the bulk of the other organ systems, the vessels and the bronchi.

Skin

The skin, the largest organ of the body and one of the most important, is a tough tissue, constantly renewed, that covers the entire body. It serves two main functions: to protect the body in the environment and to maintain nerves that convey information about that environment to the brain.

The skin's protective functions are numerous, all equally important. Over 70% of the body is water, with a delicate balance of substances in solution. Skin is watertight and keeps this internal solution intact. Unless the skin is broken by an ulcer or laceration, the bacteria that surround us cannot pass through it. Bacteria are routinely found on the skin and deep in its grooves and glands, but never beneath it.

The body derives energy from chemical reactions (metabolism) that take place within certain temperature ranges. If the temperature is too low, reactions cannot proceed, metabolism ceases, and the body dies. If the temperature becomes too high, as with severe fever, metabolism increases and permanent tissue damage can result.

The major organ for regulating body temperature is the skin. The skin cools the body through evaporation of water from its surface in hot weather (sweating) and through the constriction of skin blood vessels in cold weather. Automatically, the skin isolates us within our environment, protects us from that environment, and helps us adapt to it.

A rich supply of nerves in the skin carries information from the environment to the brain. Nerves in this organ are adapted to perceive changes in and transmit information about heat, cold, external pressure, pain and the relative position of a given part of the body in space. The skin recognizes changes in the environment or the surroundings—whether the air is hot or cold. The skin perceives pressure on a portion of the body, pain to warn us of danger as well as pleasurable stimuli.

Layers of the Skin

The skin has two layers—the epidermis and the dermis. Subcutaneous fat lies just under these layers (Fig. 16:1A).

The epidermis, the outer layer, is composed of especially durable cells. They are dead, cornified (hardened) cells that are constantly being rubbed off and replaced. This layer is the body's first mechanism of defense. It is watertight and does not admit bacteria (Fig. 16:1B). In the deeper part of the epidermis, cells of the germinal layer constantly reproduce to replace the outer cells being shed or rubbed off. Some of the cells in this deeper layer also contain pigment granules. These cells, together with the

147

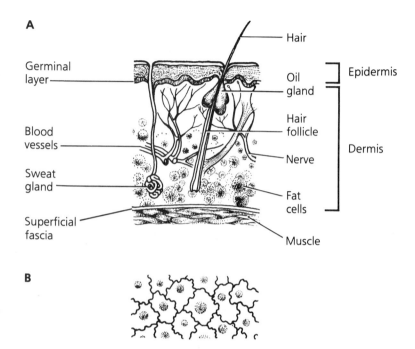

FIGURE 16:1. **A** Major structures within the skin. **B** Epidermal cells are especially durable and fit close together as a protective layer.

blood flowing in the small vessels in the skin, are responsible for skin color.

The deeper layer of skin, the dermis, is separated from the epidermis by the germinal epithelium. Within the dermis, composed of very strong elastic and fibrous tissue, lie many of the special structures of the skin: sweat glands and ducts, sebaceous or oil glands and ducts, hair follicles, blood vessels and specialized nerve endings.

Sweat glands produce sweat, discharged onto the surface of the skin through small pores and ducts, one pore for each gland. Sebaceous glands produce an oily substance called sebum, discharged along the shafts of the hairs on the head and body. It accounts for the natural oiliness of hair and skin. Sebum is important in maintaining the waterproofing of the skin and in keeping the skin supple so that it does not crack.

Hair follicles are the small organs that produce hair. There is one follicle for each hair,

connected with a sebaceous gland and a tiny muscle. The muscle serves to pull the hair into an erect position when a person is cold or frightened. All hair grows continuously and is either cut off or worn away by clothes. Blood vessels and a complex array of nerves complete the structures contained within the dermis.

Immediately under the dermis is the subcutaneous tissue. It is largely fat and insulates the body. Characteristic body curves are usually derived from subcutaneous deposits of fat.

Muscle

The great bulk of the body is made up of voluntary, or skeletal, muscle that surrounds and is attached to the skeleton. Several other types of muscle exist in the body. The heart is a single large muscular pump, the gastrointestinal tract is largely muscle, and nearly every blood vessel has its own muscle cells that give it the capability to constrict or dilate. Almost all body systems and most organs have some muscular elements. Each of these special muscular elements is considered within the system it serves.

Skeletal muscle is known by several terms and forms the major muscle mass of the body. It is called skeletal because it attaches to the bones of the skeleton. It is called voluntary because all skeletal muscle is under direct voluntary control of the brain and can be contracted or relaxed at will. It is frequently also called striated muscle because it has characteristic stripes, or striations, under the microscope. All bodily movement is a result of skeletal contraction or relaxation. Most often a given motion is the result of several muscles working together, contracting or relaxing simultaneously.

All skeletal muscles are supplied with arteries, veins and nerves (Fig. 16:2). Blood brings oxygen and food to muscles and carries away the waste produced by muscular contractions. Muscles cannot function without a continuous supply of food and continuous removal of waste. Cramps result when insuffi-

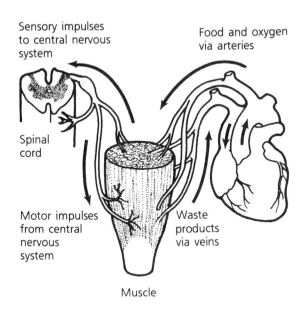

Sensory impulses to central nervous system

Food and oxygen via arteries

Spinal cord

Motor impulses from central nervous system

Waste products via veins

Muscle

FIGURE 16:2. Arterial blood carries nutrients and oxygen to skeletal muscles and venous blood removes metabolic waste.

cient oxygen or food is carried to muscles or acidic waste products accumulate.

Muscle contraction requires an energy source, adenosine triphosphate (ATP), as well as magnesium and calcium ions. ATP is a high energy phosphate-containing compound. A complex series of metabolic pathways exist for the synthesis of ATP. As ATP and oxygen are depleted and anaerobic glycolysis occurs, lactic acid is produced and an oxygen debt is created. Once exertion is finished, extra oxygen is consumed and the lactic acid is removed. The oxygen debt may be as much as six times the basal oxygen consumption. Trained athletes contract smaller oxygen debts than do untrained persons.

A muscle may contract fully or partially. It may contract isometrically (same length) or isotonically (same tension). Each individual muscle fiber contracts maximally or not at all. Increasing force of contraction of a muscle results from recruiting additional muscle fibers. A single motor neuron innervates multiple muscle fibers and constitutes a functional unit, the motor unit. Recruitment of several motor

units increases the force of contraction. A single action potential causes a muscle twitch.

Both the tension that a muscle develops when stimulated and the passive tension vary with the length of the muscle fiber. The greatest contractile force develops when the muscle is at its resting length. If the muscle is passively stretched beyond its resting length, the passive tension in the muscle increases but the active tension that the muscle can develop decreases.

There are two major types of muscle fibers: type I and type II. Whole muscles are comprised of type I (red) and type II (white) fibers of varied properties. Type I fibers, the fast-twitch fibers discussed in Chapter 14, are rich in oxidative metabolic enzymes and myoglobin, whereas type II, the slow-twitch fibers (see Chapter 14), have high concentrations of enzymes for anaerobic glycolysis and less myoglobin. Myoglobin acts as a storage site for oxygen and is believed to speed the inward diffusion of oxygen into the muscle fiber. Type I fibers have slow contraction times and are predominantly for sustained work. Type II fibers have rapid, short contraction times and fewer fibers per motor unit. Type II fibers are specialized for fine skilled movements. Some of these differences between type I and type II fibers are related to neural innervation. Experimentally, reversal of the innervation can change one type of muscle into the other type. The different quantities of type I and type II muscle fibers may explain individual differences in athletic ability, such as the sprinter versus the marathon runner.

Muscles function as agonists when they cause body movement. An antagonist causes motion opposite to the agonist muscle. An example is the biceps brachii and the triceps. Muscles must function in a coordinated manner, with synergistic muscles contracting as agonists contract and antagonists relax. Skeletal muscles cause movement by acting on bone, which functions as a lever, and across a joint, which acts as a fulcrum.

Skeletal muscles are under the direct control of the nervous system and respond to a willed command, as in the movement of an arm or leg. Nerves pass directly from the spinal cord or brain to all skeletal muscles. Movements are voluntarily initiated and involuntarily coordinated. When the normal nerve supply is lost, a voluntary muscle can neither be contracted nor relaxed and becomes limp and useless or spastic and rigid.

Most of these skeletal muscles attach directly to bones by tendons—tough, rope-like cords of fibrous tissue. Usually these attachments are at two definite points. A muscle and its tendon pass between two bony attachments called the origin of the muscle and the insertion of the muscle (Fig. 16:3). When a muscle contracts, a line of force or pull is created between the origin and the insertion, that is, between the two bones to which the muscle is connected. Most voluntary muscles pass over or across joints. Movement can take place because of these joints, the points where bones come together.

An aponeurosis is a broad, fibrous sheet attaching a muscle to another muscle. Ligaments, or fibrous bands, attach bones to

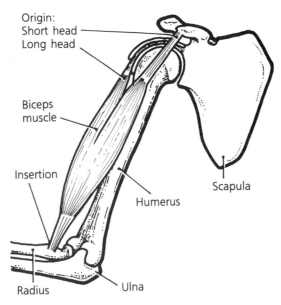

Origin:
Short head
Long head

Biceps muscle

Insertion

Humerus

Scapula

Radius   Ulna

FIGURE 16:3. The origin and insertion of the biceps muscle. Contraction of the biceps flexes the elbow.

bones. Overexertion or excessive stretching may produce an injury in which the muscle, its tendon or its aponeurosis is torn. Muscular injury, bruising or rupture may occur with or without injury of the skin. Ligamentous injury is called a sprain.

Special Muscles

The special muscles of the body are not part of the skeletal muscular system and are noted here only for completeness. The involuntary muscles carry out much of the automatic work of the body. This type of muscle is called smooth muscle from its microscopic appearance. It forms the bulk of the gastrointestinal system, the bladder and the ureters. It is found in nearly all the vessels and in bronchi. It is under involuntary nervous control and responds to stimuli such as heat or fright, the need to relieve waste or to dilate or constrict vessels. We exert no voluntary control over this type of muscle. Involuntary muscles are discussed in chapters dealing with the systems they serve.

The diaphragm is both an involuntary and a voluntary muscle. It is attached to the costal arch and the lumbar vertebrae. When we take a breath, the diaphragm flattens and its center part moves down. The volume of the chest cavity is increased, and inspiration can take place. Breathing is an automatic function that continues when we are asleep and at all other times. Automatic control of breathing can, however, be overridden by conscious will, and we can breathe faster, slower or hold our breath. We cannot do so indefinitely, however, and in the end, automatic control resumes. Hence, although the diaphragm looks like voluntary, skeletal muscle and is attached to the skeleton, it behaves like involuntary muscle most of the time.

The heart, or cardiac muscle, is a large muscle comprising a pair of pumps of unequal force, one of lower and one of higher pressure. It must function continuously from birth to death. It is a specially adapted involuntary muscle with a particularly good blood supply and its own regulatory system. It can tolerate interruption of its blood supply only for a very few minutes before severe chest pain and the signs of a heart attack develop. Like all other involuntary muscles, it is under the automatic control of the autonomic nervous system.

SOFT TISSUE INJURIES

Most injuries involve some soft tissue, skin, skeletal muscle, or fascia—the fibrous tissue enclosing muscles. An injury may be closed or open. In closed injuries soft tissue damage occurs beneath the skin with no break in the surface. In an open wound the surface of the skin or the mucous membrane that lines the major body orifices (mouth, nose, anus and vagina) is broken.

Closed Soft Tissue Wounds

A blunt object striking against the body with sufficient force crushes the tissue beneath the skin. Within this tissue, a contusion (bruise) develops (Fig. 16:4A). It is a closed injury if the skin remains intact. Subsurface damage may extend for varying depths beneath the skin. The injury is followed by the development of swelling and pain. Small blood vessels in the tissues are usually torn, and varying amounts of blood and plasma leak into the wound. The immediate leak accounts for the swelling and pain. The blood in the tissue gradually migrates toward the skin and causes a characteristic discoloration, an ecchymosis (black and blue mark).

When considerable amounts of tissue are damaged or torn or when large blood vessels are disrupted at the site of the contusion, a lump may develop rather rapidly from a pool of blood collecting within the damaged tissue. This condition is called a hematoma or, literally, a blood tumor. In all fractures, a hematoma collects about the broken ends of the bones. With a fracture of a large bone such as the femur or pelvis, more than a liter of blood collects in the fracture hematoma.

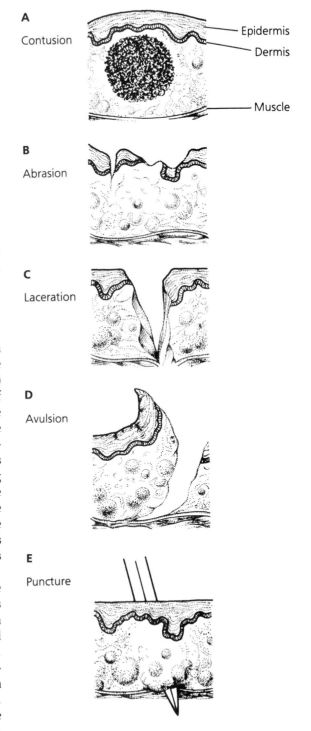

A Contusion — Epidermis, Dermis, Muscle

B Abrasion

C Laceration

D Avulsion

E Puncture

FIGURE 16:4. Soft tissue wounds

Management of Closed Wounds

Small bruises require no special emergency medical care. With severe soft tissue injuries, extensive swelling and bleeding beneath the skin may cause shock. Appying local padding and a soft roller bandage for counterpressure can partially control this bleeding in the extremities. Local applications of ice may help control initial tissue swelling. If the athlete has suffered extensive soft tissue damage, underlying fractures should be suspected. Extensive soft tissue injuries of the extremities should also be treated immediately with air pressure splints, which support the extremity and create a balanced, distributed counterpressure. When soft tissue injuries are associated with fractures, splinting is a first priority to achieve control of the bone injury and minimize soft tissue damage.

Open Soft Tissue Wounds

Open wounds cause obvious bleeding and are subject to direct contamination, and thus infection. There are four major kinds of open wounds of soft tissue.

1. An **abrasion** is a loss of a portion of the epidermis and part of the dermis from having been rubbed or scraped across a hard surface (Fig. 16:4B). It is extremely painful, and blood may ooze from injured capillary vessels at the surface, but the wound does not penetrate completely through the skin.
2. A **laceration** is a cut produced by any object that leaves a smooth or jagged wound through the skin, the subcutaneous tissue, the underlying muscles, and associated nerves and blood vessels (Fig. 16:4C).
3. An **avulsion** is an injury in which a whole piece of skin with varying portions of subcutaneous tissue or muscle is either torn loose completely or left hanging as a flap (Fig. 16:4D). Ordinarily, avulsed tissues separate at normal anatomic planes, for example, between muscle and subcutaneous tissue. Occasionally, avulsed tissue will be torn completely free and will be lying apart from the athlete. All avulsed tissue that is torn away from the athlete should be saved. Avulsions of fingers or extremities can separate portions of tissue. This amputated tissue, if readily available, should be retrieved and transported to the hospital with the patient. It should be wrapped in a sterile gauze, placed in a plastic bag, and then put in a cooled container. The tissue should not be allowed to freeze. Reimplantation of avulsed portions of the body may be feasible.
4. A **puncture** wound results from a splinter, cleat or other pointed object (Fig. 16:4E). External bleeding is usually not severe because the wound is small. However, a deep wound may injure major vessels within body cavities and require an exploratory operation in either the chest, abdomen or involved extremity. Extensive damage should always be suspected.

Management of Open Wounds

Open soft tissue wounds are treated with regard to three general rules. The order of the treatment is determined by the extent of the wound itself, the severity of bleeding and the amount of blood lost, but is usually in this order:

1. Control bleeding
2. Prevent further contamination
3. Immobilize the part and keep the patient quiet

Applying a pressure dressing directly over the wound controls bleeding. Pressure may be applied with a sterile dressing held by the hand (Fig. 16:5A), by a pressure bandage (Fig. 16:5B) or by an air splint (Fig. 16:5C).

The initial step in controlling bleeding is splinting and immobilization of the injured extremity. Frequently, splinting the extremity can help control bleeding from soft tissue wounds, whether or not they are associated with a fracture. An air splint exerts a considerable amount of gentle pressure throughout the entire length of the extremity, and may

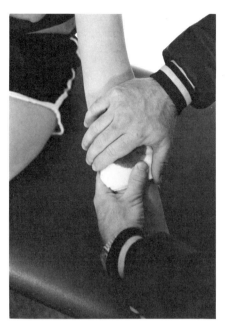

FIGURE 16:5A. Pressure applied to open wound

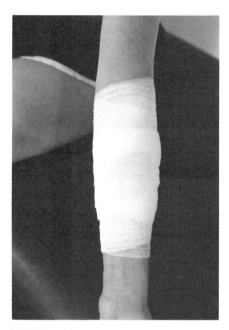

FIGURE 16:5B. Pressure bandage

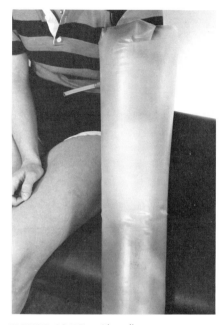

FIGURE 16:5C. Air splint

control bleeding more readily than a local pressure dressing. When bleeding is associated with a soft tissue wound accompanying a fracture, splinting is absolutely necessary for adequate control of soft tissue bleeding. Further, splinting of an extremity with severe soft tissue injury immobilizes the injury and allows the patient to be moved much more readily and more comfortably, without sustaining further damage.

Wound contamination and resultant secondary infection is less likely if the trainer can use sterile materials for the initial dressing. Every effort should be made to keep foreign matter out of the wound. Hair, clothing, dirt and fluids all increase the danger of secondary infection. However, in initial treatment, do not try to remove material embedded in the wound, no matter how dirty. Only the gross matter on the surface around the wound should be removed. A surgeon should perform the final, definitive cleaning of the wound. Much time may be lost in a fruitless attempt to clean a wound requiring surgery.

Clothing covering a wound must be removed. It is often far better to tear or cut away clothing from the wound than to try to remove normally, as motion may be painful and cause additional tissue damage and contamination. What may seem a minor movement may cause excruciating pain for the athlete.

Impaled Foreign Objects

Occasionally, an object such as a splinter of wood or a piece of glass is seen in a puncture wound (Fig. 16:6A)—an impaled foreign object. In addition to local control of bleeding, three rules should be followed in treating a patient with an impaled foreign object.

1. Do not remove the object. Its removal may cause hemorrhage or damage nearby nerves or muscles. Try to stop any bleeding from the entrance wound by direct pressure, but do not exert any force on the impaled object itself or on tissue directly adjacent to its cutting edge to avoid further tissue damage (Fig. 16:6B).

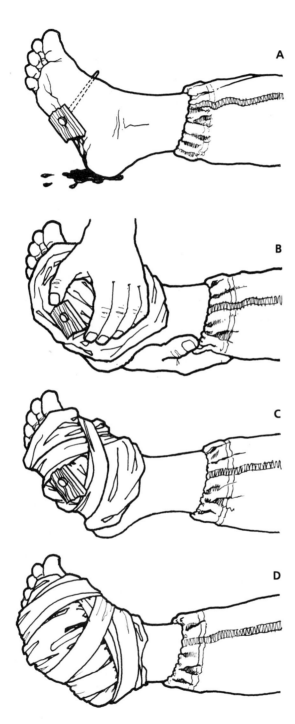

FIGURE 16:6. **A** An impaled object should be left in place. **B** Control bleeding with pressure. **C** Apply a bandage about the object to stabilize it and to maintain pressure. **D** The bulky final dressing protects the patient during transportation.

2. Use a bulky dressing to stabilize the object. The impaled foreign body itself should be incorporated within the dressing to reduce its motion after the bandage is applied (Figs. 16:6C, D).
3. Transport the athlete promptly to the emergency department with the object still in place. Ordinarily, surgery is necessary to remove the object, so the tissues immediately around it will be directly examined and treated.

If a very long impaled object must be shortened to allow transport, remember that even the slightest movement may cause severe additional pain, hemorrhage or damage of the tissue around the object. Before cutting an object, it must be made very secure, and any motion transmitted to the athlete must be minimal. Pain may aggravate shock in the athlete who has undergone severe hemorrhage and must be avoided whenever possible.

DRESSINGS AND BANDAGES

Soft tissue injuries must be bandaged and sometimes splinted. (Splinting is discussed later in this chapter.) Dressings and bandages have three main functions: to stop bleeding, to protect a wound from further damage, and to prevent further contamination and possible infection.

Universal Dressings

All training kits must carry sterile dressings. Universal dressings, conventional 4 × 4 inch gauze pads, an assortment of small, adhesive dressings and soft, self-adherent roller dressings will suffice for most wounds. A universal dressing is made of thick, absorbent material; it measures 9 × 36 inches and is packed folded into a compact size. While available commercially, it can be made at a reasonable cost. Bandage material is available in 9-inch wide, 20 yard rolls. When cut in 36-inch long pieces and folded on itself three times, from each end, each length becomes a compact dressing that fits conveniently into a number 2 paper bag. The end of the bag can be folded and stapled. The package can be sterilized by local hospital personnel and placed in a protective plastic bag with a soft roller bandage. It is an efficient, reasonably priced dressing for wounds or burns and can serve when necessary as a cervical collar or as a padding for splints.

Stabilizing Dressings

Dressings must remain in place during transport. Soft, roller, self-adherent bandages, rolls of gauze, triangular bandages or adhesive tape can stabilize dressings. The soft roller bandages are probably easiest to use. They are slightly elastic, the layers adhere to one another, and the end of the roll can be tucked back into the layers. Triangular bandages can hold a dressing in place if the ends of the bandage can be tied together. Adhesive tape can hold small bandages in place and help secure other dressings. Sucking chest wounds and abdominal wounds where organs are exposed may require adhesive tape to secure the bandage. Remember, however, that some people are allergic to ordinary adhesive tape. In any case elastic bandages should be not be used to secure dressings.

Dressings should never interfere with circulation. Always check a limb distal to a dressing after it is applied for signs of impaired circulation or loss of skin sensation.

Occlusive Dressings

A satisfactory, nonadherent, occlusive dressing for sucking chest wounds or abdominal eviscerating wounds is sterile aluminum foil. The entire roll of foil can be sterilized in its original package, and the remainder may be resterilized after each use.

Pressure Dressings

A pressure dressing is recommended to control bleeding from a wound. The universal dressing is a perfect initial layer for a pressure dressing because it can be folded or opened to adapt to most wound sizes.

After the dressing is in place, apply hand pressure on the wound through the dressing until the bleeding has slowed or stopped. Firmly applying a roller bandage to the injured part can maintain continued pressure. If bleeding continues or recurs, the original dressing and bandage should be left in place and another large dressing applied and secured with another roller bandage. Elastic bandages should not be used for pressure dressings because of possible complications from unevenly distributed pressure.

At times, bleeding will continue through the bandage. The trainer should apply yet another universal dressing and secure it with another firmly applied roller bandage. Hand pressure also may be used. The primary purpose of a pressure dressing is to stop bleeding and to do so the pressure applied must exceed the pressure in the bleeding vessels.

THE SKELETAL SYSTEM

The skeleton forms the supporting framework of the human body (Fig. 16:7). Normally it is composed of 206 bones that give form to the body and, with the joints, allow bodily motion. The skeleton also protects vital internal organs by shielding them. The brain lies within the skull; the heart, lungs and great vessels are within the thorax; much of the liver and spleen are protected by the lowermost ribs; and the spinal cord is contained within and protected by the bony spinal canal formed by the vertebrae.

Bones

Bones of the skeleton come into contact with one another at joints, where they are moved by the action of muscles. The skeleton thus is a rigid framework for the attachment of muscles and protection of organs and flexible framework to allow the parts of the body to move by muscular contraction. The skeletal framework allows an erect posture against

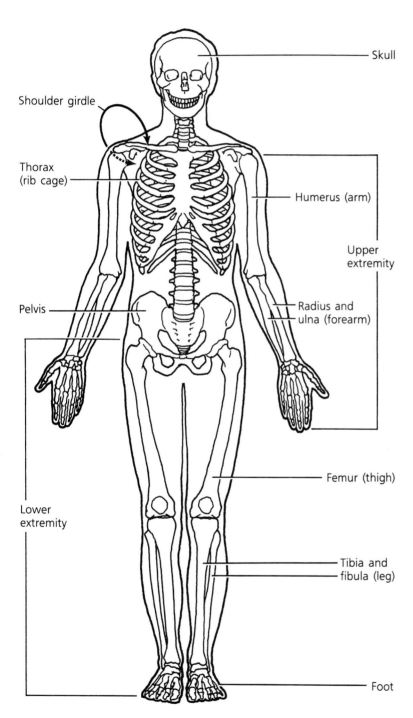

Shoulder girdle

Thorax
(rib cage)

Pelvis

Lower
extremity

Skull

Humerus (arm)

Upper
extremity

Radius and
ulna (forearm)

Femur (thigh)

Tibia and
fibula (leg)

Foot

FIGURE 16:7. The human skeleton forms the frame of the body.

the pull of gravity and gives recognizable form to the body.

Bones must be rigid and unyielding to fulfill their function, but they must also grow and adapt as the human being grows. As a rule, bone growth is complete by a person's late teens. Unless some abnormality is present, there is usually little outward skeletal change after this period. Bones in young children are more flexible than in the adult and, therefore, are less likely to be fractured. Since children are so active, however, fractures occur frequently.

Bones are just as much living tissue as muscle and skin. A rich blood supply constantly provides the oxygen and nutrients bones require. Each bone also has an extensive nerve supply primarily from the periosteum. Thus, bone fracture produces severe pain from irritation of its nerves as well as heavy bleeding from damage to its blood vessels.

Each bone is composed of a protein framework that allows its growth and remodeling. Calcium and phosphorus are deposited into this framework to make the bone hard and strong. Throughout a person's lifetime, calcium and phosphorus are constantly being deposited in bone and withdrawn from it under the control of a very complex metabolic system. This ability to grow as well as to repair by forming new bone is a phenomenon unique to bone tissue.

Anatomy of a Bone

The outer, dense layer of a bone is called the cortex, and the inner, less dense area is the cancellous bone. On the surface of the bone is the periosteum, which is composed of an outer, fibrous layer and an inner layer of cells capable of forming bone. A growing long bone has an epiphysis at each end, an adjacent physis or growth plate, a flared metaphysis, a diaphysis in the midportion and a central medullary cavity (Fig. 16:8).

Bone may be divided into nonlamellar or woven bone, which is an immature bone, and mature lamellar bone, which is arranged in layers. Lamellar bone may be further divided

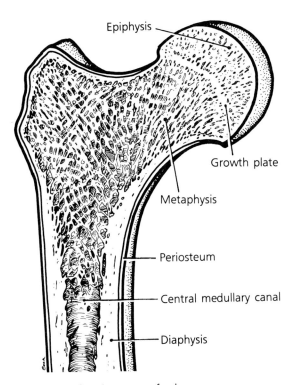

FIGURE 16:8. Anatomy of a bone

into nonhaversian and haversian bone. Haversian bone consists of lamellar bone arranged around a central canal (Fig. 16:9). This arrangement of a central canal with surrounding layers of lamellar bone is called a haversian system or osteon. The haversian bone may be primary haversian, which is bone formed in place of connective tissue, or secondary haversian, formed in place of preexisting bone.

The cells comprising bone consist of osteoblasts (which lay down new bone), osteocytes (which maintain mature bone) and osteoclasts (which resorb bone) (Fig. 16:10). The fine channels extending through the bone connecting the osteocytes are called canaliculi. They contain extracellular fluid that can transport nutrients to the osteocytes and provide a large area for the exchange of minerals. The osteoblast initially deposits unmineralized bone tissue (osteoid), which over an interval of approximately 15 days becomes mineralized. The osteoclast is present in depressions called

Howship's lacunae along calcified resorbing bone.

Depending on shape and function, parts of a bone may be designated by specific names. The head of a bone is the rounded end that allows joint rotation. The region below the head is frequently called the neck. The shaft is the long, straight, cylindrical midportion of a bone.

The condyles (called malleoli at the ankle and styloid processes at the wrist) are prominences at one or both ends of the bone that usually serve as points of ligament attachment. Tuberosities and trochanters are prominences on the bone where tendons insert.

The epiphyseal plate is a transverse cartilage plate near the end of a child's bone; it is responsible for growth in bone length.

Bone Composition and Remodeling

Bone is composed of one-third organic matrix and two-thirds mineral. The mineral is a form of amorphous tricalcium phosphate and hydroxyapatite, or $Ca_{10}(PO_4)_6(OH)_2$. The matrix is composed of 95% collagen, 1% glycosaminoglycans, 2% water and 2% bone cells.

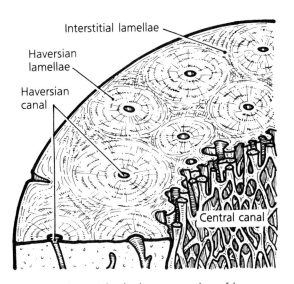

FIGURE 16:9. Histologic cross section of bone showing Haversian bone and lamellar bone around a central canal

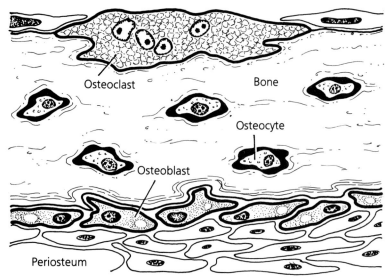

FIGURE 16:10. Bone cells

centers of ossification are formed in the epiphysis of the long bone. Each bone has a characteristic time of appearance of the secondary centers of ossification.

Bone growth and remodeling are affected by many factors, including hormones (such as parathyroid), adequacy of minerals (such as calcium and phosphorus), adequacy of vitamins (such as vitamin D), protein supply and activity level. Bone responds to physical stresses or lack of them. Bone is deposited on areas subjected to stress and reabsorbed from areas where little stress is present. This phenomenon is termed Wolff's law. A bone subjected to prolonged immobilization and thus protected from use becomes thinner, such as when a cast is worn. This loss of bone substance is osteoporosis of disuse.

Joints

Wherever two bones come into contact, they form a joint articulation. Some joints allow motion, for example, the knee, hip or elbow, whereas other bones fuse with one another at joints, producing a solid, immobile bony structure. The skull is composed of several different bones that fuse as the person grows into adulthood. The infant, whose bones are not yet fused, has soft spots called fontanelles between the bones. Many joints of the body are named by combining the names of the two bones forming that joint, for example, the sternoclavicular joint is the articulation between the sternum and the clavicle.

A joint consists of the ends of the bones and the surrounding connecting and supporting tissues. The ends of bones that articulate with each other are covered with a smooth, shiny surface called articular cartilage. The articular cartilage consists of four distinct cell zones: a superficial tangential or gliding zone, a transitional or intermediate zone, a radial zone and a calcified zone (Fig. 16:11). A thin line called the tidemark lies between the radial and the calcified zone. Adult hyaline (articular) cartilage contains fewer cells than most other adult tissues. Mature cartilage is avascular,

Bone does not grow interstitially but by apposition and resorption on its surface. Less than 5% of the adult bone surfaces are being formed or resorbed at any one time.

Bone formation and resorption occur along vertical tunnels in the bone. Most bones are formed by remodeling of a cartilage model. This is termed "enchondral ossification." The longitudinal growth of a long bone is an example. The physis grows by interstitial deposition of cartilage beneath the metaphysis. The cartilage cells die, and the cartilage is invaded by blood vessels. New bone is deposited on the cartilage model, and the cartilage is reabsorbed. Bone grows in width by apposition of new bone on the periosteal surface and remodelling of the metaphysis, a process called "funnelization."

Bone may be formed without preexisting cartilage; this is called "intramembranous ossification." The bones of the vault of the skull are formed by intramembranous ossification. Centers of ossification are places where bone begins to be laid down. The primary center of ossification of a long bone is in the diaphysis and is present by the end of the fourth month of gestation. The secondary

aneural and alymphatic. Collagen fibers in the matrix provide stiffness to the articular cartilage. Under normal adult conditions, articular cartilage cells do not undergo mitosis. Even in the presence of injury, the articular cartilage repair response is severely limited.

Articular cartilage has a high content of water (between 65% and 80%) present in the form of a gel. Collagen makes up 90% of the protein content. The cartilage contains complex large molecules called mucopolysaccharides, such as chondroitin sulfate. Also present are macromolecules called protein polysaccharides consisting of a protein core with large chains of sulfated polysaccharides. The protein polysaccharides are highly charged molecules and are important in providing resiliency to the cartilage.

Nutrients are diffused from the synovial fluid through the matrix of the articular cartilage. Very little nutrition passes from the vascular bone into the cartilage. The metabolic rate of articular cartilage, however, is high, and

the anaerobic metabolic pathway is well developed. The chondrocytes in the cartilage synthesize the protein and the polysaccharides and add the sulfate groups to the protein polysaccharide.

Inside some joints, most notably the knee, cartilaginous cushions reduce the space between the bones and aid in the joint's gliding motion. Such a cushion is called a meniscus or sometimes simply a cartilage. When injured and torn from its attachments, the meniscus can produce symptoms of locking or catching in the joint.

In joints that allow motion, the bone ends are held together by a fibrous tissue capsule. At certain points around the joint, the capsule is lax and thin to allow motion in a certain plane, while in other areas it is thick and resists stretching or bending. These bands of tough, thick capsule are called ligaments. A joint that is virtually surrounded by tough, thick ligaments, such as the sacroiliac, has little motion, whereas a joint with few ligaments, such as the shoulder, is free to move in almost any direction (and is, as a result, more prone to dislocation).

A joint's degree of freedom of motion is determined by the extent to which the ligaments hold the bone ends together and by the configuration of the bone ends themselves. The hip joint is a ball-and-socket joint allowing internal and external rotation as well as bending. The finger joints are typical hinge joints, with motion restricted to one plane. They can only bend (flex) and straighten (extend). Rotation is not possible because of the shape of the joint surfaces, and bending to the right or left is prevented by the strong ligaments on either side. Thus, while the amount of motion varies from joint to joint, all joints have a definite limit beyond which motion cannot occur. When a joint is forced beyond this limit, some structures are inevitably damaged. The bones forming the joint may break, or the supporting capsule and ligaments may be disrupted.

The inner surface of the joint capsule (the synovium) produces a fluid that nourishes and

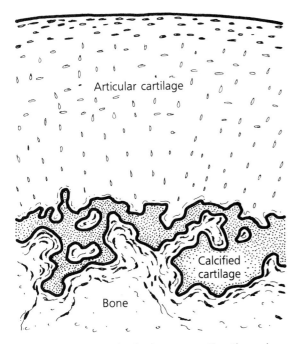

FIGURE 16:11. Histologic cross section through a gliding surface

lubricates the articular cartilage—synovial fluid. Normally only a few cubic centimeters of synovial fluid are present in a joint. The fluid is a source of nutrition for the hyaline cartilage and lubricant for the joint. With injury or disease, more fluid is produced to protect the joint, resulting in swelling inside the capsule, for example, the so-called ''water on the knee.''

Motion of a joint is produced by the action of muscles. Muscles of the extremities are attached through their tendons to two bones (Fig. 16:12A). The muscle originates from one bone, and its other end inserts into the second bone. When the muscle shortens (contracts) (Fig. 16:12B), the ends of the bones will be brought closer together, with motion at the intervening joint. Muscles on the opposite side

of the limb will relax (lengthen) to allow this motion. When motion in the opposite direction is desired, the second group of muscles contract and the first relax, rotating the joint back to its original position (Fig. 16:12C).

Skull

The skull has two major divisions, the cranium (brain case) and the face (see Fig. 33:3). The cranium is composed of a number of thick bones that fuse together to form a shell protecting the brain. The face is mostly composed of bones fused together to protect important structures as well. For example, the orbit (eye socket) is composed of two facial bones, the maxilla and the zygoma, as well as the frontal bone of the cranium, to form a solid bony rim that protrudes around the eye to protect it. The maxilla contains the upper teeth and forms the hard palate, or the roof of the mouth. The mandible, or lower jaw, is the only movable facial bone having a joint (the temporomandibular) with the cranium just in front of the ear. The nasal bone is very short, as the majority of the nose is composed of flexible cartilage.

Spinal Column

The spinal column is the central supporting structure of the body (see Fig. 33:13). The spine is composed of 33 bones called vertebrae, and is divided into five sections.

1. Cervical spine (neck)
2. Thoracic or dorsal spine (upper part of the back)
3. Lumbar spine (lower part of the back)
4. Sacral spine (part of the pelvis)
5. Coccygeal spine (coccyx, or tailbone)

The vertebrae are named according to the section of the spine in which they lie and are numbered from top to bottom. The first seven vertebrae form the cervical spine (C_1 to C_7). The next 12 vertebrae make up the thoracic or dorsal spine. One pair of ribs articulates with each of these vertebrae. The next five vertebrae form the lumbar spine, or the lower back.

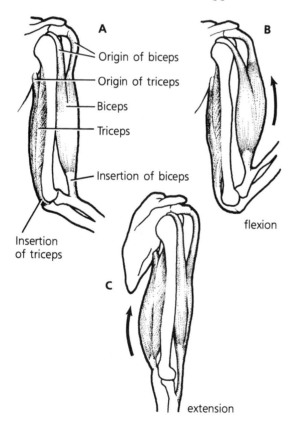

Origin of biceps
Origin of triceps
Biceps
Triceps
Insertion of biceps
Insertion of triceps
flexion
extension

FIGURE 16:12. **A** The mechanism of joint motion powered by two opposing muscles. **B** Biceps contraction flexes the elbow and **C** triceps contraction extends the elbow.

The five sacral vertebrae are fused together to form the sacrum. The sacrum is joined to the iliac bones of the pelvis with strong ligaments to form the pelvic girdle. The last four vertebrae form the coccyx, or tailbone.

The skull rests upon and articulates with the first cervical vertebra. The spinal cord is an extension of the brain composed of virtually all the nerves carrying messages between the brain and the rest of the body. The cord is contained within and protected by the vertebrae of the spinal column.

The front part of each vertebra is a round solid block of bone called the body. The back part of each vertebra forms a bony arch (Fig. 16:13). These series of arches from one vertebra to the next form a tunnel that runs the length of the spine and is called the spinal canal. The spinal canal encloses and protects the spinal cord. Nerves branch off from the spinal cord between each two vertebra to form the motor and sensory nerves of the body (Fig. 16:14).

The vertebrae are connected by ligaments, and between each vertebral body is a cushion, the intervertebral disc. These ligaments and discs allow some motion, such as turning the head or bending the trunk forward or backward, but they limit motion of the vertebrae so that the spinal cord is not injured. With a

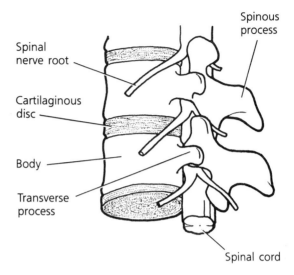

FIGURE 16:14. Relationship of the spinal nerve roots to the bony spinal column

fracture of the spine, protection for the spinal cord and its nerves may be lost. Until the fracture is stabilized, motion resulting in further injury to the spinal cord must be guarded against above all else.

The spinal column itself is virtually surrounded by muscles. However, the posterior spinous process of each vertebra can be palpated as it lies just under the skin in the midline of the back. The most prominent and most easily palpable spinous process is that of the seventh cervical vertebra at the base of the neck.

Thorax

The thorax (the rib cage) is made up of the ribs, the 12 thoracic vertebrae and the sternum (breastbone) (Fig. 16:15). There are 12 pairs of ribs, which are long, slender, curved bones. Each rib forms a joint with its respective thoracic vertebra and curves around to form the rib cage. At the front of the rib cage, the first through tenth ribs connect with the sternum through a cartilaginous bridge. For the lower five ribs, this cartilaginous bridge is called the costal arch. The sternum forms the middle part of the front of the thoracic cage.

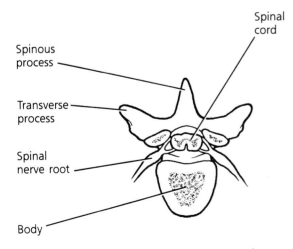

FIGURE 16:13. Top view of a thoracic vertebra showing the spinal canal protecting the spinal cord

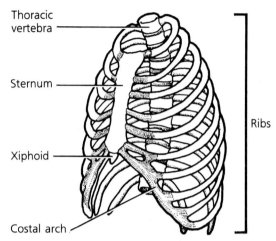

FIGURE 16:15. In the thoracic cage, twelve pairs of ribs articulate with the vertebrae in the spinal column through small joints. The first ten pairs also articulate with the sternum or the costal arch in front through a cartilaginous bridge.

This bone is approximately 7 inches long and 2 inches wide. The xiphoid process of the sternum inferiorly is cartilaginous, pointed and very tender to palpation.

Moderate pivoting of the ribs at their joints with the vertebrae allows expansion of the thorax with inspiration (breathing in). As the ribs pivot upward, the thoracic cavity becomes larger, and air is drawn into the lungs. The primary function of the rib cage is to protect the vital chest contents from injury.

Upper Extremity

The proximal portion of the upper extremity is called the shoulder girdle (Fig. 16:16) and is made up of three bones: the clavicle, the scapula and the humerus. The shoulder girdle serves to attach the upper extremity to the trunk. The upper extremity can be moved through a wide range of motion, allowing the hand to be placed in almost any position. This motion occurs at three points within the shoulder girdle: the sternoclavicular, the acromioclavicular and the glenohumeral, or true shoulder joint. Only slight motion occurs normally at the sternoclavicular and acromio-

clavicular joints, as compared to the ball-and-socket arrangement of the glenohumeral joint, which allows great freedom of motion in almost any direction.

The clavicle (collarbone) is a long, slender bone that lies just under the skin and serves as a support or prop for the upper extremity. Its medial end is attached by strong ligaments to the upper sternum, the sternoclavicular joint. Its lateral end articulates with the acromion process of the scapula at the acromioclavicular joint.

The scapula (shoulder blade) is a large, flat, triangular bone interposed between the clavicle and the humerus and held against the back of the thorax by large muscles. It has two specially named regions that form joints with the clavicle and the humerus. The acromion process anteriorly forms the scapular side of the acromioclavicular joint, and the glenoid fossa is the recess for the articulation of the humeral head laterally, forming the glenohumeral joint. The spine and medial borders of the scapula can be seen and palpated posteriorly, and the acromion process can be felt anteriorly by walking one's fingers along the clavicle and across the acromioclavicular joint.

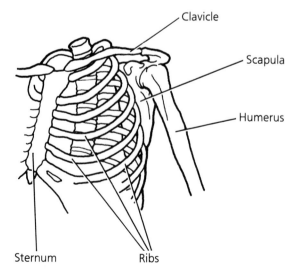

FIGURE 16:16. The shoulder girdle is composed of the clavicle, scapula, and proximal humerus.

The head of the humerus is covered by muscles forming the rounded prominence of the shoulder girdle laterally. The humerus extends from the shoulder girdle to form the supporting structure for the arm, and the distal end articulates with the radius and ulna at the elbow joint (Fig. 16:17). The humerus with its long, straight shaft serves as an effective lever for heavy lifting. The section of the upper extremity containing the humerus is called the arm.

The arm articulates with the forearm at the elbow joint. The humerus articulates with the two bones of the forearm, the radius and the ulna, in a relatively simple hinge joint. The three bony prominences comprising the elbow joint, which are all readily palpable, are the medial and lateral humeral condyles and the olecranon process of the ulna posteriorly (see Fig. 16:17).

The forearm is composed of many muscles supported by the underlying radius and ulna. At the elbow, the ulna is larger than the radius, but at the wrist the radius is the larger bone. The radius can rotate about the ulna, allowing the palm to be turned up or down. Distally in the forearm, the styloid processes of the radius and ulna lie immediately under the skin

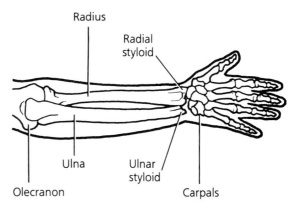

FIGURE 16:18. The forearm is made up of two bones: the radius and the ulna.

and can be easily palpated. The radial styloid is slightly longer than the ulnar styloid. The radius lies on the lateral, or thumb, side of the forearm, and the ulna is on the medial, or inner, side (Fig. 16:18).

The wrist joint is a modified ball-and-socket articulation formed by the radius and ulna proximally and several small wrist bones (the carpal bones) distally. Thus, the wrist can be flexed and extended, and also bent to each side and rotated to some degree.

Extending from the carpal bones are five metacarpals, which serve as the base for each of the digits (Fig. 16:19). The thumb (carpometacarpal) joint is a modified ball and socket, which allows the thumb to rotate as well as to flex and extend. In the thumb there are two bones beyond the metacarpal, the proximal and distal phalanges. The remaining four digits of the hand are named in order: the index, the long, the ring and the little finger. Each of these contain three phalanges. The phalanges articulate with the metacarpal and with themselves through simple hinge joints.

Pelvis and Lower Extremities

The pelvis (Fig. 16:20) is a bony ring formed posteriorly by the sacral portion of the spinal column and anterolaterally by the large, wing-like, innominate bones. Each innominate bone is formed by the fusion of three separate

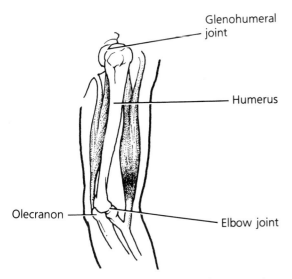

FIGURE 16:17. The upper extremity between the shoulder and elbow joint is called the arm.

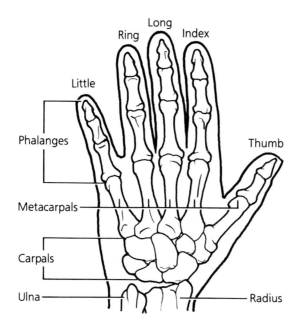

FIGURE 16:19. The bones of the wrist and hand in articulation with the radius and ulna

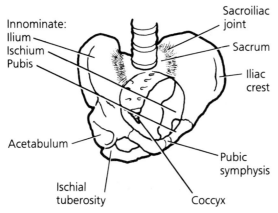

FIGURE 16:20. The sacrum firmly articulates with the two innominate bones, which are joined in front at the pubic symphysis.

bones, much as the skull is composed of several bones fused together. The three bones are: the ilium, with its iliac crest laterally; the ischium, with its ischial tuberosity palpable in the buttock; and the pubis, palpable anteriorly.

The sacrum and two innominate bones articulate at three joints: the two posterior sacroiliac joints and the anterior, midline pubic sym-

physis. All three joints allow little motion, as they are firmly held together by strong ligaments. Thus, the pelvic ring is strong and stable, designed to support the body weight and protect the structures within the pelvic cavity (the bladder, the rectum and the female reproductive organs).

On the lateral side of each innominate bone at the junction of the three component bones is the acetabulum. This is the socket portion of the hip joint, a depression into which the femoral head fits snugly.

The lower extremity consists of the thigh, the leg and the foot (Fig. 16:21). The femur (thighbone) is the longest and one of the strongest bones in the body. The femoral head proximally articulates with the acetabulum of the pelvis. This ball-and-socket joint allows flexion, extension, adduction (motion of the limb toward the midline) and abduction (motion of the limb away from the midline) as well as internal and external rotation of the lower extremity.

In the proximal, lateral thigh, the prominence of the greater trochanter of the femur can be easily palpated. This is sometimes called the "hipbone." The shaft of the femur is surrounded by muscle (the quadriceps anteriorly and the hamstrings posteriorly) and is not easily palpated. Just above the knee, however, the medial and lateral femoral condyles can be felt.

Between the thigh and the leg is the knee joint, the articulation between the distal femur and the tibia. The knee is the largest joint in the body and is essentially a hinge joint, allowing primarily flexion and extension, but also some degree of rotation. Adduction, abduction and excessive rotation are resisted by complex ligaments that are very susceptible to injury.

Anterior to the knee joint is the patella (kneecap). It lies within the tendon of the quadriceps muscle and protects the front of the knee joint from injury (Fig. 16:22A).

The leg is that portion of the lower extremity between the knee and the ankle joints (Fig. 16:22B). It has two bones, the tibia and the fibula. The tibia (shinbone) is the larger bone.

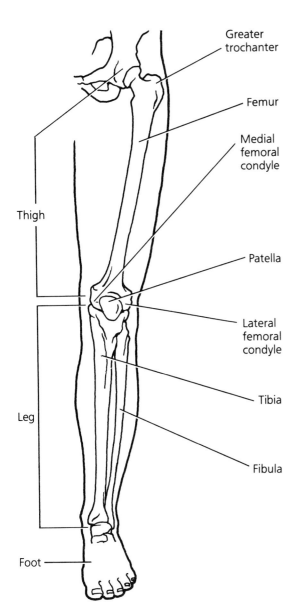

FIGURE 16:21. The lower extremity consisting of the thigh, leg and foot

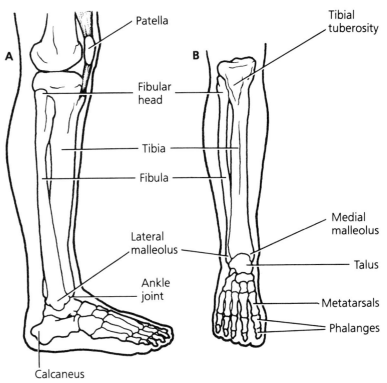

FIGURE 16:22. **A** Lateral view of the knee and leg shows the patella in the tendon of the quadriceps muscle. **B** Anterior view of the leg

It lies anterior in the leg with its anterior edge just under the skin and is easily palpable from the tibial tuberosity (the insertion of the quadriceps patellar tendon) to its medial malleolus at the ankle. The fibula lies laterally. Its head can be palpated on the lateral aspect of the knee joint, and its distal end forms the lateral malleolus of the ankle joint.

The ankle joint is a hinge that allows flexion and extension of the foot and leg. The distal end of the tibia provides a smooth articular surface for the talus (anklebone). The talus cannot rotate, abduct, or adduct because overhanging medial and lateral malleoli, along with strong ligaments, prevent such motion.

In the foot, beneath the talus, sits the calcaneus or os calcis (heelbone). The Achilles tendon inserts into the back of the calcaneus. The talus and calcaneus (as well as five other bones of the midfoot) are called tarsal bones. Five metatarsals articulate with the tarsal bones, and each gives rise to its respective toe.

FRACTURES, DISLOCATIONS AND SPRAINS

Because musculoskeletal injuries are so frequent, they must be properly evaluated and the skills necessary for their initial emergency care mastered. Appropriate emergency care of fractures and dislocations not only decreases immediate pain and reduces the possibility of shock but also improves the athlete's chances for a rapid recovery and early return to normal activity.

A fracture is any break in the continuity of a bone, ranging in severity from a simple crack to severe shattering of the bone with multiple fracture fragments (Fig. 16:23). There is no difference between a fractured and a broken bone; both terms have the same meaning.

Dislocation means disruption of a joint so that the bone ends are no longer in contact (Fig. 16:24). This can only happen if the supporting ligaments of the joint are torn, allowing the bone ends to separate.

A fracture-dislocation is a combined injury in which the joint is dislocated and a part of the bone near the joint is fractured as well (Fig. 16:25).

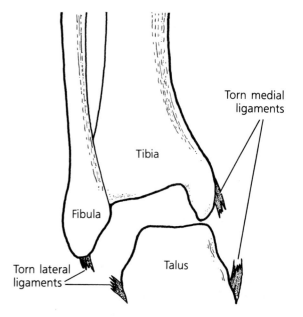

FIGURE 16:24.   Dislocated ankle joint

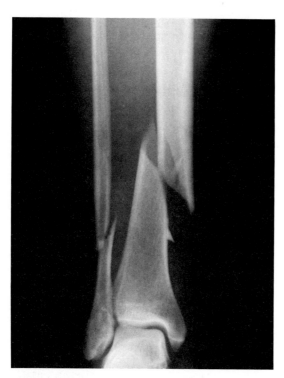

FIGURE 16:23.   X-ray of fracture fragments in a fracture of the tibia and fibula

In a sprain a joint is partially and temporarily subluxated, i.e., an incomplete or partial dislocation, and some of the supporting ligaments are stretched or torn (Fig. 16:26). The joint surfaces, however, fall back into alignment so that immediately after the injury no displacement of the joint surfaces is seen.

A strain ("muscle pull") is the stretching or tearing of a muscle. In contrast to a sprain, there is no ligament damage. The muscle fibers are partly pulled apart, producing pain and occasionally swelling and ecchymosis of the local, soft tissues.

Injury to the bones and joints is often associated with injury to surrounding soft tissue (especially the adjacent nerves and arteries) as well as to other, more remote parts of the body. Do not focus exclusively on the obviously deformed arm or leg, therefore, but make a thorough general assessment of the athlete to be certain that associated, and perhaps even more serious, injuries are not overlooked.

Causes of Musculoskeletal Injury

Substantial force is usually required to cause fractures or dislocations and may be applied

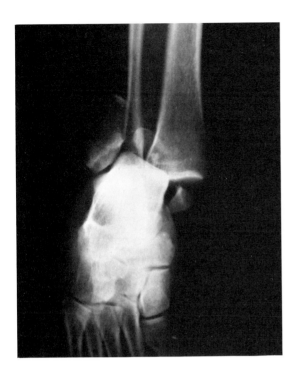

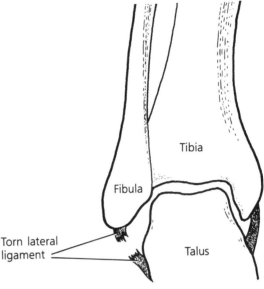

FIGURE 16:26.   Sprain of the ankle joint with one torn ligament

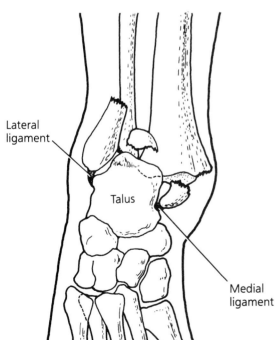

FIGURE 16:25.   Fracture-dislocation of the ankle joint. X-ray shows the talus dislocated from the distal tibia with fracture of both the medial and lateral malleoli.

to the limb in a variety of ways. Direct blows commonly cause fractures at the point of impact. For example, the patella may be fractured when it strikes a wall.

Indirect blows can also result in fracture or dislocation. In such instances, the force is applied to one part of the limb but the site of injury is some distance away from the point of impact, usually proximal. The best example is the wide range of fractures that can occur when a person falls, landing on an outstretched hand. The person may break forearm bones, the humerus or even the clavicle. Indeed, this is the most common mechanism of clavicular fracture.

Twisting forces commonly cause tibial fractures in skiers as well as knee and ankle ligament injuries. High energy injury, as in bobsled accidents or falls from heights, severely damages the skeleton, its surrounding soft tissue and the vital internal organs it protects. More than one bone in a limb may be fractured or dislocated, and multiple injuries to many parts of the body are common.

Not all fractures result from a violent force, however. Some people, especially the elderly, have weak or brittle bones, or have a localized destructive lesion, such as a cyst, that may weaken the bone so that only a slight force causes it to break.

Fractures

In the initial evaluation of a fracture the most important factor to identify is the integrity of the overlying skin and soft tissues. Thus, fractures are always classified as open (compound) or closed.

In an open fracture the overlying skin has been lacerated by the sharp bone ends protruding through the skin or by a direct blow that breaks the skin at the time of fracture. The bone may or may not be visible in the wound. The wound may be only a small puncture or a gaping hole exposing much bone and soft tissue. In a closed fracture, the bone ends have not penetrated the skin and no wound exists near the fracture.

It is extremely important to determine at once whether the fracture is open or closed. Open fractures are often more serious than closed fractures because they may be associated with greater blood loss and, since the bone is contaminated by exposure to the outside environment, they may become infected. For these reasons, all fractures should be described to emergency department personnel as open or closed so that the proper treatment can be undertaken upon arrival at the hospital.

Fractures are also described by the degree of displacement of the fragments. Nondisplaced fractures may be difficult to diagnose without x-ray films. The fracture may be thought to be only a bruise or sprain. A high index of suspicion is necessary when evaluating an injured person complaining of extremity pain. An athlete exhibiting any of the signs of fractures discussed under ''Signs and Symptoms of Fractures'' later in this chapter must be treated as if he has a fracture.

A displaced fracture produces deformity of the limb. The deformity is slight if the displacement is minimal or extreme with gross displacement of the fragments. Many different deformities may occur. Angulation and rotation of the limb distal to the fracture site are common displacements. In addition, the limb may be shortened if the fracture fragments are displaced and their ends overlap.

On occasion, special terms describe particular types of fractures.

1. A *greenstick fracture* occurs only in children, and is an incomplete fracture that passes only part way through the shaft of a bone (Fig. 16:27).
2. A *comminuted fracture* is when the bone is broken into more than two fragments (Fig. 16:28).
3. A *pathologic fracture* occurs through weak or diseased bone and is produced by minimal force.
4. A *stress* or *fatigue fracture* occurs when the bone is subjected to frequent, repeated stresses such as running or marching long distances, much as a paper clip can be broken by repeated bending back and forth.
5. An *epiphyseal fracture* occurs in growing children. It is an injury to the growth plate of a long bone that may lead to an arrest of bone growth if not properly treated (Fig. 16:29).

Signs and Symptoms of Fractures

Any athlete with a history of injury who complains of musculoskeletal pain must be suspected of having a fracture. While bone ends protruding through the skin or gross deformity of a limb makes recognizing fractures easy, many fractures are less obvious. The trainer must know the seven signs of fractures that follow. The presence of any one of these signs should arouse suspicion of a fracture, and the proper emergency treatment should be instituted.

1. *Deformity.* The limb may lie in an unnatural position, shortened, angulated or rotated at a point where no joint exists. If the deformity is unclear, the opposite limb provides a mirror image for comparison. Always compare the injured to the uninjured opposite limb when checking for deformity.

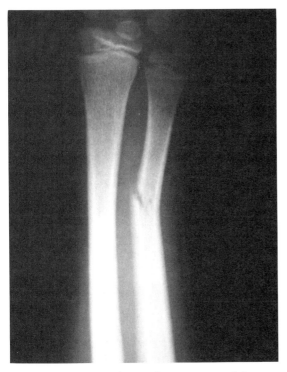

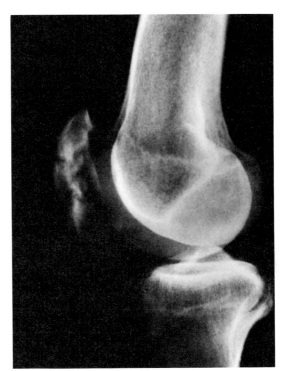

FIGURE 16:27.   An incomplete, or greenstick, fracture

2. *Tenderness.* Tenderness is usually sharply localized at the site of the break. The sensitive spot can be located by gently pressing along the bone with one fingertip. This sign is called point tenderness and is the most reliable indication of an underlying fracture.

3. *Inability to use the extremity (guarding).* An athlete with a fracture or serious injury usually guards the injured part and refuses to use it because motion increases pain. One might say that athletes attempt to splint their own fractures to minimize pain. Occasionally, nondisplaced fractures are not very painful, and some athletes may continue to use a painful limb even when fractured.

4. *Swelling and ecchymosis.* Fractures are virtually always associated with swelling and bruising of the surrounding soft tissues. These signs are present following almost any injury and are not specific for fractures. However, rapid swelling immediately after

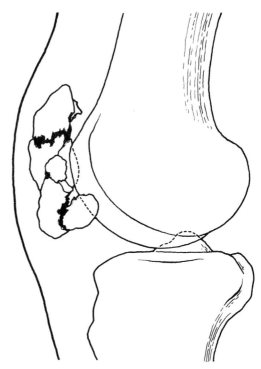

FIGURE 16:28.   A comminuted fracture of the patella. X-ray (top), line drawing (bottom)

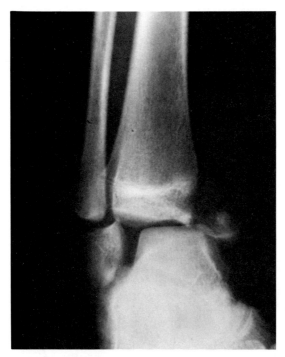

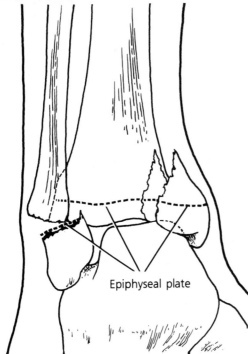

FIGURE 16:29. Transverse fracture through the growth plate of the distal fibular epiphysis and a vertical fracture through the tibial epiphysis. X-ray (top), line drawing (bottom)

Epiphyseal plate

an injury is usually due to fracture bleeding into the soft tissues from damaged blood vessels. Indeed, the swelling may mask a limb deformity produced by the broken bones. Generalized edema of the limb also occurs as a result of fracture 12 or more hours after the injury.

5. *Exposed fragments.* An open fracture's bone ends may protrude through the skin or be seen in the depths of the wound itself.

When the limb is manipulated, two additional signs of fracture may appear.

6. *Crepitus (grating).* A grating or grinding sensation called crepitus can be felt and sometimes even heard when bone ends impinge or move on one another.

7. *False motion.* Motion at a point in the limb where it usually does not occur is a positive indication of bone fracture.

Only the first five signs need to be evaluated to diagnose a fracture in the field. Crepitus and false motion are extremely painful and the limb should not be manipulated to elicit these signs. Inspection of the limb with the clothing removed reveals deformity, swelling, ecchymosis or exposed bone fragments. The athlete's unwillingness to use the affected limb indicates guarding and loss of function. Finally, palpation with one finger over the injured bone elicits point tenderness. Any of these signs is sufficient to assume limb fracture and proceed with emergency care.

Dislocation

With dislocation of a joint, injury to the supporting ligaments and capsule is so severe that the joint surfaces are completely displaced from one another. The bone ends are locked in the displaced position, making any attempted joint motion very difficult as well as very painful. Among the joints most susceptible to dislocation are the shoulder, elbow, hip, ankle and the small joints of the fingers.

The signs and symptoms of a dislocated joint are:

1. A marked deformity of the joint
2. Swelling of the joint
3. Pain at the joint, aggravated by any attempt at movement
4. Marked loss of normal joint motion (a "locked" joint)

Sprain

A joint sprain is usually produced by twisting or stretching it beyond its normal range of motion, stretching or tearing some of the supporting capsule and ligaments. A sprain is a partial dislocation. The bone ends are not completely displaced by the force of injury, and thus they can fall back into alignment when the force is removed. Therefore, the deformity of a dislocated joint is not seen with a sprain. Sprains vary in severity from a very slight injury with mild stretching of the ligaments to severe disruption of the supporting structures. Sprains are especially frequent about the knee and ankle, but any joint may be sprained. The signs of a sprain include:

1. *Tenderness.* Point tenderness can be elicited over the injured ligament just like over a fracture site.
2. *Swelling and ecchymosis.* A sprain usually results in torn blood vessels, producing immediate swelling and ecchymosis at the point of ligament injury.
3. *Inability to use the extremity.* Because of the pain of injury, the athlete cannot use the limb normally.

The signs of a sprain are the same as some signs for a fracture. Indeed, it is impossible at times to differentiate between a nondisplaced fracture and a sprain. The important point to remember is that while an injury may appear to be just a sprain, the patient must be managed as if there is a fracture.

Examination of Musculoskeletal Injuries

Three steps are essential in the examination of all athletes with injured limbs.

1. General assessment of the athlete
2. Examination of the limb
3. Evaluation of distal neurovascular function

A general, primary assessment of the injured athlete must be carried out before focusing on an injured limb. As pointed out earlier, multiple injuries occur frequently, and the athlete's general condition must first be assessed and stabilized, then the injured limb can be evaluated. Four steps should be followed.

1. *Look.* The clothing should be gently and carefully removed from the injured limb to allow a thorough inspection for:
   a. Open fracture or dislocation (remember the increased risk of open injuries)
   b. Deformity (compare with the opposite limb)
   c. Swelling and ecchymosis
2. *Ask.* Ask the athlete to move the injured limb carefully. With any major musculoskeletal injury, movement of the injured part is painful. The patient can usually localize the point of maximal discomfort. If even the slightest motion increases the pain, no further motion should be attempted. Eliminate this step when evaluating an injured person complaining of neck or back pain because even slight motion may permanently damage the spinal cord.
3. *Feel.* Gently palpate the extremities and the spine to identify point tenderness, the best indicator of an underlying fracture, dislocation or sprain.
4. *Evaluate.* The fourth, equally important, step in assessing musculoskeletal injury is a critical evaluation of the neurovascular function of the limb. Many important vessels and nerves lie close to the bone, especially around the major joints. They supply blood and nerve impulses to all the tissues distally. Any fracture or dislocation may have associated vessel or nerve injury. Neurovascular evaluation must be carried out initially and repeated every 30 minutes

until the athlete is hospitalized. It is also imperative to recheck the neurovascular status after any manipulation of the limb, such as splinting. Such manipulation might cause a bone fragment to press against or impale an important nerve or vessel. A pulseless limb may die if circulation is not restored, and such a patient must be given greater priority for emergency care.

The following neurovascular parameters should be evaluated and recorded for each injured limb.

1. *Pulse.* Palpate the pulse distal to the point of injury.
2. *Capillary filling.* Note the skin color, identifying any pallor or cyanosis. The capillary bed is best judged in the finger or toe under the nail. Firm pressure on the tip of the nail causes this bed to blanch or turn white. Upon release of the pressure, the normal pink color should return by the time it takes to say ''capillary filling.'' If the color does not return in this two-second interval, it is considered delayed, indicating impaired circulation.
3. *Sensation.* The athlete's ability to perceive light touch in the fingers or toes distal to a fracture site is a good indication that the nerve supply is intact. In the hand, check and record touch sensation on the pulp of the index and little fingers. In the foot, check and record feeling on the pulp of the great toe and on the dorsum of the foot laterally.
4. *Motor function.* When an injury is proximal to the hand or foot, muscular activity should be estimated. This can be done simply by having the athlete open and close the hand for the upper extremity and wiggle the toes or move the foot up for the lower extremity. Sometimes such motion produces pain at the injury site. If so, do not persist with this part of the examination.

In the unconscious athlete, many of the steps listed cannot be carried out because they require patient cooperation. After the primary assessment is completed and vital functions are stabilized, any limb deformity, swelling, ecchymosis or false motion should be considered evidence of a fracture and treated as such. The distal pulses and capillary filling can still be monitored in the unconscious, injured patient. Any unconscious, injured athlete should be assumed to have a spinal fracture requiring spine board immobilization.

Treatment of Musculoskeletal Injuries

Emergency management of fractures, dislocations and sprains takes place after the injured athlete's vital functions are assessed and stabilized. All open wounds should be covered completely with a dry, sterile dressing and local pressure applied to control bleeding. Once a sterile compression dressing is applied to an open fracture, it should be managed in the same way as a closed fracture—by limb alignment and appropriate splinting. Emergency department personnel should be notified of all open wounds that have been so dressed and splinted.

All fractures, dislocations and sprains should be splinted before the athlete is moved unless the athlete's life is immediately threatened. Splinting facilitates the transfer and transportation of the patient and also helps prevent:

1. Motion of fracture fragments, a dislocated joint or a soft tissue injury, thus reducing pain
2. Further damage of muscle, spinal cord, peripheral nerves and blood vessels by the broken bone ends
3. Laceration of the skin by the broken bones, converting a closed fracture into an open one
4. Restriction of distal blood flow resulting from pressure of the bone ends on blood vessels
5. Excessive bleeding into the tissues at the fracture site

A splint can be fashioned from any material. It is simply a device to prevent the injured part from moving. However, an adequate supply of standard commercial splints should be on hand (Fig. 16:30) and improvisation should only be necessary occasionally. The general rules of splinting follow.

1. It is usually best to remove clothing from the area of any suspected fracture or dislocation.
2. Note and record the circulatory and neurological (motion and sensation) status distal to the site of injury.
3. In a fracture, the splint should immobilize the joint above and the joint below the fracture.
4. In a dislocation or sprain, the splint should immobilize the bone above and the bone below the injured joint.
5. During splint application, move the limb as little as possible.
6. Straighten a severely deformed limb with constant, gentle, manual traction so that the limb can be incorporated into a splint.
7. If gentle traction increases the patient's pain substantially or if the limb resists alignment, splint the limb in the position of deformity.
8. In all suspected neck and spine injuries, correct the deformity only as much as necessary to eliminate airway obstruction and to allow effective application of a splint.
9. Cover all wounds with a dry, sterile dressing before applying a splint.
10. Pad the splints to prevent local pressure.
11. Do not move or transport patients before splinting extremity injuries.
12. When in doubt, SPLINT.

Rules 6 and 7 refer to the use of traction in managing musculoskeletal injury. Traction is defined as the action of drawing or pulling on an object. Traction, especially if excessive, can be very harmful to an injured limb. When applied correctly, however, traction stabilizes the bone fragments and improves overall alignment. Do not attempt to "reduce" the fracture

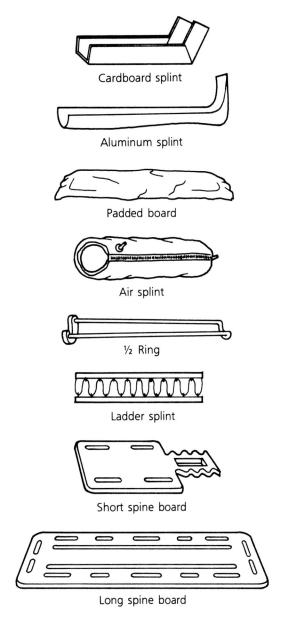

FIGURE 16:30. A good selection and adequate number of splints should be readily available.

or force all of the fragments back into anatomic alignment. This is the physician's responsibility. In the field, the goals of traction are:

1. Stabilize the fracture fragments to prevent excessive movement
2. Align the limb sufficiently to allow it to be placed in a splint

The amount of pull required to accomplish this varies but rarely will exceed 15 pounds. This is gentle traction, and the least amount of force necessary is the amount that should be employed. Hanging a weight of 10 or 15 pounds on a rope through a pulley and then pulling the weight upward 4 to 6 inches gives a feel for the force of gentle traction (Fig. 16:31).

Grasp the foot or hand firmly so that, once the traction pull is applied, it is not released until the limb is splinted. The direction of pull is always along the long axis of the limb. Imagine where the normal uninjured limb should lie and pull along the line of that normal imaginary limb. The alignment of the deformed, injured limb will then approximate this posture as gentle traction is applied (Fig. 16:32).

Grasping the distal limb and the initial pull of traction usually cause slight discomfort to the patient as the fragments move. This initial discomfort quickly subsides, and further gen-

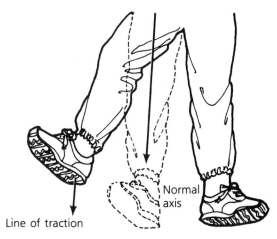

FIGURE 16:32. Apply gentle traction to the limb parallel to the normal axis of the deformed limb.

tle traction may then be applied. If the patient strongly resists this traction or if it causes more pain, stop the traction and splint the limb in the deformed position.

Splints

While splints are made from many different materials, there are three basic types: rigid, soft and traction. If no other splinting materials are available, the arm can be bound to the chest and an injured leg can be splinted to the uninjured leg to provide at least temporary stability.

Rigid Splints

Rigid splints are made from firm material and are applied to the sides, front or back of an injured extremity to prevent motion at the injury site. Common examples include padded board splints, molded plastic and metal splints, padded wire ladder splints and folded cardboard splints.

To apply rigid splints, two trainers should follow these steps.

1. One trainer gently supports the limb and applies steady traction until the splint is completely applied.
2. The second trainer places the rigid splint under or alongside the limb.

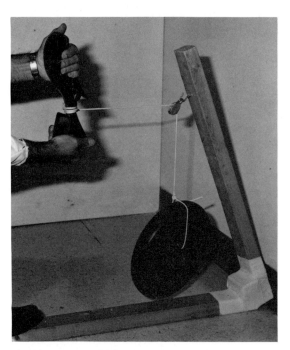

FIGURE 16:31. Pulling against a weight tied through a pulley to a shoe conveys a sense of traction force.

3. Place padding to assure even pressure and even contact between the limb and the splint, with particular attention to bony prominences.
4. Apply bindings to hold the splint securely to the limb.
5. After application, check and record distal circulation.

With severe deformities, as seen with most dislocations, or when gentle traction produces resistance or pain, the deformed limb must be splinted in the position of deformity. This can be done efficiently by applying padded board splints to each side of the limb, secured with soft roller bandages.

Soft Splints

The most commonly used soft splint is the precontoured, inflatable, clear plastic air splint. These splints are available in a variety of sizes and shapes with or without a zipper that runs the length of the splint. After application, inflate the splint by mouth, never with a pump. The air splint is comfortable to the patient, provides uniform contact and has the added advantage of applying gentle pressure on a bleeding wound.

The air splint has some disadvantages, particularly in cold weather areas. The zipper can become stuck, clogged with dirt or frozen. With extreme temperature changes, the air pressure in the splint varies, decreasing with cold and increasing with warmth.

The method of applying an air splint depends on whether it has a zipper. With either type, cover all wounds first with a dry, sterile dressing. With zipper splints hold the injured limb slightly off the ground with gentle traction, and place the open, deflated splint around the limb, zip it up and inflate it by mouth.

With the nonzipper or partial zipper type follow these steps.

1. The first trainer puts his arm through the splint, then grasps the hand or foot of the injured limb.
2. The second trainer then supports the athlete's injured limb.

3. The first trainer then applies gentle traction to the hand or foot while sliding the splint onto the injured limb.
4. Always include the hand or foot of the limb in the splint.
5. Inflate the splint by mouth.

With either type of air splint, the pressure in the splint after application must be tested. With proper inflation, a firm pinch between the thumb and index finger near the edge of the splint should just compress the walls of the splint together. As with any splint, distal neurovascular function must be checked and recorded after application.

Other soft splints such as pillow splints and the sling and swathe are used extensively and are discussed elsewhere.

Traction Splints

A traction splint holds a lower extremity fracture or dislocation immobile and exerts steady longitudinal pull on the extremity. The traction splint is usually called a Thomas splint, after the famous orthopedic surgeon, Sir Hugh Owen Thomas. Most commercial splints can be used on either lower extremity. When traction is applied to the foot through the ankle hitch, countertraction is applied by the padded half-ring, which seats against the ischial tuberosity of the patient's pelvis. Because countertraction is essential to proper function of the splint, it is not suitable for the upper extremity, as the major nerves and blood vessels in the axilla cannot tolerate countertraction.

Two trainers working together are necessary to properly apply the traction splint. It is impossible for one person to apply this splint alone. The precise technique in applying the traction splint is extremely important. The team of trainers should practice the steps over and over until the sequence and necessary teamwork are routine. Seven steps must be followed (Fig. 16:33).

1. Place the splint beside the athlete's uninjured leg and adjust it to the proper length—the ring at the ischial tuberosity

and the splint extending 12 inches beyond the foot (Fig. 16:33A). Open and adjust the Velcro support straps, which should be positioned at the midthigh, above the knee, below the knee and above the ankle.

2. Cut open the athlete's trouser leg or otherwise expose the injured lower extremity to see exactly what is being done.

3. One trainer stabilizes the injured limb to prevent motion at the fracture site, while the second trainer fastens an ankle hitch of the correct size about the athlete's ankle and foot (Fig. 16:33B). The shoe is customarily left on the foot.

4. The first trainer then supports the leg at the site of suspected injury while the second trainer simultaneously applies gentle longitudinal traction manually to the ankle hitch and foot. Apply only enough traction to align the limb grossly so that it fits into the splint. Do not try to align the fracture fragments anatomically.

5. The first trainer then slides the splint into position under the patient's limb (Fig. 16:33C), gently applies the ischial strap (Fig. 16:33D) and pads the groin.

6. While the second trainer maintains traction, the first trainer connects the loops of the ankle hitch to the end of the splint (Fig. 16:33E). Gentle traction is then applied to the connecting strap between the ankle hitch and the splint, just enough to maintain the limb alignment. Some splints come with a ratchet mechanism to tighten the strap, which can generate an excessive amount of force, overstretching the limb and injuring the patient.

7. After proper traction is applied, fasten the support straps so that the limb is held securely to the splint (Fig. 16:33F).

Traction splints are used primarily, and to the best advantage, in securing fractures of the femoral or tibial shafts. Fractures about the hip or knee can also be effectively splinted with this device if gentle traction on the limb does not decrease the distal pulse or produce pain as the limb is aligned.

Because traction splints immobilize the limb by producing countertraction in the ischium and the groin, these areas must be well padded and excessive pressure avoided, especially on external genitalia.

Commercial padded ankle hitches are readily available and must be used rather than pieces of rope, cord or tape. Such improvised hitches are painful and can obstruct circulation in the foot.

Transportation

Once the injured limb is adequately splinted, the patient is ready to be transferred to a litter and transported. The best position for the patient varies, depending upon the type of injury. With most isolated upper extremity fractures, the patient is most comfortable in a semiseated position rather than lying flat. Either position is acceptable. With lower extremity injuries, the patient should lie supine with the limb elevated slightly, about 6 inches, to minimize swelling. In all cases, the injured limb must not be allowed to flop about or dangle off the edge of the litter.

Swelling can be minimized to some degree by applying cold packs, if readily available, to the splinted injury site. Avoid placing the cold pack directly on the skin or other tissues.

Very few, if any, musculoskeletal injuries require excessively rapid ambulance transportation. Once dressed and splinted, the limb is stable, and orderly transportation can be undertaken. With the pulseless limb, a sense of urgency develops, and the patient must be given a higher priority for transport. If the hospital is only a few minutes away, reckless speeding to the emergency department makes little or no difference in the patient's eventual outcome. When the treatment facility is an hour or more away, however, evacuation of the patient via helicopter or rapid ground transportation should be given a high priority.

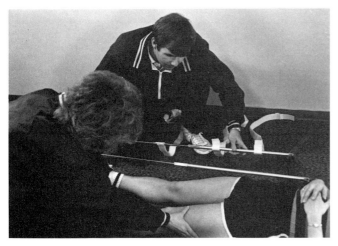

FIGURE 16:33A.

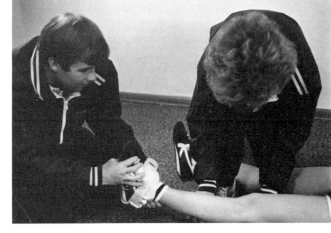

FIGURE 16:33B.

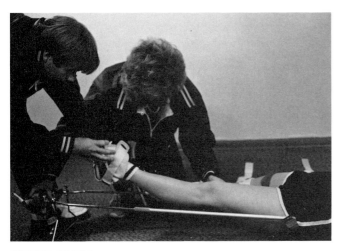

FIGURE 16:33C.

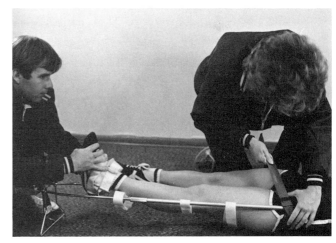

FIGURE 16:33D.

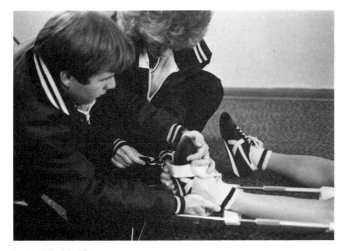

FIGURE 16:33E.

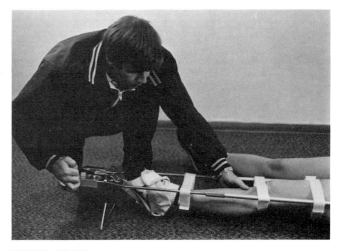

FIGURE 16:33F.

Introduction to Biomechanics

17

The athlete performing intense activity uses large muscular forces that result not only in good athletic performance but also in very large loads on bones and joints. Biomechanics relates forces and motion. Methods exist for computing muscle, bone, ligamentous and joint forces. This chapter describes some fundamental laws and definitions of biomechanics.

EFFECTS OF FORCE

When force is applied to a body, it has two effects: the first is external and causes the body to accelerate; the second is internal and produces a deformation or state of mechanical strain in the body. For example, when a tennis racket hits a tennis ball, the two effects are easily seen under high-speed photography. The external effect accelerates the tennis ball, which goes over the net into the opposite court. The internal effect, or the deformation, changes the ball's shape when the racket's strings flatten one surface of the ball. These two effects occur whenever forces are applied to bodies. In the case of a boxer struck by a heavy blow, the external effect of the force is easily seen as the boxer is knocked down and accelerated to the mat. Not so apparent is the internal effect or change in shape of the boxer's face as the glove strikes it. The acceleration and the internal deformation are caused by forces. A force is an action that changes the state or motion of a body to which it is applied.

Most of our actions involve forces acting through a lever arm, producing a moment of torque. A moment of torque is a force acting through a distance, or more precisely defined, the perpendicular distance from the line of force application to the center of motion or fulcrum of the structure. Forces are defined in terms of pound of force or in metric terms, newtons. Moments of torques are defined in terms of foot-pounds or newton-meters. The relationship between force and motion is summed up in two mathematical relationships:

$$F = ma \quad Force \text{ (F) equals } mass \text{ (m) times } acceleration \text{ (a)}$$

$$T = Ia \quad Torque \text{ (T) equals moment of } inertia \text{ (I) times } acceleration$$

Moment of inertia is defined as a measure of resistance to change. By finding the linear acceleration in the case of forces, or the angular acceleration in the case of torques, the forces about a human joint during various athletic activities can be found. For example, when someone punts a football, stroboscopic or motion pictures can help reveal acceleration. Once the moment of inertia is known, the torque can be calculated from the formula:

$T = Ia$ Where
T is the torque expressed in foot-pounds (ft-lbs) or newton-meters (N-m)
I is the mass moment of inertia expressed in newton-meters times seconds squared (N-m sec^2)
a is the angular acceleration expressed in radians per second squared (r/sec^2)

Not only is the torque a product of the mass moment of inertia and the angular acceleration of the body part, but it is also a product of the main muscle forces accelerating the body part and the perpendicular distance of the force from the instant center of the joint (lever arm). Thus:

$$T = Fd \quad \text{where}$$

F is force expressed in pounds or newtons

d is perpendicular distance expressed in feet or meters

Since T is known and d can be measured on the body part from the line application of the force to the instant center of the joint, the equation can be solved for F. When F has been calculated, the remaining problem can be solved like a static problem using simplified techniques from biomechanics to determine the minimum magnitude of the joint reaction force acting on the joint at a certain instant in time.

An example illustrates the use of dynamic analysis to calculate the joint reaction force on the tibiofemoral joint at a particular instant in time during dynamic activity, that of kicking a football. A stroboscopic film of the knee and lower leg was taken, and the maximal angular acceleration was found to occur at the instant the foot struck the ball; the lower leg was almost vertical at this instant. From the film the maximal angular acceleration was computed to be 453 radians per second squared. From anthropometric data tables, the mass moment of inertia for the lower leg was determined to be 0.35 newton-meters times seconds squared. The torque about the tibiofemoral joint was calculated according to the equation torque equals mass moment of inertia times angular acceleration ($T = Ia$):

$$(0.35 \text{ N-m sec}^2) \times (453 \text{ r/sec}^2) = 158.5 \text{ N-m}$$

After the torque was determined to be 158.5 newton-meters and the perpendicular distance from the subject's patellar tendon to the instant center for the tibiofemoral joint was found to be 0.05 meters, the muscle force acting on the joint through the patellar tendon was calculated using the equation torque equals force times distance ($T = Fd$):

$$158.5 \text{ N-m} = F \times 0.05 \text{ m}$$

$$F = \frac{158.5 \text{ N-m}}{0.05 \text{ m}}$$

$$F = 3{,}170 \text{ N}$$

The maximal force exerted by the quadriceps muscle during the kicking motion was 3,170 newtons. Thus, very large forces are produced during athletic activities.

ENERGY

Another concept of great interest to the athletic trainer is that of energy. There are three types of energy: potential, kinetic and work. Potential energy (PE) is equal to the mass times the height (h) above the base ($PE = mh$). Kinetic energy (KE) is the energy of a moving body, and it equals one half of the mass times the velocity (v) squared ($KE = \frac{1}{2}mv^2$). Work energy is the energy stored in a structure under deformation and is defined as the force times the distance a body is deformed.

During athletic activity there is a constant conversion from potential energy to kinetic energy to work energy back to kinetic energy or to potential energy. For instance, a skier standing on top of a hill has very large potential energy. He starts to come down the hill by converting his potential energy into kinetic energy. As he increases in speed he may feel uncomfortable and turn up into the hill again, converting some of the kinetic energy back into potential energy as he goes upward on the hill. Alternatively, he converts some kinetic energy into work energy by deforming his skis and deforming the snow.

Much more energy is involved in athletic and other activities than is required to break a single bone. For instance, it requires only 80 kilogram-centimeters (kg cm) of energy to fracture a tibia, although a skier going 30 kilometers per hour possesses 2,000 kg cm of energy. Large, fast athletes performing at high levels must be able to dissipate large amounts of kinetic energy without injury.

BONE STRENGTH AND STIFFNESS

All biological materials are viscoelastic; i.e., their deformation behavior is time dependent. They are also anisotropic, i.e., their properties are specific to the direction of force application. In the case of bones, this means that the strength of the material depends upon the rate that it is loaded and the direction of loading.

Strength and stiffness are the important mechanical properties of bone. These properties can best be understood for bone or any other material by examining the material under loading. When a load in a known direction is placed on a structure, the deformation of that structure can be measured and plotted on a load-deformation curve, and the strength and stiffness of the structure can be determined.

A hypothetical load-deformation curve for a somewhat pliable material is shown in Figure 17:1. When a load is applied within the elastic region of the curve (A-B area in Fig. 17:1) and is then released, the structure returns to its original shape; i.e., no permanent deformation occurs. If loading is continued, some regions of the material begin to yield permanently (B-C area in Fig. 17:1). If loading continues past this yield point and into the nonelastic region of the curve, permanent deformation results. If loading in the nonelastic region continues, an ultimate failure point for the structure is reached.

Load Deformation Curve

The load-deformation curve shows three parameters for determining the strength of a structure.

1. The load the structure can sustain before failure
2. The deformation it can sustain before failure
3. The energy it can store before failure

On the curve, the ultimate failure point indicates the strength in terms of load and deformation. The size of the area under the entire curve indicates strength in terms of energy storage. In addition, the slope of the curve in the elastic region indicates the stiffness of the structure.

The load-deformation curve is useful for determining the strength and stiffness of whole structures of various sizes, shapes and material compositions. To examine the mechanical behavior of the material that composes a structure and to compare the mechanical behavior of different materials, test specimens and testing conditions must be standardized. When samples of standardized size and shape are tested, the load per unit area and the amount of deformation in terms of length can be determined. The curve that is generated is called the stress-strain curve.

Stress and Strain

Stress is load per unit area that develops on a plane surface within a structure in response to externally applied loads. It is expressed in force units per area. The three units most commonly used for measuring stress in bone samples are newtons per centimeter squared (N/cm^2); newtons per meter squared, or pascals (N/m^2; Pa); and mega-newtons per meter squared, or megapascals (MN/m^2;

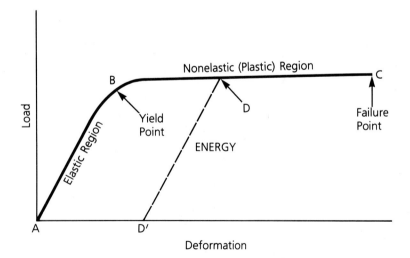

FIGURE 17:1. Load-deformation curve for a somewhat pliable material. The amount of permanent deformation that occurs if the structure is loaded to point D and then unloaded is represented by the distance between A and D. B represents the yield point at which deformation occurs.

MPa). Pounds per inch squared (psi) are also used.

Strain is the deformation at a point in a structure under loading. Two basic types of strain exist: normal strain, which is a change in length, and shear strain, which is a change in angle. Normal strain is the amount of deformation (lengthening or shortening divided by the structure's original length). It is a non-dimensional parameter expressed as a percentage (for example, centimeter per centimeter). Shear strain, under conditions of torque loading, is the amount of angular deformation in a structure, i.e., the amount that the original angle of the structure changes. It is expressed in radians (one radian equals approximately 57.3°).

Stress-Strain Curve

Stress and strain values can be obtained for bone by placing a standard specimen of bone tissue in a testing jig and loading it to failure

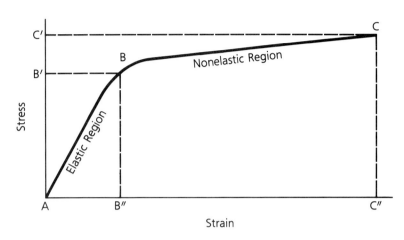

FIGURE 17:3. Stress-strain curve for cortical bone tested in tension.
Yield point (B)—point past which some permanent deformation of the bone occurs
Yield stress (B')—load per unit area that the bone sample sustained before nonelastic deformation
Yield strain (B")—amount of deformation that the sample sustained before nonelastic deformation. The strain at any point in the elastic region of the curve is proportional to the stress at this point.
Ultimate failure point (C)—the point past which the sample failed
Ultimate stress (C')—load per unit area that the sample sustained before failure
Ultimate strain (C")—amount of deformation that the sample sustained before failure

(Fig. 17:2). The strain that results can be illustrated in a stress-strain curve (Fig. 17:3). The regions of the stress-strain curve are similar to those of the load-deformation curve. Loads in the elastic region do not cause permanent deformation or strain. Once the yield point is exceeded, however, permanent deformation occurs. The stiffness of the material is represented by the slope of the curve in the elastic region. The strength in terms of energy storage is represented by the area under the entire curve, and this is called the toughness of the material.

Stress-strain curves for metal, glass and bone illustrate the differences in mechanical behavior among these materials (Fig. 17:4). Variations in stiffness are reflected by differences in the slope of the curve in the elastic region. Metal has the steepest slope and is thus the stiffest material. A value for stiffness is obtained by dividing the stress at any point in the elastic portion of the curve by the strain

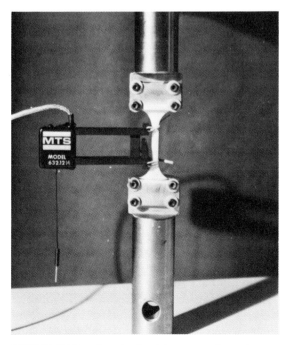

FIGURE 17:2. Standardized bone specimen in a testing machine. The strain between the two gauge arms is measured with a strain gauge. The stress is calculated from the total load measure.

at that point. This value is called the modulus of elasticity (Young's modulus). Stiffer materials have higher moduli.

The elastic portion of the stress-strain curve for metal is a straight line, indicating linearly elastic behavior. Precise testing has shown that the elastic portion of the curve for bone is not straight but curves slightly, indicating that bone is not linearly elastic in its behavior. Some yielding may occur when the bone is loaded in the elastic region. The difference in nonelastic behavior for the two materials is due to differences in micromechanical events during mechanical yielding. Yielding in bone (tested in tension) is caused by debonding of the osteons and microfracture and the role of the organic components. Yielding in metal (tested in tension) is caused by plastic flow and formation of slip lines. Slip lines are formed when the planes of atoms of the atomic lattice structure dislocate relative to one another.

Materials are classified as brittle or ductile depending on the amount of deformation they undergo before failure. Glass, a typical brittle material, deforms little before failure as indicated by the absence of a nonelastic (plastic)

region on the stress-strain curve (see Fig. 17:4). Soft metal, a typical ductile material, deforms extensively before failure, as indicated by a long, nonelastic (plastic) region on the curve (see Fig. 17:4). The fracture surfaces of the two types of material reflect this difference in amount of deformation (Fig. 17:5). A ductile material that is pieced together after fracture will not conform to its original shape, whereas brittle material will.

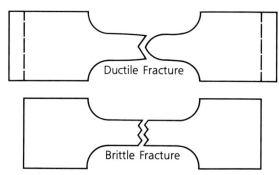

FIGURE 17:5. Fracture surfaces of a ductile and a brittle material. The dotted lines on the ductile material indicate the original length of the structure, before deformation. The brittle material deformed very little before fracture.

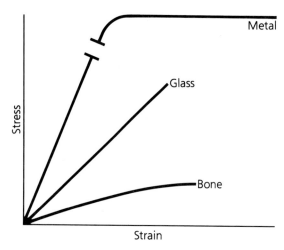

FIGURE 17:4. Stress-strain curves for three materials: metal, glass and bone. The elastic portion of the graph for bone is slightly curved, indicating that bone is not linearly elastic in its behavior. Soft metal is a ductile material and therefore has no plastic region.

SOFT TISSUES UNDER LOADING

The soft tissues that make up ligaments, tendons and capsules exhibit a specific type of behavior under loading. When a ligament is subjected to loading, microfailure takes place even before the yield point is reached. When the yield point is exceeded, the ligament begins to undergo gross failure, and simultaneously the joint begins to displace abnormally. Because failure of a ligament leads to a large joint displacement, the surrounding structures such as the joint capsule and other ligaments may also be damaged. In a clinical test, the anterior drawer test, force was applied to a cadaver knee up to the point of anterior cruciate ligament failure and a ligament-bone preparation was tested. Figure 17:6 depicts the progressive failure of this ligament and displacement of the joint. At maximum load the joint had dis-

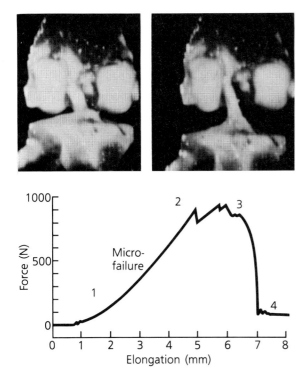

FIGURE 17:6. Progressive failure of the anterior cruciate ligament. Almost 8 mm of joint displacement took place before the ligament reached complete failure. Courtesy of Frank R. Noyes, M.D. and Edward S. Grood, Ph.D.

placed several millimeters. The ligament was still in continuity even though it had undergone extensive macro- and microfailure and extensive elongation. The force-elongation curve generated during this experiment indicates where microfailure of the ligament begins.

The results of this in vitro test can be correlated with clinical findings. In Figure 17:7, the curve for the experimental study is divided into three regions. The first region corresponds to the amount of load placed on a ligament during tests of joint stability performed clinically. The second region corresponds to the amount of load placed on the ligament during physiological activity. The third region corresponds to the amount of load imposed on the ligament from the beginning of microfailure to complete rupture.

Ligament Injuries

Ligament injuries fall into three categories depending on their severity. Injuries in the first category produce negligible clinical symptoms. Some pain is felt, but no joint instability can be detected clinically. However, microfailure of the collagen fibers may have occurred.

Injuries in the second category produce severe pain and some joint instability if detected clinically. Progressive failure of the collagen fibers has taken place, producing partial ligament rupture. The strength and stiffness of the ligament may be decreased by 50% or more. Often the joint instability produced by a partial rupture of a ligament is masked by muscle activity, and thus the clinical test for joint stability is usually performed under anesthesia.

Injuries in the third category produce severe pain during the course of trauma with less pain after injury. Clinically the joint is found to be completely unstable. Most collagen fibers have ruptured, but a few may still be intact, giving the ligament the appearance of continuity although it is unable to support any loads.

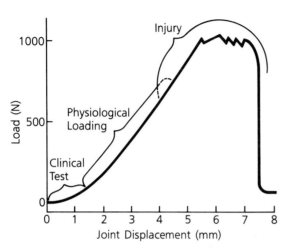

FIGURE 17:7. The curve in Figure 17:6 converted to a load-displacement curve and divided into three regions that correlate with clinical findings.

Loading of a joint that is unstable due to ligament or joint capsule rupture produces abnormally high stresses on the joint cartilage. This abnormal type of loading of the cartilage in the knee has been correlated with osteoarthritis in humans and animals.

MUSCLES UNDER LOADING

The strength of bone is influenced not only by the loading rate and loading direction, but also by muscle activity. When bone is loaded in vivo, contraction of the muscles attached to the bone substantially alters the magnitude and type of stress within the bone. This muscle contraction can decrease or eliminate tensile stress in the bone by producing compressive stresses that either partially or totally neutralize the tensile stresses.

The effect of muscle contraction can be illustrated in a tibia subjected to three-point bending. Figure 17:8A represents the leg of a skier who is falling forward, subjecting his tibia to a bending moment. High tensile stress is produced on the posterior aspect of this tibia, and high compressive stress acts on the anterior aspect. Contraction of the triceps surae muscles produces a high compressive stress on the posterior aspect (Fig. 17:8B), neutralizing

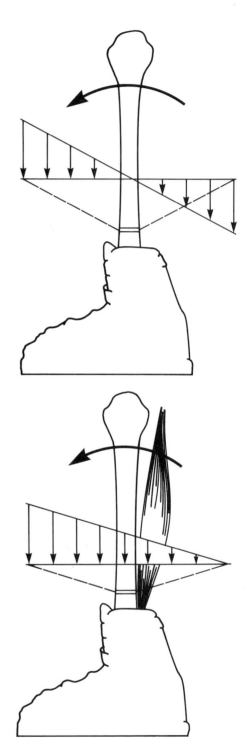

FIGURE 17:8. **A** Distribution of compressive and tensile stresses in a tibia subjected to three-point bending. **B** Contraction of the triceps surae muscle produces high compressive stress on the posterior aspect, neutralizing the high tensile stress.

the high tensile stress and thereby protecting the tibia from failure in tension. This muscle contraction may result in a higher compressive stress on the anterior surface of the tibia. Adult bone can usually withstand this stress, but immature bone, which is weaker, may fail in compression.

Muscle contraction produces a similar effect on the hip joint (Fig. 17:9). During locomotion, bending moments are applied to the femoral neck, and tensile stress is produced on the superior cortex. Contraction of the gluteus medius muscle produces compressive stress that neutralizes this tensile stress, with the net result that neither compressive nor tensile stress acts on the superior cortex. Thus, the muscle contraction allows the femoral neck to sustain higher loads than would otherwise be possible.

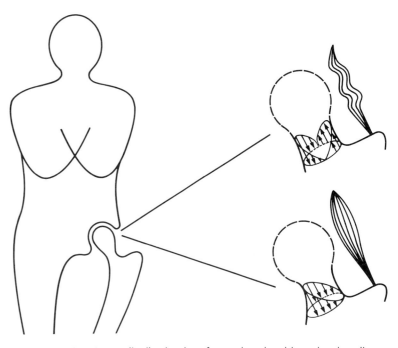

FIGURE 17:9. Stress distribution in a femoral neck subjected to bending.

FRACTURE OF BONE UNDER REPETITIVE LOADING

Bone fracture that occurs after many loading cycles is called a fatigue fracture. Fatigue fractures occur when terrain, foot wear or exercise regimen changes. To understand fatigue fractures one must understand the interrelationships of the mechanical properties of bone, the properties of muscle, the effect of muscle activity on loading of bones and the cyclic properties of loading. Under excessive compression loading, bone fails because many small microcracks are produced. Under excessive tensial load of the bone, the osteons are debonded at the cement lines. Either tension failure of bone, compression failure or combinations of these will take place.

Fractures can be produced by a single load, or the repeated application of a smaller load. A fatigue fracture is typically produced by either a few high loads or many small or normal loads.

The interplay of the load and repetition for all materials can be plotted on a fatigue curve (Fig. 17:10). For some materials (some metals, for example), the fatigue curve is asymptotic, indicating that if the load is kept below a cer-

tain level, the material will remain intact, no matter how large the number of repetitions. For bone tested in vitro, the curve may not be asymptotic. Fatigue microfractures may be created in bone subjected to low repetitive loads.

Testing of bone in vitro also reveals that bone fatigues rapidly when load or deformation approaches the yield strength of the bone; that is, the number of repetitions needed to produce a fracture greatly diminishes.

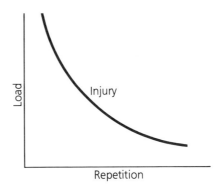

FIGURE 17:10. The interplay of load and repetition represented on a fatigue curve.

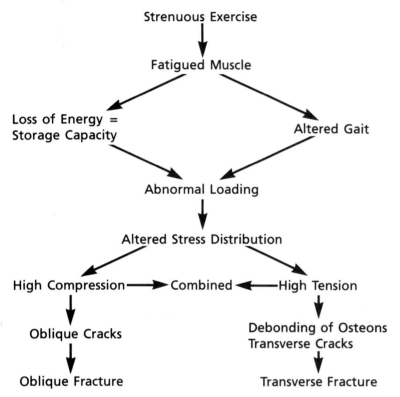

FIGURE 17:11. Schemata for effective exercise of bone fatigue

or both sides of the bone. Failure on the tensile side results in a transverse crack, and the bone may proceed rapidly to complete fracture. Fatigue fracture on the compressive side appears to be produced more slowly; the remodeling is less easily out-paced by the fatigue process, and the bone may not proceed to complete fracture. A schemata for effective exercise of bone fatigue is shown in Figure 17:11.

KINEMATICS

Kinematics data are used to analyze motion in a joint. Internal joint function can be determined with an instant center analysis. For more complex joints a complex rotation or a screw axis must also be determined. The instant center technique permits the center of motion to be determined for a joint in any range of motion.

In the knee, surface joint motion occurs between the tibia and femoral condyles and between the femoral condyles and the patella. The instant center locations for the range of knee motion for 0 to 90° have been determined. Tangential sliding at the joint surface was found in all cases. An investigation of the instant center pathway for the tibiofemoral joint in knees with internal derangements found that in all cases the instant center was displaced from the normal position during some portion of the motion examined. The abnormal instant center pathway for one subject, a 35-year-old man with a bucket handle derangement, is shown in Figure 17:12. If the knee is extended and flexed about a displaced instant center, the tibiofemoral joint surfaces do not slide (tangentially) throughout the range of motion but become either distracted or compressed (Figs. 17:13A, B). Such a knee is analogous to a door with a bent hinge, which no longer fits into the door jamb.

If the knee is continually forced to move about a displaced instant center, it will gradually adjust to this situation by either stretching the ligament and supporting structures of the joint or exerting abnormally high forces on the articular surfaces.

In repetitive loading of living bone, not only does the amount of load and the number of repetitions affect the fatigue process, but also the frequency of loading. Since living bone is self-repairing, a fatigue fracture only results when the remodeling process is outpaced by the fatigue process, that is, when the frequency of loading precludes the remodeling necessary to prevent failure.

Fatigue fractures are usually sustained during continuous, strenuous physical activity. Such activity causes the muscles to lose their tone or become fatigued. When muscles "fatigue," their ability to contract is reduced; as a result, they are less able to store energy and thus to neutralize the stress imposed on the bone. The resulting alteration of the stress distribution in the bone causes abnormally high loads to be imposed on the bone, and a fatigue fracture may be produced. Failure may occur on the tensile side, the compressive side,

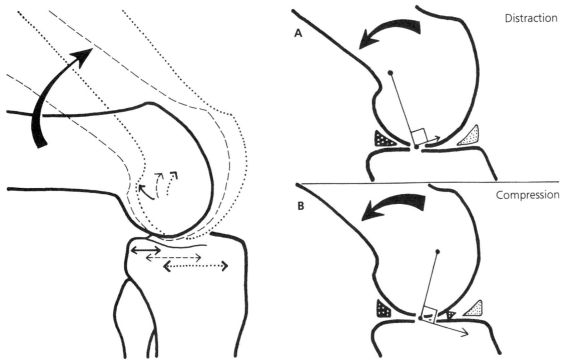

FIGURE 17:12. In this "bucket handle" derangement, the abnormal center jumps at full extension of the knee.

FIGURE 17:13. Surface motion in two tibiofemoral joints with displaced instant centers. The right angle lines indicate the direction of displacement of the contact points. **A** With further flexion the tibiofemoral joint is distracted (arrow). **B** With further flexion the joint is compressed (arrow).

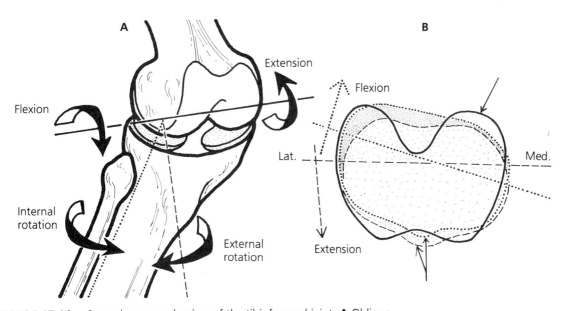

FIGURE 17:14. Screw-home mechanism of the tibiofemoral joint. **A** Oblique view of the femur and tibia. Shaded area indicates the tibial plateau. **B** Top view showing the position of the tibial plateau on the femoral condyles in knee flexion and extension. The light shaded area indicates the position of the plateau in knee flexion; the dark shaded area shows its position during knee extension. Adapted from Helfet, 1974

Internal derangements of the tibiofemoral joint may interfere with the so-called screw-home mechanism, a combination of knee extension and external rotation of the tibia (Fig. 17:14). The tibiofemoral joint is not a simple hinge joint but has spiral, or helical, motion. The spiral motion of the tibia about the femur during flexion and extension results from the anatomical configuration of the medial femoral condyle. In a normal knee this condyle is approximately 1.7 cm longer than the lateral femoral condyle. As the tibia slides on the femur from the fully flexed to the fully extended position, it descends and then ascends the curve of the medial femoral condyle and simultaneously rotates externally. This motion is reversed as the tibia moves back into the fully flexed position. The screw-home mechanism gives more stability to the knee in any position than would be possible if the tibiofemoral joint were a simple hinge joint.

During activities such as walking and running, the knee, hip and ankle joints experience very high loads. In level walking the forces on the hip, knee and ankle joints are three to five times body weight. With running and more rigorous activities the forces may rise. The hip joint has the characteristic force pattern during normal gait, with a high force at heel strike and at toe-off. Even during stance phase the forces are at least body weight. During walking the knee forces have three peaks, all associated with contraction of the various muscles. Obviously, the higher the muscle contraction force the higher the joint reaction force.

The Shoulder and Upper Extremity

SHOULDER

The shoulder is a complex structure that actually comprises four separate articulations: glenohumeral, acromioclavicular, sternoclavicular and scapulothoracic (Fig. 18:1). Motion of the arm on the trunk involves coordinated movements at all these joints.

Skeleton

The shoulder bony anatomy is composed of the scapula, the humerus and clavicle. Between these three bones, two true joints exist, the glenohumeral and acromioclavicular. In addition, there are two other joints intimately associated with shoulder motion, the scapulothoracic joint, in which the scapula itself is held to the body through muscular attachments to the ribs and spine, and the only true bony attachment to the axial skeleton, the sternoclavicular joint between the clavicle and the sternum.

Joints

The glenohumeral, the shoulder joint proper, is a relatively unstable mechanism with a large humeral head articulating with a shallow glenoid socket (Fig. 18:2). However, this arrangement allows a remarkable range of motion, which is necessary for throwing and other upper extremity activities. Joint stability is increased by a fibrocartilaginous rim around the glenoid, called the labrum, which slightly widens and deepens the concavity. The main stabilizers of the glenohumeral joint are the capsule and the cuff of musculotendinous

units that reinforce the capsule, called the rotator cuff. This rotator cuff is composed of the subscapularis muscle anteriorly, the supraspinatus muscle superiorly, and the infraspinatus and teres minor muscles posteriorly. The biceps tendon runs under the rotator cuff in the bicipital groove between the anterior and superior rotator cuff muscles. The acromion acts as a roof over the glenohumeral joint, with the subacromial bursa separating it from the rotator cuff. This roof is also reinforced anteriorly by ligamentous structures from the coracoid process to the acromion, the coracoacromial ligament.

The acromioclavicular joint is capable of only small rotatory movements. The joint is

18

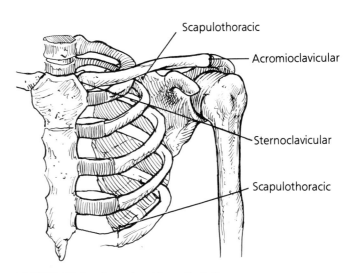

FIGURE 18:1. Four shoulder articulations

189

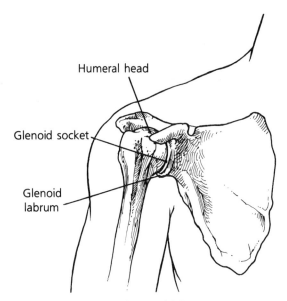

FIGURE 18:2. Glenohumeral joint

made up of a weak capsule reinforced by ligaments interposed by a fibrocartilaginous meniscus. Further support is given by the trapezius and deltoid muscles overlying the joint. The main support for the joint is supplied by the coracoclavicular ligaments, which run from the coracoid process to the outer, inferior surface of the clavicle. These ligaments prevent the clavicle from riding superiorly on the acromion (Fig. 18:3).

The sternoclavicular joint is the only true articulation between the upper extremity and the trunk, and includes a portion of the first rib near its sternal attachment. The sternoclavicular joint has motion in all planes, but with limited excursion. The stability is maintained by a capsule reinforced by ligaments between the medial aspect of the clavicle, first rib and sternum. There is also an interposed meniscus.

Although not a true joint, as there are no bony articulations, the scapulothoracic functions as a joint in shoulder motion. The scapula glides in the posterior thoracic rib cage and is stabilized on the thorax by muscular attachments.

Muscles

The shoulder girdle is enveloped superficially by three muscles: anteriorly, the pectoralis major; superiorly and laterally, the deltoid; and posteriorly, the trapezius (Fig. 18:4).

Four muscles comprise the rotator cuff of the shoulder. The subscapularis arises from the deep surface of the scapula and inserts on the

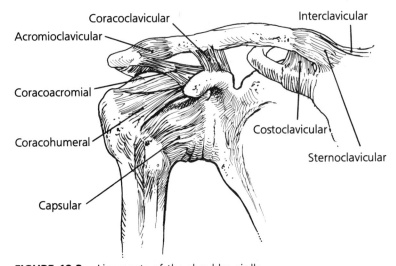

FIGURE 18:3. Ligaments of the shoulder girdle

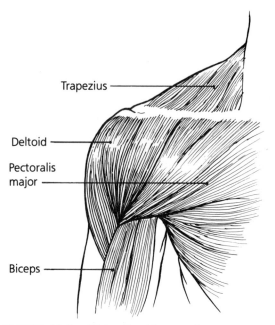

FIGURE 18:4. Major shoulder muscles

lesser tuberosity. The supraspinatus, infraspinatus and teres minor arise from the posterior surface of the scapula and insert on the greater tuberosity, from superior to inferior, respectively (Fig. 18:5).

The biceps brachii muscle has two heads of origin. The long head arises from the superior rim of the glenoid, passes through the shoulder joint under the rotator cuff to run in the bicipital groove between the tuberosities on its way to the forearm. The short head arises from the coracoid process and joins the long head in the arm.

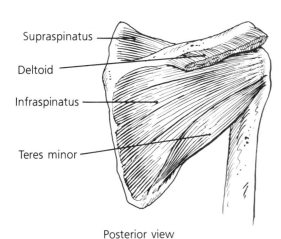

Posterior view

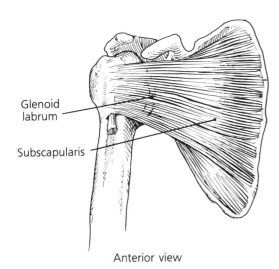

Anterior view

FIGURE 18:5. Rotator cuff muscles and insertions

Motion

The movements of the shoulder are (Fig. 18:6):

1. *Flexion,* in which the arm starts at the side and elevates in the sagittal plane of the body anteriorly
2. *Extension,* in which the arm starts at the side and elevates in the sagittal plane of the body posteriorly
3. *Adduction,* in which the arm moves toward the midline of the body
4. *Abduction,* in which the arm moves away from the midline of the body
5. *Internal rotation,* in which the arm rotates medially, inward toward the body
6. *External rotation,* in which the arm rotates laterally, or outward from the body
7. *Horizontal adduction,* in which the arm, starting at 90° of abduction, adducts forward and medially toward the center of the body
8. *Horizontal abduction,* in which the arm starts in 90° of abduction and moves outward, away from the body

Motion of the upper extremity involves movement in all four joints of the shoulder complex. The deltoid muscle is the primary abductor of the arm, with assistance from the supraspinatus. However, all of the rotator cuff muscles are essential for effective abduction of the arm, as they must stabilize the humeral head in the glenoid during abduction.

The infraspinatus, teres minor and posterior deltoid muscles are the prime external rotators of the shoulders. External rotation of almost 90° is necessary to prevent impingement of the greater tuberosity on the acromion during abduction. Elevation of the lateral aspect of the scapula is necessary for full forward flexion and abduction. This is accomplished by the upper part of the trapezius muscle and the underlying serratus anterior muscle. Forward flexion is mainly accomplished by the anterior deltoid clavicular, part of the pectoralis major and the biceps brachii muscles. Extension is primarily the function of the posterior deltoid

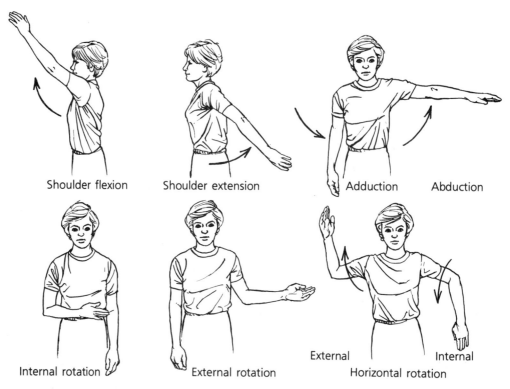

Shoulder flexion   Shoulder extension   Adduction   Abduction

Internal rotation   External rotation   External   Internal

Horizontal rotation

FIGURE 18:6.   Movements of the shoulder

and latissimus dorsi muscles. Adduction is accomplished primarily by the pectoralis major and latissimus dorsi. Internal rotation is primarily a function of the subscapularis muscle, with assistance from the pectoralis major and latissimus dorsi muscles as they adduct, flex or extend.

The function of the various muscles of the shoulder changes, depending on the position of the shoulder itself. For example, in the act of throwing when the arm is brought into abduction, extension and external rotation, the primary internal rotators of the shoulder change from the subscapularis to the pectoralis major and latissimus dorsi muscles.

Nerve Supply and Circulation

While a number of peripheral nerves pass through the shoulder area, the fifth cervical is the basic nerve root that supplies the shoulder girdle. Four peripheral nerves supply most of the shoulder musculature. The suprascapular

nerve innervates the supraspinatus and infraspinatus muscles, while the axillary nerve supplies the teres minor and the deltoid muscle. The subscapular nerve supplies the subscapularis and teres major muscles, and the long thoracic nerve innervates the serratus anterior muscle.

The primary artery traversing the shoulder region is the axillary artery, which is divided into three parts by the pectoralis minor muscle (Fig. 18:7). On occasion, this artery can be damaged by repetitive trauma from the pectoralis minor, particularly in throwing sports.

Biomechanics

With the arm at the side, the deltoid exerts an upward and outward force, whereas the rotator cuff exerts a downward and inward force. The rotator cuff muscles, acting independently, depress the humeral head and may cause subluxation of the humeral head inferiorly. Acting together, the vertical forces cancel each other and combine to stabilize the humeral head in the glenoid. The slight horizontal force of the deltoid acts below the center of rotation of the humeral head, and is opposite in direction to the horizontal force of the rotator cuff, which is applied above the center of rotation. These forces that act synergistically to effect smooth abduction are known biomechanically as a "force couple."

Examples of altered biomechanics are seen in a variety of pathologic states. When abduction is attempted with a rotator cuff tear, the greater tuberosity of the humeral head tends to rise and impinge on the undersurface of the acromion. Abduction is laborious up to a point of 90°. Conversely, in axillary nerve lesions where the deltoid muscle is nonfunctional, abduction cannot be initiated or sustained. Thus the dominant muscle in the shoulder region for abduction is clearly the deltoid, but in the absence of the rotator cuff muscle, its effectiveness is markedly diminished.

If the scapula is restrained from movement, the humerus can only abduct to 120°. Also, the posterior deltoid, teres minor and infraspinatus must externally rotate the humerus to allow the greater tuberosity to rotate posterior to the acromion. The simultaneous movement of both the scapula and the humerus, producing a smooth, rhythmic motion, is called "scapulohumeral rhythm." For every 30° of abduction, 20° of the motion occurs at the glenohumeral joint and 10° is due to the scapula rotating on the thorax.

The motion of the humerus on the glenoid can be described in terms of the center of rotation, which is the pivot point about which the humerus appears to rotate. Using x-ray and graphic analysis, the instant center of rotation for any movement can be determined. As long as the rotator cuff exerts a compression force, the glenohumeral joint is stable and the humeral head rotates on a fixed center of rotation. Excessive movement of the humeral head in a vertical or horizontal direction results in varying instant centers of rotation. This occurs if the conformity of the joint is disturbed, as when the labrum is torn with a shoulder dis-

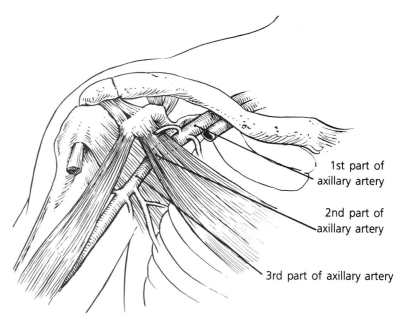

1st part of axillary artery

2nd part of axillary artery

3rd part of axillary artery

FIGURE 18:7. Axillary artery divided into its three parts by the pectoralis minor muscle

location. Among other factors causing this variance is an imbalance of forces between the deltoid and the rotator cuff, as in a rotator cuff tear, when severe shoulder pain disturbs the muscle coordination of the scapulohumeral rhythm, or, if a single rotator cuff muscle is weak compared to the others, in the case of entrapment of the suprascapular nerve in baseball pitchers.

Mechanism of Injury

Shoulder injuries can be caused by acute trauma or by chronic repetitive movement.

Acute Trauma

Direct Forces. While in many instances it is difficult to differentiate between direct and indirect blows in a specific injury, certain injuries about the shoulder joint are usually the result of a more or less unidirectional force. Classically, acromioclavicular joint dislocations are caused by a direct blow on the shoulder, forcing the acromion inferiorly and leaving the clavicle in place.

In addition, posterior glenohumeral dislocations are most likely due to direct blows to the

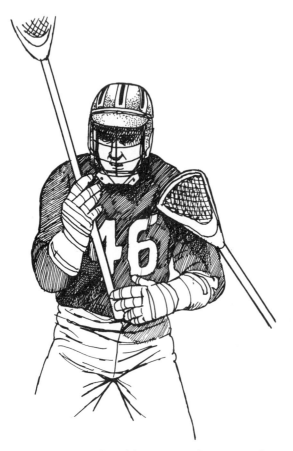

FIGURE 18:8. Direct blow on anterior aspect of the shoulder with arm held in internal rotation

Chronic Repetitive Movements

Repetitive movements that individually do not cause acute pathology frequently cause shoulder problems because of their cumulative nature. Pitching a baseball is a prime example. The pitcher is working near maximum stress level, and is very susceptible to micro tears in the soft tissue, tears that accumulate with repeated episodes of submaximal trauma—known as an overuse syndrome. A second problem arises when a swelling and scarring in the rotator cuff and in the subacromial bursa impinge on a fairly small space. This leads to the impingement syndrome in which the rotator cuff, the long head of the biceps and the bursal structures are impinged under the anterior lateral rim of the acromion and the coracoacromial ligament. In most cases, this is the cause of rotator cuff tendonitis and bicipital tendonitis and bursitis, and may eventually lead to tears in these structures. Overuse can also cause problems with the posterior shoulder structures. When a pitcher does not adequately follow through, the resulting abrupt deceleration produces repetitive tugging on the posterior capsule and teres minor muscles.

anterior aspect of the shoulder with the arm held in internal rotation (Fig. 18:8). This forces the humeral head posteriorly and out of its shallow glenoid. Direct blows are instrumental in producing fractures, particularly those of the scapular body and the clavicle.

Indirect Forces. Indirect forces can and do cause the same injuries as direct forces, but are classically involved in the anterior shoulder dislocation. Here the humeral head is levered anteriorly as the arm is brought into extremes of abduction, extension and external rotation. A good example of this mechanism of injury is an arm tackle in football. A further example of indirect injury to the shoulder is a fall on the outstretched hand with subsequent fracture of the humeral head region (Fig. 18:9).

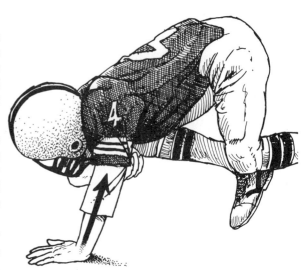

FIGURE 18:9. Fall producing fracture of the humeral head region

Pathology and Treatment

When the upper extremity is subjected to abnormal forces, the resulting injuries may be bony or soft tissue, depending primarily on three elements: the direction of the force, the magnitude of the force, and the rapidity with which it is applied. The shoulder girdle generally has the rich blood supply necessary for rapid healing, and bony injuries heal well even in the face of some movement at the fracture site. Ligaments and tendons are less well vascularized, however, and even in the shoulder region their healing time is prolonged.

Sternoclavicular Dislocation

Generally, in the mature athlete, there is no fracture when the sternoclavicular joint is injured, rather a soft tissue injury with a tear of the sternoclavicular joint capsule. The injury may range from a mildly symptomatic sprain to a complete dislocation with disruption of the entire anterior capsule and its restraining ligaments. By far the most common type of sternoclavicular dislocation is the anterior dislocation. This dislocation is easily recognized clinically by prominence of the proximal clavicle anteriorly on the involved side. Radiographic documentation of a sternoclavicular joint dislocation is difficult but can be confirmed by the Rockwood view, where the x-ray tube is angled 50° from the plane with the patient lying on his back. A cassette is placed behind the patient's shoulder and back.

While dislocation of the sternoclavicular joint may cause considerable distress initially, usually the symptoms rapidly subside with no functional loss to the shoulder. A variety of treatments have been advocated, both closed and open. Little evidence suggests that surgery improves the functional results, and the procedures have significant complications. Closed treatment modalities vary from a sling alone to attempts at closed reduction. While closed reduction can be successful initially, it is difficult to maintain.

In contrast to the anterior dislocation of the sternoclavicular joint, posterior displacement, although much less common, has a higher morbidity with potential injury to the great vessels, the esophagus and the trachea (Fig. 18:10). Presenting symptoms may vary from mild to moderate pain in the sternoclavicular joint region to hoarseness, difficulty in swallowing or severe respiratory distress. Subcutaneous emphysema from tracheal injury may be seen. Again, the Rockwood radiographic view confirms the dislocation.

In most instances, particularly when performed early, closed reduction of a posterior dislocation is successful and stable. To achieve reduction place a pillow under the upper back of the supine patient and apply gentle traction on the shoulder with 90° of abduction and in maximum extension. Occasionally, open reduction or surgical manipulation under general anesthesia is required.

In athletes under 25 years of age, sternoclavicular dislocations may not be true dislocations but rather fractures through the growth center of the proximal clavicle. These fractures, which present similarly to true dislocations, can be treated conservatively without growth deformities. Inasmuch as they represent a growth center fracture, remodeling occurs readily. The problem presents most commonly as a gradually enlarging mass at the

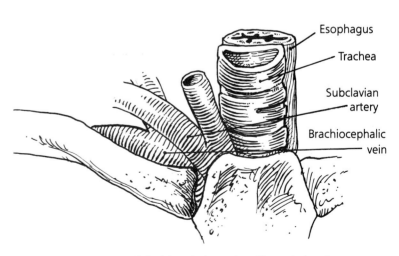

FIGURE 18:10. Potentially injured elements with posterior sternoclavicular joint dislocation

sternoclavicular joint that is firm and not reducible. It is seen in throwers and tennis players in the under 25 age group. This fracture is difficult to diagnose by x-ray films because there is no calcification in the area distal to the epiphysis. It appears as a true dislocation rather than a slipped epiphysis. Repeated attempts to reduce this "dislocation" fail. This injury should be treated symptomatically with a reduction in activities.

Clavicle Fractures

Despite the proximity of vital structures, the clavicle fracture is rarely associated with arterial or nerve damage. Accompanying soft tissue pathology is also uncommon. Because of the shape of the clavicle and the type of forces applied to it, midclavicular breaks account for 80% of clavicular fractures (Fig. 18:11), distal fractures account for 15%, and proximal for 5%. The routine success of conservative treatment in preadolescent midclavicular fractures contrasts strongly with the potential difficulty encountered in treating the older athlete with a clavicle fracture.

Because the clavicle is a single, bony structure fixing the shoulder girdle to the thorax,

its loss allows the shoulder to sag down and forward. The pull of the sternocleidomastoid muscle displaces the proximal fragment superiorly. In the older child or adult, the size of the bone and the muscular development hinders the initial reduction and maintenance of reduction. In addition, fractures of the distal clavicle, more common in older age groups, may involve tears of the coracoclavicular ligament. Such a tear allows the proximal clavicle to ride up superiorly, creating an increased possibility of a delayed union. Clavicular fractures in all age groups are usually treated with a figure-of-eight strapping, tightened periodically to maintain good shoulder position. In addition, in the adult a sling may be used on the affected side to prevent excessive sagging. Rare but serious neurovascular complications, such as a tear of the subclavian artery or injury to the brachial plexus, must be kept in mind when treating these injuries.

Acromioclavicular Joint Injuries

Acromioclavicular separations or "shoulder point" injuries vary in severity because the acromioclavicular ligament across the joint is not all that tethers the clavicle to the scapula. Also at work are the conoid and trapezoid components of the coracoclavicular ligament, which holds the distal portion of the clavicle to the coracoid process.

If the blow producing the injury is mild, usually only a strain or partial tear of the acromioclavicular ligament occurs, producing a first-degree injury. When the acromioclavicular ligament is completely torn but the coracoclavicular ligament remains intact, the second-degree injury involves subluxation or partial displacement. Not always obvious, the diagnosis can be confirmed by an x-ray of the shoulder with the shoulder girdle weighted.

When the force is severe enough to tear the coracoclavicular ligament, a third-degree injury, the resulting total displacement of the joint is often obvious upon observation, and can also be demonstrated by a weighted shoulder x-ray. When obtaining the weighted shoulder x-ray, attach 10 pound weights to

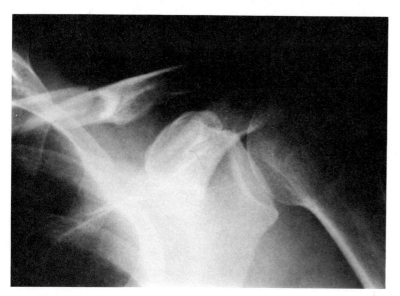

FIGURE 18:11. Midclavicular fracture on x-ray film, the most common clavicular fracture

both wrists rather than have the patient hold them in his hands. When the weight is held in the hand, the increased muscular effort required to hold it may mask the degree of separation (Fig. 18:12). An anteroposterior x-ray of the entire upper thorax allows the vertical distance between the coracoid and the clavicle on both the involved and uninvolved sides to be compared. An increase in this distance indicates incompetence of coracoclavicular ligaments and categorizes the injury as a third-degree separation.

Management of acromioclavicular joint injuries depends upon their severity. First-degree sprains of the joint can be successfully managed with a sling alone until discomfort dissipates, usually within two to four weeks. The more severe, second-degree acromioclavicular sprain implies that the acromioclavicular joint is seriously injured but without dislocation and cosmetic deformity. It can be managed conservatively either with a sling alone or by one of the commercial devices such as the Kenny Howard sling (Fig. 18:13).

The treatment of third degree sprains or complete dislocations is controversial. At one extreme are physicians who advocate open reduction of all such cases and at the other end of the spectrum are those who believe that all should be treated conservatively. Inasmuch as some athletes can and do function well with complete dislocation of the acromioclavicular joint, treatment can be tempered with judgment and reasonable expectations. Treatment, by and large, remains at the discretion of the attending surgeon.

Rotator Cuff Injuries

When the detailed anatomy of the shoulder region is considered, the mechanisms of injury to the rotator cuff become obvious. The rotator cuff is the flat structure that extends from the scapula to its insertion, lateral to the articular surface of the humerus. It does this by passing beneath the overhanging ledge of the acromion and the strong transverse band of the coracoacromial ligament. With prolonged, repetitive activities such as with pitching, the

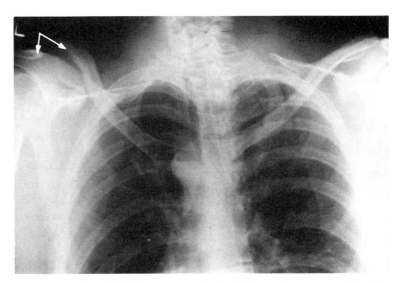

FIGURE 18:12. Third-degree acromioclavicular sprain on x-ray film with weights. Note space between acromion process and distal clavicle.

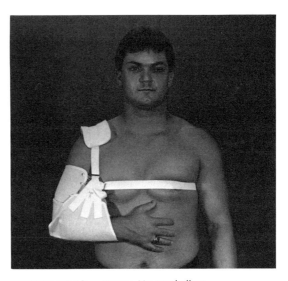

FIGURE 18:13. Kenny Howard sling

tennis serve or swimming, the rotator cuff impinges on the acromion and the overlying coracoacromial ligament which may produce microtrauma to the cuff, with local inflammation, edema, softening and pain. Blood supply to this tendon is precarious, just as in any tendinous structure, diminishing the capability for healing. The pathology may include changes within the rotator cuff musculature.

An impingement syndrome is a pain syndrome that is characteristically produced by repetitive overhead activity. Physical findings are few but the history of debilitating pain during and following swimming, throwing and serving is highly suggestive. Usually the pain is poorly localized but is accentuated by placing the arm in abduction and external rotation. X-ray reveals that the bony anatomy is essentially normal.

Conservative treatment in the form of restricted activities, heat–cold, occasional steroid injection, rest and, most important, stretching exercises in abduction and external rotation while healing is going on frequently relieves symptoms. Only after extensive observation and with debilitating symptoms should surgery be considered. Sectioning the coraco-acromial ligament and removing the anterior, under-portion of the acromion can, in selected athletes, produce gratifying results.

Rotator cuff tears may be divided into two categories, acute traumatic and chronic.

Acute Traumatic Tears

Occasionally, the indirect force on the abducted arm is sufficient to tear a normal rotator cuff muscle and tendon, most often in the young athlete engaged in a violent sport. The presenting symptoms include acute pain and often the patient heard the cuff tear. Strength is diminished in abduction at varying levels. Many athletes with strong shoulder musculature can lose a major percentage of their strength with no clinically apparent diminution. While a high index of suspicion is required clinically, confirmation by arthrogram is helpful. If arthrography confirms the clinical signs and symptoms, surgical repair is mandatory for optimal recovery and return to sports.

Chronic Rotator Cuff Tears

In the older age group, the cuff degenerates and gradually thins, resulting in final rupture, sometimes with minimal trauma. The chronic tears seen in the younger age group are an indirect result of the impingement syndrome and are usually caused by continuation of repetitive trauma. There need not be any single episode of giving way. The patient describes a gradual loss of strength in abduction and external rotation with persistent pain in this range. The pain is difficult to locate, but is usually described as being deep in the shoulder and present at night. Confirmation of the diagnosis by arthrogram is desirable, but if the tear is incomplete and involves only a few thicknesses of the rotator cuff, the arthrogram may prove unproductive. If the tear is small, a long period of rest allows healing. If the patient returns to his previous sport, however, and again the area impinges on the acromion, the symptoms as well as pain and weakness may recur.

The whole healing process can take a considerable amount of time out of an athlete's career. Surgery for rotator cuff repair commits the athlete to a long-term rehabilitation program before returning to pitching, swimming or serving at tennis. It is now well established that cuff repair requires at least one year for full return of integrity. This is especially true in a sport where maximum stress is applied to the repaired area. The success of surgery may be predicted by the size of the tear. If the tear is large and repair requires a great deal of anatomical change, the prognosis is less optimistic than with a small tear. Here, the margins can be excised and normal tendons sutured to normal tendons. Rehabilitating the shoulder following this type of surgery is almost a full time job for at least a year.

Bicipital Tendonitis

Bicipital tendonitis occasionally results from rupture of the transverse ligament that holds the tendon in the bicipital groove. The tendon then subluxates with overhead activity.

The symptoms of bicipital tendonitis, whether due to overlying cuff disease or associated with tendon subluxation, are essentially the same. Pain is localized to the proximal humerus and shoulder joint. Resistive supination of the forearm aggravates pain since the biceps' primary function is supination.

The long head of the biceps extends through the cuff approximately to its intra-articular insertion at the top of the glenoid, and is encased in a tendon sheath with connection to the joint itself. The same mechanism that initiates the impingement syndrome symptoms in the rotator cuff can inflame the sheath, producing bicipital tendonitis. Often this is the earliest phase of the impingement syndrome.

If bicipital tendonitis is associated with the shoulder impingement syndrome, therapy directed to the impingement syndrome can result in spontaneous resolution of the bicipital tendonitis. If subluxation of the tendon within its groove is the cause, conservative treatment by restricting activities and heat may be warranted. Steroid injections are hazardous since they can be detrimental to the integrity of the tendon. If symptoms are persistent, tenodesis of the biceps tendon directly into bone or transplantation of the long head into the short head of the biceps may be considered.

Bursitis of the Shoulder Joint

Bursitis of the shoulder joint is a nonspecific term more commonly applied to the middle-aged athlete than the young athlete. Although the subacromial bursa may be thickened and chronically inflamed, generally it is only one of several structures showing these changes. Bursal enlargement may be seen in the young adult with impingement syndrome stemming from chronic, repetitive trauma. Here, however, the bursitis is the result of the impingement and is not the primary pathology.

Scapular Fractures

Scapular fractures may be divided into three groups—those involving the glenohumeral joint, those of the spine and acromion process, and those of the body. They occur in approximately that descending order of frequency. Fractures of the glenoid usually involve the rim and are associated with dislocation and subluxation of the shoulder. They are usually minimally displaced, and the treatment is dictated by the shoulder subluxation and not by the scapular fracture. Fractures of the acromion may occur in connection with the acromioclavicular separations. These minimally displaced fractures are likewise treated as the acromioclavicular separation. Occasionally a markedly displaced acromion fracture with substantial acromioclavicular disruption requires surgical treatment. Fractures of the body and spine of the scapula can be treated in the same manner as the surrounding soft tissue, that is, by cold applications for the first 48 hours to minimize bleeding followed by heat and early mobilization. Considerable displacement is compatible with a good result and can be accepted.

Shoulder Dislocation

The glenohumeral joint exists not for stability but for mobility. Not only is there minimal bony articular contact, but the capsular ligaments are lax in all but the extremes of shoulder motion. Consequently, control of the joint is provided primarily by the dynamic action of muscles. When the forces driving the glenohumeral joint toward the limits of its normal range of motion exceed the restraining strength of the shoulder muscles and capsular ligaments, the humeral head may tear out of the joint and lodge outside. The majority of dislocations are anterior or inferior to the glenoid rim; only about 2% are posterior.

Anterior Dislocation. When external rotation/abduction force on the humerus or a direct posterior or posterolateral blow on the shoulder is great enough to displace the humeral head, the anterior capsule is either stretched or torn within its substance, or torn from its attachment to the anterior glenoid. The head may be displaced into the subcoracoid, subglenoid, subclavicular or intrathoracic position.

Two gross pathological lesions are typical. One is an anterior capsule injury with a tear of the labrum, known as the Bankart lesion (Fig. 18:14). The second is an indentation or eroded area on the articular surface of the humeral head created by the sharp edge of the anterior glenoid known as the Hill-Sachs lesion (see Fig. 18:14). Both of the lesions pre-

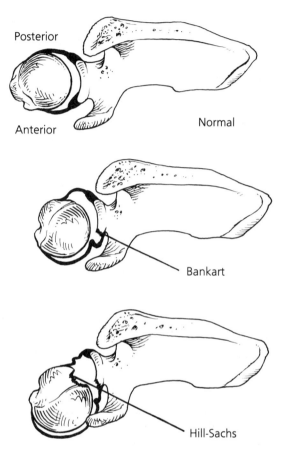

FIGURE 18:14. Gross pathological lesions in anterior shoulder dislocation

Anterior dislocation is common in athletes and some distinction should be made between first and recurrent dislocations (Fig. 18:15). The athlete with a first dislocation has been subjected to considerable trauma. The possibility of associated fractures and nerve injuries requires a complete examination, including x-ray. In these instances, reduction is not recommended, and the arm should be immobilized in a simple sling and the patient transferred to a medical facility for roentgenographic evaluation.

On the other hand, massive trauma is not usually required with recurrent dislocations. Furthermore, when seen at the time of injury, they can be reduced with minimal effort. Attempted reduction of a recurrent dislocation at the time of repeat injury is reasonable. If force is required, the arm should be placed in a sling and the patient transferred to a medical facility for a more complete evaluation.

Anterior glenohumeral dislocations can be reduced by several techniques. Longitudinal traction can be exerted on the affected arm with slight external followed by internal movement of the arm. The patient should be counterbalanced by a sheet or towel in the axilla and care taken to avoid neurovascular injury or fracture. With another technique, the Stimson technique, the patient lies between two tables with his head resting on one and his body on the other. The affected arm is between the tables with a 5 to 10 pound weight tied to it. As the musculature relaxes about the shoulder from the force of the weight, spontaneous reduction takes place.

Following the initial dislocation, it is advisable to immobilize the shoulder in internal rotation for three to six weeks. The athlete will probably not return to competition prior to six weeks; certainly, he should regain normal strength without pain before returning. With recurrent shoulder dislocations, immobilization seems not only unnecessary but, in many instances, detrimental to the athlete's career. Treatment should be symptomatic until the symptoms subside and range of motion and strength return.

dispose to recurrent dislocations. There is no restraining force when the arm is placed in abduction and external rotation. Likewise, the indentation of a crushed trabecular bone and hyaline cartilage on the posterior surface may act as a fulcrum, so that if subluxation causes the glenoid rim to slip into it, the humeral head is then more easily levered out of place.

Two other associated injuries occur with some frequency in the young athlete. One, the greater tuberosity may be avulsed from the humerus by traction from the rotator cuff. The second involves the axillary nerve, which branches into the deltoid. This nerve may be bruised or torn during an anterior dislocation, and deltoid function should be documented at examination.

For recurrent dislocation, multiple restraining devices are available to prevent the arm going into abduction, extension and external rotation. These devices can be effective, but all will substantially hinder the athlete's participation in the sport. In most instances, these patients can be nursed through a season but surgical reconstruction of the shoulder joint is advisable if the athlete has sustained more than one dislocation.

The type of surgical procedure is left to the judgment of the surgeon. The type of activity the athlete hopes to continue, the amount of damage to the rim of the anterior glenoid and the surgeon's skill with any particular procedure all influence the choice. Although the orthopedic literature presents a wide variety of shoulder repairs, the recurrence rate for the various repairs is approximately the same, with few exceptions. With the professional athlete many physicians would consider surgical reconstruction of a dislocated shoulder after a single anterior dislocation. Results with this approach have not yet been fully documented.

Posterior Dislocation. Although the posterior shoulder dislocation results from a different set of forces, in many ways the pathology is similar to that of the anterior. The posterior capsule is either stretched, torn or disrupted from the posterior glenoid. A reverse Hill-Sachs lesion is created on the anterior articular surface by the posterior lip of the glenoid. Although with an anterior dislocation the rotator cuff or its bony attachment at the greater tuberosity may be injured by stretching, with a posterior dislocation the subscapularis or its insertion on the lesser tuberosity may be injured.

Posterior dislocations of the glenohumeral joint are reduced by applying traction in the line of the adducted deformity and concomitant direct posterior pressure on the humeral head. If the maneuver is done gently after total body relaxation, reduction should be atraumatic.

In diagnosing shoulder lesions in athletes, the posterior shoulder dislocation is perhaps

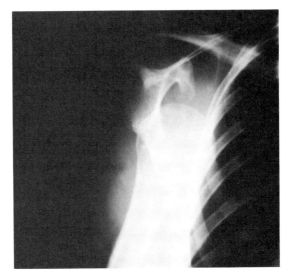

FIGURE 18:15. Anterior shoulder dislocation on x-ray film

one of the major pitfalls. In contrast to anterior shoulder dislocation where the deformity is easily visible and the position of the arm is extreme, posterior dislocation presents with a normal anterior contour. Chest muscles appear intact and, in the well-developed individual with a large deltoid, it is difficult to see that the shoulder is depressed. A cardinal sign of a posterior shoulder dislocation is prominence of the humeral head posteriorly in the shoulder; again, this can be masked by heavy deltoid musculature. What cannot be masked, however, is that the shoulder is held in internal rotation and cannot be externally rotated.

All shoulder injuries on the playing field should be evaluated first by observation, by gentle palpation and by attempts at bringing the joint carefully and gently through a full range of motion. Restriction of the joint motion is an indication for transfer to a medical facility and radiographic examination. Even with radiographic documentation, posterior dislocations have been, and probably will continue to be, missed. They should not, however, be missed if a careful physical exam notes the shoulder's inability to externally rotate. Several roentgenographic views can be obtained if the diagnosis is in question. These include an axillary, a West Point view or the Rockwood view of the shoulder.

Initial treatment following posterior dislocation is the same as for anterior dislocation. For an initial dislocation, immobilization for three to six weeks is warranted. The recurrent dislocation should be treated symptomatically, and surgical treatment considered. In some instances, the posterior shoulder dislocation simply does not present a major functional problem to the athlete.

Recurrent Anterior Subluxation

An interesting entity is recurrent anterior subluxation of the glenohumeral joint. The basic pathology closely parallels the pathology in current dislocations. The difference is degree. Clinically, these athletes do not undergo a frank dislocation. Rather, they have pain when bringing the arm into abduction/extension in internal rotation. Various examiners have described this as a "positive apprehension" sign. As in recurrent shoulder dislocations, it is a reliable clinical finding in anterior shoulder instability or recurrent anterior subluxations.

Roentgenographically, these patients differ from patients with dislocations in that the classic Hill-Sachs lesion is not present, although small flecks of bone avulsed from the anterior glenoid are occasionally seen. The basic treatment of recurrent subluxation is the same as for recurrent dislocation: surgical repair, the procedure depending on the judgment of the attending surgeon.

Fractures of the Proximal Humerus

Fractures of the proximal humerus are less frequent than the more common shoulder girdle sports injuries. When they do occur, however, they may create one or more fragments in the following locations: the joint surface and anatomical neck; the greater tuberosity, which is the attachment site for the rotator cuff; the lesser tuberosity, which is the attachment site for the subscapularis; the shaft or surgical neck fracture.

The articular surface may also be dislocated out of the glenoid, creating either an anterior or a posterior fracture dislocation of the proximal humerus. Depending on the number of fragments, that is, the amount of soft tissue attachments with their accompanying blood supply that have been disrupted, these proximal humeral fractures may be easily treated. On the other hand, they may pose a major problem with permanently decreased function of the glenohumeral joint. In the young athlete, multiple fragment, proximal humeral fractures are not uncommon. The separate growth centers of the articular surface, the greater and lesser tuberosities, coalesce into a single center by age 7. The remaining growth plate does not close until 20 or 22 years of age. Fracture separations of this area can occur at any age until the growth plate is closed. Fractures in this area usually do not cause growth arrest. In the mature athlete, primary healing with conservative treatment is usually the rule unless, of course, the articular surface is a free fragment or the tuberosities are displaced significantly. Stiffness, even in young people, remains a threat because the soft tissues that envelope the shoulder joint lose their range of excursion with injury and immobilization.

Adhesive Capsulitis (Frozen Shoulder)

Adhesive capsulitis is a clinical entity that presents with shoulder pain occurring both day and night, but primarily at night, associated with progressive limitation of the range of motion of the shoulder joint. The disease as classically described moves through three phases. The first, or active phase, begins with the production of intra-articular scar tissue that progressively matures. During this phase, the patient is uncomfortable, again primarily at night, and shoulder motion becomes progressively limited.

The second, more mature phase occurs when the shoulder has essentially undergone a fibrous arthrodesis. During the maturing phase, the shoulder motion is markedly limited, although arm abduction is still possible due to motion of the scapulothoracic joint.

Pain progressively diminishes as the shoulder becomes stiffer.

The third phase is resolution, when the shoulder becomes progressively supple and gradually returns to normal. During the third phase, symptoms are minimal. The overall time from onset to resolution varies, but 18 months is a good approximation.

Diagnosis in the early phases of adhesive capsulitis is often difficult. Clinical signs include inability to bring the arm up the back to the same level as the opposite, normal shoulder. In women, this generally means inability to reach their bra fasteners. Examination of the shoulder with the arm abducted to 90° shows varying degrees of loss of internal and external rotation, but especially external rotation. Similar findings may be noted when the adducted arm is examined.

Radiographic confirmation of adhesive capsulitis may be obtained through arthrography when a small capacity joint is identified. Often the affected shoulder will not take more than 2 to 3 cc of dye, although normal shoulder capacity is approximately 12 cc.

Treatment modalities vary, but most patients can be managed conservatively with heat, progressive range of motion exercises and, in a few instances, intra-articular steroids. More rarely, surgical manipulation under general anesthesia may be warranted.

Brachial Plexus Traction Injury

This injury does not technically belong under shoulder lesions, since it is not a lesion of the shoulder but rather of the brachial plexus itself and its parent nerve roots from the cervical spinal cord (Fig. 18:16). The mechanism of injury is thought to be depression of the shoulder or adduction of the arm with head and neck forced to the contralateral side.

If the injury is minimal, symptoms may be transient. More severe injuries can produce persistent neurological deficits which, if they do not resolve within three weeks, require further medical evaluation, usually in the form of an electromyogram with nerve conduction studies. Despite the extent of the injury, most

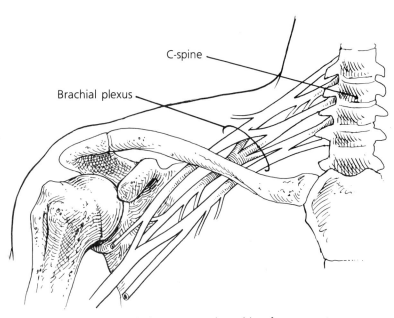

C-spine

Brachial plexus

FIGURE 18:16. Brachial plexus nerves branching from parent nerve roots on cervical spinal cord

patients can be successfully managed conservatively and symptom resolution is the rule, not the exception.

Initial Examination and First Aid

The initial examination should consist of a history of the mechanism of injury followed by removal of clothing and protective equipment. The examiner should determine if there is any neurovascular compromise. The radial and ulnar arterial pulses should be palpated and assessed, and a sensory examination of the entire upper extremity done, especially in obvious glenohumeral dislocations, since from 5% to 20% of patients are reported to have neurological deficits following dislocation. The most common nerve deficit involves the axillary nerve. Following this, motor function should be assessed. With any evidence of neurovascular compromise of the upper extremity, the patient requires immediate transportation to a medical facility.

After assessing neurovascular status, observe the shoulder area for any obvious deformity, lacerations, abrasions, hemorrhage, ecchymosis or swelling. These signs indicate the location of damaged underlying structures. Then palpate the area of injury to determine the location of tenderness and any crepitus indicative of a fracture. Lastly, if possible, take the shoulder through a complete range of motion passively and actively, including abduction, adduction, internal and external rotation, flexion and extension. Note any limitation of motion or movement that causes pain.

The shoulder is best immobilized with a standard, triangular bandage sling and ice applied to the injured area to decrease pain.

Evaluation of a Painful Shoulder

Many times an athlete complains of a painful shoulder of several hours' to weeks' duration. The examination on this occasion is different from the evaluation of an acute injury on the field.

History

1. Exact location of pain
2. Associated with acute trauma or gradual onset
3. Character of pain (e.g., throbbing, aching, sharp, stabbing, burning)
4. Duration
5. Associated symptoms (e.g., tingling, weakness, snapping, radiation, catching)
6. Factors that aggravate and relieve the pain (e.g., pain with throwing, pain with placing arm behind back, pain with neck movements)
7. Prior treatment

Inspection

1. Deformity:
   a. Acromioclavicular joint: chronic dislocation
   b. Scapula wen: long thoracic nerve palsy
   c. Deltoid atrophy: disuse, axillary nerve palsy

Palpation

1. Skin temperature

2. Swelling: interstitial fluid, tumor, abscess
3. Tenderness
4. Crepitus: joint, tendon, subcutaneous

Range of Motion

1. Active range of motion: coordinated motion
2. Passive range of motion: difference between active and passive

Strength

1. Resistive motion: weakness

Stress Test

1. Apprehension test: anterior costal stability
2. Acromioclavicular distraction test
3. Yergason test: biceps, tendon subluxation

The examiner should perform each of these sections in a systematic fashion, not eliminating any of the vital steps. Remember that pain in the shoulder is often referred from other areas, i.e., neck, heart, abdomen (spleen, gall bladder).

Rehabilitation

Shoulder rehabilitation, like with any other joint, involves two phases—restoration of motion and re-establishment of strength. Motion is the prime goal in shoulder rehabilitation, as the shoulder joint is designed for mobility rather than stability. The function of the upper extremity is severely limited without full shoulder motion.

The primary exercise to restore scapulohumeral motion is the Codman pendulum exercise. The patient bends over and lets his arm hang like a pendulum. He then makes approximately 100 circles in a clockwise direction, and 100 circles in a counterclockwise direction, repeating the series two or three times a day, gradually making the circles larger each day. After this loosens up the shoulder, the patient can do further stretching with the aid of a broomstick or long stick. Grasping the stick in both hands, he lifts it as high as possible in forward flexion and abduction. He does the same thing in internal and external rotation. He also performs sawing motions in the sagittal and coronal planes. After he can perform these movements easily, the athlete can start on a shoulder flexibility program to increase the range of motion further.

Shoulder Flexibility Exercises

Shoulder flexibility exercises concentrate on three major movements, abduction-adduction, flexion-extension and internal-external rotation. These exercises are generally held 10 to 20 seconds and are repeated two to three times.

Adduction-abduction exercises stretch the latissimus, deltoid and rotator cuff areas.

1. *Sky reach.* Standing straight up, lift arms vertically above head. Grasp hands directly above head with elbows straight and push hands toward the sky. Hold 10 to 20 seconds. Bring arms down and grasp hands behind back. Lift arms up as high as possible toward head. Be sure to stand straight while doing this. Hold 10 to 20 seconds. Grasping hands behind back, bend over at the waist and lift arms as high as possible (Figs. 18:17A, B, C).

2. *Double shoulder stretch* (anterior shoulder muscles). Standing erect, hold arms straight in front at shoulder height. Turn palms out and slowly bring arms behind. Lift arms backward as far as comfortable without leaning forward and hold for 10 to 20 seconds. A partner can assist.

3. *Crossover arm stretch* (posterior rotator cuff). Standing erect, hold right arm in front of chest with hand near the left shoulder. Place left hand just above the elbow and gently pull right arm into left shoulder, keeping right arm as straight as possible. Pull as far as comfortable, hold 10 to 20 seconds, then repeat on the other side.

Flexion-extension exercise stretches the upper back muscles. One example is the wall twist for the horizontal adductors and interior

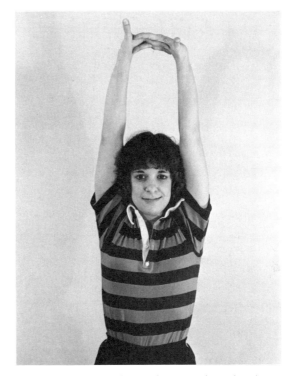

FIGURE 18:17A. Sky reach: arms above head

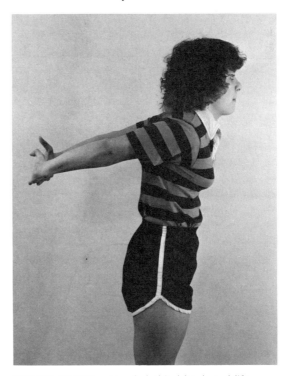

FIGURE 18:17B. Hands behind back and lift

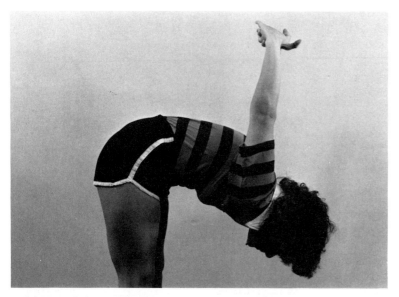

FIGURE 18:17C.   Bend over and lift

shoulder joint. Stand sideways, grasp the corner of a wall or stable object with the arm extended straight out at shoulder height. Keeping the arm in stationary position, slowly rotate body away from arm. Go as far as possible and hold the position for 10 to 20 seconds. Then, turn in the opposite direction, toward the arm, going as far as comfortable. Hold for 10 to 20 seconds and then repeat with the opposite arm.

Strength Training

A strength training program builds up and maintains muscular strength, endurance and flexibility. For building programs, the athlete must participate three days a week, and these should be alternating days. To develop a habit, exercise on Monday, Wednesday and Friday. During the season, if strength gains have already been achieved, a maintenance program is recommended. For athletes playing regularly, only one day a week is sufficient. If the athlete wants to do more, he can continue on the three-day program without substantially increasing the weights. The athlete who does not play regularly should work out on the strength program at least two days per week. Two programs are suggested, depending on the availability of equipment.

Nautilus Program: Begin with light weights to insure that the athlete is executing the exercises properly. How the athlete lifts the weight is very important. The program is designed to be done in repetitions of 8 to 10 to 12; then the weight is increased and repetitions are begun again. Be sure the athlete stresses the complete range of motion.

Free Weight Exercise Program: When using free weights or the Universal Gym, select a weight that allows at least 10 but no more than 12 repetitions. Increase the weight when the athlete can do more than 12 repetitions. The following program provides exercises for each of the major muscle groups. Start with two sets of 10 for each exercise; increase the number of repetitions and weights as tolerated.

1. *Straight flexion* (straight flexors). Hold dumbbell in one hand, lift arm forward above head. Keep palm down. Repeat 10 to 12 times, with each repetition taking four to six seconds. Repeat exercise with opposite arm (Fig. 18:18A).
2. *Lateral raises* (adductors/abductors-deltoid suspraspinatus). Holding dumbbell in each hand, lift both arms up sideways to slightly above shoulders. Keep palms down. Each repetition should take four to six seconds (Fig. 18:18B).
3. *Bend-over lateral raises* (rotator cuff). Holding dumbbell in each hand, bend over at the waist and lift arms up toward shoulders, palms down. Hold at the highest point for two seconds and then slowly lower to a starting position (Fig. 18:18C). Keep elbows straight. This can also be done lying face down on the table. Start with the arms hanging straight down, then lift as high as possible, making sure not to rotate arms backward or forward. The motion must be straight, up and down with the palms down.
4. *Flys* (adductors-pectoralis). Lie flat on back (preferably on a table) with knees bent.

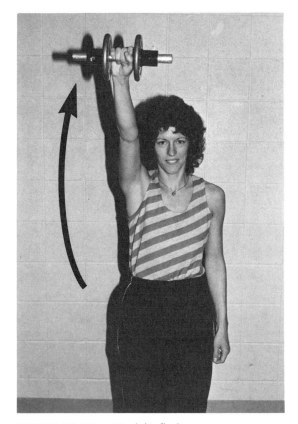

FIGURE 18:18A. Straight flexion

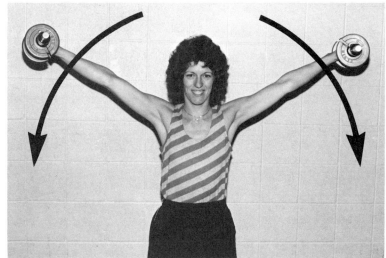

FIGURE 18:18B. Lateral raises

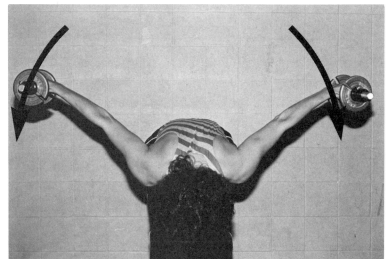

FIGURE 18:18C. Bend-over lateral raises

Holding dumbbells in each hand, bring arms straight up in front, then lower back to starting position (Fig. 18:18D). If table is narrow enough, arms can be lowered beyond table top. Care must be taken not to overstretch the muscles. Each repetition should take between four to six seconds.

5. *Upright row* (abductors-deltoid, supraspinatus and arm flexors-biceps). Standing erect, lift barbell (or Universal Gym) up to chin with elbows out and back straight, then lower back to starting position (Fig. 18:18E).

6. *Pullovers* (shoulder extensors). Lying on back and holding a barbell with the arms extended above head, slowly raise the barbell to a position straight above chest (Fig. 18:18F); then slowly lower back to starting position (barbell behind head).

Exercises After Surgery

After shoulder surgery, shoulder motion is decreased from the surgical dissection, postoperative immobilization and pain. A patient must usually start on Codman pendulum exercises for two to three weeks before he can

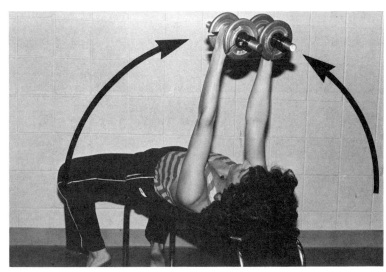

FIGURE 18:18D. Flys

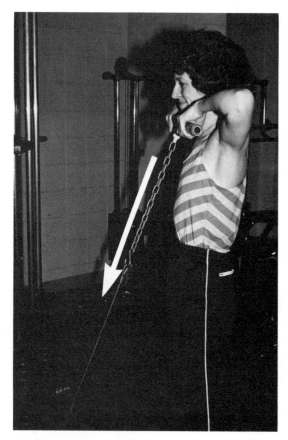

FIGURE 18:18E. Upright row

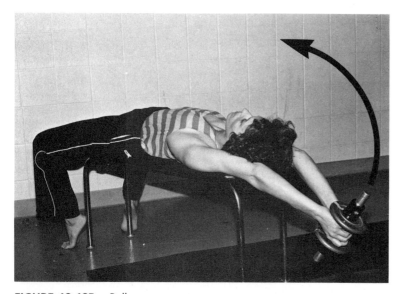

FIGURE 18:18F. Pullovers

tolerate further stretching. Up to three to six months may be necessary to regain maximum shoulder motion.

Recurrent Anterior Dislocation. After a Bristow procedure for recurrent anterior shoulder dislocation, the arm is placed in a sling postoperatively and the athlete may start on Codman pendulum exercises within a few days. After three weeks, the sling is removed and the athlete can begin a stretching program. Usually external rotation of the shoulder is markedly decreased, and the internal rotator muscles, including the subscapularis, pectoralis major and latissimus dorsi, must be stretched to obtain full motion.

Four to six weeks after surgery, the athlete can begin to stretch these internal rotators. At six to eight weeks, he can begin shoulder strengthening. All of the muscles of the shoulder girdle are usually weak at this time. However, exercises 3 and 4 under Strength Training will help strengthen the rotator muscles of the shoulder.

After Bankart, Magnusson-Stack, Putti-Platt and other surgical procedures, two to three weeks of immobilization in internal rotation may be required before starting the exercise program. After that, the patient follows essentially the same program.

With chronic shoulder subluxations not requiring surgical intervention, treatment involves standard modality routines and emphasis on strengthening the rotator cuff muscle group.

Rotator Cuff. After rotator cuff surgery, the arm is also placed in a sling and the athlete started on Codman exercises. The trainer begins with passive abduction and external rotation to restore motion on the first day following surgery. No active abduction-external rotation, however, is allowed for approximately six weeks following surgery to protect the repair of the rotator cuff and the deltoid muscle. The athlete continues with Codman exercises and passive stretching of the shoulder in abduction-external rotation for four to six weeks. At six weeks, the sky reach and crossover arm stretch are emphasized to stretch the rotator cuff area. At three months following surgery, a strengthening program can begin. Strengthening exercises should begin slowly and progress slowly so as not to damage the repair. Exercises 2 and 3 (lateral raises and bend-over lateral raises) in the strengthening program are especially helpful.

Pitchers who have undergone shoulder surgery (usually rotator cuff repairs or impingement procedures) often require special consideration. They usually need at least three months to regain full shoulder motion. They are then placed on a shoulder strengthening program consisting of isotonic and isokinetic exercises. If the pitcher is progressing satisfactorily without pain, he can begin to toss the baseball. The athlete tosses every other day and, when this feels comfortable, progresses to half speed, then three quarter and, finally, full speed. This progression usually takes six to eight weeks, and the time in each stage is divided, based upon the pitcher's continued improvement. The pitcher may return to competitive pitching eight to twelve months following surgery.

Exercises for Pitchers and Throwers

For pitchers and athletes involved in throwing activities, the "fungo routine" allows return to a normal throwing motion. However, no throwing is allowed until a full range of motion is obtained. This routine is used primarily after minor shoulder problems have been treated nonsurgically. The athlete begins with long, easy throws from the outfield so the ball just barely reaches the fungo hitter. He does this for 30 minutes on two consecutive days and then rests for one day. He then progresses to stronger throws, getting the ball back on four or six bounces for 30 minutes on two consecutive days and rests a day. He then makes strong, crisp throws on a relatively straight trajectory from the short outfield on one bounce to the fungo hitter, again for 30 minutes on two consecutive days. After resting a day, he can start on the pitcher's mound, or his usual throwing activity.

Exercises After Shoulder Joint Sprains

With injuries to the acromioclavicular and sternoclavicular joints, treatment includes standard modalities and a general strengthening program for the entire shoulder girdle. Athletes with this type of injury frequently encounter difficulty when attempting to resume lifting heavy weights. Therefore, it is recommended that rehabilitation emphasize high repetitions with low weights to avoid aggravating the injured area.

For the impingement syndrome, strengthening exercises should concentrate on the rotator cuff muscle group, emphasizing the restriction of abduction.

Deltoid group strengthening activities should be de-emphasized to avoid further aggravating the area of impingement. For overuse syndromes, appropriate rest is required to allow inflamed tissues to heal. Rest should be followed by a total restrengthening program, taking care to avoid recurrence of the initial inflammation.

UPPER ARM AND ELBOW

Upper extremity injuries caused by acute trauma or recurrent overuse are common in the athletic population. The function of the upper arm, elbow and forearm depends upon musculotendinous units having their origin proximal to the shoulder joint and insertion attaching distally near the wrist and hand. An appreciation of the anatomy of these adjacent regions is essential to complete understanding of upper extremity problems.

Skeleton

The humerus, distal to the humeral head, is cylindrical in its proximal and midportion and then becomes flattened in the anteroposterior direction just proximal to its distal articulating surface (Fig. 18:19). At the elbow, the humerus has two articulating areas: the convex capitellum laterally, and trochlea medially, which has a spool-shaped depression articulating with the ulna. Extending proximally

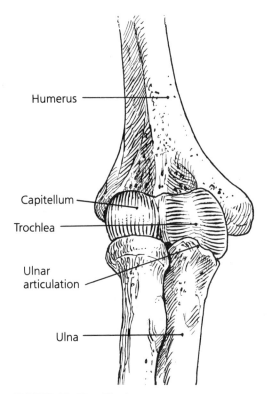

Humerus

Capitellum

Trochlea

Ulnar
articulation

Ulna

FIGURE 18:19. The humerus

from these humeral condyles are the medial and lateral epicondylar ridges, to which the forearm flexor pronator muscles attach medially, and the extensor supinator laterally. The medial epicondyle is more prominent than the lateral, and has a cartilaginous apophyseal growth plate that does not close until 16 or 17 years of age.

The ulna is a large bone proximally but becomes narrower as it extends distally toward the wrist. The proximal ulna has a deep, semilunar notch that articulates with the trochlea of the humerus as a hinged joint. This is a very stable articulation that allows flexion and extension only. The olecranon process of the ulna extends posteriorly, preventing hyperextension of the elbow, and the coronoid process of the ulna extends anteriorly, preventing hyperflexion. The oblique inclination of the trochlear articulation with the ulna produces a valgus-carrying angle of 5° to 20°.

The radius is much larger distally at the wrist and narrows as it extends proximally to the radial neck and the radial head. The radial head is a round, concave disc that articulates with a convex capitellum of the humerus. The radius rotates over the ulna, allowing pronation and supination of the forearm. A strong ligament extends around the head and neck of the radius, allowing motion along the longitudinal axis but restricting anteroposterior motion. The radius is closely approximated to the ulna distally and proximally. However, it has a radial bow in its midportion, separating it from the ulna. An interosseous membrane connects the two bones in the forearm and separates the anterior flexor compartment from the posterior extensor group.

Ligaments

The medial collateral ligament of the elbow consists of anterior, posterior and oblique components (Figs. 18:20A, B). A portion of the anterior fibers is tight throughout the range of motion of the elbow. The more anterior fibers are tight in extension, whereas the posterior portion is tight in flexion. This anterior band extends from the medial epicondyle to the medial aspect of the coronoid process. The posterior fibers of the medial collateral ligament are fan-shaped and thin compared to the anterior fibers. They are tight only beyond 90° of flexion. They originate on the medial epicondyle and extend down to the medial side of the olecranon. The oblique portion of the medial collateral ligament is less important clinically and extends from the medial side of the olecranon to the medial side of the coronoid process.

The lateral collateral ligament consists of a capsular thickening extending from the lateral epicondyle to the annular ligament.

Muscles

The biceps muscle extends from its two origins, one in the superior region of the glenoid and the other on the coronoid process, distally to attach into the tuberosity of the radius. The brachial muscle originates on the humerus, extends anteriorly across the elbow joint, attaching into the ulna. The extensor muscle, the triceps, originates from both the inferior-posterior aspect of the glenoid fascia and the posterolateral aspect of the humerus and extends into its attachment on the olecranon.

The flexor pronator muscle group of the forearm and wrist have their origins on the medial epicondyle and then extend along the epicondylar ridge. They extend down the forearm anteriorly into their attachments at the wrist and fingers. The extensor supinator muscle group originates on the lateral epicondyle and extends down the forearm dorsally into the wrist and hand.

Nerves, Vessels and Bursae

The brachial artery and median nerve extend medially down the upper arm and course across the anterior aspect of the elbow joint. The radial nerve begins superiorly and medially in the upper arm and winds around the humeral shaft, covered by the triceps, and then extends over the lateral epicondylar ridge, across the anterior aspect of the elbow joint. The ulnar nerve runs posteriorly in a bony groove behind the medial humeral epicondyle and then extends into the muscle groups of the forearm (Fig. 18:21). Knowing the relationships of these vessels and nerves is important in assessing possible neurovascular complications of upper extremity injuries.

The olecranon bursa of the elbow separates the skin from the underlying ulna. It allows the soft tissue to glide smoothly over this bony prominence. The radial humeral bursa is located anteriorly between the radial head and the lateral epicondyle.

Upper Arm Injuries

Contusions

Contusions to the upper extremity are common in contact sports. Direct blows sustained

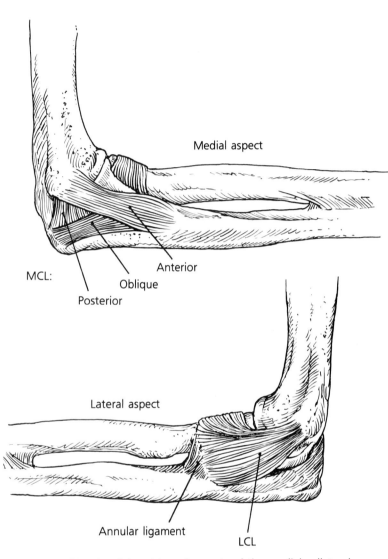

FIGURE 18:20. Medial and lateral aspects of the medial collateral ligament

while tackling and blocking can produce bleeding within muscle groups and also subperiosteally along the humerus. Contusions within the muscle groups, particularly the triceps, biceps and brachial muscles, can be painful and result in restricted motion and disability. A common site of contusion in the upper arm is over the lateral aspect of the humerus, just distal to the attachment of the deltoid and lateral to the biceps muscle. Here,

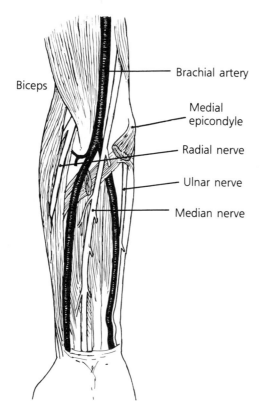

FIGURE 18:21. Arteries, nerves and bony structure of the upper arm and elbow

Labels on figure: Biceps, Brachial artery, Medial epicondyle, Radial nerve, Ulnar nerve, Median nerve

Depending on the severity of the injury, ice applications, compression bandages and immobilization either singly or all together can be used. A sling or a posterior splint may be necessary to restrict motion and relieve pain for the first 48 hours. A compressive bandage of sheet wadding and elastic bandages is often helpful, extending from the fingertips to the axilla. Avoid putting a constricting bandage around the elbow since venous return may be obstructed.

Ice applications are generally continued for 48 to 72 hours, or at least until the inflammatory response and swelling appear under control. Thereafter, initiate gentle, active range of motion exercises. Heat may be helpful after 48 hours.

Strengthening exercises to rehabilitate the upper extremity can be done within the pain-free arc of motion. Avoid passive stretching and massage. A vigorous rehabilitation program to strengthen the triceps and biceps muscle groups should wait until a painless full range of motion is achieved. Use protective padding when the athlete returns to contact sports.

either a severe single blow or repeated injuries from blocking and tackling can cause subperiosteal hematoma formation with subsequent myositis ossificans, tackler's exostosis. The lower edge of a poorly fitted shoulder pad can contribute to trauma in this area.

The clinical symptoms are pain, stiffness and associated weakness within the involved muscle groups. On examination, the site of the tenderness and swelling must be localized carefully. In contusions of the upper extremity, any neurological impairment must be noted. Hematoma formation within the muscle groups can lead to calcification and permanent restriction of motion and function. Consequently, careful diagnosis and prompt treatment are important. The typical tackler's exostosis does not involve the adjacent muscle group but presents as a painful, firm mass just distal to the deltoid insertion.

Radial Nerve. The radial nerve winds around the posterolateral aspect of the humerus, protected by the triceps muscle. It then extends over the lateral epicondyle, where it is more subcutaneous and vulnerable to injury. Contusions in this region of the arm may injure the radial nerve.

The clinical symptoms of radial nerve injury are pain in the arm extending down the forearm toward the wrist. Numbness and tingling may be noted in the dorsum of the wrist. The first dorsum web space of the hand may be numb and the wrist extensors weak, producing the characteristic wrist drop.

Initial treatment consists of immobilization in a cock-up splint in dorsiflexion and a sling. Ice can be used to relieve the swelling and the patient should be referred to a physician for further evaluation. The ice should not be placed directly over the nerve, as nerve lesions from application of ice have been reported.

Although many of these lesions are self-limiting and recover spontaneously, others may result in serious hemorrhage within the nerve sheath, resulting in permanent loss of function. Consequently, a physician should see these patients promptly, assess the neurological status and initiate appropriate care.

Fractures

Humeral shaft fractures in the athletic population result from direct force as well as indirect rotary torque. A fall on a flexed elbow can result in a humeral shaft fracture. A sudden, severe rotary force extending through a fixed forearm and elbow, such as in arm wrestling, can produce a spiral fracture of the humeral shaft. In addition, the growing child can fracture his humerus in the act of throwing, particularly if there is a weakened area in the growth plate or a bone cyst. Such bone lesions in children may be asymptomatic until fracturing during an athletic event. The clinical symptoms are pain and weakness in the upper extremity, perhaps extending along the entire course of the upper extremity and into the elbow. Clinical examination often shows swelling and tenderness along the shaft of the humerus. The ability to flex or extend the elbow does not rule out a fractured humerus. Again, because of the proximity of the radial nerve to the humeral shaft, neurological assessment must be carried out to be sure the nerve is not injured (Fig. 18:22).

The initial treatment consists of splinting. A sling and a swathe can be used effectively if the individual is not comfortable by making a posterior splint out of plaster. Refer the patient to a physician for definitive treatment. Closed reduction and a plaster cast are usually required.

Elbow

Contusions

Contusions about the elbow resulting from falls or direct blows are common. The olecranon and epicondylar ridges are particularly vulnerable to direct trauma. The medial

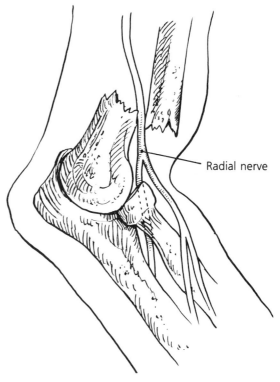

FIGURE 18:22. Radial nerve subject to injury in humeral shaft fracture

epicondyle is the more protected of the two. The lateral epicondyle is often contused and remains painful if not appropriately treated. Treatment of these contusions is similar to that described for the upper arm. Applications of ice and compression bandages for 24 to 48 hours help prevent swelling and pain, taking care not to apply ice directly over the ulnar nerve. A sling may be used when motion at the elbow joint is painful. When the acute inflammatory response has subsided, heat may aid the rehabilitation program. Appropriate protection can help avoid recurrent injuries.

Ulnar Nerve. The ulnar nerve runs subcutaneously in a groove in the posteromedial aspect of the medial epicondyle. Consequently, it is vulnerable to a direct blow in this area. Such a blow may produce numbness and tingling in the forearm and hand, as when the so-called funny bone is hit. A fascial sheath holds the ulnar nerve within its groove. Occasionally, this sheath is injured, causing subluxation of the nerve from the groove. Flexion and extension of the elbow with a valgus force may irritate the nerve as it subluxes in its groove.

The symptoms of ulnar nerve contusions are pain and numbness extending into the fourth and fifth fingers of the hand, perhaps with associated weakness. On clinical exam, the ulnar groove is often tender directly over the nerve. Pressure in this area may produce symptoms extending down into the hand. Sensation along the fourth and fifth fingers should be carefully assessed as well as strength of the muscles, particularly the adductor of the little finger and abductor of the index finger.

The initial treatment for contusions of the ulnar nerve consists of rest and cold. The elbow may be immobilized with a sling. If a nerve injury is suspected, the athlete must be referred to a physician for further evaluation. Many of these lesions are incomplete tears and will subside spontaneously. However, more severe injuries result in hemorrhage within the nerve fibers and sheath. This can produce permanent scarring with loss of nerve function

and can require surgical decompression and anterior transposition of the nerve.

Bursitis

The olecranon bursa of the elbow is equally traumatized by a fall on the flexed elbow or by recurrent irritation, such as in wrestling. Swelling and hemorrhage develop within the bursal sac, producing sensations of pain and stiffness posteriorly. On clinical exam, there is often local swelling and tenderness over the olecranon bursa (Fig. 18:23). Initial treatment consists of compression and ice to reduce the swelling and inflammation. Immobilization and a splint or sling may be indicated in severe cases. When swelling is marked, aspiration of the fluid within the bursa can be helpful and speed recovery. In chronic cases, infection manifested by heat and redness can develop within this bursa. When athletes with olecranon bursitis return to competition, this area should be protected with padding. Those individuals with chronic olecranon bursitis may require surgical excision.

Strains

Strains of the musculotendinous units of the upper extremity vary from mild, first-degree injuries to severe, third-degree with total disruptions. An elbow forced into extension produces a load on the contracting biceps and brachial muscles that can result in partial or complete tears to these musculotendinous units. Similarly, a flexion force against the contracting triceps can result in similar injuries to the extensor muscle groups attaching on the olecranon. In addition to acute injury resulting from violent force, these musculotendinous units can be injured by repeated microtrauma, as in the act of throwing or rowing. Symptoms from such chronic trauma, including pain, stiffness and restricted motion, are gradual in onset but can be equally disabling. The patient often has a history of hyperextension injury to his elbow. On clinical examination, swelling and tenderness should be carefully localized. Although most of these injuries are partial tears, a complete tear with avulsion

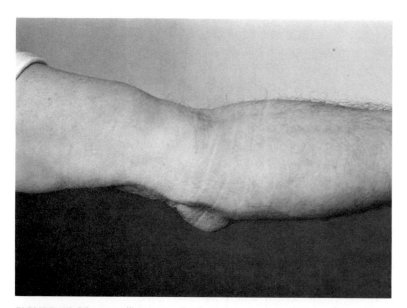

FIGURE 18:23. Swelling over olecranon bursa indicating bursitis

of the biceps or brachial muscles from their attachments on the radius and ulna, respectively, is possible. Careful palpation and comparison with the normal side helps determining the presence of a complete tear. Resistive flexion in the elbow will cause pain. If either the biceps or brachial is intact, the patient may still be able to flex his elbow. Since this mechanism of injury is often associated with avulsion fractures or injuries to the coronoid process, it is important to obtain x-ray films of these injuries. Neurological status must also be carefully assessed.

Initial treatment of a strain includes application of ice, compression bandages and immobilization. In mild, first- and second-degree injuries, the ice and immobilization can generally be discontinued after the first 48 hours. Heat treatment with whirlpools or hydrocolator packs may be helpful after the inflammatory response and swelling subsides. Stretching exercises, resistive exercises or massage must not be done with these acute injuries. Rest is essential until a pain-free range of motion is achieved. Exercising these musculotendinous units prematurely can result in calcification within the muscle mass, with permanent restriction of elbow motion. Myositis ossificans, particularly in the brachial muscle, is not an uncommon sequela. The athlete who returns to competition may benefit from protective taping to prevent hyperextension forces at the elbow.

Third-degree injuries to these muscle groups should be referred promptly to a physician. Avulsion of the biceps from the radial tuberosity requires surgical reattachment of the tendon. Certainly, complete avulsion of the triceps from the olecranon is a surgical emergency. A prolonged period of disability follows surgical repair of these injuries because several months are required to regain strength and range of motion.

Epicondylitis

Epicondylitis is an inflammatory response to overuse of either a flexor or extensor muscle group attaching into the medial and lateral epicondyle of the humerus. Tennis elbow, or lateral epicondylitis, is perhaps the most common of these injuries. Similar symptoms on the medial epicondyle are frequent in the throwing sports. Repeated overload of these musculotendinous units attaching into the epicondyle is the most accepted cause of these conditions. The typical lateral epicondylitis, or tennis elbow, produces pain along the lateral epicondyle, extending down the forearm extensor muscle group. The pain is intensified by resistive extension of the wrist and fingers as well as shaking hands. Pressure or contact over the lateral epicondyle is painful. Although tennis elbow is frequently associated with the weekend tennis player, it occurs regularly in experienced tennis players, as well. Factors influencing this condition include faulty techniques, particularly the backhand, excessive pronation forces and an inadequate racquet. Loss of tissue fluids, prominence of the radial head and relative weakness of the extensor muscle group compared to the flexors have also been incriminated. The condition is also seen in golfers and bowlers.

Athletes such as baseball pitchers and tennis players with a vigorous overhead motion may have symptoms along the medial epicondyle as a result of valgus forces through the elbow joint. The ulnar nerve must be examined to rule out subluxation or entrapment of that nerve in the groove behind the medial epicondyle.

The treatment of epicondylitis, whether medial or lateral, initially is rest, ice and nonsteroidal and anti-inflammatory medications. Injections of soluble, cortical steroids into acute lesions is often helpful but the extremity must be rested for at least two weeks following injection. Steroid injections into muscle or tendon may cause necrosis of tissue that must heal before the athlete can participate in vigorous activities. Heat may be helpful once the acute inflammatory response subsides. A rehabilitation program to strengthen the extensor muscle groups is indicated when pain has subsided sufficiently. Since injuries to these structures can decrease flexibility, stretching must be part of rehabilitation. Because faulty technique may cause the injury to recur, the athletic trainer should view the athlete's serve or delivery with the coach to correct any biomechanical faults. Although most cases of epicondylitis subside with conservative programs over a 6- to 12-month period, some become chronic and disabling. In these cases, surgical intervention may be indicated to release the aponeurotic attachments of the involved muscle group at the epicondylar level. This must be done on the medial side to avoid substantial weakening of this flexor group.

Sprains

Falls on the outstretched hand produce a hyperextension or varus/valgus forces that injure the ligamentous structures of the elbow as well as the musculotendinous unit. Partial or complete tears to medial ligamentous structures of the elbow can occur from a fall or violent force such as in a throwing sport. Most of these injuries occur along the medial collateral ligament due to valgus and extension forces resulting in pain and stiffness within the elbow joint. The athlete often is unable to throw or grasp with adequate force.

Physical examination shows local tenderness over the medial collateral ligament. Possible injury to the muscular attachments of the flexor muscle groups must also be carefully assessed. Since the elbow is stable in extension, the elbow should be stressed into 20° to 30° of valgus flexion to determine whether the ligament is completely disrupted. Since avulsion injuries of the medial epicondyle are not uncommon with this mechanism of injury, x-ray evaluation is generally indicated. In addition, the ulnar nerve should be carefully examined to rule out possible subluxation or contusion to the nerve. A first- or second-degree partial sprain of the medial collateral ligament should be treated with ice, applications of compressive bandages and immobilization in a sling. After 48 hours, heat may help relieve further swelling and pain. Apply ice in the medial aspect of the elbow cautiously to avoid cold injury to the ulnar nerve.

Dislocation

Dislocation of the elbow is a severe, traumatic injury that can be caused by either a fall on the fully extended elbow or a sudden, violent, unidirectional blow to the elbow. Pain is immediate and severe, with total loss of function in the elbow and obvious deformity (Fig. 18:24). Numbness, especially along the ulnar nerve, is frequently present, indicating injury to this structure. Frequently there are associated fractures of either the forearm bones or the radial head or coranoid process of the ulna. Hence, immediate transportation to a medical facility for x-ray films and further evaluation is mandatory. Closed reduction with general anesthesia is necessary. The elbow should be splinted unless it causes the patient too much pain.

Dislocations of the radial head may occur with and without associated ulnar fractures. If the displacement is severe, incarceration of the ruptured annular ligament of the radius within the joint may block closed reduction, necessitating surgery.

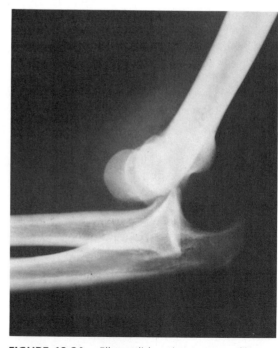

FIGURE 18:24. Elbow dislocation on x-ray film

Fractures

Elbow fractures are some of the most severe problems the athlete can encounter. Stiffness, limitation of motion, angular deformities, growth disturbances and neurovascular problems frequently result. Except for undisplaced fractures, surgical intervention is often necessary.

Supracondylar fractures of the humerus are usually caused by falls on the outstretched arm. Diagnosis is easy in the displaced fracture because of the severe pain and deformity (Fig. 18:25). Neurovascular status of the hand and forearm should be assessed. Immediate referral to a medical facility for further treatment is mandatory.

Fractures of the olecranon are usually the result of direct trauma. If displaced, these fractures generally do not respond to conservative treatment as the pull of the triceps further distracts the fragments, and surgical treatment is indicated.

Undisplaced fractures of the radial head generally respond to conservative care with pain and swelling controlled by ice, sling and a short period of splinting followed by gentle active exercise until the fracture is healed. Displaced fractures require surgical intervention.

Fractures in children's elbows are complicated by the problem of growth deformity resulting from malalignment of the reduction or injury to the growth center. Open reduction with pin fixation is almost always needed in the displaced fracture.

The avulsion fracture of the medial epicondyle is peculiar to young and adolescent age groups. Because the tension from the extensor supinator group of muscles may displace even the undisplaced fracture, open reduction and pinning may be necessary.

The most dangerous and, many times, subtle complication in supracondylar fractures is ischemic necrosis of the forearm muscles, known as Volkmann's contracture (Fig. 18:26). It can be caused by compression or damage to the vascular supply at the elbow or in the upper forearm, and emergency surgery is required to prevent irreversible damage to the forearm muscles. Coldness, stiffness and numbness of the fingers and severe pain in the forearm aggravated by passive extension of the fingers are warnings that treatment must be instituted immediately. The presence of a radial pulse is not a reliable indicator of adequate circulation to the forearm muscles.

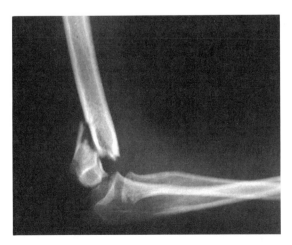

FIGURE 18:25. Supracondylar fracture on x-ray film

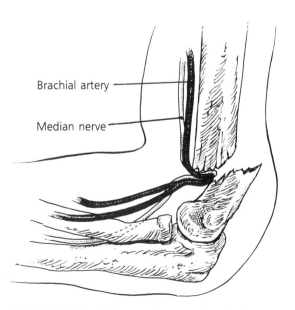

Brachial artery

Median nerve

FIGURE 18:26. Volkmann's contracture: ischemic necrosis of the forearm muscles

FOREARM

Forearm injuries include fractures, soft tissue contusions, nerve entrapment syndromes and tendonitis. The radius and ulna anatomy is described in the previous section on the elbow. The important soft tissues include the flexor-pronator muscle group that originates from the medial humeral epicondyle and extends along the volar side of the forearm to the wrist.

The extensor supinator muscles originate from the lateral epicondyle of the humerus and course distally into the wrist and fingers. The median nerve crosses the anterior aspect of the elbow and descends into the forearm between the two heads of the pronator teres muscle. It then courses toward the wrist between the flexor sublimis and profundus muscles, entering the palm of the hand from beneath the transverse carpal ligament.

The ulnar nerve passes behind the medial epicondyle at the elbow and extends into the forearm between the two heads of the flexor carpi ulnaris muscle. At the wrist, it passes around the side of the pisiform bone.

The radial nerve crosses the elbow anteriorly and passes down the forearm under the supinator muscle. A major terminal branch of the nerve, the posterior interosseus nerve, winds around the radius to the dorsal side of the forearm under the supinator muscle. The radial and ulnar arteries accompany their respective nerves along the distal half of the forearm (Fig. 18:27).

Fractures

Children frequently break the forearm bones, the radius and ulna, during athletic competition. The mechanism of injury is a fall on the outstretched arm or a direct blow. One or both bones may be fractured, or one bone may fracture and the other dislocate at the adjacent elbow joint. A Monteggia fracture is a dislocation of the radial head in association with an ulnar fracture; a dislocated ulna with a fractured radius is a Galeazzi fracture. These are serious injuries and require prompt treatment by a physician.

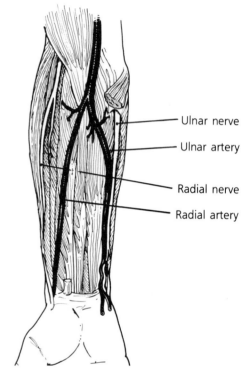

Ulnar nerve

Ulnar artery

Radial nerve

Radial artery

FIGURE 18:27. Arteries and nerves of the forearm

A fracture must be suspected whenever the forearm is severely injured. Initial inspection may reveal an obvious deformity, particularly when the middle or distal third of the forearm is fractured. The bones must be gently palpated, looking for tenderness and crepitus. Neurovascular status must be observed and recorded before applying a splint to immobilize the fracture, since progressive swelling may produce a compartment syndrome. It is essential that the physician who sees the patient later knows whether the nerves and vessels were damaged by the initial injury or by subsequent swelling. Pressure within the closed spaces of the forearm can produce ischemic necrosis of the forearm (Volkmann's contracture) or damage to the posterior interosseus nerve, with weakness in the hand and wrist.

Contusions of the forearm are common during athletic competition. These injuries should be treated with ice, rest and elevation in a sling. Fractures must be carefully ruled out and the complication of compartment syndromes avoided. Myositis ossificans is not very commonly seen following forearm injuries.

Acute tenosynovitis involving the extensor and flexor tendons of the wrist is seen in certain athletic activities. Particularly in oarsmen, repeated dorsiflexion of the wrist while "feathering" the oar leads to extensor tenosynovitis. Similarly, a prolonged tight grip on the oar may result in flexor tendonitis, not only in the forearm but often extending down into the fingers. Examination reveals tenderness, swelling and crepitus over the involved tendons. Treatment includes rest, ice and oral anti-inflammatory drugs. Injections of cortisone may be attempted, but the needle must be inserted into the tendon sheath and not the tendon itself. Since this is a self-limited condition, it is best to treat the tendonitis conservatively and avoid injections.

In athletes, most nerve injuries are the result of direct trauma, associated with either a contusion or fracture. However, repeated muscular activity may result in nerve entrapment.

The median nerve may be compressed by hypertrophy of the pronator teres through which it passes. Pain may be felt in the forearm, but numbness and weakness may extend distally into the hand. This condition occurs in tennis players from overuse or an abnormal technique of gripping the racquet. The median nerve may also be compressed at the wrist (carpal tunnel syndrome) after injuries and produce similar symptoms in the hand and forearm. On examination, tenderness proximally in the forearm suggests the pronator teres syndrome. Weakness in the thenar muscle group and numbness in the median nerve distribution of the hand are present in both of these conditions. Electromyography and nerve conduction studies help to localize the site of nerve entrapment. Treatment consists of ice, rest and oral anti-inflammatory drugs. Occasionally, a persistent nerve compression requires surgical decompression. In those cases related to an abnormal grip, the coach and player should carefully assess techniques and equipment.

HAND AND WRIST

The bones of the hand and wrist are connected by joint capsules and ligaments. Each bone, except the carpals, is joined by tendons that flex or extend the joints on the dorsal and palmar surfaces (Fig. 18:28). At the proximal levels, intrinsic muscles of the hand also produce motion to either side. The same possibilities for motion are provided at the wrist with muscles and tendons that produce flexion, extension, abduction, adduction, rotation or combinations thereof. The thumb, in addition, has the power of opposition. This entire unit is the most versatile, functional unit that has evolved in animals.

An anastomosing network of branches of the radial and ulnar arteries and their accompanying veins supplies blood to the hand.

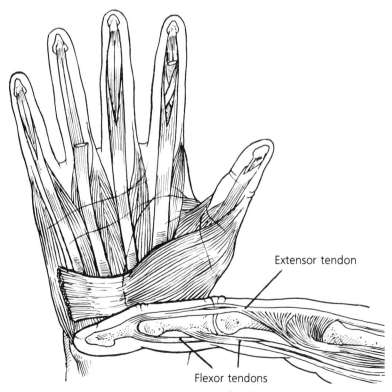

Extensor tendon

Flexor tendons

FIGURE 18:28. Tendons of the hand and wrist

After entering the hand, the radial and ulnar arteries divide into two branches, forming the superficial and deep volar arches, which anastomose and send common branches to the fingers. The nerve supply to the hand is mediated by the radial, ulnar and median nerves, which innervate the muscles and provide a sensory distribution to the hand in a fairly regular pattern, subject to many variations (Fig. 18:29). The ulnar nerve innervates the little finger and ulnar side of the ring finger on the dorsal and volar surfaces, the median nerve innervates the remainder of the volar surface of the hand and fingers, and the radial nerve innervates the dorsum of the hand. The radial nerve supplies the muscles that extend the fingers at the knuckles or metacarpophalangeal (MCP) joints. The median nerve controls the muscles that oppose the thumb to the fingers, while the ulnar nerve supplies the intrinsic muscles that move the fingers apart or together when they are held in full ex-

tension. The radial and ulnar nerves control extension of the wrist while the median and ulnar nerves control flexion.

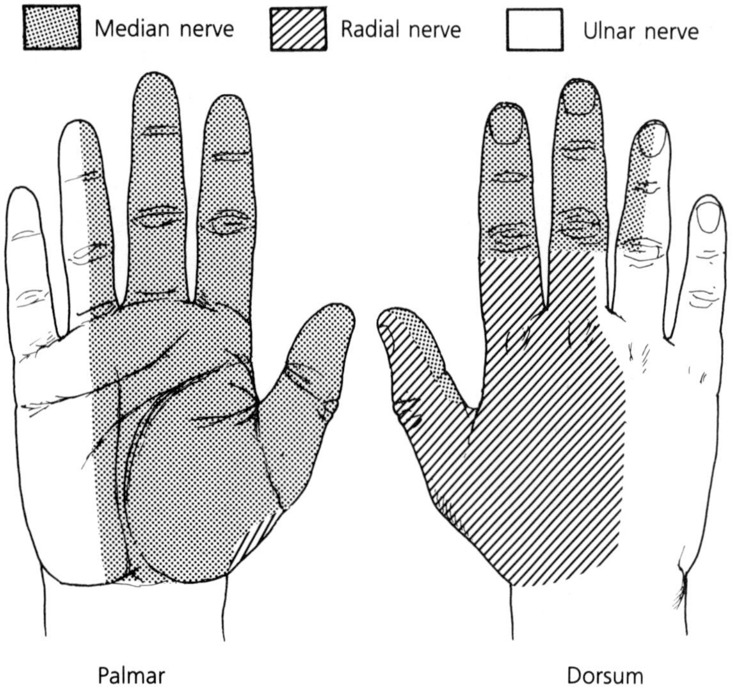

When describing injuries of the hand, nomenclature can be confusing. The problem arises because the first finger rests on the second metacarpal. To avoid confusion, it is best to describe metacarpal injuries by their numbers, that is, first, second, third, fourth and fifth metacarpals, and digital injuries by their names, i.e., thumb, index, middle or long, ring and little fingers.

Finger, Hand and Wrist Injuries

In general, injuries to the fingers that require immobilization should be splinted with the interphalangeal joints held in full extension. The few injuries that require immobilization in flexion must be closely supervised to prevent the development of flexion contractures (Fig. 18:30). The ligaments of the interphalangeal joints are tightest in extension and more relaxed when the joint is flexed. Because of this, a joint that has been fixed in a fully straight position for several weeks is usually easy to mobilize, whereas a finger joint that has been held in flexion for a prolonged period may be very difficult to straighten.

Fingertip Injuries

The most common injuries to the fingertips are direct contusions, such as a blow with a hard missile like a baseball or a jamming of the fingertip against an object, and crush injuries, as when the fingers are stepped on. Subungual hematomas, a collection of blood beneath the nail, often form. In treating this injury, be certain that there is no underlying fracture. Soak the finger in ice water for 10 to 15 minutes for analgesia and to reduce the swelling from additional bleeding. Then drain the hematoma by cutting a hole through the nail either with a rotary drill or a number 11 surgical blade, or melt a hole through the nail with the end of a paper clip heated to cherry red in a flame (cigarette lighter or alcohol lamp) or a disposable electrocautery.

Median nerve   Radial nerve   Ulnar nerve

Palmar   Dorsum

FIGURE 18:29. Medial, radial, and ulnar nerve distribution to the hand. Pattern is subject to many variations.

The nail may be avulsed by being caught in an object or in an opponent's clothing. A partially avulsed nail can be restored to near anatomical position by manipulation and held in place by clear tape after a hole is drilled in the nail. This affords a protective layer to a very sensitive nail bed. The nail should be removed only if absolutely necessary. With a complete avulsion, apply a protective dressing of fine mesh vaseline gauze and change it regularly. A plastic "cage" over the affected fingertip provides additional protection and often allows the athlete to participate. Disruption of the nail bed, either by laceration or crush injury, should be brought to the immediate attention of the physician for repair.

A paronychia is an infection along the edge of the nail and can cause purulent drainage. Treatment is by warm water soaks, germicide, protection with a dry, sterile dressing and referral to a physician for possible drainage or antibiotics.

A felon is an infection of the pulp of the fingertip and may follow a puncture wound of the fingertip from a needle or even a severe contusion. As a closed space infection it causes extreme tenderness and firmness of the fingertip. If treatment is delayed, infection may spread to the adjacent area, and osteomyelitis of the terminal phalanx may develop.

The "mallet" or "baseball finger" is caused by a sudden flexion force on the distal interphalangeal (DIP) joint while the finger is actively extended, such as when the player is poised to catch a ball (Fig. 18:31). The extensor tendon ruptures at or near its insertion on the terminal phalanx and can no longer actively extend the terminal joint. The terminal phalanx is usually held in partial flexion and cannot be actively extended. Early after the injury, the finger may be extended passively with external pressure. A physician should evaluate all serious mallet injuries and obtain x-ray films to reveal fracture of the distal phalanx or subluxation of that joint. Initial treatment is ice and elevation, followed by splinting of the terminal interphalangeal joint in full extension. Surgery is usually not re-

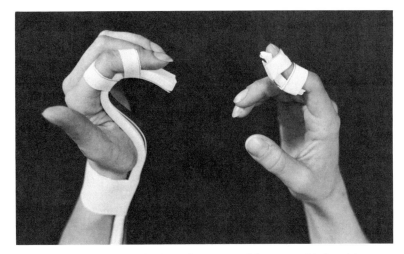

FIGURE 18:30. Left: Splinting of metacarpal fracture with hand in functional position. Right: Slight hypertension of DIP joint when splinting a mallet finger

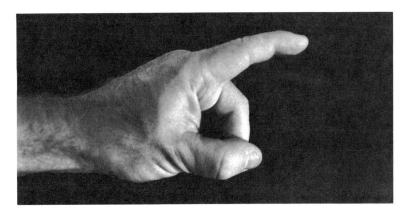

FIGURE 18:31. Mallet finger injury. Distal phalanx is no longer able to extend in index finger.

quired unless there is a large fracture of the joint or subluxation.

The counterpart of the mallet finger, the "jersey finger," is caused by a sudden, forceful extension of the DIP joint while held in flexion, typically when a tightly held jersey is torn out of the grasp of a would-be tackler. An avulsion of the long flexor tendon to the distal joint can result. The athlete cannot flex this joint, although it can be passively flexed. This critical injury must be recognized early, as delay in treatment may compromise repair and require tendon graft surgery.

Proximal Finger Joint Injuries

Injuries of the proximal finger joint can occur in the same manner as described for the fingertips. In addition, forceful twisting injuries may occur as a result of grabbing or being grabbed, or catching fingers on opponents' clothing or equipment.

Hyperextension Injury. One of the most common injuries of the proximal interphalangeal (PIP) joint is the hyperextension injury, where the finger is bent forcibly backward, stretching or rupturing the volar plate on the palmar side of the joint. In very severe injuries, dorsal dislocations, rupture of the collateral ligaments or fractures may occur. Often with a simple hyperextension injury, the joint swells. The palmar side of the joint is tender, and attempts to hyperextend the joint cause pain. A physician should evaluate significant injuries and obtain x-ray films to locate an associated fracture or dislocation. Evaluation should include a stress examination of the collateral ligaments to be certain they are intact.

Initial treatment is ice and elevation, and the whole finger should be splinted with both joints in full extension to prevent a flexion contracture from developing. Failure to splint and supervise these injuries satisfactorily until fully healed results in a painful, stiff finger with a fixed flexion deformity or ''coach's finger.'' Surgery is rarely required except with large fractures involving the joints, subluxation or marked instability of the collateral ligaments.

Dislocations. In dislocations of the PIP joint the middle phalanx usually dislocates dorsally on the proximal phalanx. The cause is most often a hyperextension force and the dislocation is an extension of the simple hyperextension injury. Ordinarily, the finger is foreshortened with obvious deformity and swelling.

In athletics, many of these dislocations are treated at the sidelines with simple, longitudinal distraction that produces successful and prompt reduction. Despite this, a physician should evaluate the integrity of the collateral ligament, and obtain x-ray films to check for associated fractures and to assure that the reduction is satisfactory. The finger should be splinted with the involved joints in extension for at least three weeks to prevent a flexion contracture. Thereafter, active motion is begun, splinting the finger at night in extension for an additional three weeks. Surgery is rarely required, except with serious fracture of the joint surface or persistent subluxation.

Collateral Ligament Tears. Hyperextension injuries can also cause tears of the collateral ligaments but are more commonly associated with a force applied to the sides of the fingers. Swelling of the joint is common, but obvious deformity is rare. To assess the integrity of the collateral ligaments, apply a lateral force to the joint, first fully extended and then flexed approximately 30°. Minor tears may imbue a joint laxity up to 10° and a definite end point is felt. With complete ruptures, there is no resistance to lateral forces and no end point is felt. Stress after an acute injury may be too painful to tolerate and anesthesia may be required to assess instability adequately. On careful examination, tenderness is usually localized to the side of the ligament rupture, and the ligament itself may be palpable in the subcutaneous tissue, rolled up on one side.

Minor tears may be treated by simple splinting with the joint extended. More severe or complete ruptures may require surgical repair.

Boutonnière Deformity. The boutonnière deformity is caused by rapid, forceful flexion at the PIP joint (Fig. 18:32). The central slip of the extensor tendon of the middle phalanx ruptures with associated separation and palmar displacement of the lateral band. This injury leaves no effective, active extensor mechanism of the middle joint. As a result, the proximal joint flexes and the distal joint tends to hyperextend.

Initial treatment is splinting the finger in full extension, but surgical repair may be required to regain full function. For this reason, early evaluation by a physician and x-ray films are recommended.

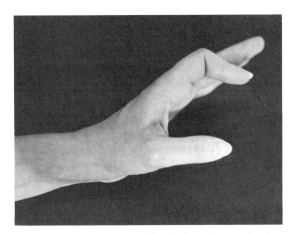

FIGURE 18:32. Boutonnière deformity. Proximal joint flexes while distal hyperextends.

Finger Fractures

In general, x-ray films are required to diagnose and evaluate all fractures of the hand, and physician consultation is recommended. Treatment is often complex and the functional result may depend on the expertise of the person managing these injuries. The clinical diagnosis may be obvious if there is gross deformity. However, in the case of occult, or nondisclosed, fractures, diagnosis may be difficult. The most reliable sign of clinical injury is localized tenderness, but this does not indicate whether soft tissue or bone is injured. Diagnosis may be simplified where the bone is prominent or superficial. However, the safest course is to x-ray the involved part whenever a fracture is suspected. The old adages of "It's not broken if you can move it" or "If it doesn't swell" are unreliable.

Perhaps fractures of the proximal and middle phalanges and their associated joints are the most difficult to manage. The four fingers must move as a unit. Failure to maintain the longitudinal and rotational alignments severely hampers grasping or manipulating small objects within the palm. The most difficult alignment to evaluate and maintain is rotation. Failure to correct a malrotation causes one finger to overlap the other when a fist is made. The easiest way to assess rotation is to flex all the fingers, bringing them as close together as possible, remembering that the fifth finger should point toward the middle of the wrist. If in doubt, compare the alignment with the unaffected hand, or your own hand.

Thumb Injuries

The thumb is a unique digit because it has only two phalanges and one interphalangeal joint. Generally, all of the injuries described for the fingers can also affect the thumb, except for the boutonnière deformity.

Gamekeeper's Thumb. Because the MCP joint of the thumb is more exposed than its counterparts in the fingers, it is subject to an injury peculiar to this joint known as the "gamekeeper's thumb." This is a rupture of the ulnar collateral ligament of the thumb (Fig. 18:33). While originally described in gamekeepers, it is seen in many contact sports such as football and wrestling as well as in skiing. It is caused by forceful abduction of the thumb away from the hand, with the MCP joint in extension. On examination, there is usually local tenderness on the ulnar side of the MCP joint. Diagnosis is confirmed by stressing the joint laterally in extension and then in 30° of flexion, looking

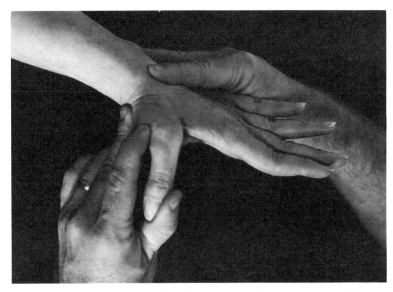

FIGURE 18:33. Rupture of the ulnar collateral ligament can be exhibited by laxity when stressing the MCP joint laterally.

for laxity of the joint on the ulnar side. With partial ligament tears, a definite end point is felt, and only modest lateral laxity is noted. In the more severe, or complete, tears, laxity of 45° or more is noted, and no discrete end point is felt. In all cases, the laxity of the involved thumb must be compared with the uninvolved thumb to determine what is normal for that patient.

Stability of the ulnar collateral ligament is critical to normal hand function, particularly fine pinching, or grasping a key, between the thumb and index finger. Therefore a physician should evaluate all mild cases of collateral ligament injuries in the thumb. An x-ray film should be obtained to reveal fractures or volar subluxation of the joint. Incomplete tears should be placed in a thumb spica cast for four to six weeks. However, severe cases require surgical repair to gain an effective result. Generally, undisplaced, avulsion fractures at the site of injury heal with conservative treatment.

Palm and Dorsum Injuries

Simple Contusions. Simple contusions of the hand produce a soft, painful, bluish discoloration of the dorsum of the hand, and must be differentiated from metacarpal fractures. Treatment is ice, compression and elevation of the hand. Disability seldom lasts longer than two or three days.

Thenar and Hypothenar Eminence Contusions. Contusions of the thenar and hypothenar eminence are seen especially in baseball, hockey and handball players. They follow trauma and appear as tender, painful swelling of the fleshy areas at the base of the thumb or the little finger. These contusions can be confused with a tendon sheath infection or a carpal or metacarpal fracture. Treatment is ice, compression, elevation and protective padding, such as a sponge rubber doughnut. Local heat is used after 24 to 48 hours, and disability may last four days, or longer if the injury is severe.

Dislocation of MCP Joints. MCP dislocations usually follow hyperextension injuries, with the proximal phalanx dislocating dorsally in respect to the metacarpal head (Fig. 18:34). The joint remains hyperextended and foreshortened, with obvious deformity. Simple injuries may be reduced by closed means. Occasionally, a dimple may be apparent on the skin of the palm, which indicates a "complex" or irreducible dislocation. This will not respond to closed manipulation because the metacarpal head is entrapped by the surrounding soft tissues of the volar plate, which is interposed within the joint. These injuries ordinarily require open surgical reduction because a simple dislocation may be converted into a complex and fixed dislocation by incorrect attempts at reduction. A physician should treat all of these injuries definitively.

Rupture of the Transverse Metacarpal Ligament. Rupture of the transverse metacarpal ligament is an unusual but very disabling injury caused by a spreading force to the fingers, such as a faulty catch, that forces the fingers apart and spreads the interior metacarpal joints. The intrinsic muscle attachments can also be ruptured. Diagnosis is made by flexing the metaphalangeal joint and spreading it apart. When the transverse metacarpal ligament is torn, the joint spreads excessively.

Metacarpal Fracture. Metacarpal fractures, particularly of the neck of the fifth metacarpal, are relatively common. They are caused by a direct blow to the MCP joint with a clenched fist, as when striking a hard object. Ordinarily, the MCP joint is depressed and there is tenderness, swelling and angulation on the back of the hand. X-ray films and referral to a physician are important. Axial compression, twisting stress or direct blows can also cause metacarpal fractures. In general, the metacarpal shafts are splinted to one another and are more stable when fractured than the phalanages. However, external splinting in flexion and, occasionally, surgical fixation are required to maintain alignment and length.

First Metacarpal Fracture. The metacarpal of the thumb is not inherently stable, and fractures of the first metacarpal often need special care, including internal fixation. The metacarpal may fracture along its shaft or at the carpal/metacarpal joint. Bennett's fracture occurs in the base of the first metacarpal with a dislocation of the carpal/metacarpal joint. It is a severe disabling injury, usually produced by the same forces as the gamekeeper's thumb. It may be treated by closed manipulation and casting, closed manipulation and percutaneous pinning or by open reduction and internal fixation.

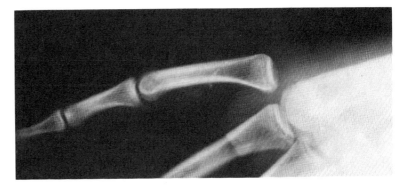

FIGURE 18:34. Dislocated metacarpal-phalangeal joint

Wrist Injuries

Injuries to the wrist that present pitfalls in diagnosis are considered here. These injuries may produce pain and disability but the seriousness of the injury can be easily overlooked.

Carpal Scaphoid Fracture. The carpal scaphoid fracture usually can be diagnosed by an x-ray film. Occasionally, however, these fractures are occult, that is, cannot be seen on the film. The fracture becomes obvious a week to ten days later when bone resorption occurs around the fracture line. For this reason, any patient with a fall on the wrist, tenderness of the anatomical snuff box and pain in the wrist should be initially treated by casting for seven to ten days and then another x-ray done out of plaster, including special scaphoid views or x-ray on mammographic film.

Base of Second and Third Metacarpal Fractures. Although other metacarpal fractures were discussed with the hand, fractures of the base of the second and third metacarpals are considered with the wrist, as symptoms are closely involved with wrist function. These fractures are often associated with subluxation of the carpal/metacarpal joint and are tender in this area. The patient probably fell on the volar-flexed wrist. X-ray films may or may not show a small flake of bone just dorsal to the base of the metacarpal. Casting for six weeks in the position of function is necessary.

Rotary Dislocation of the Radioulnar Joint. Rotary dislocation of the radioulnar joint is a hyperpronation injury whose only signs are pain and disability of the wrist and a shift of the ulnar styloid to the center of the bone on an anteroposterior x-ray view of the wrist. There may be a click on supination of the wrist. The wrist should be casted in supination for four weeks.

Hamate Hook Fracture. Hamate hook fractures occur with a strong, twisting force or from a direct blow (Fig. 18:35). Tenderness over the hypothenar eminence and inability to perform twisting motions, such as a golf swing, persist. Only a tunnel x-ray view of the wrist discloses this disabling fracture.

Radiocarpal Joint Injuries. The radiocarpal joint can be sprained, but it is rarely dislocated except at the distal radioulnar joint (see above). If the force applied, often from a fall on the outstretched arm with hand extended, is severe, usually the radius fractures, frequently with the tip of the ulna as well, a Colles' fracture (Fig. 18:36). This same mechanism produces other injuries in the upper extremity, as already noted. In the growing child, the epiphyseal plate can be injured, which is only differentiated by x-ray films. These injuries must be diagnosed and treated, or growth or angular deformity may result. A sudden twisting injury to the wrist may also tear the articular disc, a small, fibrocartilaginous structure located between the distal end of the ulna

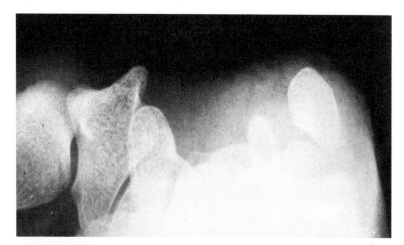

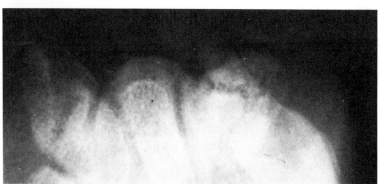

FIGURE 18:35.   Hamate hook: normal (top) and fracture (bottom)

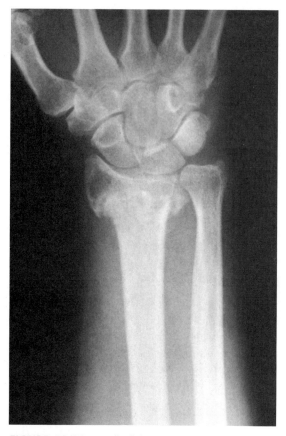

FIGURE 18:36.   Colles' fracture

and the carpus. Point tenderness in this area accompanied by pain on wrist motion is evidence of this injury. Routine x-ray films are normal, and an arthrogram is necessary for diagnosis.

SKIN

Hand abrasions should be completely cleaned and all foreign matter removed. The entire hand should be scrubbed with surgical soap for at least ten minutes and the abrasion washed with a prepared iodine solution. Remove imbedded foreign matter, perhaps with a prepackaged sterile brush impregnated with water-soluble iodine compounds. Dress the abrasion with a nonadherent dressing and inspect it daily for signs of infection. Keep the dressing dry. Air drying after 24 hours often greatly helps the healing process. Abrasions resulting from contact with synthetic playing surfaces should be treated promptly and checked daily because incidence of infection is increased.

Superficial lacerations of the fingers and the back of the fingers and hand may be treated with careful scrubbing, removal of debris and closing, using butterfly tapes. If the laceration crosses a joint on the dorsal surface, it may spread with motion and splinting, in addition, may be required. All lacerations, particularly those of the palm of the hand, should be referred to a physician promptly.

Evaluating the extent of injury, including nerve, vascular and tendon injury, expedites proper care. Evaluation should include sensory testing using a pin on each side of the involved digit to determine whether the palmar and digital nerves are intact. In most cases, evaluation using touch only is deceptive, as the patient thinks he feels touch when the sense is actually transmitted through proprioceptive elements within the joints. The same patient may not feel the sharpness of a pin. As previously noted, sensory innervation of the hand varies. Each of the three nerves has autonomous areas, namely, the base of the thumb for the median nerve, the base of the fifth finger for the ulnar nerve, and the web space between the thumb and index finger on the thumb and dorsal side for the radial nerve.

To assess the integrity of the tendons, observe the hand in the resting position. Normally all fingers flex slightly at rest. With loss of a flexor tendon, one or more fingers remain extended. To test (Fig. 18:37) for continuity of the long flexors of the thumb or fingers, hold the proximal joints straight, and ask the patient to bend the distal joints. He can do this only if the long flexor tendon is intact. To check for the short flexor tendons (flexor sublimis), hold all but one finger extended, and ask the patient to flex this digit. The long flexors will remain tethered, and only the flexor sublimis of the finger being examined will be able to move. Assess each of the four fingers separately.

Puncture wounds often appear trivial initially, but may cause serious injury to deeper structures and have a high incidence of infection. Carefully check for disturbance of nerve and tendon function, particularly in puncture wounds of the palm. Treatment is thorough cleaning with soaks in warm water and appropriate germicidal agents followed by a sterile dressing and referral to a physician. A tetanus toxoid booster should be given when indicated. Puncture wounds of the fingertip can produce a felon (see Fingertip Injuries).

Human bites most commonly occur on a knuckle, when a closed fist strikes a human tooth. The severity of human bites must be recognized, as these injuries are heavily contaminated and require special and intensive treatment. In addition, the extensor tendon of the MCP joint may be severed.

Rehabilitation of Hand Injuries

Rehabilitation of the injured hand is as important to the functional outcome as any other component of treatment. In complex injuries, failure to follow through with rehabilitation may lead to stiffness and limited function despite perfect primary care and surgery.

In general, the goals of rehabilitation are to minimize swelling and mobilize the hand as soon as the injured parts permit. Initially, simple, active motion is begun while protecting the area of injury from stress. Thereafter, resistance and strengthening exercises are added progressively. A specific exercise routine lasting only five to ten minutes is prepared for each patient. In many cases, a splint may be removed for these exercise periods and replaced when completed. Short periods of active motion permit early return of function

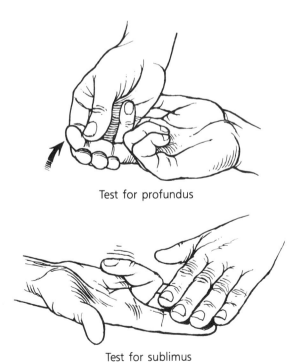

Test for profundus

Test for sublimus

FIGURE 18:37. Test for integrity of tendons of the fingers

without adding swelling or injury. Protective splinting and taping together with padding in selective instances may allow the athlete to participate. Fractured metacarpals, especially the third and fourth, can be taped together and protective sponge rubber or Styrofoam padding used.

Fractures of the second and fifth metacarpals are less stable, and this form of treatment is not as effective. The phalanges may be taped to their adjacent fingers and splinted with Styrofoam or rubber protective splints, and the thumb may be fitted with an adhesive tape checkrein to protect a gamekeeper's thumb.

The Pelvis

PELVIC INJURIES

The pelvis is commonly fractured as a result of direct compression in which it is literally crushed by a heavy impact. Injuries of the pelvic area are often seen after falls from heights and similar accidents. Indirect forces acting on the femur through the hip joint can also produce pelvic injury, as when the knee strikes a wall, driving the femoral head into the pelvis and fracturing it. Even a simple fall can fracture the pelvis.

Fracture of the pelvis may be associated with blood loss severe enough to cause hypovolemic shock and death. Remember the possibility of shock as a result of the fracture and take steps to combat it. Open fracture of the pelvis with obvious external bleeding is uncommon because heavy musculature surrounds the pelvis. The extent of blood loss in a closed pelvic fracture may not be apparent because the hemorrhage occurs within the pelvic cavity and into the retroperitoneal space and thus is not visible. Evaluate the athlete's vital signs as soon as possible and carefully monitor them during stabilization and transport.

The patient usually complains of pain in the pelvic region. Frequently, the only visible deformity is diffuse swelling in the pelvic region. There may be a contusion or abrasion over the iliac crest if the fracture resulted from a direct blow. The most important signs in diagnosing pelvic fractures are pain, felt when the iliac crests are compressed together, or tenderness on palpation of the pubic symphysis. Injuries of the genitourinary system, such as rupture of the bladder or a laceration of the urethra, are frequently associated with these fractures and must be suspected. Always check for abdominal pain and tenderness as well as hematuria—blood in the urine or blood around the urethral opening.

Patients with a suspected pelvic fracture should be monitored closely for changes in vital signs. The fracture is splinted by immobilization on a long spine board. Mild shock can be minimized by elevating the foot of the spine board 6 to 12 inches.

19

The Hip and Thigh

20

HIP

Anatomy

The articulation of the femur with the pelvis forms the hip joint—a ball and socket joint. The acetabulum, or socket, is deepened and reinforced by a fibrocartilaginous rim, the acetabular labrum. The joint is encased in a tough fibrous capsule lined by synovial tissue that nourishes the joint. Three extremely strong ligaments, the iliofemoral, pubofemoral and ischiofemoral, surround the joint anteriorly and posteriorly and reinforce the capsule (Fig. 20:1).

Of numerous bursae about the hip joint, the two most important are the trochanteric bursa,

located just behind the greater trochanter and deep to the gluteus maximus and tensor fascia femoris muscle, and the iliopsoas bursa, located between the capsule and the iliopsoas muscle anteriorly (Fig. 20:2).

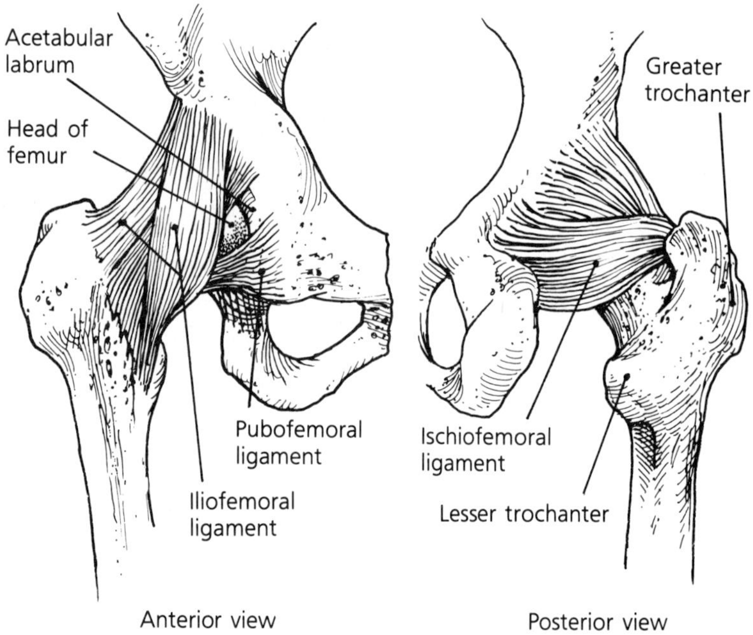

Motion of the hip joint includes flexion, extension, abduction, adduction, circumduction and rotation. The primary flexors of the hip are the iliopsoas, rectus femoris and adductor muscles. The primary extensors of the hip are the gluteus maximus and hamstrings. Adduction is primarily from the adductors and medial hamstrings. The primary abductors are the tensor fascia femoris and gluteus maximus and medius muscles. The internal rotators are the gluteus medius, tensor fascia femoris, adductors and iliopsoas muscles. The external rotators include the gluteus maximus, piriformis, obturator and gemellae muscles (Fig. 20:3).

Overuse Injuries

The trochanteric and iliopsoas bursae may become inflamed from overuse, such as in jogging. If the trochanteric bursa is involved, usually there is aching pain after running. If the iliopsoas muscle is involved, the pain is more medial and anterior in the groin.

Treatment includes rest of the hip joint and daily use of ice packs and oral anti-inflammatories. Examine the athlete carefully for any biomechanical problem, such as leg length discrepancy or muscle contracture, that predisposes to the bursitis.

Synovitis

Synovitis is a generalized nonspecific inflammatory condition of the hip. It may be

Acetabular labrum

Head of femur

Pubofemoral ligament

Iliofemoral ligament

Greater trochanter

Ischiofemoral ligament

Lesser trochanter

Anterior view

Posterior view

FIGURE 20:1. Hip joint: articulation of femur with pelvis

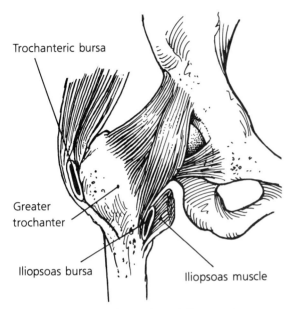

FIGURE 20:2. Trochanteric and iliopsoas bursae

caused by direct injury, such as a blow or twisting, or by overuse. Bacterial infections can also cause synovitis. The pain in the hip joint sometimes radiates down the medial aspect of the thigh to the knee via the obturator nerve. Any type of motion generally causes pain and the patient has an antalgic gluteus medius gait. The cause of the synovitis must be determined. Frequently the patient requires complete bed rest or must be totally nonweight bearing on crutches until the synovitis has been properly diagnosed and treated. He should be referred to an orthopedist for complete examination.

Hip Joint Sprain

Hip joint sprain is readily diagnosed by a history of a twisting injury to the hip. Circumduction of the leg always causes pain. Treatment consists of rest and protected weight bearing with crutches until walking is no longer painful.

Groin Strain

The muscles of the anterior groin, the adductor groups—the iliopsoas and rectus femoris—are frequently injured during athletics. Strains can occur with any stretch activity such as running, jumping or twisting. The injuries range from very mild causing only minor pain after exercise to severe, incapacitating tears. A sharp pain in the groin area, usually while twisting, running or jumping, is followed by increased pain, stiffness and weakness on hip flexion.

The proper muscle tests or stretching the affected muscle can determine which muscle group is involved. If straight leg raising against resistance causes pain, the rectus femoris group is probably involved. Pain on flexion of the hip with the knee bent on resistance above the top of the knee indicates iliopsoas injury. Adduction of the leg against resistance causes pain if the adductors are involved.

Treatment includes ice packs and rest, followed by several days of whirlpool and gentle range of motion exercise. Active stretching and progressive resistance exercises are begun

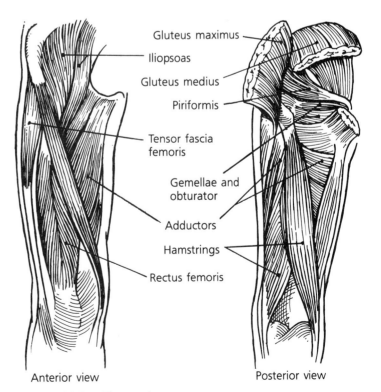

Anterior view   Posterior view

FIGURE 20:3. Hip muscles

Gluteus maximus
Iliopsoas
Gluteus medius
Piriformis
Tensor fascia femoris
Gemellae and obturator
Adductors
Hamstrings
Rectus femoris

when the muscle is no longer painful. Running is also allowed when range of motion and strength are adequate.

Pelvis and Hip Injuries

Injuries of the pelvis, hip region and bones of the lower extremity usually result from very severe trauma. Injury patterns vary with age. Violent trauma can cause severe, sometimes permanently disabling, injury in young, healthy individuals.

The general principles of splinting should always be followed (see Chapter 16). A general, primary assessment of the patient should be performed and serious problems stabilized before the limb injury is evaluated and splinted. Distal neurovascular function must be evaluated immediately and monitored frequently. All obvious bleeding must be controlled and open wounds protected from further contamination by applying a dry, sterile dressing.

Hip Dislocation

Posterior hip dislocation is commonly caused by a direct impact to the flexed knee and hip. There is immediate onset of pain and inability to walk or even move the hip. The hip remains in a flexed and internally rotated position, and the pain is usually severe. First-aid measures include supporting the injured part manually or with pillows and transporting the patient to the nearest medical facility immediately. This injury can damage the sciatic nerve and this must be considered on examination. Dislocations require hospitalization and general anesthesia to reduce pain.

Fractures

Hip fractures are rare in young athletes. When they occur, they are often caused by a severe impact while the foot is planted and the hip twisted. A slipped capital femoral epiphysis can occur in an older child or younger teenager. Ordinarily, symptoms of this serious injury develop over a period of time, starting with aching pain. Gradually the athlete begins to limp after activities and progresses to walking with an antalgic gait with the foot externally rotated.

Examination reveals fixed external rotation and inability to internally rotate, with some loss of flexion and extension. In about 10% of cases, the slipped epiphysis occurs acutely, perhaps while the individual is taking part in sports. Pain is severe and the patient should be referred to an orthopedist for immediate treatment.

THIGH

Anatomy

The femur is the largest, longest and strongest bone in the body and is almost perfectly cylindrical in shape. The shaft is bowed slightly outward and forward to accommodate the stress of locomotion and weight bearing.

There are four major groups of muscles in the thigh: flexors, extensors, abductors and adductors. The strongest group are the knee extensors (quadriceps) on the anterior aspect. The quadriceps consist of the rectus femoris, vastus intermedius, vastus medialis and the vastus lateralis. The rectus femoris originates on the anterior inferior iliac spine; the others arise from the shaft of the femur. They all converge to form the quadriceps tendon, inserting into the patella and extending on as the patella tendon to the tibial tuberosity. In addition, the rectus femoris acts as a hip flexor.

The hamstrings on the posterior aspect of the thigh are composed of the biceps femoris, semitendinous and semimembranous muscles. All three originate on the tuberosity of the ischium. The biceps has two heads: the long head arises from the medial aspect of the ischial tuberosity, and the short head arises from the linea aspera of the femur. It inserts on the head of the fibula and lateral condyle of the tibia. The biceps courses along the lateral side of the posterior thigh, while the semitendinous and semimembranous muscles course along the medial aspect of the femur.

The gracilis and the sartorius muscles, while not technically hamstring muscles, contribute to the medial hamstrings through a conjoined tendon called the pes anserinus (goose foot), which inserts onto the upper medial aspect of the tibia. The hamstrings are strong decelerators (flexors) of the knee and major extensors of the hip.

The adductor group consists primarily of the adductor magnus, brevis and longus muscles and the gracilis. The adductors arise from the pubic ramus and insert along the medial aspect of the distal femur, the gracilis attaching to the tibia through the pes anserinus tendons. They adduct the hip and help in hip and knee flexion.

The hip abductors consist of the tensor fasciae latae and gluteus medius muscles, which originate along the crest of the ilium. The gluteus medius inserts on the greater trochanter, and the tensor fasciae latae courses along the outer aspect of the thigh as the iliotibial band, inserting on the lateral aspect of the femoral condyle and tibia.

The extensor muscles of the thigh are supplied by the femoral artery and nerve. The hamstrings are innervated by the sciatic nerve and nourished by the femoral artery. The adductors are supplied principally by the obturator nerve. The muscles of the thigh are covered and divided into groups by a heavy, fibrous sheath, the fascia.

Soft Tissue Injuries

Injuries to the thigh muscles are among the most common in sports. Because of their large size and accessibility, they are subject to numerous stresses and strains. Contusion to the anterior and lateral thigh is very common in contact sports.

Contusion

A contusion results from a direct impact against the quadriceps muscle. It may vary from a mild bruise to a large, deep hematoma that may take months to heal. Usually loss of function, severe pain and progressive swelling and stiffness immediately follow impact. A localized area of exquisite tenderness appears and the athlete is unable to flex the knee. There is often an associated tear of muscle fibers.

Hemorrhage should be immediately controlled, initially with a compression dressing and ice applied directly to the area of trauma. Daily ice packs, very gentle active stretching of the muscle within the athlete's pain limits, and isometric exercises encourage early rehabilitation. Heat, ultrasound and massage after several days are sometimes advocated, but may intensify the inflammatory reaction if used too soon. As knee range of motion is gained, a progressive resistive quadriceps program and gradual return to jogging and running are instituted. Anti-inflammatory drugs may be very useful. Some physicians use oral or injectable enzymes with varying degrees of success. Enzymes are only effective in the first 24 to 48 hours postinjury, if at all.

Myositis Ossificans

In traumatic myositis ossificans, bone is deposited within a muscle as a result of contusion and subsequent resolution of the hematoma. The most common sites for bone proliferation in soft tissue are the quadriceps and the brachialis muscle of the arm. The process usually starts within one to two weeks after a severe contusion and may be palpated as a very hard mass within the soft tissue within three to four weeks after injury. At this time, x-ray films reveal fluffy, immature bone in the soft tissue. Over a period of months, the bone matures to typical cortical type bone (Fig. 20:4). This condition must be recognized early, as the process is self-limiting if the muscle is not irritated by active exercise or vigorous massage.

Treatment consists of rest and ice packs to reduce the swelling. The process is generally followed to maturity within six to 12 months by periodic x-ray examination. Usually the bony mass is no handicap once it has matured and no treatment is required other than padding. The bony mass may be excised surgical-

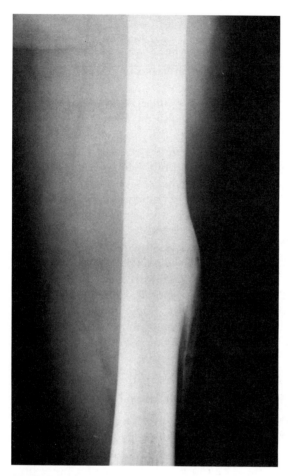

FIGURE 20:4.   Late myositis ossificans on x-ray. Note formation of cortical type bone.

ly if it causes some functional disability, such as pain or limitation of motion. Excision of the bone before it has matured simply results in its reforming, sometimes larger than before.

Any severe contusion of the thigh should be treated as impending myositis ossificans. Passive stretching and massage should be avoided and the injured part rested until painless range of motion has been restored. Myositis ossificans can sometimes be prevented by this program of rest.

Muscle Strain

Muscle strains (pulls) are very common injuries in all sports that involve running. They may range from mild first-degree strains to third-degree tears of the muscles. Hamstring strains are among the most feared injuries to athletes, as they tend to be nagging injuries that recur. They have been the demise of many great athletes. Hamstrings are particularly vulnerable to pulls because of the nature of their action and because they are opposed by the stronger quadriceps muscle. Individuals whose quadriceps are more than twice as strong as their hamstrings, or who have a significant imbalance between the strength of one leg and the other, are particularly vulnerable to tears.

Poor posture, inflexibility, fatigue and poor coordination also tend to lead to strains. Quantitative assessment of quadriceps to hamstring strength and comparison between the two extremities are valuable in detecting potential candidates for hamstring problems. As in most other injuries, it is much easier to prevent a hamstring strain through proper preventive rehabilitation and strengthening than it is to treat it once it has occurred. Athletes with tight, inelastic hamstrings and low back problems should follow a vigorous program of static stretching exercises. Those with markedly weaker hamstrings on one side compared with the other should undertake a progressive resistance exercise program to balance their muscles.

Hamstring strains are easily diagnosed. The athlete feels an immediate pain locally in the posterior thigh, usually while in full stride. In milder cases, this may simply lead to some tightness of the muscle. In third-degree tears, the patient is unable to walk. There is local tenderness and pain with any attempt to do a stretching maneuver. Large hamstring tears frequently result in profuse hemorrhage and ecchymosis that show up a few days postinjury. Severe muscle disruption and avulsions may require open repair.

Immediate treatment consists of ice and a compression dressing, followed by gradual active stretching and progressive exercise. Third-degree tears of the muscle are severe injuries and usually require crutches for ambulation.

Very mild injuries may heal within ten days to three weeks while the severe injuries may take two to six months to heal.

Because these injuries tend to recur due to inelasticity of the scar tissue in a torn muscle, the athlete should not be allowed to resume full activity until he can demonstrate complete flexibility and return of strength and muscle balance.

Fractures

Stress Fractures

Stress fractures of the femur may occur, particularly in runners. They generally present clinically as a chronic, nonspecific soft tissue pain about the groin and thigh. Examination usually reveals mild tenderness about the mid to proximal portion of the thigh with palpation. Diagnosis is confirmed by x-ray films, which may show a periosteal reactive bone formation several weeks after the onset of symptoms. In early cases a bone scan may be necessary to diagnose a stress fracture. Treatment consists of rest until symptoms subside.

Femoral Shaft Fractures

Fractures of the femur usually result from direct, very forceful impact. They may occur in any part of the shaft, from the hip region to the femoral condyles just above the knee joint. Diagnosis is usually easily made since the athlete will often lie with the leg in marked deformity, severely angulated or rotated at the fracture site, frequently with shortening of the limb.

Fractures of the femur are often open. Closed or open, they are always associated with severe blood loss. It is not unusual for a patient with a fracture of the femur to go into hypovolemic shock. Patients must be handled extremely carefully, since any extra movement or fracture manipulation increases the blood loss. An open fracture of the femur should, like any other open fracture, be treated with appropriate sterile pressure dressings applied over the wound.

Vascular injuries may accompany femoral fractures with impaired circulation distally, causing a pale, cold and pulseless foot. Gentle, longitudinal traction in line with the long axis of the limb, gradually restoring the overall alignment of the limb, and splinting the limb in that position usually restores circulation. If signs of circulation return are not seen after appropriate alignment and splinting, a serious vascular injury may have occurred and prompt transportation to a medical facility is indicated.

A fracture of the femoral shaft is best immobilized with a traction splint. (The technique for applying a traction splint is described in Chapter 16.) The precise sequence of steps to properly apply this splint must be thoroughly known, understood and practiced frequently to maintain the skill.

The Knee

21

The key to understanding the knee joint is in realizing that its movement is helicoid or spiral in character and not that of a simple hinge joint. The joint consists of large, rounded condyles of the femur (Fig. 21:1) and the much flattened condyles of the tibia. The fibula does not take part in the joint. The patella articulates with the patellar surface of the femur and thus the knee joint consists of three joints in one: a joint between the patella and the femur and between each tibial condyle and femoral condyle. The anatomical axis of the lower extremity, shown in Figure 21:2, differs from the mechanical axis, which is a line drawn from the center of the hip, knee and ankle joints. With a wider pelvis, as in women, the inward angulation of the femur is greater, as is the outward angulation of the tibia. This is referred to as genu valgum, or knock knees. The opposite condition, genu varum, refers to bowed knees.

ANATOMY

Skeleton

The femoral condyles are two rounded prominences of the distal femur that are eccentrically curved. The anterior portion is part of an oval and the posterior portion a section of a sphere. The condyles project very little in front of the femoral shaft but markedly behind. The groove that runs anteriorly between the condyles (see Fig. 21:1) is the patellofemoral groove or trochlea, which accepts the patella. Posteriorly, the condyles are separated by the intercondylar notch. The articular surface of the medial condyle is longer from front to back than the lateral condyle, but the lateral condyle is wider. The long axis of the lateral condyle is oriented essentially along the sagittal plane, but the medial condyle is usually at approximately a 22° angle to the sagittal plane.

The expanded proximal end of the tibia is formed by two rather flat surfaces, or plateaus, that articulate with the femoral condyles. They are separated in the midline by the intercondylar eminence with its medial and lateral intercondylar tubercles. Anterior and posterior to the intercondylar eminence are attachment sites for the cruciate ligaments and menisci.

The lateral tibial plateau is flatter and more convex, shorter from front to back, and more oval. The anatomy for the tibial plateau is such that, in order to properly visualize the plateau

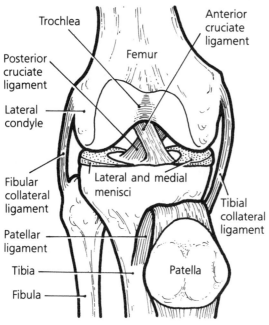

FIGURE 21:1. Knee joint

Labels on figure:
- Trochlea
- Posterior cruciate ligament
- Lateral condyle
- Fibular collateral ligament
- Patellar ligament
- Tibia
- Fibula
- Femur
- Anterior cruciate ligament
- Lateral and medial menisci
- Tibial collateral ligament
- Patella

on an anteroposterior roentgenogram, the x-ray tube must be angled about 15° inferiorly because the tibia slopes in a downward direction from front to back.

The patella is a rounded, triangular bone, wider at the upper (proximal) end than at the bottom (distal) end. The articular surface of the patella is divided by a vertical ridge (see Fig. 21:1) that creates a smaller medial and a larger lateral articular facet or surface. A smaller vertical ridge that lies even more medially separates the extreme medial "odd facet," which begins to contact the femur at around 135° knee flexion.

Quadriceps Tendon

The quadriceps tendon inserts into the top end of the patella. There are four components of the quadriceps muscle (Fig. 21:3), the vastus medialis, vastus lateralis, vastus intermedius and rectus femoris. A broad fibrous expansion on either side of the patella (see Fig. 21:3), made up of extensions of the vastus medialis and vastus lateralis, continues anteriorly over the knee joint to insert onto the tibia. These are called medial and lateral patellar retinacula. The retinacula are important and help extend the knee joint even when the patellar tendon is ruptured. The fibers of the medial retinaculum, formed from the aponeurosis of the vastus medialis obliquus plus the vastus medialis muscle itself, insert directly into the medial side of the patella. This is the dynamic medial restraint that may prevent lateral displacement of the patella. Thus the extensor mechanism is a complex interaction of muscles, patellar ligaments medially and laterally that stabilize the patellofemoral joint and the patellar ligament (tendon) that inserts onto the tibial tubercle.

Medial Aspect

The major structures on the medial aspect of the knee are the medial retinaculum, the medial collateral ligament, the medial capsular ligaments and the pes anserinus, which consists of the sartorius, gracilis and semiten-

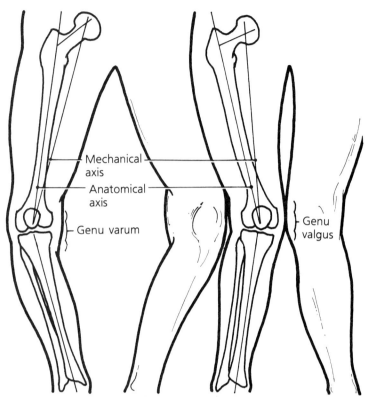

FIGURE 21:2. Anatomical and mechanical axis of lower extremity. Genu valgum and genu varum

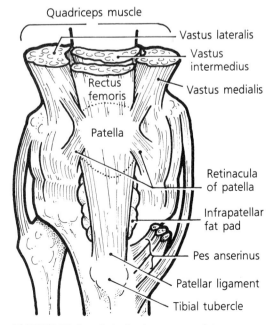

FIGURE 21:3. Anterior knee musculature

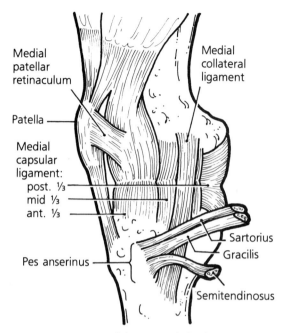

FIGURE 21:4. Medial aspect of the knee

dinous muscles (Fig. 21:4). Starting anteriorly, the patellar ligament is evident, attaching to the anterior surface of the tibia. The medial retinaculum attaches along the medial border of the patella. Its function is primarily to hold the patella medially. The medial collateral ligament is composed of long parallel fibers overlying the joint capsule. Further posterior are the three tendons of the sartorius, gracilis and semitendinous muscles coursing inferiorly to attach as the pes anserinus to the anteromedial aspect of the tibia. These muscles help protect the knee against rotary and valgus stress.

The parallel fibers of the superficial medial (collateral) ligament as a whole form a well delineated, band-like structure inserting proximally into the medial femoral epicondyle and distally about a hand's breadth below the joint line onto the medial aspect of the tibia. It glides anterior in extension and posterior with flexion. The specific functions of this ligament are discussed later in this text.

The mid third of the true capsule of the knee joint is sometimes called the deep medial collateral ligament. The medial capsular ligament

extends from the femur to the midportion of the meniscus and then to the tibia. The attachments of this deep structure to the medial meniscus are termed the meniscofemoral and meniscotibial (or coronary) ligaments. They limit excessive motion of the meniscus.

Posterior Aspect

The hollow area that appears on the posterior surface of the knee is the popliteal space (Fig. 21:5). Superiorly, the popliteal space is bounded by the tendon of the biceps femoris muscle laterally and the semimembranous and semitendinous tendons medially. Inferiorly the popliteal space is bounded by the two heads of the gastrocnemius muscle.

Some of the more important structures in the popliteal space are the nerves, which are the most superficially located. The division of the sciatic nerve into the common peroneal and tibial is easily seen and the branches of the common peroneal (lateral sural cutaneous and peroneal communicating) arise on the medial side of this nerve. Motor branches to the plantaris and gastrocnemius muscles arise from the

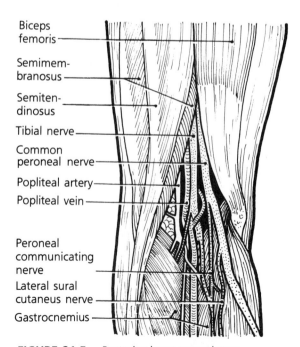

FIGURE 21:5. Posterior knee musculature

tibial nerve. The tibial nerve disappears from view as it courses deep to the gastrocnemius muscle, while the common peroneal nerve disappears by piercing the peroneus longus muscle and winding around the fibula to the anterior surface of the leg.

If the nerves are pulled to one side, the main popliteal vein appears anterior to the nerve. The femoral artery, as it courses through the tendon of the adductor magnus muscle, enters the popliteal fossa as the popliteal artery and is in contact with the capsule of the knee joint. With any knee surgery, such as removal of a meniscus, the artery must be protected from injury as it lies directly behind the knee joint capsule.

Another muscle that appears deep to the artery is the popliteus muscle (Fig. 21:6). This muscle is unusual in that it has three distal origins—the posterior tibia proximally, the posterior aspect of the fibular head and the posterior horn of the lateral meniscus. It inserts on the lateral femoral condyle just below the fibular collateral ligament. Its primary function is internal rotation of the tibia on the femur. It provides dynamic stability to the posterolateral capsular complex of the knee (popliteal-arcuate complex shown in Fig. 21:6). The popliteus also pulls the posterior horn of the lateral meniscus posteriorly with knee flexion.

Medially, the semimembranous muscle is an important stabilizing structure to the posterior aspect of the knee. The posterior capsule is pulled tightly around the femoral condyles in extension and helps to stabilize the knee in this position.

Lateral Aspect

The patellar ligament is shown anteriorly in Figure 21:3. The iliotibial tract is superficial to the capsule of the knee joint (Fig. 21:7).

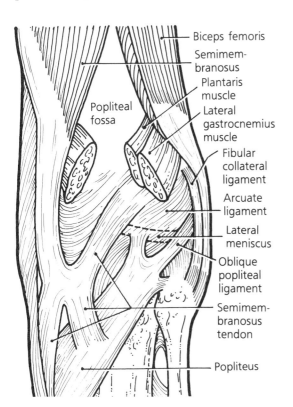

FIGURE 21:6. Popliteus and semimembranous muscles

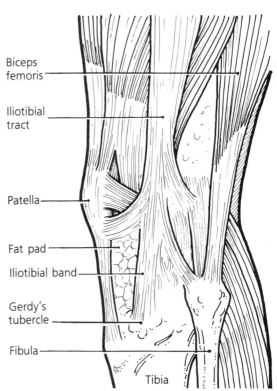

FIGURE 21:7. Lateral knee musculature

Posterior to this are the fibular collateral ligament and, finally, the tendon of the biceps femoris muscle. The common peroneal nerve can also be seen at this location as it winds around the lateral head of the gastrocnemius and the fibula to pierce the peroneus longus muscle.

The fascia lata or iliotibial tract envelops the lateral aspect of the thigh as it originates from the lateral iliac crest region, continues as a fibrous expansion over the vastus lateralis and into the lateral intermuscular septum and continues over the lateral aspect of the knee. One major extension goes into the lateral soft tissue restraining structures of the patellofemoral joint. The iliotibial band is a thickening of the iliotibial tract that inserts directly into the lateral tubercle of the tibia (Gerdy's tubercle, see Fig. 21:7). The proximal attachment of this band is at the distal intermuscular septum. With knee flexion the iliotibial band moves posteriorly and with knee extension it moves anteriorly.

Underneath the fascia lata and iliotibial band is the capsule of the joint. The capsule provides meniscus attachments as shown in Figure 21:6. The posterior third of the lateral capsule together with the popliteus attachments previously described form the arcuate ligament. This muscular structure provides considerable stability to the posterolateral corner of the knee.

The lateral collateral ligament of the knee inserts from the femoral condyle to the fibular head. The insertion of the biceps muscle completely envelops the fibular insertion of the ligament.

Deep to the lateral collateral ligament lies the short collateral ligament (see Fig. 21:6). If there is a sesamoid bone (fabella) deep to the lateral head of the gastrocnemius, this latter ligament is attached to it and is then called the fabellofibular ligament. It runs parallel to the lateral collateral ligament and attaches to the fibular head posterior to the tendon of the biceps. It reinforces the posterior capsule and contributes to the lateral stability of the knee (Fig. 21:8).

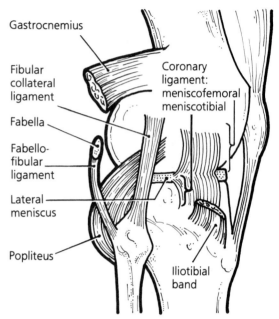

FIGURE 21:8. Lateral ligament complex

Internal Knee Anatomy

The cruciate ligaments and meniscus structures guide the movements of the knee. The menisci are cartilaginous and tough when compressed between the femur and tibia. Both the medial and lateral menisci are C-shaped and conform to the shapes of the tibial surfaces on which they rest. The intricate anatomy of the menisci is discussed later when tears to these structures are considered.

Cruciate Ligaments

The anterior and posterior cruciate ligaments function in both anteroposterior and rotatory stability. They are so named because they cross each other like the limbs of an X. The anterior cruciate attaches to the posterior medial aspect of the lateral femoral condyle. It has a fan-shaped attachment that corresponds to the curve of the medial margin of the lateral femoral condyle. This is a difficult attachment to reach in performing ligament repairs. The tibial attachment is more compact and easily visualized.

The posterior cruciate is attached behind the intercondylar area of the posterior surface of the tibia. It is shorter, thicker, stronger and less oblique than the anterior cruciate ligament. From its tibial attachment it is directed in a superior, anterior and medial direction to its femoral attachment on the lateral surface of the medial femoral condyle. Technically, both ligaments are outside the synovial cavity of the joint. As shown in Figure 21:9, ligament tears occur within the synovial envelope, and the ligament can sometimes appear normal at surgery, only to be found to be torn when the envelope is opened. The different types of cruciate tears are also shown in Figure 21:9. Most commonly, the anterior cruciate is torn in its substance. The mop-end tear is nearly impossible to repair, so commonly a tendon graft or other material is added. Tears at the bony attachment involve reattaching the bone, with the prognosis for function often good. The anterior cruciate blood supply through the middle geniculate artery and fat pad is usually interrupted, with tears making healing even more difficult.

The infrapatellar fat pad (see Fig. 21:3) extends from the lower pole of the patella to the level of the tibia, behind and on each side of the patellar tendon. The pliable fat pad is a relatively mobile structure. The pad has connections with the front ends of the semilunar cartilages which are attached and which it overlaps. The blood supply to the patellar tendon courses through it.

Plica

The advent of diagnostic and surgical arthroscopy has created increased recognition of the presence of knee plicae (Fig. 21:10). In embryonic development, a septum separates the suprapatellar pouch from the knee joint. This septum usually disappears but, in approximately 20% of knees, it persists into adult life as a fibrous band and may be clinically significant. The synovial fold begins on the medial wall of the knee joint and proceeds obliquely downward to insert into the synovia covering the infrapatellar fat pad. Most of these plicae are soft and pliable and remain asymptomatic. A large, thick medial patellar plica may act as a fibrous shelf and irritate the medial femoral condyle. The athlete with a symptomatic plica may give a history of medial joint pain, but usually without antecedent trauma. The symptoms often increase with activity, but the plica may also produce knee pain when the knee is

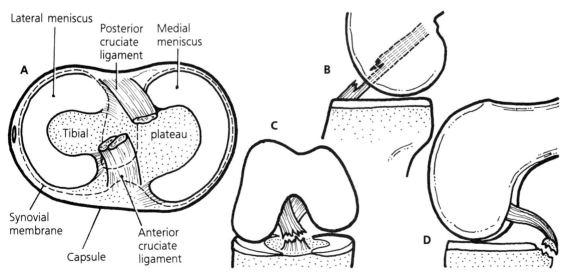

FIGURE 21:9. **A** Tibial attachments of the anterior and posterior cruciate ligaments (ACL, PCL) in relationship to the synovial cavity. **B** Partial tear of the ACL. **C** Midsubstance mop-end tear of the ACL. **D** Bony avulsion of the PCL

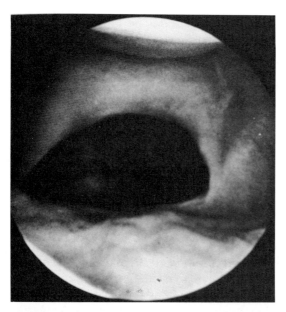

FIGURE 21:10. Patella plica is the synovial curtain at the top of the image (arthroscopic view).

kept in one position for prolonged periods, as in sitting. There may also be snapping or pseudolocking that may mimic a torn meniscus. In some cases, the medial plica can be palpated on physical examination, especially with the knee flexed to approximately 45°. As the examining thumb is rolled over the medial shelf, tenderness may be produced and the shelf may be clinically palpable.

Diagnosis can rarely be made by arthrogram, but is best made arthroscopically, at which time treatment can be rendered. In symptomatic plica, excision of the shelf is recommended, although some feel that division of the shelf is sufficient.

EVALUATION OF KNEE INJURY

The knee is one of the most vulnerable joints of the body and has an intricate and complex anatomy. Correct diagnosis of the exact structure that has been injured is often difficult. Practical guidelines for analyzing knee injuries are presented here. Most knee injuries are first evaluated by the trainer or primary care physi-

cian. Therefore, potentially serious injuries must be differentiated from minor injuries. More serious knee injuries with severe ligament damage and gross instability are easy to diagnose and require immediate treatment. On the other hand, subtle, benign-appearing or less common injuries are sometimes underestimated, but may later seriously impair knee stability. The common error is to assume a knee ligament injury is less severe than it actually is. Certain features about the patient's history and physical findings should alert the trainer or physician as to the seriousness of the acutely injured knee, particularly where gross instability or fracture is not immediately obvious.

The secret of accurate diagnosis in the acutely injured knee is a standardized, systematic approach designed to elicit key symptoms and physical findings that alert the examiner to the need for further tests, immediate treatment or surgery. Although the examination of the acutely injured knee differs markedly from that of the chronically unstable knee, many examination techniques do not distinguish between them. With the chronic knee, the examiner can perform a variety of different tests to fully bring out the subtleties of the instability. With the acute knee injury, pain and muscle spasm may prevent a precise examination, necessitating examination under anesthesia and, in certain instances, arthroscopy.

The trainer and primary care physician have five goals in the initial evaluation of an acute knee injury. The first is to exclude immediately a limb-threatening disorder such as interruption of blood supply to the extremity or serious fracture or dislocation. Second, they must record the details associated with the injury that may facilitate the physician's diagnosis. Third, they must carry out gross stability tests to indicate the severity of the injury. Fourth, they must provide immediate splinting and first-aid care to the extremity and, fifth, arrange immediate transport and triage for definitive medical care. In the less acute knee injury, such as where swelling has occurred over three to four days without a specific injury, the initial examiner can perform more diagnostic tests. In the chronically unstable knee, a variety of diagnostic tests are available to arrive at the correct diagnosis.

This section initially considers the evaluation of an acute knee injury. More sophisticated instability tests as performed in the physician's office or under anesthesia on the less acute injured knee or on the chronically unstable knee are detailed later in this chapter.

History

Knee evaluation begins with a detailed history of the most recent injury and subsequent developments. The history itself very often leads to a presumptive diagnosis which the physical examination then substantiates and qualifies.

1. Did the injured knee swell acutely? This is an extremely important fact to determine along with appropriate qualifying factors of location of swelling, rate of accumulation and amount of swelling. Rapid swelling is an ominous sign. It suggests hemorrhage within the knee joint and the high likelihood of a cruciate ligament tear, osteochondral fracture or patellar dislocation.
2. What was the mechanism of injury? A medial or lateral blow causing an abnormal joint opening to the opposite side of the knee suggests injury to the collateral ligament and associated capsular ligaments, the adjacent meniscus or a fracture at the site of impact. Anterior cruciate injuries are much more common than originally suspected, as will be discussed. Such injuries may follow a hyperextension and internal tibial rotation injury, although they more commonly result from any twisting or deceleration injury. Additional mechanisms include a posterior blow to the proximal tibia, such as an illegal clip in football. Associated mechanisms of injury that may produce particular ligament tears are described under ligament function.
3. Has the knee sustained a serious injury before this last accident? On occasion a prior injury to a meniscus or cruciate ligament has led to an internal derangement and unstable knee. The first examiner may be misled by thinking that the instability is secondary to an acute injury.
4. Was the patient able to continue playing after his knee injury? This important question helps determine the extent of injury. Over 80% of patients with serious ligament injuries are unable to continue playing after the injury. Because approximately 20% are able to continue playing after the injury, however, the ability to walk from the playing field does not signify the lack of a serious injury.
5. Did the patient's knee "give way" or "go out of place" at the time of injury? There are many causes for the knee's giving way. This symptom is often found in chronic cases of instability. However, the giving way episode may reflect an acute injury. The patient's sensation of knee instability without actual giving way may also indicate a ligament problem. The knee actually "going out of place" or the "joint separating" at the time of injury may indicate a serious injury.

The extent of historical evaluation depends upon the circumstances surrounding the injury. On the playing field, the examiner may readily assess how the injury occurred and the anatomical site of the injury. Later, in a more relaxed atmosphere, time allows the close scrutiny of all historical details.

Physical Examination

The physical examination is designed to methodically and specifically test all of the major components of the knee joint, including the major ligaments of the knee, menisci structures, patellofemoral joint and muscles about the knee. The examiner should always compare the injured knee with the opposite side. The techniques for performing the tests are described in a later section.

A few points of caution in examining the acute injury must be emphasized. First and foremost you are dealing with an injury. The initial evaluation of any injury should exclude more serious or life-threatening associated injuries.

The second note of caution deals specifically with the examination of the knee joint. The examiner must realize the limitations of clinical examination in an acutely injured knee. Always remember: be gentle. Do not force the knee joint through any sudden motions. Determine the severity of injury and pain without producing more discomfort. Do not place great reliance on a negative test. A joint effusion and even slight muscle spasm may block any of the laxity tests, giving a false negative test for knee stability.

The initial examination includes obtaining a history, observing the limb, as indicated in Figure 21:11, and palpating the joint for local tenderness. Gently perform a simple antero-posterior drawer test and simple abduction-adduction stress test. If the knee is grossly unstable, do not carry out any further stability tests. Rather, immobilize the limb and immediately transfer the athlete to a medical facility for a definitive diagnosis and treatment. With a chronically unstable knee without the

effects of an injury, a variety of stability tests can be used. In the acutely injured knee, the treating physician will eventually have to perform similar tests, but necessarily under ideal conditions with the patient relaxed. Not infrequently stability tests and knee evaluation must be done under general anesthesia. Therefore, the trainer need only initially determine gross laxity by simple anteroposterior drawer tests and abduction-adduction stress tests. These tests are best done with the knee at 30° flexion, usually the least painful position. Negative test results, as previously discussed, do not exclude major injury. Any knee injury that disrupts an athlete's play or performance, no matter how trivial it may appear, needs comprehensive evaluation by the treating physician.

Always examine the patellofemoral joint for a tendency for subluxation or dislocation. Symptoms caused by subluxation of the patellofemoral joint can resemble those of meniscus or ligamentous origin, including giving way episodes, generalized pain and swelling.

Again, an acute hemarthrosis is extremely important to note. It can be confirmed during the examination comparing the peripatellar re-

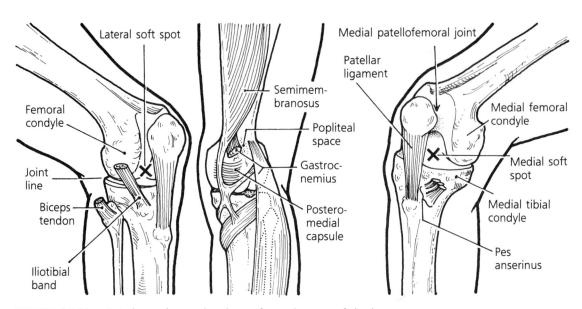

FIGURE 21:11. Anterior and posterior views of prominences of the knee

cesses to the normal knee. Also the patella will ballott to digital pressure, indicating joint swelling. The knee also has decreased range of motion.

Observation

Before adequate examination can take place, the patient must be as relaxed as possible and the extremities bare from the toes to the groin. If possible, begin the examination by observing the patient's gait, limp and functional range of motion. Tailor the examination to the injury. In the chronic condition, observe the patient's use of the knee joint through a variety of activities, including jumping and squatting, to note a functional deficit. Many other aspects of a comprehensive knee evaluation by the treating physician are not covered. However, the outline of the physical examination lists the essentials for initial evaluation.

1. History
   A. When injury occurred
   B. Mechanisms of injury
   C. Previous injuries
   D. Swelling
   E. Knee "gave way" or "went out of place"
   F. Continued participation after injury
   G. Felt or heard a "pop"
2. Observation
   A. Skin color
   B. Swelling (total vs. confined)
   C. Assumed position
   D. Ecchymosis
   E. Alignment (tibia/femur; patella/femur)
   F. Q-angle
3. Palpation
   A. Pulses
   B. Pain/tenderness
   C. Swelling (ballottable patella)
   D. Temperature
   E. Sensation
   F. Integrity of collateral ligaments
4. Movement
   A. Total painless range of motion
   B. Patella mobility
   C. Patella grating, crepitus
5. Stability Testing
   A. Abduction/adduction
      0° Flexion
      30° Flexion
   B. Anteroposterior drawer
      20°–30° Flexion (Lachman's test)
      90° Flexion
   C. Genu recurvation test
   D. Posterior cruciate gravity test
   E. Patellar apprehension test
   F. Others:
      Slocum rotatory tests
      Flexion–rotation drawer test
      Jerk test
      Pivot shift test
      Anterolateral rotatory instability test
      Manual muscle test, quadriceps and hamstrings
      Plica test
6. Meniscus Tests
   A. McMurray's test
   B. Apley's compression test

Palpation

Palpation is performed ideally with the patient seated or supine. Palpation for localized tenderness can detect injury to the structure felt. Always begin palpation of the area distal from the suspected injury. This promotes the patient's cooperation and prevents the examiner from overlooking a concomitant injury (Fig. 21:11). For example, if a lesion on the medial aspect of the knee is suspected, begin by palpating all of the lateral structures: the lateral femoral condyle, the lateral aspect of the patellofemoral joint, the soft spot lateral to the patellar tendon that gives access to the lateral joint line, the entire joint line progressing to the posterolateral corner, the iliotibial band, the biceps tendon and the lateral head of the gastrocnemius muscle. In a cooperative patient with legs crossed, the lateral collateral ligament can be easily palpated. Then proceed to the medial aspect of the joint, palpating the medial femoral condyle, medial tibial condyle, medial portion of the patella, patellar tendon and medial soft spot. Examine the joint line progressing anteriorly to posteriorly to the region of the posteromedial capsule semimembranous and gastrocnemius muscle.

Finally, palpate the popliteal space. In the anterior aspect of the knee, palpate the quadriceps attachment to the patella for a defect or localized tenderness that may indicate rupture. Tenderness directly to the patella may indicate a fracture. Pain on palpation of the patellar tendon at its attachment to the inferior pole of the patella or tibia may indicate tears. Next test the movement or range of motion in the chronic knee but not in an acute knee injury. Ask the patient to extend the knee and palpate the integrity of the extensor mechanism, looking for rupture of the quadriceps tendon, patella fracture, patellar tendon disruption or tibial tubercle avulsion. This is done only after palpation excludes a gross disruption where any active motion would be contraindicated. Inability to extend the knee fully may be due to rupture of the extensor mechanism or due to pain and joint swelling.

The patellofemoral joint needs to be thoroughly examined at some point in the evaluation. Palpate for localized tenderness to the en-

tire extensor mechanism as just discussed. The ''apprehension'' test involves lateral displacement of the patella (Fig. 21:12). Attempt to subluxate the patella laterally to see if apprehension or pain is elicited. Often localized tenderness about the medial retinacular and ligamentous supports to the patella indicates tearing of these tissues due to subluxation or dislocation. Patella grating and crepitus are also noted during movement of the patellofemoral joint.

Stability Testing

The initial examiner of an acute injury need only determine gross ligamentous instability. The treating physician will perform more specialized stability tests. First, perform a gentle anteroposterior drawer test with the knee joint at 20° to 30° of flexion. Flexion to 90° is usually not possible due to pain and swelling. Additionally, the test at 30° is considered more accurate in detecting anteroposterior laxity. Second, carry out an abduction/adduction stress test with the knee at 30° of flexion; this may be repeated at full knee extension. This test may be gently done on the field of play. Later, more comprehensive testing may follow, depending upon the patient's injury and pain. These tests are described more thoroughly later in this chapter.

Meniscus Tests

In evaluating the acutely injured knee, the goal is to exclude a significant fracture or ligamentous injury requiring immediate treatment. Tests for meniscus structures are inaccurate with acute injury due to pain and swelling. What's more, they are not required, and the diagnosis of a meniscus tear is not an emergency. Later, if there is no serious injury, perform the McMurray test and Apley's compression test (Fig. 21:13). In this latter test, place the patient in a prone position and flex the knee to 90°. Rotate the knee joint by rotating the leg while pressing the knee joint together. The test is positive if pain is produced. This test may or may not be positive with a meniscus tear. The maneuver presses

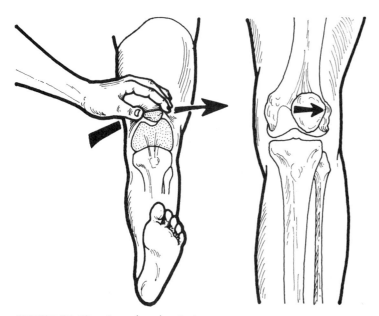

FIGURE 21:12. Apprehension test

a dislodged portion of the meniscus or puts excess pressure on a damaged meniscus attachment, thereby producing pain. The pressure on the meniscus structures is relieved by repeating the test with the joint distracted, and the pain is typically diminished or absent.

A modification of this test can detect some meniscus tears. By gently flexing and extending the knee with the patient supine, first place a valgus load on the knee joint, producing increased compression to the lateral joint. Alternatively, produce varus or adduction to the knee, creating increased compression to the medial aspect of the joint. Note crepitus and pain while taking the knee through 0 to 90° of motion. Crepitus palpated and heard at the joint may be due to either a torn meniscus or surface deterioration indicating early joint arthritis.

In the well-known McMurray's test for a major disruption of the posterior horn of either the medial or lateral meniscus, with full flexion externally rotate the leg, then extend the knee. The desire is to trap the displaced portion of the medial meniscus in the joint, producing an audible and palpable click or thud. Alternatively, with full flexion and marked internal rotation, attempt to dislodge a portion of the lateral meniscus into the joint, producing a similar sign. In the presence of injury this test may or may not be positive. In fact, negative results are more common in knees with meniscus tears. Actually, meniscus tears in the chronically unstable knee are best diagnosed by the history and finding of localized tenderness to the joint line.

Pain

The occurrence and location of pain, particularly elicited on palpation, indicates the severity of the injury. However, in some cases pain symptoms are unreliable. In certain injuries, severe capsular disruption prevents the accumulation of blood under pressure and there may be a surprising lack of pain. Also, a few patients may continue their sport immediately after injury despite having sustained

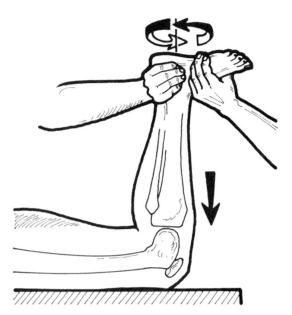

FIGURE 21:13. Apley's compression test

a major ligament tear. The athlete may only complain of a slight wobbliness to the knee while the knee may show gross instability on examination. Therefore, the lack of considerable pain in an acutely injured knee does not eliminate the possibility of a serious injury. On the other hand, the finding of severe pain and inability to walk suggests a major intraarticular problem.

In the adolescent, pain and swelling may indicate a distal femoral or proximal tibial epiphyseal fracture. In the latter case, routine radiographs may not confirm the diagnosis and stress radiographs must be obtained. A clue to an epiphyseal fracture is the finding of localized tenderness above the joint line in the region of the medial or lateral femoral condyle. Alternatively, similar tenderness below the joint line in the region of the tibial growth plate may indicate a fracture.

Swelling

When swelling in the knee joint is established, either by history or examination, it is important to document the following.

1. *Location of swelling.* Restricted swelling to one side of the knee or the other does not indicate intra-articular fluid, but usually means local tissue disruption. It may indicate tearing of the medial or lateral collateral ligaments. Swelling confined to the femoral condylar areas above the knee in an adolescent may indicate an epiphyseal fracture. Discrete swelling can also mean hemorrhagic bursitis, such as a contused pre-patellar bursa. The ominous sign is a true bloody effusion or hemarthrosis after injury, that is, an intra-articular accumulation of blood.

2. *Rate of accumulation.* A rapid accumulation of intra-articular fluid after injury indicates a hemarthrosis. However, intra-articular swelling after 24 hours may not be secondary to blood. An aspiration may be required.

3. *Quantity of blood.* Generally speaking, a large amount of blood with tense swelling of the knee is presumptive evidence of more severe damage. However, the amount of blood is not a reliable indicator of severity.

4. *Characteristics of blood aspirated.* In the past, the character of the blood aspirated was often incorrectly used to make a presumptive diagnosis. If fat globules were present in the blood when examined under direct vision, a presumptive diagnosis of an intra-articular fracture was made. This sign can certainly be present with articular fractures; however, it can also be present secondary to synovial or fat pad injury and therefore is unreliable. The term "cruciate blood" has been used to describe the grossly bloody aspirate from knees with anterior cruciate tears. This structure is vascular and tends to bleed profusely when injured. Meniscus tears do not cause a large hemarthrosis. Menisci blood supply is at their synovial attachments, which usually do not bleed much when torn. Bright red blood can occur from osteochondral fractures or dislocation of the patella. Generally, aspiration of an acutely injured knee where swelling has occurred within only two to three hours is

not necessary except to relieve severe pain associated with a tense hemarthrosis. Aspiration should be avoided when possible since it potentially introduces bacteria and may in rare cases lead to joint infection (pyarthrosis). A local anesthetic may be instilled on aspiration to obtain a more reliable stability examination.

Roentgenograms

Radiographic studies of the knee should include routine anteroposterior, lateral and axial patellar views. Additionally, condylar tunnel views and medial and lateral oblique views may be required to exclude an intra-articular fracture. Routine stress views are generally of little help unless the patient is an adolescent with open epiphyseal growth centers. In this instance, varus or valgus stress views may be included to rule out an epiphyseal plate injury. The radiographs will show opening at the growth plate of the femur or tibia rather than at the joint line (Fig. 21:14).

In summary, routine evaluation of the acute knee injury establishes, in most cases, significant injury requiring immediate treatment and definitive diagnostic evaluation. If the approach outlined is performed consistently and systematically with proper emphasis on historical and clinical findings during initial

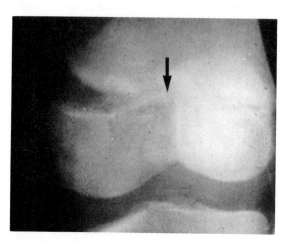

FIGURE 21:14. Epiphyseal plate injury showing opening at growth plate of femur

evaluation, the majority of serious injuries will be detected. This initial triage can identify those knee injuries that are emergencies, but signs of severe injury may be subtle and the severity may not be detected initially. Swelling the next day or continued pain or stiffness indicates the need for comprehensive evaluation. Therefore, all knee injuries diagnosed as minor absolutely require repeat evaluation after 24 and even 48 hours. Further evaluation is required to document return to normal function. One final point requires emphasis. Marked swelling in the knee joint within 24 hours of injury is an ominous sign indicating hemorrhage and a potential for a significant intra-articular injury. A review of 85 knee injuries found a disruption of the anterior cruciate ligament in almost three fourths. Despite an acute hemarthrosis the stability examination did not reveal gross instability. The knees appeared similar to the common knee sprain usually treated symptomatically except that swelling developed within 24 hours of injury due to an acute hemarthrosis.

Acute Treatment

An acute knee injury should be treated immediately with a soft compression dressing combined with coaptation splinting, designed to decrease knee mobility, following the initial evaluation and pending further disposition. Commercial knee splints and knee immobilizers are also available.

At no time should the patient be allowed to bear weight on an acutely painful or swollen knee. He should remain supine with the involved leg elevated and ice packs applied to the knee initially and after the compression dressing. The patient should be shown how to conduct his own neurovascular examination. The foot and toes should always have active movement with normal color and warmth. The patient should report any increase in pain immediately.

In referring a patient to the treating physician, a detailed report must be included. A verbal description of the events surrounding the injury and immediate treatment is best, if at all possible. Because of developing muscle spasm and joint swelling, sometimes the initial examination is more reliable than a subsequent examination. If a knee dislocation is suspected, hospitalization and close observation must be considered. A number of associated neurovascular complications are common in knee dislocations and require emergency hospitalization.

Testing for Knee Instabilities

Testing for knee laxity is the final phase of the examination. Unfortunately, controversy exists over which ligament structures are tested and, therefore, competent examiners may interpret identical findings differently. Each examiner should develop an individual approach and refine the techniques continuously on the basis of experience and developing concepts. The information here is the basis for evolving such an individualized testing program.

For many years straight anterior and straight posterior instability were well appreciated. Additionally, a straight medial and straight lateral opening of the knee may exist. In 1968, the concept of rotatory instability was first described. What appeared to be a straight anterior drawer was in fact the medial aspect of the tibia externally rotating out from underneath the medial femoral condyle. Since this time, other forms of rotatory instability have been described.

Testing for knee instability must be conducted with precision and meticulously. The first observation may be more valid than subsequent ones due to additional pain and muscle spasm. The test for varus or valgus instability is initially done with the knee in 20° to 30° of flexion because full extension is often impossible. Even when full extension can be achieved, it is often better to conduct the test first with the knee flexed to prevent initiating muscle spasm that will distort any further information obtained. Even one positive test, such as extensive medial opening, indicates a laxity and, therefore, there may be little reason to proceed with further initial testing. This knee requires a comprehensive evaluation and a physician will repeat the tests under anesthesia, as required. A negative test result does not necessarily exclude damage to the ligament in question because remaining secondary restraints may block the opening of the knee. Additionally, muscle spasms may block stability testing. During testing the patient should be reassured, relaxed and made as comfortable as possible in a fully supine position with a pillow under the head.

Straight Anterior Laxity

True anterior instability is demonstrated by a straight forward motion of the tibia on the femur and cannot occur unless the anterior cruciate ligament has been damaged (Fig. 21:15). The anterior cruciate ligament provides some 85% of the resisting force to anterior movement of the tibia on the femur. All of the remaining medial and lateral ligamentous structures provide a small force and are thus classified as secondary restraints. On rare occasions following medial collateral ligament

and capsular ligamentous damage, a mild anteromedial rotation of the medial aspect of the tibia may give the false impression of an anterior drawer. This anteromedial rotatory instability is discussed later.

A subtle anterior laxity is often difficult to see in an acutely injured and swollen knee. The anterior drawer test conducted at 30° flexion (see Fig. 21:16) is often more reliable than at 90° flexion because the secondary ligamentous restraints are less tight at 30° flexion and therefore allow more anterior tibial displacement when the anterior cruciate ligament is torn. The anterior drawer test at 30° knee flexion is sometimes referred to as the Lachman test and is extremely useful in acute knee injuries (Fig. 21:16). The Lachman drawer test can be performed without lifting the extremity. The patient must be relaxed. Gently grasp the lower thigh just above the patella while the other hand gently grasps the proximal aspect of the tibia. The thumb may extend over the tibial tubercle to palpate the joint line. While stabilizing the thigh, carry out an anteroposterior drawer motion with the hand holding the proximal tibia. Subtle changes in

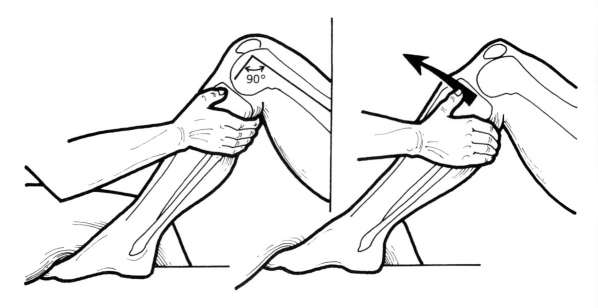

FIGURE 21:15. Anterior drawer test determines anterior cruciate instability. Flex knee to 90° and stabilize foot. Note forward shift of tibia.

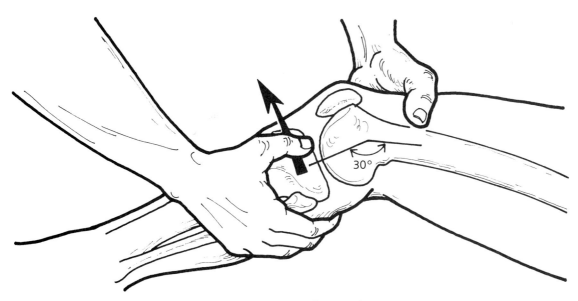

FIGURE 21:16. Lachman drawer test for knee is at 30° flexion. The extremity does not have to be lifted or foot stabilized.

anteroposterior displacement of the tibia can thus be detected. When this test proves positive, subsequent anterior lateral rotatory instability tests are performed as described later. An increase in anteroposterior laxity means either anterior cruciate or posterior cruciate damage. On occasion, both ligaments may be damaged. Because of this, any positive drawer test should be followed by a gravity drawer test to determine the status of the posterior cruciate ligament. When the anterior cruciate ligament is torn, anterior lateral rotatory instability also occurs. This should not be confusing. The anterior cruciate ligament provides both straight anterior stability and anterior lateral rotatory stability. Ligaments typically provide stability in both a straight and a rotatory plane of motion. Remember also that the amount of laxity depends on the tightness of the remaining secondary restraints. Some knees may have only a small initial laxity. With time, the weaker secondary restraints stretch and a grossly positive anterior drawer motion develops. Thus, the laxity of an acute knee may differ from that in the chronic knee.

Occasionally, the anterior cruciate ligament may be partially torn. The anterior drawer sign may or may not be positive in such situations. When only a portion of the anterior cruciate ligament seems to be ruptured, as noted at arthroscopy, the remaining portion of the ligament usually has also sustained some microfailure.

Straight Posterior Laxity

With posterior straight laxity, the tibia can be displaced posteriorly in a neutral position, i.e., without any rotation. The posterior cruciate ligament is the primary ligamentous restraint, providing some 95% of the resisting force for posterior displacement of the tibia. All of the structures provide a small remaining contribution. However, these less effective structures may still block the drawer test in acute knee injuries. Later, when stretching occurs, the amount of posterior displacement of the tibia may substantially increase.

A posterior laxity can be confused with an anterior laxity. The neutral point for the knee joint for anteroposterior laxity must be established. A posterior sag or dropping back of the tibia can often be observed with the knee flexed to 90°. If the tibia has dropped backward in the drawer test, the examiner brings the tibia forward and may mistakenly believe the anterior drawer test is positive. In fact, the tibia started from a dropped back position and the real injury is to the posterior cruciate ligament. It is recommended that the gravity drawer test be performed as a routine procedure (Fig. 21:17). In this test a ruler or straight edge is placed across the front of the knee. Any concavity compared with the normal side indicates a posterior dropping back of the tibia and a posterior cruciate tear is suspect. The test is not accurate with long-standing Osgood-Schlatter disease since the height of the tibial tubercle may be different from one side compared with the other.

Posterior lateral rotatory instability, as will be discussed, may give a false appearance of dropping back of the tibia when in fact the tibia is actually externally rotating. In posterior lateral rotatory instability, the posterior cruciate may be intact or only partially damaged.

In the acutely injured knee the posterior cruciate ligament may be completely disrupted but the posterior drawer test is often negative. The posterior capsular structure prevents dropping back of the tibia. In the chronic posterior cruciate injury, the weak secondary

restraints gradually stretch and the test becomes grossly positive. However, the time for acute repair is lost if the diagnosis is not initially made. As previously indicated, the mechanism of injury may often suggest a posterior cruciate tear. Any loading on the front of the tibia which drives it backward suggests a posterior cruciate injury.

Straight Medial Laxity

In straight medial laxity there is medial opening to the joint, or valgus laxity. This is different from anteromedial rotatory instability where the tibia rotates anteriorly and there is an associated medial opening. To examine for medial or valgus laxity, place the knee in 30° flexion (Fig. 21:18). Be sure to palpate for the physical integrity of the medial collateral ligament while the valgus stress is applied. The knee can actually be rocked in an abduction/adduction position, testing both the medial and lateral sides at the same time. Placing the finger at the joint line may increase the accuracy of this test. Estimate the amount of joint opening in millimeters to classify the amount of laxity, as discussed.

Increased medial opening at 30° knee flexion indicates damage to the primary restraint, the medial collateral ligament. This ligament supports about 80% of the force applied to the knee joint at 30° flexion. Since isolated failure does not occur, opening also indicates damage to the secondary restraints, namely the medial capsular structures. As the knee is taken toward extension, the posterior medial capsule progressively becomes tighter and accounts for a greater force in resisting joint opening. Therefore, opening with the knee in extension also indicates damage to the posteromedial capsular structures. If the opening of the medial joint is large (over 10 mm), then damage to the anterior or posterior cruciate structures should also be suspected. After sequential rupture of the collateral ligament and capsular structures, full reliance is placed on the cruciate structures. Therefore, with significant medial opening these structures may be damaged, as well. With the knee in full

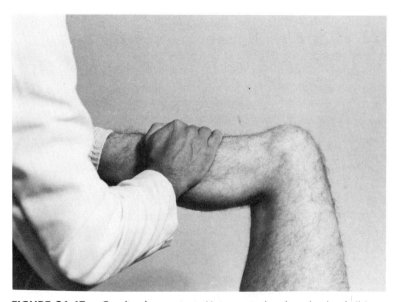

FIGURE 21:17.   Gravity drawer test. Note posterior drop back of tibia.

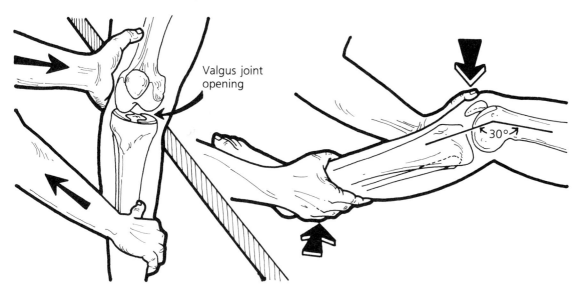

FIGURE 21:18. Valgus test in 30° flexion

hyperextension, the cruciate ligaments alone lock the femur into the tibia and no medial opening is possible. Therefore, any finding of medial opening with the knee in hyperextension suggests a severe injury involving all of the medial structures plus the cruciate ligaments.

An alternative way to examine medial laxity is to hold the lower leg cradled against your side with the thigh supported (Fig. 21:19). To examine the right knee, gently place your left hand over the patient's posterior lateral thigh, supporting the thigh. Place your right hand over the medial joint line of the knee. Support the foot and leg by your right arm against the side and resting on the hip. At 30° of knee flexion apply a gentle valgus force with the left hand. Place the fingertips of the right hand directly over the joint line to estimate the millimeters of joint opening. In the severely swollen knee, locate the medial joint line by palpating the lower pole of the patella and proceeding directly medial and posterior to where the fingertips locate the joint line. The physical integrity of the medial collateral ligament can also be palpated. Both positions, the cradled one and the leg over the side of the examining table, are recommended.

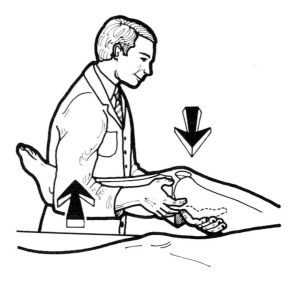

FIGURE 21:19. Alternate test for straight medial laxity

Straight Lateral Laxity

The techniques for determining lateral or varus laxity are identical to those for medial laxity. Apply a varus force to produce straight lateral opening of the joint. Varus laxity with the knee in 30° flexion indicates an injury to the fibular collateral ligament and lateral capsular structures. The lateral collateral ligament is the primary ligamentous restraint to the lateral aspect of the joint, accounting for some 70% of resisting force during the testing procedure. The lateral capsular structures and underlying anterior and posterior cruciate ligament also provide varus stability. Again, when the knee is extended, the posterolateral capsular structures tighten, just as on the medial side, and any opening indicates capsular and posterior capsular damage in addition to collateral ligament damage. With the knee fully extended, significant joint opening indicates cruciate damage as discussed for the medial side. With the knee fully extended or hyperextended, significant lateral opening indicates damage to the cruciate ligaments, as well. Additionally, any time the lateral opening is large—for example, increased 1 cm or more over the opposite side—involvement of the cruciate ligaments should be suspected no matter what the knee flexion position tested. However, cruciate laxity is verified best by a Lachman or drawer test.

Genu Recurvatum

Genu recurvatum is not classified as a true instability. However, it is not uncommon and therefore some discussion is indicated (Fig. 21:20). Three types of genu recurvatum are possible. The first type is physiologic, related to generalized laxity of the knee joint. Hyperextension to 15° may be seen in the loose-jointed individual. An individual with this amount of hyperextension generally does poorly after sustaining a ligamentous injury because the knee joint lacks additional supporting ligamentous structures. Rarely, increased recurvatum may be due to chronic stretching of the posterior capsular and ligamentous structures, and may be an infrequent reason for excluding an individual from participating in strenuous sports activities. The importance of examining both extremities is underscored in that recurvatum due to a ligamentous injury may be diagnosed, whereas the other knee shows a similar amount of recurvatum. Additionally, other joints may show generalized laxity in loose-jointed individuals.

A second type of genu recurvatum gives this appearance, but it actually is a posterolateral rotatory instability as will be discussed. Instead of pure hyperextension of the joint, the tibia rotates posterolaterally.

The third type of recurvatum is due to posterior capsular and associated cruciate ligament damage. Severe hyperextension injuries to the knee joint can damage capsular and cruciate structures. Either the anterior cruciate, posterior cruciate or both can be injured, depending on the type of hyperextension injury. In the true hyperextension injury, the posterior capsule and posterior cruciate ligament are first injured. If the hyperextension continues or if there is any component of the force directing the tibia forward, then the anterior cruciate ligament is also injured. Sometimes hyperextension is described but instead the tibia is actually being displaced forward similar to an anterior drawer. This causes damage predominantly to the anterior cruciate ligament. Hyperextension injuries are often associated with damage to the neurovascular system in the popliteal space.

Anteromedial Rotatory Instability

In anteromedial rotatory instability the medial plateau of the tibia rotates anteriorly. Additionally, joint opening on the medial side can be detected. The classical form of this in-

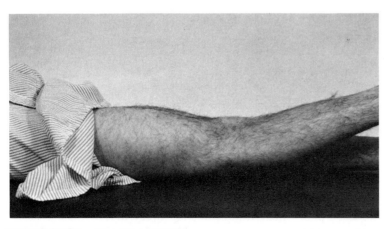

FIGURE 21:20.   Genu recurvatum

stability involves a disruption of the superficial medial collateral ligament, adjacent capsular structures including the posterior medial complex and medial capsule and, as well, the anterior cruciate ligament. In a more subtle form of this injury the predominant injury is to the superficial medial collateral ligament and associated medial capsular structures without major involvement of the anterior cruciate ligament. In this case, there is more external rotation of the tibia and medial opening. However, since the anterior cruciate ligament is intact, anterior tibial displacement is less.

There are two tests for anteromedial rotatory instability. The first is the Slocum external rotation test (Fig. 21:21), which is conducted with the hip flexed to approximately 45° and the knee to approximately 80° while the foot rests on the examining table. The normal knee is tested first for comparison with the injured leg. Sit on the side of the table, trapping the patient's foot with your upper thigh, and gently place both hands about the upper lower leg. With the index finger, palpate the hamstrings to be certain they are lax and then apply a gentle forward symmetrical pull. Record the degree of anterior drawer in the in-

jured knee as compared with the normal knee, noting the amount of laxity in 5 mm increments. With a simple anterior drawer test the neutral rotation is essential to focus on the movements of both the medial tibial condyle and the lateral tibial condyle to learn whether asymmetrical rotation is involved with the anterior tibial displacement. Also, if the patient is cooperative, the basic rotational elements of the anterior drawer can also be tested. With the patient's foot in neutral rotation apply a pure rotational force to the medial tibial condyle and note the anterior medial rotation. A similar procedure can be done on the lateral tibial condyle to reveal the amount of anterolateral rotatory instability.

After the neutral anterior drawer and rotational components are established, repeat the test at intervals of approximately 10° of progressive external rotation. The normal knee shows very little change in the amount of anterior drawer for the first 10° to 15° of external rotation. Actually, the cruciates are unwinding and the amount of anterior drawer may increase slightly. Thereafter, the amount of anterior drawer should progressively diminish as the amount of tibial rotation on the

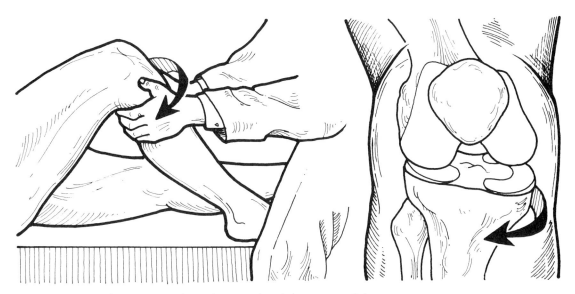

FIGURE 21:21. Slocum external rotation test showing anteromedial instability as the medial tibial plateau shifts forward and externally rotates.

femur tightens the medial ligamentous sleeve. Predominantly, this tightens the medial collateral ligament, but all of the medial capsular structures are tightened. An increasing amount of external rotation eventually blocks the amount of anteromedial excursion of the tibia since some medial structures are tightened no matter how much damage has been produced. Thus, the amount of anteromedial excursion must be gauged in comparison with the opposite side.

The second common test for anteromedial rotatory instability uses the same position as in the test for medial instability where the extremity is dropped from the side of the table (Fig. 21:22). In testing for straight medial instability only a straight valgus force is applied. In other words, only straight medial opening in one plane is elicited. In the test for anteromedial rotatory laxity, however, apply external rotation to the tibia while also applying the valgus distraction force. Therefore, increased external rotation and medial joint opening are produced together. In many knees this may be a more sensitive test for anteromedial rotation than the Slocum external rotation test because both medial opening and increased ex-

ternal rotation occur simultaneously. Thus, the rotation component as well as the medial opening component is being tested which increases the test's sensitivity. Since rotation is also occurring, be careful not to overestimate the amount of true medial opening. Also this test is more accurate with the knee partially flexed. With full extension other ligamentous structures tend to tighten, which may block the findings.

Note that in Figure 21:23, the tibia rotates about an axis that is shifted to the lateral side. If the rotation axis were straight through the center of the tibia, then normal external rotation would occur. However, with the axis shifted to the lateral aspect, both anterior displacement of the tibia and increased rotation occur—anteromedial rotatory instability.

To summarize, the primary ligamentous restraint for anteromedial rotatory instability is the medial collateral ligament, which resists external tibial rotation and medial joint opening, assisted by secondary restraints consisting of the capsular structures. The anterior cruciate ligament provides the primary restraint for the anterior drawer component of this instability. Therefore, if marked laxity is present, there is

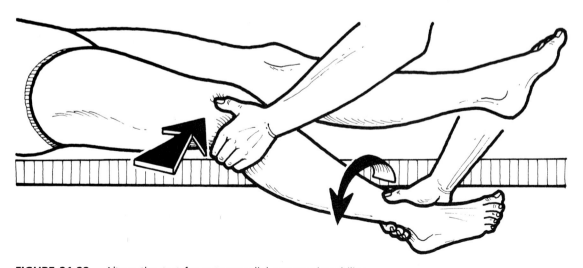

FIGURE 21:22. Alternative test for anteromedial rotatory instability. External rotation is applied to the tibia while applying valgus stress in slight flexion.

a defect in both ligaments. The midmedial capsule was initially thought to be an important stabilizer; however, it is now known as a secondary restraint.

Anterolateral Rotatory Instability

Anterolateral rotatory instability is characterized by an anterior internal rotational subluxation of the lateral tibial condyle on the femur (see Fig. 21:23). The lateral pivot shift test is used for diagnosing this laxity. The lateral tibial condyle subluxates anteriorly from underneath the lateral femoral condyle. This is particularly likely to occur when an athlete makes a sudden change in direction, such as in a cutting movement or while decelerating. This subluxation is assisted by the anterior pull of the quadriceps mechanism. Also, the iliotibial band passes anterior to the flexion axis of the knee joint as the knee extends and therefore its ability to resist the anterolateral subluxation is lessened.

The most frequent rotatory instability encountered in the knee is anterolateral. A number of clinical laxity tests can reproduce the subluxation of the lateral tibial plateau: the lateral pivot shift test, the jerk test, the Slocum anterolateral rotatory instability test and the flexion rotation drawer. All tests produce an anterolateral subluxation of the joint followed by a reduction. The reduction is usually accompanied by a thud, jump or jerk within the joint.

More recently, it has been recognized that approximately one out of five anterior cruciate deficient knees have mild anterolateral laxity that may be difficult to detect. These knees have no obvious jump, jerk or thud, and the classical pivot shift test may be negative. The flexion rotation drawer test and the Lachman anterior drawer test are often more sensitive, indicating subtle anterior cruciate laxity. These cases must be diagnosed for two reasons. First, this form of laxity is very common in the athlete. Rehabilitation and modification of strenuous activities may overcome symptoms and markedly improve knee function. Second, mild symptoms of swelling and giving way

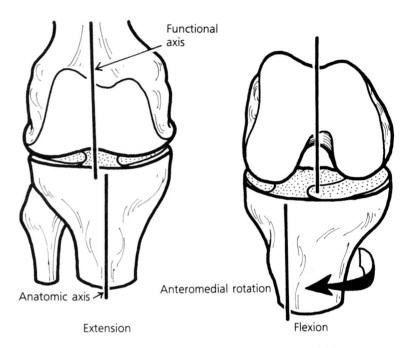

FIGURE 21:23. Tibia rotating about an axis shifted laterally in anteromedial rotatory instability

may be incorrectly attributed to a torn meniscus when the gross pivot shift sign tests are negative.

In summary, there are a battery of tests for anterolateral laxity. In the acutely injured knee there may be inadequate relaxation and many of the tests may be negative. Under anesthesia a variety of tests should be performed. Each examiner will develop those tests most sensitive to arrive at a diagnosis of this laxity. For completeness all of the tests are briefly described.

The primary restraint for anterolateral rotatory stability is the anterior cruciate ligament. The iliotibial band and, less so, the lateral capsule provide a secondary restraint. Biomechanical studies have shown that rupture of the anterior cruciate as the primary lesion results in a mild to moderate laxity. For a severe laxity the lateral structures must show associated laxity. This laxity may be (1) due to a physiologic laxity without injury to the lateral structures or (2) a result of actual injury to the lateral structures. In acute injuries hemorrhage

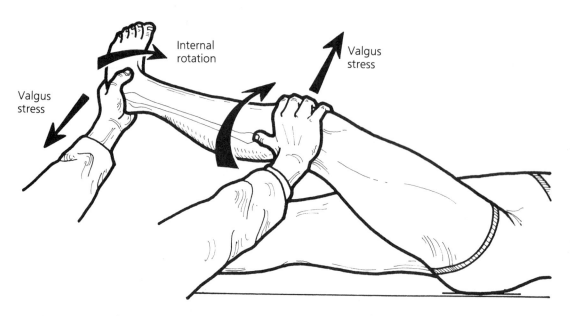

FIGURE 21:24. Lateral pivot shift test

may be noted in the lateral capsule. Damage to the iliotibial band is often difficult to detect. In the loose-jointed athlete with physiologic laxity to the supporting ligaments, including the lateral structures, the rupture of the anterior cruciate alone results in severe third-degree anterolateral rotatory instability. In the more tight-jointed athlete, rupture of the anterior cruciate ligament initially results in only a mild to moderate laxity, since the lateral structures provide a restraining force. If the lateral structures subsequently stretch, then in time a severe rotatory laxity may develop. The spectrum of knees that presents with this laxity underscores the need for performing more than one of the tests for anterolateral laxity.

In the lateral pivot shift test, the patient should be supine and relaxed (Fig. 21:24). Place the heel of the involved leg in the palm of your hand. To test the left knee, place your left hand under the left heel. Place your right hand over the lateral tibia with the thumb behind the fibular head. Take the knee to approximately 5° of flexion and use both hands to internally rotate the lower leg on the femur. At the same time, push the proximal tibia an-

teriorly with the proximal hand. Lifting the fibular head gently with the thumb will help. At this point in a markedly positive test, the lateral tibial plateau subluxates anteriorly out from under the femoral condyle. Use the right hand as a fulcrum to apply a gentle valgus stress with the left hand. This compresses the lateral compartment. The iliotibial band acting as an extensor in this position becomes a flexor as it passes over the lateral femoral condyle at about 20° of flexion. In a positive test, the tibia markedly reduces, which is visible and palpable. The key elements of a positive lateral pivot shift test are internal rotation of the lower leg on the femur, lateral compartment compression and excursion of the knee from an extended to flexed position.

The anterior lateral rotatory instability test is a modification of the lateral pivot shift test (Fig. 21:25). The patient lies on his side, with the uninvolved leg flexed at the hip while the knee and the pelvis are permitted to fall back. This position automatically produces internal rotation and a gentle valgus stress to the knee. To test the right knee, place your right hand on the proximal tibia to provide further internal rotation and to take the knee out of hyper-extension. Place your left hand on the femoral condylar region and with both hands gently increase the valgus stress on the joint. As the knee goes into about 20° of flexion, the subluxation reduces visibly, palpably and audibly. In a markedly positive test, the lateral tibial condyle is easily seen going from a subluxated position in extension to a reduced position in flexion.

In the Hughston jerk test for anterolateral rotatory instability the patient lies supine, with the knee flexed approximately to a right angle and the hip at about 45° of flexion (Fig. 21:26). To test the left knee, hold the left foot with your left hand and apply an internal rotational force. Simultaneously, place your right hand over the proximal tibia and fibula to aid the internal rotation and act as a fulcrum for the application of a valgus stress. While these forces are maintained, gradually extend the knee. Subluxation of the lateral femoral tibial articulation occurs at about 30°. The positive test produces a snap and a pop. If the knee is carried to complete extension, reduction again occurs.

The flexion rotation drawer test described is a modification of the pivot shift test and the

Lachman test (Fig. 21:27). This test has proved extremely sensitive in detecting mild and moderate anterolateral rotatory instability. Again, as indicated for severe forms of instability, the pivot shift test and other tests are used.

In the flexion rotation drawer test, the leg is held in neutral rotation at 20° of knee flexion. The quadriceps must be relaxed. With anterior cruciate laxity, the weight of the thigh results in a posterior dropping back of the femur—the drawer component of the test. Very importantly, however, the femur also externally rotates—the rotational component of the test. This increased external rotation of the femur produces the anterolateral subluxation of the lateral femoro-tibial articulation (see Fig. 21:27). Thus, simply holding the leg produces the subluxated position of the lateral femoral tibial joint. A gentle flexion movement of approximately 10° combined with a downward push on the tibia produces a fully reduced position. The tibia moves posteriorly into a normal relationship with the femur. One gently goes between the subluxated, extended position and reduced flexed position. In essence, the tibia or leg is used as the handle to flip the femur in an up-down motion. The test

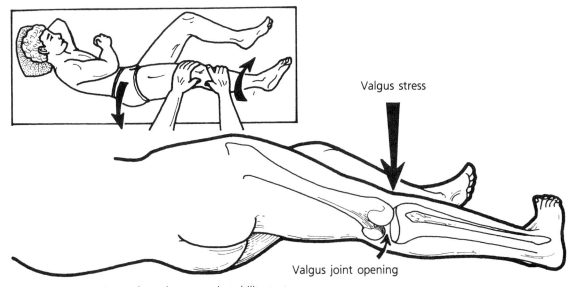

FIGURE 21:25. Anterolateral rotatory instability test

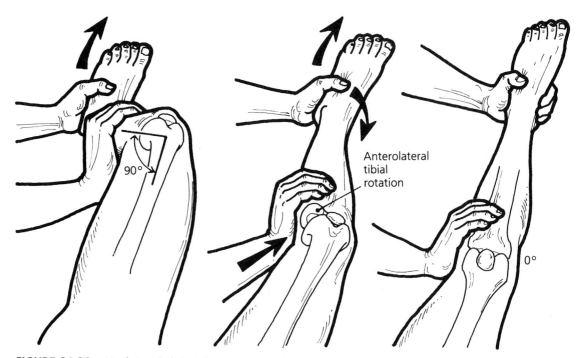

FIGURE 21:26. Hughston jerk test for anterolateral rotatory instability

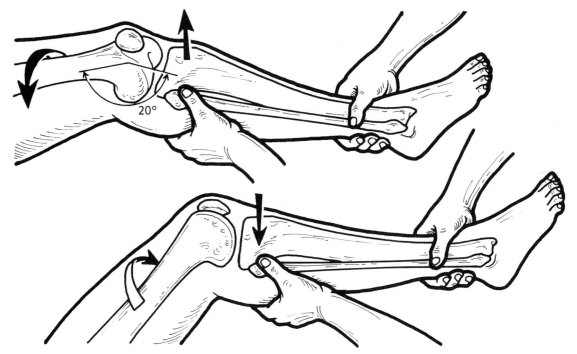

FIGURE 21:27. Flexion rotation drawer test

brings out both anteroposterior tibial translation and the rotatory motions of the femur; therefore it can help detect the more subtle anterior cruciate laxity. It is also highly diagnostic under general anesthesia in detecting anterior cruciate tears. With the up-down rocking and gentle extension-flexion of the knee, the normal concavity of the infra-patellar tendon and tibial region is less in the subluxated position and increased in the flexion position exactly as in the Lachman test. However, the femoral rotation motion can also be seen and felt by watching the femur rotate during the test. A lateral valgus compressive force may or may not be applied, depending on the examiner.

In summary, tests for anterolateral rotatory instability all produce a subluxation of the lateral tibial condyle anterolaterally with the knee in a near-extended position followed by reduction in flexion. The jerk test is a slightly different aspect of the subluxation-reduction event in that it moves from reduction to subluxation rather than from subluxation to reduction. The rotatory tests can also detect anterolateral rotatory instability, as previously described, by carefully noting the increase in anterior lateral excursion of the lateral tibial plateau. The flexion rotation drawer and Lachman drawer may be more sensitive in subtle anterior cruciate laxities.

Posterolateral Rotatory Instability

In this laxity, the lateral tibial plateau rotates posteriorly in relationship to the femur. A force directed from the anteromedial aspect against the extended knee can cause a rupture of the posterolateral ligamentous structures, usually involving a tear in the arcuate ligament complex, the associated popliteal tendon or its ramifications into the posterolateral capsule and, as well, the lateral collateral ligament. Some knees may also have partial or complete tears of the posterior cruciate ligament. The exact pathology in this instability is still confusing. Additionally, clinical tests for this laxity are complex. Hughston clarified the diagnosis of posterolateral rotatory instability and described the external rotation recurvatum test (Fig. 21:28). For this test, lift the affected extremity by the foot and evaluate the external rotation of the lateral tibia on the femur and

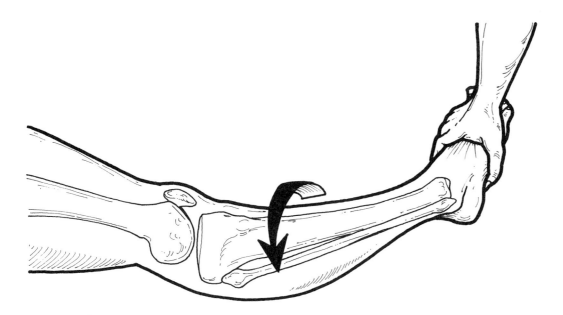

FIGURE 21:28. External rotation recurvatum test

any associated appearance of recurvatum to the knee and tibia varum.

Another helpful test in determining posterolateral rotatory instability is the gravity external rotation test described by Noyes (Fig. 21:29). This test is performed very similarly to the gravity drop-back test where the knee is flexed to 90° as well as at the hip joint. When examining the right knee, with the right hand grasp the foot and ankle of the patient while the left hand holds the thigh with the thumb at the fibular head. Rotate the tibia and foot externally and note the excursion of the fibular head and tibial tubercle. When posterolateral rotatory instability is present, the fibular head travels farther than the normal side and proceeds posteriorly and slightly inferior to its original position. In severe cases, it may rotate into the popliteal space and not be visible. Increased external rotation of the leg can also be compared with the normal side. This test also helps detect associated injuries to the posterior cruciate ligament, since the amount of straight posterior drawer of the tibia can be distinguished from the amount of posterolateral rotation of the tibia during the test.

Posteromedial Rotatory Instability

In this laxity, the medial tibial plateau rotates posteriorly on the femur with associated medial opening. This is a severe injury. Structures involved are the superficial medial collateral ligament and associated medial capsular structures plus the cruciate ligaments. There still exists confusion in reference to this laxity. A significant valgus force to the limb can disrupt all the medial structures, plus both cruciate ligaments. In such severe laxities, the posterior medial corner of the tibia sags on the femur with valgus opening. Actually in such an injury the tibia can be rotated into a number of different positions, and global instability of the knee joint is common.

Anteromedial/Anterolateral Instability

Although combined anteromedial/anterolateral is a common laxity, there is no agreement as to the exact structures involved. The tests previously discussed can demonstrate extensive anteromedial rotatory instability as well as excessive anterolateral rotatory instability. This instability is commonly thought to develop as a result of an anterior cruciate tear. With recurrent giving way episodes, both the lateral and medial ligamentous structures stretch. Commonly, the medial or lateral meniscus, or both, tear resulting in meniscectomy. The second most common cause of this instability is involvement of the anterior cruciate ligament in medial ligamentous injuries. In such cases, there is complete anteromedial rotatory instability. The degree of anterolateral rotatory instability may differ when the anterior cruciate is torn, and the amount of this latter laxity depends on the tightness of the lateral restraining structures. Again, after repeat giving way episodes or with chronic stretching of the remaining lateral structures, further rotatory instability develops.

In the presence of this combined instability, the anterior cruciate ligament has lost its integrity. There is associated stretching, injury or laxity of lateral structures that contribute to anterolateral rotatory stability and of medial ligamentous structures that contribute to anteromedial rotatory instability. Reports recognizing this complex instability relate to the surgical procedures employed. Both the medial and lateral ligamentous structures must be restored, either alone or concomitant with anterior cruciate reconstructive surgery.

Anterolateral/Posterolateral Rotatory Instability

With anterolateral/posterolateral laxity the lateral tibial plateau rotates excessively in a posterior direction as described for posterolateral rotatory instability. It also rotates excessively in an anterolateral direction as described for anterolateral rotatory instability. It is extremely difficult to define the neutral point for this rotatory instability. Therefore, take care that cases of gross anterolateral rotatory instability, in which excessive rotation of the tibia is demonstrable, are not incorrectly diagnosed

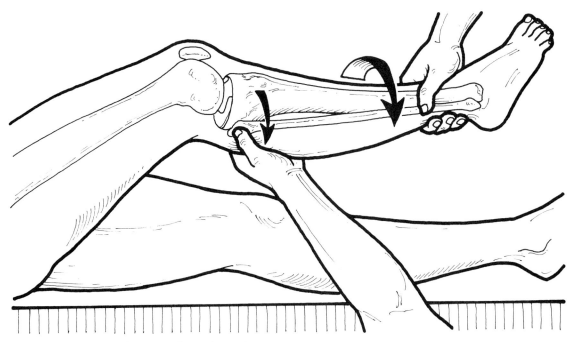

FIGURE 21:29.   Gravity external rotation test

as having a posterolateral rotatory component. How to determine a neutral point between excessive anterolateral rotation of the tibia and excessive posterolateral rotation of the tibia is confusing. In true combined rotatory instability, most structures on the lateral side of the knee are extensively damaged and the anterior cruciate ligament is disrupted. Initially, it was thought that rotation occurred about an intact posterior cruciate ligament. However, it is now appreciated that different degrees of injury may also involve this ligament.

Anteromedial/Posteromedial Rotatory Instability

In anteromedial/posteromedial laxity there is excessive anteromedial excursion of the tibia on the femur and, as well, excessive posteromedial excursion of the tibia on the femur. There is also medial opening of the knee joint. This severe injury involves all of the medial structures in combination with the anterior and posterior cruciate ligaments. With dislocations, global instabilities can also occur.

KNEE LIGAMENT INJURIES

The stability of the knee depends on three anatomical systems. First is the passive system comprising the ligament and capsular structures linking the femur, tibia and patella. Second is the active system comprising the muscles acting through a functioning nervous system. The neuromuscular system coordinates muscle forces at the right time required for activity. Muscle forces provide stability to the joint, protecting ligaments from injury. Sudden turning or twisting, or a blow to the side of the knee, requires counteraction by muscle forces to keep the joint from collapsing. An athlete in superb condition in terms of muscle strength, coordination and agility obviously responds much better to sudden and jarring movements. In contrast, an athlete with a recent injury or residual weakness from prior injury may be at risk for repeat injury or even worse injury. This point cannot be overemphasized and stresses the need for proper rehabilitation of all the muscles of the extremity after injury. Neuromuscular coordination is the keystone for stability of the knee joint. Therefore whether defects exist from the standpoint of strength, endurance and neuromuscular coordination (agility) must be determined.

The third anatomical system providing stability relates to the actual geometry of the joint itself. Some joints are exceptionally stable, such as the elbow with its interlocking bone ends. The knee joint has much less inherent stability. The joint has to have more freedom for motion. Besides flexion and extension, the knee rotates internally and externally. Still, the geometry of the knee joint does provide considerable stability. The femoral condyles are literally pressed into the tibial surface. The meniscus structures add concavity to the tibial surface, helping to contain the femoral condyles. The tibial intercondylar notch sweeps upward, providing a bumper stop for excessive inward or outward femoral rotation about the tibia. The meniscus structures add a restraining peripheral ring. This increases the concavity of the tibial surface, particularly of the lateral tibial plateau where the convex surface slopes backward in contrast to the concave medial side.

With activity, forces much larger than commonly realized are placed across joints. For example, in walking about three times body weight is placed across the knee joint (also hip and ankle joints). A person weighing 70 kg places up to 210 kg across the knee joint. In jumping and other strenuous activity, the forces may be as large as six to eight times body weight, or easily a half ton in a large individual. Where do the large forces come from? Principally from the muscles. Each muscle contraction exerts a large force that moves the joint about a certain axis (e.g., flexion or extension). The muscle forces also compress the joint, which provides stability. It forces the femur into the tibia and therefore makes it harder for a jolt or sudden movement to dislodge the femur off the tibia. The body's weight above the knee joint provides additional joint compressive forces. Activities increase compressive forces, as in sports involving jumping.

There are three determinants of joint stability. Activity generates large external forces that act on the knee joint. These forces must be balanced and resisted by internal forces in ligaments, muscles and joint geometry (compressive forces across the joint). If the external forces are too high and cannot be properly resisted, then ligaments or muscles may be injured, and bones fractured (Fig. 21:30). With sudden external forces, such as in a clipping injury or in an unexpected fall, the muscles may not have time to contract and resist the injury forces. Full resistance is then placed on the ligaments, with ligament injury all too frequent. As soon as a ligament tears, the joint can separate even farther. If the femoral condyle rocks off, then the stabilizing effect of the interlocking bone ends is lost, resulting in increased instability and probably complete collapse. Stability of the knee and any other joint is a dynamic balance between external forces and internal forces. The rationale for many treatment programs, therefore, aims at increasing stability of the joint. All three systems for joint stability are required for proper functioning.

Mechanisms of Ligament Injury

The mechanism of injury includes all details of the injury. Of importance is the position of the knee joint at the time of injury. The direction in which the knee displaces or rotates may tell which ligaments have been torn. The trainer may actually observe the injury; obviously, this is best. Did the knee bend to the inside (medial opening, abduction or valgus position) or to the outside (lateral opening, adduction or varus position)? Did the knee bend backward (hyperextension)? Did the femur rotate over a fixed tibia (internal or external) or vice versa? Did it feel as if the knee was coming apart? If so, it probably did, with tearing of the ligaments.

The athlete may remember only a few details of the injury but this still gives important diagnostic clues. For example, most anterior cruciate tears occur in noncontact injuries, as

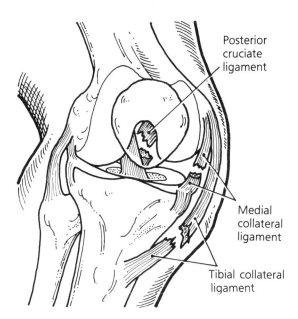

FIGURE 21:30. Sudden external forces may result in multiple disruptions to the ligamentous structures.

Labels in figure: Posterior cruciate ligament; Medial collateral ligament; Tibial collateral ligament

with a sudden turning or twisting of the femur to the outside. The athlete may feel a pop. Swelling within 24 hours, often within two hours, means joint hemorrhage and implies a serious injury. Posterior cruciate injury may be suspected with a sudden blow to the front of the tibia, driving it backward. This commonly occurs in auto accidents where the knee strikes the dashboard. The same mechanism can occur during a fall in any sporting activity. Remember, in cruciate injuries, the laxity examination may be entirely normal. All aspects of the injury mechanism, symptoms and other data must be compiled to make a tentative diagnosis.

Table 21:1 lists common mechanisms of injury and the ligament structures that may be injured. In describing rotation of the knee, it is customary to refer to the tibia as the part that moves. Thus, a valgus external rotation injury means that the femur is fixed and the tibia is placed in a valgus position (medial joint opening) and externally rotates. Actually, in most injury situations the reverse motion occurs. The femur and upper body rotate about the

fixed tibia and planted foot. The convention has always been to refer to the tibia moving, and this is actually what is done in the clinical laxity exam. The tibia is moved while the femur is stationary. Thus, there is some justification for keeping this system. Remember, the same joint position is reached and the same ligaments are stretched whether the tibia externally rotates on a fixed femur or the femur internally rotates on a fixed tibia. In describing an injury, the femur is fixed and the position of the tibia is being described, unless otherwise stated.

Classification of Ligament Injuries

Four different classification systems denote the type and extent of injury to the ligament and capsular structures of the knee. Each system is somewhat separate and provides additional information.

Severity of Sprain

The AMA standard nomenclature of athletic injuries classifies ligament injuries into mild sprains (few fibers torn), moderate sprains (a

TABLE 21:1. Common Mechanisms of Knee Injury

Mechanism of Injury (Knee Position*)	Ligament Injury
Valgus (straight medial opening)	Medial collateral plus capsular ligaments†
Valgus external rotation	Medial structures, medial meniscus, anterior cruciate, "terrible triad"
Varus (straight lateral opening)	Lateral collateral plus capsular ligaments†
Varus internal rotation	Lateral ligaments plus anterior cruciate
Varus external rotation	Lateral ligaments plus posterior cruciate
Hyperextension	Posterior capsule and posterior cruciate‡
Direct blow driving tibia backward	Posterior cruciate
Direct blow driving tibia forward	Anterior cruciate

*Tibia moving with femur fixed.
†Severe opening implies injury to either one or both cruciates.
‡Severe hyperextension may also injure the anterior cruciate ligament.

definite tear in some component of the ligament), and severe sprains (ligament torn completely across). The classification is based on the symptoms, signs and severity of the injury (Table 21:2). The AMA classification provides an overall diagnosis of the degree of ligamentous injury. There is one criticism of this system. A sprain of a ligament is defined in medical dictionaries as only a partial tearing without complete disruption. Also, a sprain commonly denotes no subluxation or dislocation of the joint. This is correct only for the first-degree, or mild, sprain. Note in the AMA classification that a second-degree sprain indicates moderate motion or joint laxity and a third-degree sprain indicates marked abnormal laxity. There is no laxity by definition with a first-degree sprain where there is only minor tearing of ligament fibers. If laxity is present, then there is by definition either a second- or third-degree sprain.

Amount and Direction of Laxity

With laxity to the knee joint, a ligament restraint has been functionally disrupted to one degree or another and the injury is significant. This injury can be further classified by amount of laxity (Table 21:3) and by direction of laxity (Table 21:4). The amount of laxity may not correlate in every case with the degree of ligament damage. In some ligament injuries, there may be a complete tear of a ligament (functional capacity lost) but little laxity. This is because other ligaments may block the amount of joint distraction or opening even though a primary ligament restraint is torn. This is discussed elsewhere in greater detail. However, an accurate grading by amount of joint opening is a useful index for defining the injury and treatment.

The classification by the direction of the laxity (see Table 21:4) is divided into the four straight laxities and the four rotatory laxities, discussed under clinical tests for laxity.

Specific Ligaments Disrupted

The injured ligaments must be classified. A simple classification is given in the following list. The structures involved in the injury are specified based on the laxity exam, thus simply

TABLE 21:2.   Clinical Diagnosis of Ligament Injury

	First-Degree Sprain	Second-Degree Sprain	Third-Degree Sprain
Synonym	Mild sprain	Moderate sprain	Severe sprain
Etiology	Direct or indirect trauma to joint	Same	Severe direct or indirect trauma to joint
Symptoms	Pain; mild disability	Pain; moderate disability	Pain; severe disability
Signs	Mild point tenderness; no abnormal motion; little or no swelling	Point tenderness; moderate loss of function; slight to moderate abnormal motion; swelling; localized hemorrhage	Loss of function; marked abnormal motion; possible deformity; x-rays: stress films demonstrate abnormal motion
Complications	Tendency to recurrence, aggravation	Tendency to recurrence, aggravation; persistent instability; traumatic arthritis	Persistent instability; traumatic arthritis
Pathology	Minor tearing of ligament	Partial tear of ligament	Complete tear of ligament

Standard Nomenclature of Athletic Injuries, American Medical Association defining injury by the ligament involved. Remember some laxities can be rather complex when one or two ligaments are torn.

   A. Medial ligament injuries
      1. No associated anterior cruciate tear
      2. Associated anterior cruciate tear
      3. Associated anterior and posterior cruciate tear
   B. Lateral ligament injury
      1. No associated anterior cruciate tear
      2. Associated anterior cruciate tear
      3. Associated anterior and posterior cruciate tears
   C. Anterior cruciate injury: as the primary injury
   D. Posterior cruciate injury: as the primary injury

In this classification the injury to the medial and lateral sides is easily identified in terms of seriousness. If the injury is confined to the medial or lateral collateral ligaments and capsular structures, the prognosis for healing and functional stability is good. If, however, the anterior cruciate is included in the injury (A-2 or B-2 in the classification), the prognosis is less favorable. In this context, an anterior cruciate injury in association with any other major ligament structure disruption has an overall poor prognosis. The presence or absence of the anterior cruciate tear therefore immediately defines the seriousness of the injury. With an associated posterior cruciate tear, the injury is actually a dislocation of the knee. The prognosis for return to athletic activities after tears of both cruciate ligaments is even more dismal. In severe injuries, with one or both cruciates torn, an athlete is fortunate to have a stable knee for recreational activities. If a stable knee is achieved, as is becoming possible with modern surgical reconstruction, more vigorous activities may not be advisable. A repeat injury potentially means major disability for any activity.

Tears involving predominantly the anterior or posterior cruciate ligament have separate categories. These tears are not isolated in the strictest sense. Associated injuries to the cap-

TABLE 21:3. Classification of Ligament Injury

	Straight Laxity	Rotatory Laxity
First-degree	Mild (less than 5 mm distraction)	Mild
Second-degree	Moderate (5–10 mm distraction)	Moderate
Third-degree	Severe (over 10 mm distraction)	Severe

TABLE 21:4. Direction of Laxity

Straight*	Rotatory
Medial	Anteromedial (anterior external rotation)
Lateral	Anterolateral (anterior internal rotation)
Anterior	Posteromedial (posterior internal rotation)
Posterior	Posterolateral (posterior external rotation)

*Denotes position of knee joint with tibia moving on fixed femur.

sular ligaments, meniscus and joint are frequent. However, the predominant injury in terms of joint stability is the cruciate ligament. An anterior cruciate tear is extremely common under these circumstances, as will be discussed.

Functional Capacity of Injured Knee

Biomechanical information on the functional capacity of ligaments and their mechanisms of failure allows classification of injury based on the functional capacity of the injured ligament (Table 21:5). Here the residual ability of the damaged ligament to provide joint stability is gauged. This is correlated with the extent of damage, degree of sprain and the amount of joint laxity as contained in the other classification systems. In addition, the residual strength, length and functional capacity of the ligament are correlated. This provides the final index for treatment. In short, the estimate of functional capacity of a ligament defines the treatment. If the extent of ligament damage is minimal with failure of less than one third of fibers, the residual functional capacity is retained. The ligament can still provide stability

TABLE 21:5. Functional Capacity of Injured Ligament

Extent of Failure	Sprain	Damage*	Amount of Joint Laxity†	Residual Strength	Residual Functional Length	Residual Functional Capacity	Treatment
Minimal	First degree	Less than ⅓ of fibers failed; includes most sprains with few to some fibers failed; microtears also exist	None	Retained or slightly decreased	Normal	Retained	Rest until acute symptoms subside; active rehabilitation; early return to activity
Partial	Second degree	⅓ to ⅔ ligament damage; significant damage but parts of the ligaments are still functional	0–5 mm increased opening, fibers in ligament resist opening	Marked decrease	Increased, still within functional range but may act as a checkrein	Marked compromise, requires healing to regain function	a) When laxity is minimal, risk to complete the tear is minimal; treated by early rehabilitation and no plaster immobilization
		Microtears may exist	5–10 mm opening when damage is more considerable	At risk for complete failure			b) When laxity approaches higher values (5–10 mm) treated by plaster immobilization to allow healing; rehabilitation; delayed return to activity
Complete	Third degree	a) Over ⅔ to complete failure; continuity remains in part between fibers	If 10 mm opening, remaining fibers are torn, incontinuity & complete failure exist	Little to none	Severely compromised but may provide late checkrein function	Severely compromised or lost	a) Plaster immobilization, protection for healing when laxity increased 10 mm; continuity of ligament is assumed
		b) Continuity lost and gross separation between fibers	Depends on secondary restraints to limit amount of laxity, but they later stretch out	None	Lost	Lost	b) Surgical repair required when continuity of ligament is functionally lost; usually exists when medial or lateral opening increased 10–12 mm

*Estimate of damage is often very difficult. However, the different types listed can usually be distinguished.
†Anterior and posterior cruciate tears are included with the exception that acute tears commonly exist with little to no laxity. Thus the clinical laxity exam is less accurate. In the medial and lateral exam the grading is more accurate for collateral tears.

even though healing must take place. This is an important point. There is no joint laxity in this category. The remaining intact ligament fibers resist joint opening. In fact, the seriousness of the injury can be easily underdiagnosed. The ligament has sustained a real injury requiring healing and remodeling. Return to activity is allowed only after symptoms subside and after adequate rehabilitation to overcome disuse and injury effects that produce muscular weakness. Overall, risk for completing the ligament tear or for producing further ligament damage is minimal as long as rehabilitation is complete.

Damage to the cruciate or collateral ligament structure is classified as a significant injury in which laxity of the joint can be detected. The laxity may not correspond with the degree of damage. For example, in anterior cruciate tears, the ligament observed at arthroscopy may have a rupture in one half of its fibers, a second-degree sprain. The functional capacity is markedly compromised. Yet the increase in anterior laxity may only amount to a few millimeters since the remaining ligament fibers still provide a resisting force. Thus in the anterior and posterior cruciate ligaments, the amount of laxity may not be a reliable indicator of the extent of damage or residual functional capacity of the ligament. In fact, either cruciate ligament can undergo complete functional disruption with little or no laxity initially on the physical examination. Weak secondary restraints block the laxity but later stretch out and a gross laxity is then detected. In this instance, the time for acute repair has been lost.

In the second-degree sprain or partial ligament injury, there are actually two different types of injuries to the medial or lateral ligament complex (collateral plus capsular structures): those knees where the damage is partial with 0 to 5 mm increased laxity; and those knees in which the partial ligament injury is nearly complete, with 5 to 10 mm increased laxity. The latter knees require protection for the remaining ligament and to prevent the injury from becoming a complete tear. Additionally, some stability (decrease in joint opening) may be regained from protection.

The clinical laxity examination is subjective and, at times, to accurately define the true amount of laxity may be difficult. The second-degree sprain may not be easy to distinguish from a third-degree sprain with complete ligament disruption. In the second-degree sprain, the laxity determination is first made based on the best estimate of straight medial or lateral opening with the knee flexed to about 30°. This relaxes the posterior capsule at the medial and lateral corners of the knee so that the amount of opening more truly reflects damage to the collateral ligaments. However, the capsular structures still provide some resistance to medial or lateral opening. A laxity of over 10 mm implies complete functional disruption. At knee extension, joint opening is always less as the posteromedial or posterolateral capsule tightens. If joint opening is the same at knee extension, major added damage to these capsular structures has occurred. Also, remember that any time the laxity is increased over 10 mm (over the opposite, normal side), one or both cruciate ligaments may have partial or complete tears. Thus other tests for the cruciate ligaments should be performed as discussed elsewhere. With the knee at full hyperextension, the cruciates lock or jam the femur into the tibia and no medial or lateral joint opening is possible, even though there

may be a severe collateral ligament injury. Therefore, any opening at full knee hyperextension means a serious injury also involving the cruciate ligaments.

There are two types of complete failure (see Table 21:5). In the first case failed ligament fibers are still in continuity, touching each other, even though ligament function is lost. In the second case, there is a gross separation between the ligament ends. The two conditions should be distinguished for two reasons even though in both the ligaments' functional capacity is lost. First, ligament fibers in continuity may heal, whereas if the ligament ends are separated, surgery is required to restore continuity for healing. Second, a ligament is out of continuity only with significant displacement of the joint. This means that other structures including the capsule, meniscus and cruciates may also be damaged. The amount of laxity depends on secondary restraints, such as the capsule, after the collateral ligament is disrupted. Thus, the greater the laxity the greater the chance for concomitant injury and loss of ligament continuity.

A tear in continuity probably cannot be distinguished from a tear out of continuity with certainty before surgery. If the laxity is in the range of 10 to 12 mm increased over the opposite side, then immobilization is an option. However, each knee injury must be evaluated individually and many factors considered in determining the need for surgery. Greater laxity implies a severe loss of continuity requiring surgery.

Functional Stability of Injured Knee

All three stabilizing systems (active, passive and joint geometry compressive forces) are required for proper function of the knee joint. A defect in one system, such as an anterior cruciate laxity or weak quadriceps muscle, may lead to pain, swelling and giving way and therefore loss of functional stability. If the symptoms prevent activity, then a functional disability is said to exist. Some ligament injuries lead to a marked functional disability and others do not. Highly coordinated athletes can compensate to a degree for a ligament laxity. The muscles contract at just the right time, providing knee stability. Still, a word of caution must be sounded. After serious ligament injuries, many competitive and recreational athletes have a residual laxity of the knee joint, most commonly following an anterior cruciate tear. Some athletes compensate and take part in sports. In the past it was thought that if activity could be resumed, the athlete had "functional stability" and all was well. The ability to return to play was used to judge the success of treatment. In fact, in many knees, arthritis of the joint slowly developed only to be discovered some 5, 10 or 15 years later.

This underscores the need for great caution about who should and should not return to competitive athletics after a major ligament injury. We now know that even minor to moderate symptoms of pain, swelling or giving way, over time, may lead to joint arthritis. Even an occasional giving way episode every two to three months, such as when jumping or twisting with anterior cruciate laxity, may, within a few years, lead to arthritis. Joint arthritis, or wear and erosion of the cartilage surface, is often initially occult and may be totally unsuspected. Although wearing unevenly, the cartilage functions normally until it wears out, much as an out of alignment tire. Arthroscopy of the knee joint after serious ligament injuries often provides important information about joint arthritis and the overall condition of the knee joint. Arthroscopy is being performed earlier in symptomatic athletes to detect occult abnormalities.

The point is not to be misled about joint arthritis and the ability of an athlete to perform. Any athlete who sustains a serious ligament injury or even a meniscus removal is at risk for joint arthritis. The percentage of risk varies according to the nature of the injury and many other factors and may be difficult to predict. The criteria for the athlete with a prior injury returning to competitive and recreational activities must include an analysis of the risks for future joint arthritis. The "football knee" is commonly seen today in the middle-aged athlete who is paying the price for a few added years of competitive sports. The ability of an athlete to compensate for an injury is highly individual. A "trial of function" is usually given after injury and rehabilitation to determine if the knee joint can withstand the rigors of competition. If symptoms such as pain, swelling or giving way—the "big three"—occur, a functional disability exists. The athlete should not play with these symptoms. The symptoms may be minor, initially ignored, or perhaps do not prevent activity. However, they are usually persistent and may be first evidence of joint arthritis. The "red flags" for beginning arthritic symptoms signal the need for caution and orthopedic consultation.

1. Persistent, low-grade swelling in the joint, usually the first symptom
2. Persistent stiffness in a joint after activity, often 24 hours later, signaling hidden joint swelling
3. Any major joint swelling after strenuous activity. This requires rest and diagnosis. An athlete should never compete with joint swelling.
4. Persistent minor pains in the knee joint, initially only after activity but usually progressive, limiting activity more and more
5. Any giving way episodes. Initially, this may be a complaint of weakness or feeling of instability rather than full giving way
6. Any grating in the knee joint, which means surface erosions and wear

The "red flags" are not specific for arthritis but may also occur due to other joint disorders. Persistence of any of the symptoms indicates the need for a specific examination as to the cause of the disorder. Causes may include a meniscus tear, ligament laxity, patellofemoral abnormalities or joint arthritis.

Knee dislocation is an infrequent but very serious orthopedic emergency. Damage to the major vessel (popliteal artery) occurs in at least 50% of cases despite the fact that peripheral pulses may be palpable. A physician should attempt immediate reduction by extension and longitudinal traction. If a physician or emergency medical facility is not readily accessible, the certified trainer may attempt reduction. In addition to definitive orthopedic treatment, follow-up vascular evaluation, including arteriography, is done. Anticipation of such serious emergencies is the reason for the health care team formulating an action plan, especially for times when the team physician is not in attendance.

PATELLOFEMORAL DISORDERS

Pathology related to the patella is the single most common cause of knee pain seen in orthopedic offices. The discomfort may be a result of direct trauma, repetitive direct pressure (i.e., constant kneeling), constant repetitive motion with a bent knee against resistance (i.e., crew, biking), malalignment or combinations of these factors. A sound understanding of patellofemoral anatomy and biomechanics is required for proper diagnosis, treatment and rehabilitation of patellofemoral disorders.

Anatomy and Biomechanics

The patella is a sesamoid bone formed in the quadriceps tendon. Acting as a fulcrum, its primary function is to increase the extending moment of the quadriceps muscle (Fig. 21:31). Forces transmitted from the patella to the femoral sulcus increase as knee flexion increases. The patellofemoral compression forces are less than body weight during walking and increase to 2.5 times body weight with activities such as stair climbing.

Normal function depends upon adequate stabilization that is provided by both active and passive elements of the extensor mechanism. The bone contours of the femoral sulcus and the configuration of the patella as well as thickening of the capsule provide passive stabilization. The depth of the patellofemoral groove and height of the lateral femoral condyle buttress against lateral dislocation. The

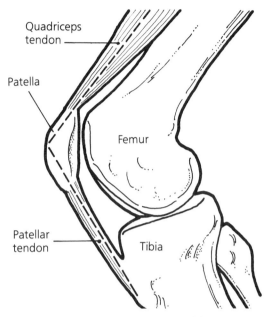

FIGURE 21:31.   The patella acts as a fulcrum, increasing the extension moment of the quadriceps muscle.

patella is held in the groove superiorly by the quadriceps tendon and anteriorly by the patellar tendon as the quadriceps muscle contracts. The passive ligamentous stabilizers consist of thickenings of the capsule extending from the midportion of the patella to the medial and lateral femoral condyles and are termed patellofemoral ligaments. The most important of these is the medial patellofemoral ligament. This ligament helps prevent lateral displacement. The lateral patellofemoral ligament is part of the lateral retinaculum, which is composed of two layers. The first of these is a longitudinal layer of superficial fascia. The second is a distinct, deep layer consisting of transverse fibers that form the bulk of the lateral patellofemoral ligament. These fibers are an expansion into the retinaculum of the vastus lateralis and iliotibial tract. In certain situations these ligamentous structures may be excessively tight, contributing to lateral patellar tilt, malalignment and excessive patellofemoral compressive forces.

The chief active stabilizer of the patella is the vastus medialis obliquus muscle. The importance of this muscle to knee function and patellar position was first described in the middle nineteenth century. More recent studies found that the primary function of the vastus medialis obliquus is patellar alignment. From anatomical dissections a definite cleavage line was reported between the larger vastus medialis muscle and its smaller component, the vastus medialis obliquus. Investigators believed that the two muscle masses should be identified as separate muscles in the total quadriceps mass. Later, electromyogram studies found the action potential count of the vastus medialis obliquus was consistently two times greater than that of the other quadriceps muscle components, indicating continuing vastus medialis obliquus muscle effort to help keep the patella centralized in its groove.

A remote stabilizer of the patellofemoral joint is the pes anserinus group of muscles: the sartorius, gracilis and semitendinous. Through its internal rotatory action on the proximal tibia, the pes anserinus helps to maintain alignment of the tibial tubercle with the femoral sulcus.

As previously noted, stability provided by the femoral groove through the patella depends primarily on the shape of the groove and concomitant patellar configuration. Six types of patellae have been described (Fig. 21:32). The type I and II patellae are most stable with equal distribution of forces over the well-formed medial and lateral patellar facets. The other types of patellae are more prone to unequal stresses and thus lateral luxation. Patella type and femoral sulcus anatomy can be determined by axial radiographic views of the patella.

In 1840 Cruveilhier observed that a contracting quadriceps muscle seeks the shortest route between origin and insertion and stated, "The tendon of the triceps femoris is directed slightly downward and inward and the ligamentum patellae downward and slightly outward, so that the tendon and the ligamentum patellae form an obtuse angle open laterally." This has subsequently been referred to as the "Q angle" and is determined by drawing one line in the middle of the patella to the center of the tibial tubercle and a second line from the center of the patella to the center of the anterior-superior iliac spine on the pelvis (Fig. 21:33). An increase in the Q angle above 15° may increase the tendency for lateral patellar malposition, but by itself is not diagnostic. An increased Q angle, associated with another deficiency of the extensor mechanism, may, however, allow the patella to subluxate more easily.

The Law of Valgus

With the consistent valgus Q angle and the considerably stronger and more fibrous lateral patella stabilizers, this aspect of the physiology and biomechanics of the patellofemoral joint was so important to understanding both normal and abnormal knee function that it was elevated to the level of a "law." The law of valgus helps explain nearly all the pathophysiology involved in this joint, as well as how the delicate balance compatible with symptom-free function might be restored. Morphologically, this law is based on the pre-

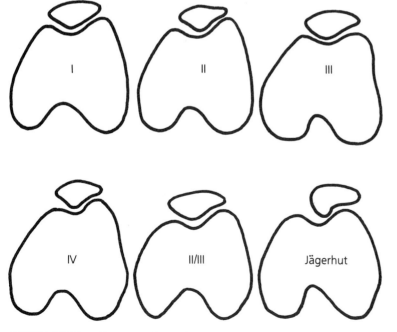

FIGURE 21:32.   Six types of patella

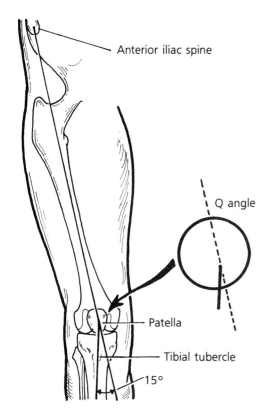

FIGURE 21:33. Q angle and valgus angulation

Labels in figure: Anterior iliac spine; Q angle; Patella; Tibial tubercle; 15°

dominant lateral trochlear surface. The more frequently found patellar form (Wiberg, type II) has a larger lateral facet than medial. The lateral soft tissue elements reinforced by the fascia lata are balanced by similar medial soft tissue stabilizers. These medial soft tissue stabilizers, along with the congruence of the contact surfaces of the joint, offer further stability and thus tend to negate the existing valgus vector. The orientation of the lateral trochlear facet offers further impediment to lateralization of the patella. With this understanding, then, we can discuss the pathogenesis of patellar malalignment.

Extensor Mechanism Deficiencies

Because of the law of valgus, any stabilizing deficiency in the extensor mechanism leads to patellar malposition manifested by lateral patellar subluxation or dislocation. Deficiencies of the extensor mechanism can be divided into three categories: (1) abnormalities of the patellofemoral configuration; (2) deficiencies of the supporting muscles or guiding mechanisms; and (3) malalignment of the extremity relating to knee mechanics. Often deficiencies in more than one category contribute to the patellar malalignment.

Under abnormalities of the patellofemoral configuration, a combination of a low profile of the femoral sulcus and deficiency of the medial patellar facet predisposes to patellar instability. Usually these deficiencies are developmental, caused by deficiency of the supporting muscle or malalignment that did not allow the patella and sulcus to develop normally. These deficiencies are best evaluated by roentgenographic studies. The lateral condyle is higher than the medial and projects anteriorly an estimated 7 mm or more, preventing lateral patellar displacement. The patellofemoral joint can undergo further development during the last several years of growth; thus the sulcus angle and patellar configuration can improve during treatment. This is one of several reasons why conservative treatment in the adolescent is strongly suggested. Thus, when an unstable patellar mechanism demands surgery, it should, if possible, be delayed until skeletal maturity.

Deficiencies of the supporting muscles and guiding mechanisms that allow the patella to subluxate or dislocate laterally include weakness of the anterior medial retinaculum, weakness of the vastus medialis obliquus muscle, hypermobility of the patella due to poor muscle tone after injury, congenital genu recurvatum with a resultant laxity in the extensor mechanism, patella alta and tightness of the lateral retinaculum. Lack of development of the vastus medialis obliquus muscle, which is normally attached to the proximal one third of the patella, allows overpull of the vastus lateralis during walking and running activities, particularly between midstance and take off, thus enhancing lateral subluxation or dislocation of the patella. In patella alta, only the more vertically oriented fibers that attach to the proximal portion of the medial patella are present, diminishing control of lateral patellar displacement.

The association of generalized joint laxity in recurrent patellar dislocation has been noted. Familial joint laxity is commonly the cause of recurrent dislocation. One study found a 10% incidence of patients with recurrent patellar dislocation and a relative who also had the condition, while another report found that 25% of patients had relatives with the same abnormality.

A wide variety of structural abnormalities of the lower extremity may influence patellar tracking in the patellar groove and account for malalignment of the extremity. Certainly, genu valgum increases the valgus vector to the knee, thus setting the stage for patellar subluxation or dislocation. Likewise, lateral displacement of the tibial tubercle in relationship to the anterior superior iliac spine enhances the tendency for the patella to displace laterally.

Femoral anteversion and internal femoral rotation cause the femoral sulcus to be more medially placed in relation to the tibial tubercle and thus give, functionally, a more lateral insertion to the patellar tendon, enhancing the lateral pull of the quadriceps contraction or valgus vector. It is not uncommon for patients with patellar malalignment problems to have a history of having been treated as children for lower extremity malalignment with special orthopedic shoes and leg braces.

Foot mechanics may also alter patellar tracking. During the foot strike of a running gait, the foot pronates with subsequent external rotation of the tibia on the femur as the knee extends. Quadriceps contraction with either foot pronation or external tibial rotation enhances the lateral forces acting on the patella. For less active people who run short distances, this problem usually does not appear. However, in the long distance runner who logs hundreds of miles per year, the abnormal lateral forces directed at the patella may lead to "runner's knee" or patellofemoral arthralgia.

The deficiencies discussed above are usually compensated for in the normal knee by the triangular shape of the patella, depth of the patellofemoral groove and the restraining action of the passive ligamentous structures. However, when bone or soft tissue deficiencies occur by themselves or in combination, the potential for an unstable patella exists, particularly when the knee suffers a secondary insult. The resultant muscle atrophy and weakness associated with even the slightest knee injury tips the delicate scales of the extensor mechanism in favor of malalignment. Pain, usually the first sign of patellofemoral difficulties, further adds to muscular atrophy and disuse. Voluntary or imposed rest to control pain and inflammation creates further muscular imbalances. Once patellofemoral arthralgia has subsided with rest, the mistake is usually to resume full activities without proper reconditioning and restoration of muscle balance. Failure to appreciate this important principle is perhaps the most common cause of failure of conservative treatment of patellofemoral malalignment.

Lateral Patellar Compression Syndrome

The lateral patellar compression syndrome is being recognized more often by physicians and trainers. Essentially, either the lateral retinaculum that holds the lateral facet of the patella firmly to the femoral condyle is tight or the muscles are imbalanced so that the patella is pulled laterally. In either case, excessive pressure develops on the lateral facet and the lateral tissues about the patellofemoral joint and pain occurs. The source of the pain is not well understood as is sometimes true with other patellar disorders. The lateral retinaculum, being under tension, can become tender. Also, the amount of lateral compression on the articular cartilage and underlying subchondral bone of the lateral facet may explain the pain symptoms. On evaluation, the cardinal finding is the inability to displace the patella medially more than 1 cm.

Additional findings in lateral patellar compression syndrome include tenderness of the lateral facet and swelling with synovial irritation. Subluxation can coexist with this syndrome. The athlete complains of pain, usually dull and aching, in the "center of the knee." The knee is swollen, tender as described above and can give way, presumably due to avoidance of pain. Treatment consists of ice, rest and rehabilitation. This syndrome is not as responsive to therapy as others and often leads to either cessation of athletics or surgery. Degeneration of the articular cartilage is not uncommon, and the athlete needs to be followed carefully for this. Again, arthroscopy helps determine the condition of the joint surface.

Preventative measures are the same as for any patellofemoral joint problem. These include the use of mild anti-inflammatory medications during the season, flexibility and adequate warm-up prior to sports, patella supports, alteration of the training program and ice after activity to reduce swelling and pain. Many athletes can get through a season this way, but they should be carefully followed to avoid irreversible damage to the articular surface.

Patellar Tendonitis

The patellar tendon can become inflamed and tender, usually due to an overuse syndrome. Recurrent forces probably produce microfailure of the collagen bundles, and pain with inflammation follows. This occurs in the jumping athlete, thus the term "jumper's knee." Specifically, the athlete complains of pain over the tendon, difficulty jumping or running and pain with many of the prescribed exercises. The fat pad may even become inflamed and contribute to the symptoms. Evaluation reveals tenderness and swelling along the patellar tendon, usually concentrated along the upper portion of the tendon, but not necessarily. In the chronic case, a nodule of scar tissue, often very tender, can be palpated within the tendon or near its insertion site into the patella. Acutely, treatment is the same as for the other problems. Rest may be required initially until acute symptoms subside. Quadriceps strengthening enhances the muscles' absorption of strain. Flexibility, warm-up and icing after practice are all important. A floor that absorbs some of the stress is also important— running on concrete or asphalt increases symptoms. In the chronic case, when a nodule is present and tender, surgical resection of the nodule decreases symptoms. Also, patellar subluxation or the lateral patellar compression syndrome can co-exist with this syndrome. Remember that a subtle lateral subluxation may be the cause for overloading the patellar tendon.

Patellar Subluxation

While not so dramatic as patellar dislocation (discussed later), the patellar subluxation syndrome can be just as disabling and is more common. Here, the patella repetitively subluxates laterally and places strain on the medial restraints and excessive stress on the patellofemoral joint. Symptoms are related to the amount of activity. The condition is commonly brought out by running and jumping sports that place large forces on the patellofemoral joint. Patellar subluxation was once thought to occur mainly in women due to the frequency of genu valgum and lax ligaments. However, now the frequency of this condition in any athletically active person, man or woman, is apparent.

Commonly, the athlete complains of pain and giving way episodes that suggest ligament or meniscal problems. True locking does not occur but stiffness of the patellofemoral joint is common. Evaluation shows tenderness of the medial restraints, swelling of the knee with synovial irritation, disuse atrophy of the quadriceps muscles, in particular the vastus medialis obliquus, and increased "looseness" of the patella, usually, with an excessive Q angle.

The treatment is the same as for patellar dislocation, except cast immobilization is rarely used. If, following an appropriate rehabilitation program, symptoms still occur, surgical realignment of the patellofemoral joint may be necessary. Arthroscopy can be used to view the articular surface directly. Sometimes the symptoms are only mild yet the arthroscope shows serious cartilage erosion, fibrillation and wear. Here again, rehabilitation should emphasize strengthening of the vastus medialis obliquus, since this muscle holds the patella medially to prevent subluxation. Patellar support braces or taping are extremely helpful. Most patients with mild lateral patellar subluxation do well with proper rehabilitation. Often, decreasing activity is enough to cause symptoms to subside. In other knees, the condition can be progressive, with increasing patellofemoral crepitus and continuing symptoms despite all treatment. The trainer must be aware of symptoms indicating chronicity, even though they are seen in only 1 out of 15 patients.

Patellar Dislocation

Acute patellar dislocation can simulate a major collateral ligament injury of the knee. The athlete is usually cutting from the involved knee when a violent giving way episode occurs, often with an audible pop. Usually, the patella spontaneously reduces, leaving a painful, swollen and tender knee. The trainer should palpate to detect a defect in the medial retinaculum and vastus medialis insertion before swelling obscures it. This "rent" occurs as the patella dislocates laterally, tearing the medial restraints. Also, pain along the lateral femoral condyle is suggestive. Obviously, if a ligament examination can be done, normal results exclude the possibility of a ligament disruption. Finally, examination of the opposite knee may reveal a tendency for patella dislocation (hypermobile patella, loose patellofemoral ligaments), another clue for a correct diagnosis. Immediate care consists of ice, elevation, compression and a splint, with physician evaluation to follow.

Treatment is usually one of three modes. First, in recurrent cases of dislocation, attention is directed toward rehabilitation to better provide dynamic stability, patellar support brace and modification of activities. A second treatment regimen calls for cast immobilization if this is the first episode or if medial patellar restraints have torn. This allows healing of the soft tissue restraints. Occasionally, surgery is necessary to repair the restraints or remove an osteochondral fracture. This is followed by rehabilitation and a support brace. Special x-ray films are often required, e.g., axial or oblique views to exclude a fracture of the patella or lateral femoral condyle. Arthroscopy can determine the diagnosis and evaluate the entire knee, if necessary. Rehabilitation is aimed at decreasing the symptoms initially, followed by strengthening the quadriceps muscles, especially the vastus medialis obliquus, to hold the patella in place. When the athlete is ready to return to activity, a patella support brace or, better yet, taping is absolutely required with all activities to decrease the risk of another dislocation. Each dislocation does more damage to the patellar cartilage surface. With multiple episodes, traumatic arthritis can be expected. Therefore, if dislocation occurs more than twice, despite taping and rehabilitation, either the athlete should give up activity or undergo surgical correction.

Surgery for Patellofemoral Malalignment

The objective of surgical treatment is realignment of the extensor apparatus and stabilization of the patella in the trochlea during function. Patients with recurrent subluxations and patellar dislocations often have a congenital deficiency, such as ligamentous laxity. When conservative therapy fails to correct the patient's difficulties, and when multiple deficiencies of the extensor mechanism exist with major disability, then surgical procedures are generally necessary. The determination of which surgical procedure to use must take into account the complexities of the extensor mechanism, the biomechanics of the patellofemoral joint and the particular deficiencies. The key to success in surgery for patellofemoral malalignment lies not in applying a single technique to all patients, but in selecting the proper combination for a given individual.

The number of techniques for patellar realignment and stabilization reported in the literature is astonishing. In 1959, one report counted 137 surgical methods directed at solving the problem of the unstable or malaligned patella. Despite the fact that many of these techniques did not enjoy great success, a large number of variations are still practiced today. Many of these procedures are relatively minor variations or different combinations of other procedures. This multitude of surgical procedures has been categorized for purposes of reviewing them. For our purposes, essentially, those procedures directed at correcting persistent or recurrent patella malalignment prior to the development of serious patella chondromalacia or patellofemoral arthrosis can be considered "reconstructive" rather than "salvage" procedures, and can be divided into three general areas as far as surgical technique and postoperative rehabilitation.

Lateral Retinacular Release

Lateral retinacular release, or capsulorrhaphy, is the simplest of all surgical procedures and may be sufficient for many patients. In this procedure the lateral retinaculum is simply weakened by surgical release to allow the patella to move more centrally in the groove. Lateral release is particularly valuable in the adolescent since it is a relatively simple procedure and does not involve any bony structures in which surgery may interfere with growth. The procedure may be done at arthrotomy in a "z-plasty lengthening" technique, or subcutaneously either by direct vision through the arthroscope or indirect vision using digital palpation.

The lateral release is extensive and includes the entire lateral retinaculum extending from the patellar tendon superiorly as well as the majority of the vastus lateralis tendon (Fig. 21:34). Lateral retinacular release lessens the

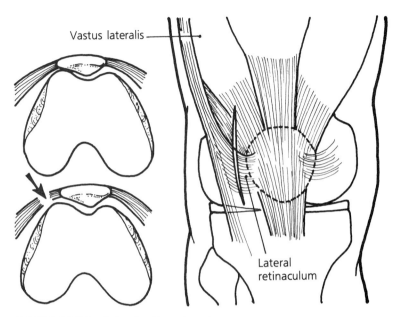

FIGURE 21:34. Lateral retinacular release

compressive forces on the articular surface of the patella and allows a more longitudinal force of the vastus lateralis. Lessening the resistance of the lateral patellofemoral ligament reduces the valgus vector and augments the function of the vastus medialis obliquus muscle due to the improved alignment.

Simple lateral retinacular release, by itself, has only recently become popular. The long-term results of this procedure are yet to be compiled, but early reports are encouraging. The key to success with this procedure lies in preventing postoperative hemarthrosis as well as vastus medialis obliquus strengthening and re-education.

Proximal Realignment

Proximal soft tissue reconstruction is designed to align the muscle pull on the patella and thus enhance the active action of the vastus medialis obliquus. It also tightens the medial capsule, which includes the medial patellar ligament. Meticulous surgical technique is mandatory when the vastus medialis obliquus muscle is to be changed dynamically. Those procedures employing proximal realignment combine lateral retinacular release with reimplantation of the vastus medialis obliquus muscle laterally and distally on the patella.

A multitude of other soft tissue procedures designed to "dynamically" as well as "statically" control patellofemoral alignment have been described. These procedures mainly use the individual hamstring tendons such as the sartorius, gracilis, or semitendinous tendon. These tendons are left attached to their tibial tubercle insertion site and then transferred to the medial border of the patella. Most of these procedures produce erratic results and have not met with great enthusiasm.

Distal Realignment of the Extensor Mechanism

When the patella is not centralized in the femoral sulcus with a lateral retinacular release, or if the tibial tubercle is anatomically lateral to the femoral sulcus producing a large valgus vector, the patellar tendon may need realignment. Several procedures are commonly being done, and in the mature adult essentially employ moving the patellar tendon along with its bony attachment to a new site on the tibia. However, detachment of the tibial tubercle is not recommended in the adolescent because of the potential for growth disturbance.

An association of chondromalacia with recurrent or persistent patellar malalignment is well known. This association is important because the chondromalacia has a great tendency to progress after surgery. The effects of immobility and lack of cartilage nutrition are well documented in the literature, and protecting the patella and its compromised cartilaginous surface during the early rehabilitation phases is of primary concern. This is why a postoperative rehabilitation program for the knee must begin with straight leg raising exercises and then progress slowly to bent leg, progressive resistive exercises. In the bent knee position, the patellofemoral forces are greatest and the softened, compromised cartilage is at greatest risk. Should signs of increasing chondromalacia occur, such as anterior patellar aching, re-

current swelling, palpable synovitis or increasing patellofemoral crepitance, patellofemoral forces should be decreased immediately. This includes cessation of running and jumping activities, abandonment of bent-knee progressive resistive exercises, and re-initiation of straight leg raising and isometric exercises.

Potential Complications

The trainer treating patellofemoral disorders may well be the first to recognize any of the potential complications after patellofemoral joint surgery. Instituting appropriate measures can prevent further disability.

Decreased knee flexion has been reported in virtually all series. Any procedure that transplants the distal patellar tendon attachment should be suspect for this complication. Prolonged immobility, poor patient cooperation and persistent and unrelenting pain have all been attributed to knee flexion contractures. Should the therapist detect a plateau in knee motion during the immediate postoperative weeks, he should alert the operating surgeon as to the need for a possible anesthetic manipulation. Early recognition of this problem usually results in a successful outcome.

Occasionally, medial instability occurs after a medial tubercle transplant. The patella may actually sublux or dislocate medially. This distal advancement may increase the compressive forces on the patella, producing increased patellar wear and discomfort. The common features of this complication are:

1. Immediate disability following surgery
2. Retropatellar pain and crepitation
3. Limitation of motion
4. Distal displacement of the patella confirmed by physical examination and x-ray

The symptoms are caused by pressure of the patella on the underlying femur, fat pad and tibial surfaces. Early recognition and revision of the transfer are necessary to prevent irreversible damage.

Recurvatum occurs as a result of tibial tubercle transplant in the immature skeleton. Most authors recommend that bony procedures involving the proximal tibial epiphysis not be done prior to age 14. Distal migration of the tibial tubercle has also been reported due to patellar tendon transplantation in the growing skeleton.

The patella may rotate in the femoral groove when the vastus medialis obliquus is advanced distally past the midline of the patella. If the vastus medialis is advanced too far distally, undue pressure on the medial facet might result, causing either discomfort or limitation of flexion. Signs of increasing chondromalacia despite cautious rehabilitation may be the first clue to this problem.

Other complications include detachment of the tibial bone block or rupture of the patellar tendon, infection, perineal nerve palsy or numbness along the distribution of the saphenous nerve, thrombophlebitis and anterior compartment syndrome.

Prognosis

Most series report 80% to 90% good results with procedures to prevent recurrent subluxation and dislocation. While short-term results may be good, length of follow-up must be considered. Chondromalacia and osteoarthritis have been found to develop in most series when treatment was followed over a long term. Because of the erratic and uncertain results produced by patellofemoral joint surgery, conservative treatment with proper rehabilitation cannot be overemphasized.

MENISCUS DISORDERS

The menisci are triangular, C-shaped intraarticular structures wedge-shaped in cross section. Macroscopically they are opaque, firm and fibrous. Microscopically the menisci are composite structures that contain fibrous collagen bundles for strength imbedded in homogeneous ground substance typical of articular cartilage. These cells in the meniscus have the appearance of chondrocytes. The collagen fibers in the meniscus are basically arranged in circumferential direction although some are perpendicular and radial in orientation. Circumferential fibers aid in resisting the hoop stresses to which a meniscus is subjected. The femur pushes the curved meniscus outward like a washer being pushed out of place. The greatest tensile strength is in the circumferential fibers.

The peripheral 2 to 3 mm of the menisci are nourished directly by blood supplied from the branches of the medial and lateral inferior geniculate arteries (Fig. 21:35). Menisci seem to have the same nutritional diffusion pattern as articular cartilage. The critical depth of nutrition to articular cartilage by physiologic diffusion is 3 mm. Work on the consistent anatomical relationships in the menisci demonstrates that the medial meniscus varies in width and thickness from anterior to posterior. The lateral meniscus does not vary much in width, but does increase in thickness as it progresses from anterior to posterior. This increased thickness becomes important when analyzing a cross section of this segment for nutrient supply. The central portion of this segment is at, or

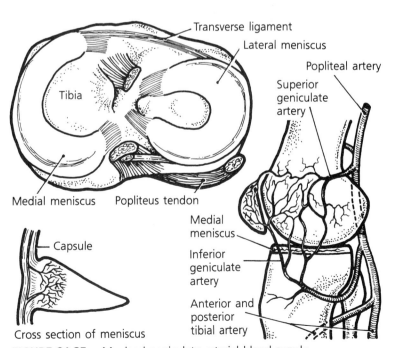

FIGURE 21:35. Meniscal geniculate arterial blood supply

above, the upper limits for efficient diffusion of nutrients. This could explain the high incidence of early microscopic tears in this region.

Gross Anatomy

Medial Meniscus

The anterior horn of the medial meniscus is usually attached to the nonarticulating area of the tibia, just anterior to the anterior horn of the lateral meniscus and the anterior cruciate ligament. The second attachment is known as the transverse ligament. It extends from the anterior horn of the medial meniscus to the anterior border of the lateral meniscus, or it may extend posteriorly into the attachment area of the anterior cruciate ligament (see Fig. 21:35).

The midportion of the meniscus is attached to the tibia and the femur at its periphery via the meniscofemoral and the meniscotibial ligaments. The posterior horn is attached firmly to the nonarticular area of the tibial plateau, between the tibial spine and the origin of the posterior cruciate ligament. As mentioned, the width of the medial meniscus changes. The anterior half is narrow, and the posterior half is very broad.

Lateral Meniscus

The anterior horn of the lateral meniscus is attached to the tibia directly anterior to the intercondylar eminence. Additionally, it may have an attachment to the anterior cruciate ligament.

The midportion of the lateral meniscus is also attached at the periphery by the meniscofemoral and meniscotibial ligaments. An opening in these peripheral attachments allows passage of the popliteus tendon.

In the posterolateral portion of the lateral meniscus the arcuate complex is attached to the meniscal border. The popliteus is strongly attached to the arcuate ligament and the meniscus. These two attachments aid in posterior displacement of the posterior segment during medial rotation.

The posterior horn is firmly attached in the medial portion of the tibial plateau, between the spines of the tibia. There is a second group of attachments from the posterior convex border of the lateral meniscus and the posterior horn. They insert on the tibia just anterior and posterior to the posterior cruciate ligament. These attachments are the ligaments of Humphry and Wrisberg, respectively. The width of the lateral meniscus is greater and more uniform throughout, when compared to the medial meniscus, and the periphery is thicker.

Some differences between the menisci must be detailed. The lateral meniscus is more mobile than the medial meniscus, as explained by careful anatomic assessment. The attachments of the anterior and posterior horns of the lateral meniscus are close together. This allows more mobility than in the medial meniscus with its widely spaced end attachments of the anterior and posterior horns. The increased mobility results in less stress on the lateral meniscus, thus leading to a decreased incidence of injury.

Contour differences are found between the menisci. The lateral meniscus is almost the entire circumference of a small circle. By comparison, the medial meniscus is a small section of a larger circle.

The menisci divide the knee joint into two compartments. In flexion, extension and rotation of the knee joint, the menisci move with the tibia. Most motion of the knee joint occurs in the upper compartment, between the menisci and the femur. Still, some motion does occur between the tibia and the menisci in the lower compartment, particularly with rotation. The final motion of the femur before full extension is medial rotation—which is commonly known as the "screw home" movement (Fig. 21:36). The motion is due to the larger medial femoral condyle rotating around the tibial spine after full excursion of the lateral condylar articular surface. This terminal rotation may be blocked if a portion of the meniscus is caught in the joint, as discussed later in this chapter.

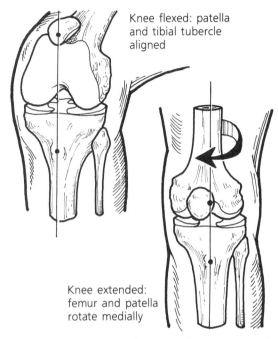

Knee flexed: patella and tibial tubercle aligned

Knee extended: femur and patella rotate medially

FIGURE 21:36. Screw-home mechanism. Femoral condyle rotates around tibial spine.

Function

The functions of menisci are accepted generally as being nutritional, weight-bearing, stabilizing and movement. The nutritional function aids in spreading a thin film of synovial fluid over the articular cartilage and in circulating that fluid throughout the joint.

From 30% to 55% of joint weight is carried by the menisci, and the menisci form a major portion of the weight-bearing surface of a joint. Following meniscectomy, between two and three times more compressive deformation occurs than in a normal joint. The menisci aid in joint function by deepening the tibial articular surfaces. This fills in potential dead spaces at the periphery of tibio-femoral contact, increasing joint stability.

The menisci, because of their figure-of-eight arrangement on the tibia, participate in joint movement. They guide the femur and assist in its tracking during the final screw home motion of extension.

Classification of Meniscus Tears

Meniscal tears can be classified according to age, location and axis of orientation (Fig. 21:37). If the degenerative horizontal tear is more common, the acute longitudinal tear that occurs in youth is more disabling. The usual history is a twisting injury to the knee when the foot is fixed and the knee is flexed, producing compression and rotation on a meniscus trapped in the joint. This injury usually demands immediate attention and urgent surgical intervention. These lesions will therefore be considered first.

In order to have a longitudinal tear, the posterior medial segment of the meniscus must be displaced to some extent. Longitudinal tears are of two types, peripheral or extra-peripheral. The meniscus can remain intact during compression and rotation, and the tear can occur through the posterior peripheral attachment or in the substance of the meniscus itself. These tears can be partial (confined to the posterior segment only) or complete. With a partial tear through the substance of the meniscus, central displacement of the medial fragment is temporary. Repeated episodes may lead to multiple partial tears of the posterior segment or progression of the tear into the anterior segment. With a complete tear, the entire central segment is again displaced medially during the injury. The complete longitudinal or bucket handle tear of the meniscus may produce locking of the knee joint, or the meniscus may return to its normal position in the knee joint following injury.

Locking occurs when the meniscus or a segment of a meniscus becomes interposed between the femur and the tibia at a point anterior to the coronal plane of the knee. Locking occurs in only about one third of complete tears of the meniscus.

Longitudinal tears limited to the anterior segment of a meniscus are rare. They occur most often in the lateral meniscus. The anterior horn of the lateral meniscus is situated more posteriorly than the corresponding portion of the medial structure. It is therefore more prone to trapping in hyperextension and rotation.

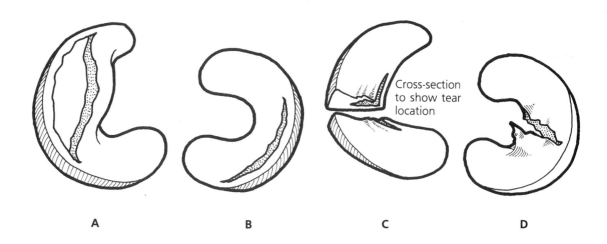

Cross-section
to show tear
location

A   B   C   D

FIGURE 21:37. Four types of meniscal tears. **A** Bucket handle. **B** Longitudinal tear of lateral meniscus. **C** Horizontal tear. **D** Radial tear

Horizontal tears of the menisci are basically due to fibrocartilage degeneration. Presumably, nutrition of the central portion of the meniscus decreases with age. Rotation in the knee joint also causes shear forces between the superior and inferior surfaces of the meniscus. The initial tears can be entirely in the substance of the meniscus, not visible on the meniscal surface. Repeated traumatic episodes may complete the single tear or cause multiple tears in the horizontal plane. The tears may occur in the substance rather than the meniscal surface because of less nutrition and the less tightly woven arrangement of collagen fibrils in the interior as compared to the surfaces.

Horizontal cleavage lesions are most frequent in the posterior medial portion of the meniscus. They can be confined to the posterior segment alone, or can extend to the anterior segment. Once cleavage is complete, the inferior portion can detach, usually posteriorly, which can lead to episodes of momentary locking with associated pain and instability.

The parrot beak tear of the lateral meniscus is listed under horizontal cleavage lesions, but is different for several reasons. It is usually a traumatic tear of youth and is almost always located in the middle segment of the lateral meniscus. Usually, it is associated with previous pathology and is actually a combination of tears.

The parrot beak tear occurs in the thicker portion of the lateral meniscus. This area has usually been previously traumatized and the meniscus has become fixed at its periphery, due to cystic degeneration or some other fibrosis-producing pathology. Because of the fixation and cartilage thickness, two horizontal tears occur. The relative increased mobility of the lateral meniscus during flexion and extension causes the central medial portion between the two tears to attenuate and, finally, to connect. The meniscal superior and inferior surfaces finally attenuate, and a transverse connecting tear occurs, thus completing the complex parrot beak tear.

The acute tears can be traumatic or degenerative in origin. A traumatic tear is usually not an isolated knee injury, and is generally associated with moderate to severe pain, swelling and disability. The degenerative tear generally is an isolated injury and has less pain, disability and reactive swelling. Chronic tears that extend are usually related to episodes of minimal trauma and may have almost no pain or swelling. This decreased swelling is due to less synovial reaction following a smaller injury but also indicates the minimal or complete absence of hemorrhage seen in degenerative and chronic meniscal extended tears. If the central fragment of the meniscus is displaced into the joint, the joint will lock as extended, usually 10° to 40° short of full extension. Once impingement has occurred, further extension is achieved at the expense of the medial portion of the femoral condyle. If the fragment is dislocated into the notch, the normal "screw home" mechanism of the knee is disrupted.

The terminal rotation is regained by stretching the anterior cruciate ligament. This stretching by fragment impingement in full extension and medial rotation can lead to chronic instability. Repeated episodes of joint impingement by fragment displacement can lead to damage of the cartilage surfaces. This accelerated wear can progress through all the stages of chondromalacia. It is not possible to predict which knees will have deterioration of the cartilage surfaces. In many chronic instances of locking, arthroscopy has surprisingly shown no surface deterioration.

In a knee with a torn meniscus, pain can be a variable finding. Chronic meniscus tears without any degenerative joint disease may have point tenderness only over the site of the lesion. With associated degenerative joint disease, the chronic pain increases with activity and there is more local tenderness at the site of the lesion, particularly at night. The etiology for night pain in meniscus tears is uncertain. It may be caused by unguarded knee rotation while turning in bed. Since little joint compression occurs in bed, the fragment can more easily displace, becomes trapped and thereby produces pain. Chronic local inflammation is often more painful at night, or more easily perceived at night when there are fewer distractions. Of interest, some report the weight of the bed sheet increases local pain.

Discoid Meniscus

An anomalous (congenital) variation of the normal semilunar meniscus is the discoid meniscus, which probably is found more often in women than men. This condition may become symptomatic in childhood but may not cause problems until later. The lateral meniscus is more often the discoid (Fig. 21:38). Classically, persons with this condition have a loud "clunking" at the lateral joint line.

Cystic degeneration and tears develop without the usual mechanism of meniscal tears due to its abnormal discoid shape and consequent stresses and forces absorbed. Diagnosis is confirmed by arthrography or arthroscopy. Surgical excision is performed in symptomatic cases.

Diagnosis of Meniscus Tears

Diagnosis of an internal derangement of the knee involving a meniscus can be very difficult. Several physical findings are helpful.

1. *Effusion.* This is usually due to synovial inflammation. It can be associated with an acute injury but usually is seen with chronic meniscal lesions.
2. *Locking.* True locking of the knee joint is a restriction of knee joint extension, generally secondary to a displaced bucket handle tear

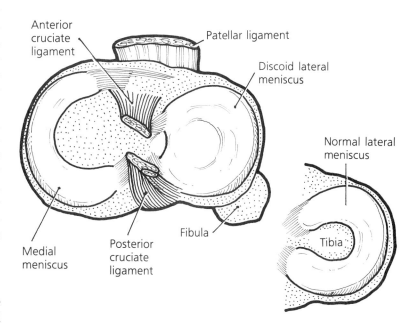

FIGURE 21:38. Lateral discoid and normal medial meniscus

of the meniscus. Usually about 10° of extension is lacking and joint motion is painful. An episode of locking may follow severe or apparently insignificant trauma. If it follows minor trauma, there have usually been multiple episodes of minor trauma. The effusion associated with locking in this knee may be correspondingly small.

3. *Joint line tenderness.* In a person who has had repeated episodes of minor meniscal tears, this may be the only positive sign.
4. *Quadriceps atrophy.* This is usually present in acute or chronic injuries.
5. *Sensation of giving way.* This subjective complaint by the patient indicates a meniscal tear. When the torn portion becomes momentarily caught in the knee joint, pain ensues and giving way occurs due to reflex inhibition of the quadriceps.
6. *Incomplete flexion.*
7. *Tibiofemoral clicking on stairs.*
8. *Reproduction of a click by a McMurray test.*

This is a valuable diagnostic tool for a major bucket handle tear. These clicks should not be confused with flexion-extension clicks secondary to the patella or quadriceps mechanism.

The click caused by a McMurray test is usually secondary to a posterior horn tear. In the McMurray test, place the patient on a table in a supine position, then flex the hip and knee acutely and palpate the posteromedial joint line (Fig. 21:39). Externally rotate the foot and extend the knee. A click is felt as the medial femoral condyle passes over the tear. Note the location of a click, its painfulness and point of occurrence in the arc of motion. To test the lateral meniscus, flex the hip and knee again acutely, and this time internally rotate the foot before extending the knee.

In order to test anterior horn tears, have the patient stand and perform internal and external rotatory movements with the knee extended. This weight bearing causes anterior impingement.

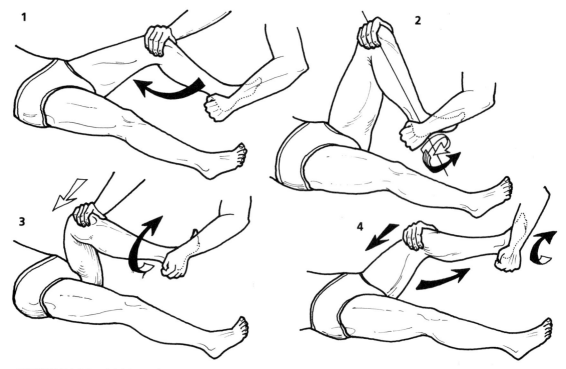

FIGURE 21:39. McMurray's test to produce click

Another test, the Apley grind test, can separate meniscal tears from other internal derangements. Place the patient in a prone position with the knee flexed to 90°. Then rotate the foot internally and externally, first with upward distracting force, then with a compression force. Generally, pain only on compression is due to a meniscal lesion. To modify the test first apply a varus force to the knee to compress the medial joint space. Flex and extend the knee, feeling for any grinding or clicking. This is a valuable test for detecting meniscus tears in the middle portions. A clicking is felt, sometimes heard at around 45° to 60° knee flexion. Test the lateral meniscus in a similar way but apply a varus force during flexion and extension. This test also brings out crepitus to the lateral or medial joint indicative of surface arthritis. This crepitus is usually present throughout a large arc of motion so can be distinguished from the meniscus click.

Treatment

Once a meniscal tear has been diagnosed, treatment must be considered. If the patient has a locked knee, the dislodged meniscus must often be removed if spontaneous reduction assisted by rotation or joint dislocation is not successful. If the patient only has pain and effusion, the standard program for knee effusion is undertaken—rest, ice, compression, elevation and early rehabilitation. Ice should be applied immediately following injury. A bulky pressure dressing from the toes to the inguinal region provides compression. Elevation controls swelling. If the joint is painfully swollen, aspiration for patient comfort may be performed. The patient is placed on crutches and isometrics started. As soon as major pain subsides, weight bearing and quadriceps exercises are increased. Return to full weight bearing is not recommended until swelling has resolved and range of motion and exercise are pain free.

Surgical Treatment

Surgery is indicated for torn menisci that are causing symptoms, i.e., pain, effusion, giving way and/or locking. In contrast to past literature, recent investigations of the function, biomechanics and blood supply of the menisci, as well as clinical observations with arthroscopic surgery, have shown that partial meniscectomy is preferable, if possible, to total meniscectomy. Additionally, certain peripheral meniscal tears seem amenable to surgical repair, as opposed to excision, in late as well as acute cases. Meniscal repair is most often performed as open surgery, although an arthroscopic procedure is coming into use. Preoperative arthrography is helpful in defining the tear and planning the surgical repair.

In bucket handle tears, excision of the bucket handle segment only is preferred. Meniscal regeneration does not follow excision of the centrally displaced portion of a longitudinal tear. Morbidity and rehabilitation time following meniscectomy is lessened with partial meniscectomy. With the advent of arthroscopic surgery, a partial or total meniscectomy can be performed with little morbidity. If the knee joint must be opened, the incision is smaller and less traumatic because arthroscopy prior to arthrotomy defines all of the pathology in the joint. Thus, exploratory surgery is now relegated to history and arthroscopy establishes the diagnosis before surgery.

Long-Term Results

Three radiographic changes may follow meniscectomy: (1) marginal osteophytes (spurs) at the old meniscus site, (2) flattening of the marginal half of the femoral condyle, and (3) narrowing of the joint space on the side of the operation.

Current literature implies that meniscectomy should not be performed simply when a tear exists. With pathologic changes in the joint or major interference with normal function, meniscectomy is indicated. Menisci have important stabilizing and weight-bearing functions. Continued wear, instability and joint pain following meniscectomy have markedly changed the approach to meniscus lesions. Further, arthroscopy can now often define the exact diagnosis. Future studies of meniscectomy will be based on arthroscopic diagnosis and follow-up, and will undoubtedly answer some of the remaining questions.

A note of caution is warranted. There is an extremely high association of meniscus tears with deficient anterior cruciates. The cruciates are the guardians of the menisci. With acute cruciate damage and after chronic laxity, the frequency of meniscus damage is in the 50% to 75% range. Perhaps some of the poor results after meniscectomy were due to unrecognized concomitant anterior cruciate laxity.

BURSITIS

Athletes frequently develop inflammation of the bursae about the knee. Bursitis is usually recognized without difficulty but because of the close proximity to tendons and ligaments, the diagnosis may be confusing at times. Bursae are closed, fluid-filled sacs lined with synovium, similar to that lining the joint space. Their elegant but simple function is to reduce the friction between adjacent tissues, such as where skin and tendons pass over a bony prominence.

Anatomy

Although many bursae are found about the knee, problems with only a few are consistently encountered (Fig. 21:40). The bursae are subject to a variety of conditions including trauma, infection, metabolic abnormalities, rheumatic afflictions and neoplasms. Athlete bursitis can usually be classified as acute or chronic. The cause is usually trauma, although an acute infectious bursitis requiring vigorous treatment and antibiotics must always be considered.

Acute traumatic bursitis occurs in those bursae subject to direct injury. A typical example is prepatellar bursitis. The bursal sac becomes distended, often with a bloody effusion.

Chronic traumatic bursitis is encountered more frequently than the acute type. Because of repeated insults to the bursa, the bursal wall becomes thickened and the sac volume in-

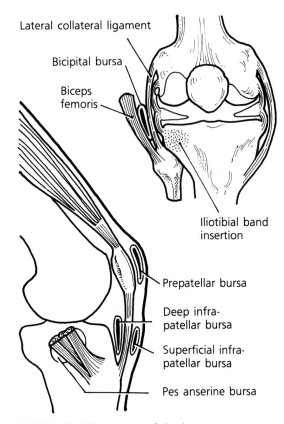

FIGURE 21:40. Bursae of the knee

creases so that the bursa extends far beyond its usual confines.

Acute bursitis secondary to infection is seen in the athlete who sustains a penetrating injury. Bacteria are innoculated into the bursa and rapidly produce a clinical picture of swelling, erythema and exquisite tenderness. Infectious bursitis differs from the traumatic variety because of the added constitutional symptoms of fever and malaise. However, there can be local inflammation, redness and pain in both the acute traumatic and infectious bursitis. Since it may be very difficult to distinguish between the two, a high index of suspicion is necessary to diagnose the infectious type early. Usually, with infection, more redness and inflammation is present. A scratch or break in the skin may precede the onset of symptoms. If there is any question, a physician should be consulted immediately. Bacteria can spread by way of the lymphatics to the joint, causing a pyarthrosis. This highlights the necessity for prompt first aid of lacerations to prevent a deep-seated infection, in this case an infectious bursitis. Also, extensive laceration of a bursa, such as the prepatellar bursa over the knee, requires formal cleansing, irrigation and closure, often over a drain, as outpatient surgery.

Prepatellar Bursitis

The prepatellar bursa lies anteriorly between the skin and the outer surface of the patella (Fig. 21:41). This location makes it particularly susceptible to direct trauma. Acute prepatellar bursitis presents as a tender, erythematous area of swelling over the patella. With knee flexion, increased skin tension directly over the bursa produces pain. Direct pressure over the bursa is also be painful. The localization of signs and symptoms in front of the patella allows prepatellar bursitis to be distinguished from problems within the knee joint. Again, the first principle is to make the correct diagnosis and exclude an infectious cause of the swelling.

For acute traumatic bursitis, treatment consists of ice packs if bursal swelling arises within 24 hours after injury, followed by compression and rest until acute symptoms subside. On occasion, the bursa requires aspiration. When aspiration is performed, cultures should be taken. Rarely, operative drainage or excision is necessary. Recurrence of an effusion is likely in any knees subjected to direct trauma. For this reason, athletes should wear protective knee padding to prevent reinjury.

Chronic prepatellar bursitis is more frequent than the acute type. It results from repeated episodes of slight trauma, and the inflammation is usually recalcitrant to conservative therapy. Treatment consists of fluid aspiration and application of a pressure bandage. Again, padding is required to prevent recurrent trauma. Infrequently, the bursa becomes so distended that nothing short of surgical exci-

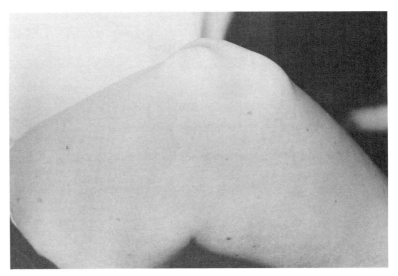

FIGURE 21:41. Chronic prepatellar bursitis that did not respond to conservative measures. Surgical excision is the treatment of choice.

sion will suffice. As with the acute inflammation, the hallmark of effective treatment is to prevent direct trauma through protective padding. Local corticosteroid injection is reserved for those bursae that are inflamed due to trauma, where infection can be absolutely excluded, and where all other means of treatment have not decreased inflammation. Corticosteroid is administered into the bursa itself, with care to prevent injection into any neighboring structure. Steroids seriously weaken tendons, so they are not injected close to or about any tendon or ligament structure.

Deep Infrapatellar Bursitis

The deep infrapatellar bursa is positioned beneath and behind the patellar tendon and in front of the infrapatellar fat pad that lies on the anterior surface of the tibia. These neighboring structures make direct injury to the bursa difficult. Infrapatellar bursitis may be an overuse syndrome due to friction between the patellar tendon and bone. Due to its deep location, this bursa is probably only rarely the cause of symptoms. Localized pain and tenderness in this region are more frequently due to Osgood-Schlatter disease. The diagnosis is by local palpation to find the area of maximum tenderness. Treatment is as previously described.

Superficial Infrapatellar Bursitis

The superficial infrapatellar bursa rests between the skin and the anterior surface of the infrapatellar tendon. It becomes inflamed secondary to direct trauma, and may be clinically indistinguishable from Osgood-Schlatter disease. The symptoms of bursitis are localized pain and tenderness just over the patellar tendon and the tibial tubercle. Treatment is as described, with local protection to prevent recurrent trauma.

Anserine Bursitis

The anserine bursa lies between the pes anserinus tendons (sartorius, gracilis and semitendinous) and the medial collateral ligament on the medial aspect of the tibia. Bursitis develops because of friction or from direct injury. Pain and tenderness are localized to the anteromedial aspect of the tibia. Rotation motion and contraction of the pes anserinus muscles aggravate symptoms. Anserine bursitis must be distinguished from an injury to the medial collateral ligament, medial tendons or tear of the medial meniscus. Crepitus can be elicited (a feature of bursitis), and there is tenderness beneath the pes tendons. A valgus stress usually produces much more pain in a medial collateral ligament injury than in bursitis. With meniscus tears, there is localized tenderness directly at the joint line. The pes bursa lies about 2 cm or so distal to the medial joint line so that the exact side of the tenderness is palpated below the joint line. Treatment is principally symptomatic, consisting of ice, anti-inflammatory agents and steroid injections as indicated.

Bicipital Bursitis

The lateral aspect of the knee contains many small bursae that reduce friction between the interdigitations of the biceps tendon and the lateral collateral ligament and other lateral structures. While most of these bursae are inconstant in location, the bicipital bursa consistently lies between the lateral collateral ligament and the fibular attachment of the biceps tendon. Inflammation ensues after overactivity and infrequently after direct trauma. The diagnosis again rests with excluding ligament or meniscus injuries. Local swelling, so typical of bursitis, is the only real differential. Treatment is symptomatic as previously described.

Iliotibial Band-Friction Syndrome

An acute inflammatory condition occurs where the iliotibial band repeatedly rubs against the bony prominence of the lateral femoral epicondyle. This is frequent with running or any activities with repetitive flexion and extension of the knee. Symptoms are worse climbing hills or stairs. The band drops posteriorly with knee flexion and rubs against the femoral epicondyle. The person often walks with the knee in full extension, preventing knee flexion.

While standard anatomy texts do not describe a bursa over the bony prominence, this has been reported on dissection of one cadaver. Also clear, yellow, viscous fluid has been aspirated from a bursa in one patient who had localized swelling in this region. It is more common not to find a swollen bursa, and the exact site of inflammation is often in the soft tissue, presumably due to the mechanical friction. Treatment is symptomatic with rest or decrease in activities, ice and use of anti-inflammatory medication. In persistent conditions, a local corticosteroid injection is occasionally prescribed. With lateral knee pain on running, a malalignment problem, such as knee varus, that places stress on the lateral tissues may be present.

Baker's Cyst

The term ''Baker's cyst'' is a catch-all for cystic disease in the posterior fossa of the knee.

Such inflammation may be due to actual bursitis (such as seen in the semimembranous bursa) or a structural defect in the posterior capsule that permits synovial herniation. There may be as much as a 50% incidence of communication between the joint space and the popliteal (semimembranous) bursa in asymptomatic individuals. With chronic knee effusions, torn menisci or swelling due to any cause within the knee, synovial fluid accumulates within the communicating bursae.

Most patients with a ''Baker's cyst'' complain of a mass behind the knee that may or may not be painful. The mass is particularly bothersome at full flexion and extension. Furthermore, many patients report periods during which the mass disappears. It is of utmost importance to exclude other causes of a popliteal mass. Rarely, rheumatoid arthritis, arterial aneurysm, anteriovenous fistula, thrombophlebitis and tumors may be present.

The treatment of the cyst rests on correcting the underlying cause of joint swelling, after which the cyst often disappears. Arthrography or arthroscopy can often help diagnose the cause of chronic joint effusion. Occasionally, in long-standing cases, the ''cyst'' requires excision after the primary internal derangement of the knee has been corrected. In general, cyst aspiration and injection, as well as joint immobilization, are not regarded as satisfactory modes of treatment since they do not treat the primary cause of the cyst. In children, the cyst may appear spontaneously, with no intra-articular abnormality, and later disappear without recurrence. However, in adults, the presence of the fluid-filled bursa often denotes intra-articular abnormalities (meniscus tear, arthritis, etc.) as described.

OSGOOD-SCHLATTER DISEASE

Osgood-Schlatter disease was first described in 1903 by Osgood as a partial avulsion of the tibial tubercle causing painful swelling in the knee of the adolescent (Fig. 21:42). Several months later, Schlatter described the same condition and concluded that it was an apo-

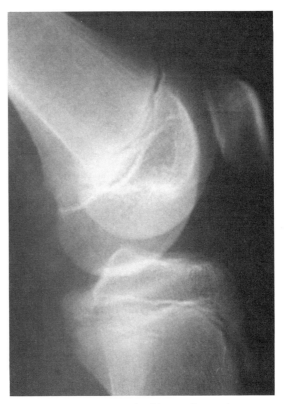

FIGURE 21:42. Osgood-Schlatter disease is epiphyseal inflammation of the tibial tubercle, which is often irregular, enlarged or pulled away on x-ray.

physitis (inflammation) of the tibial tubercle rather than a true bone avulsion fracture. Opinion since then has been divided. Traumatic separation is a distinct injury and often gives identical clinical findings. Most commonly, the condition represents an apophysitis that develops and is aggravated by activity.

This entity is commonly seen by coaches and trainers. It develops during the period of most rapid growth, between the ages of 9 and 13, and is more common in boys than in girls. Bilateral involvement is noted in 20% to 30% of the cases.

Osgood-Schlatter disease is characterized by a painful swelling over the tibial tuberosity, exacerbated by activity, relieved by rest, and usually of several months' duration. Tenderness is most marked at the insertion of the patellar tendon. In cases of long duration, the anterior aspect of the knee appears enlarged and a bony prominence may be palpated—so-called "knobby knees." The range of knee motion is not affected. However, pain may be elicited toward the end of active extension or forced flexion.

X-ray films may show an irregularity and fragmentation of the tibial apophysis. Many believe the diagnosis is roentgenographic, but fragmentation can also be seen in adolescents without symptoms.

Treatment

Treatment is symptomatic. In persistent or moderately painful knees, restrict sports activities until the pain subsides. If the pain is particularly disabling, the knee may be immobilized in a plaster cylinder cast for four to six weeks. Knee pads are used to avoid contusion to the prominent tibial tubercle. The symptoms usually occur from overuse or vigorous activity. Symptoms stop after growth ceases; however, the bony prominence remains.

Very rarely, tumors and acute avulsion fractures may present with similar complaints and findings and must be differentiated from Osgood-Schlatter disease. Infrequently, persistent pain and failure to respond to treatment requires surgery, but only in severe cases after all other treatment modalities are exhausted. In such knees often an extra bony fragment is imbedded within the patellar ligament at the tibial attachment. Surgery consists of removing the accessory bone fragment and associated scar tissue. This lesion probably represents an old fracture of the patellar ligament attachment.

OSTEOCHONDRITIS DISSECANS

Osteochondritis dissecans is a condition of adolescents and young adults in which a part of the articular surface of a joint separates because of a cleavage plane through the subchondral bone.

The true cause of the condition is not definitely known, and several theories have been proposed. Although a familial tendency and an association with certain skeletal or endocrine abnormalities have been noted, in most cases a combination of factors including trauma, nonunion of a fracture line and ischemic necrosis seems to be involved. Clinically and experimentally, osteochondral fractures are seen wherever osteochondritis dissecans is seen. Either direct exogenous trauma to the articular surface or indirect endogenous trauma from one bony surface forcefully striking another produces an acute osteochondral fracture. Some feel that a very prominent tibial spine may impinge against the intercondylar portion of the medial femoral condyle, producing the fracture. This is the classic and most common site for the lesion. More recently, in the hyperflexed knee the odd facet of the patella has been shown to impinge against this region and, with enough force, can cause a fracture. The fracture may be undiagnosed and, with repeated trauma, it fails to unite. The fracture fragment becomes walled off from the remainder of the epiphysis by fibrous tissue. As a result of this, the blood supply becomes interrupted and the bone dies. The cartilage of the articular surface remains alive, however, because it receives nutrition from the synovial fluid. This results in the typical lesion of osteochondritis dissecans—viable articular cartilage with underlying dead subchondral bone, separated from the remainder of the epiphysis by a layer of fibrous tissue.

Two additional observations may explain the particular association of this lesion with the adolescent age group. First, an adult joint has a junction between calcified and uncalcified cartilage called the tide mark, where the cartilage surface gains attachment to the underlying bone. This is absent in the juvenile joint. When shearing forces are applied in the adult, they are transmitted through the tide mark, causing a chondral fracture but sparing the subchondral bone, resulting in the typical osteochondral fracture. Secondly, irregular ossification centers frequently occur in normal children. Minor trauma may cause a cleavage plane that interrupts an already tenuous blood supply and results in the typical lesion.

Pathology

The typical lesion consists of a separated fragment of dead subchondral bone covered by live cartilage. A cleavage plane of fibrous and inflammatory tissue separates the dead bone from the underlying normal, viable epiphyseal bone. Three stages of lesions are based on the degree of separation from the underlying epiphysis: (1) nondisplaced with continuity of the articular cartilage; (2) partially displaced with disruption of the articular cartilage; and (3) completely detached (i.e., loose body in the joint). The non- or partially separated lesion may heal. Capillaries invade from the periphery, bringing in viable osteoclasts and osteoblasts that remodel and lay down new bone on top of the necrotic trabecular bone. In the totally detached lesion, the raw bony surface of both the loose body and the cavity are covered with a fibrous tissue that becomes fibrocartilage.

Clinical Presentation

The peak incidence is in the adolescent and young adult. Males are more commonly affected than females. About half of the patients give a history of trauma. In 10% of cases additional sites may be involved, including the other knee, elbow or ankle. The occurrence of many anatomical sites supports the theory of anomalous ossification or disturbances in growth.

The clinical presentation is usually chronic knee pain and/or swelling with exertion. The pain is aching and poorly localized. If there is a loose body, the knee may momentarily lock.

Physical examination reveals signs of chronic limitation and disuse, perhaps with synovial thickening and atrophy of the quadriceps muscles. With the classical lesion on the lateral portion of the medial femoral condyle, this region may be tender to palpation when the knee is acutely flexed.

In some patients a clinical sign (Wilson's) may be specific for the classical lesion of osteochondritis. To perform this test flex the knee to 90°, internally rotate the tibia and then extend the knee. At approximately 70° of flexion pain is elicited about the region of the medial femoral condyle. About 25% of patients show alignment deformities of the knee such as genu valgum (knock knee), genu varum (bowleg) or genu recurvatum (back knee). The significance of these growth abnormalities is not known.

The definitive diagnosis can only be made by roentgenograms. A well circumscribed area of sclerotic (dense) subchondral bone is separated from the remainder of the epiphysis by a radiolucent line. Since most lesions are noted in the intercondylar notch region of the medial femoral condyle, a tunnel view often shows this area to best advantage.

Arthroscopy and arthrogram are two additional diagnostic procedures if routine roentgenograms are inconsistent or to stage the lesion and determine the correct treatment.

Treatment

For the early, nonseparated symptomatic lesion, immobilization by casting and diminished weight bearing is usually adequate. The leg is casted in a position that protects the lesion from tibial-femoral contact. Plaster immobilization for six to eight weeks followed by refraining from strenuous activities is the prescribed treatment until roentgenograms demonstrate satisfactory healing. The younger the child and the shorter the duration of symptoms, the more likely is satisfactory healing. Occasionally, an entirely asymptomatic patient may have a small osteochondral defect on a roentgenogram taken for another reason. Here, treatment is close follow-up and repeat roentgenograms, but plaster immobilization is unnecessary.

In the older patient or the more chronic lesion, surgery is frequently the treatment of choice. Certainly surgical removal of a loose fragment is necessary. For the lesion still attached, treatments available include simple drilling, curettage and drilling and pinning in situ by metallic pins or cortical bone pegs. Some procedures can be performed by arthroscopic surgery. Whatever method is used, cast immobilization for six to eight weeks follows. A second operative procedure is required to remove the metallic pins if used.

The overall prognosis is generally good to excellent, depending on the size of the lesion. Older patients have less favorable results, especially when degenerative joint changes have already developed before surgery.

CHONDRAL AND OSTEOCHONDRAL FRACTURES

An osteochondral fracture is an intra-articular fracture in which part of the articular surface is separated from the remainder of the epiphysis by a fracture line through the subchondral bone (Fig. 21:43). The fracture may result from exogenous trauma with a direct, tangential blow to the knee or from endogenous trauma where one bony structure hits another as a result of forceful rotation and axial compression.

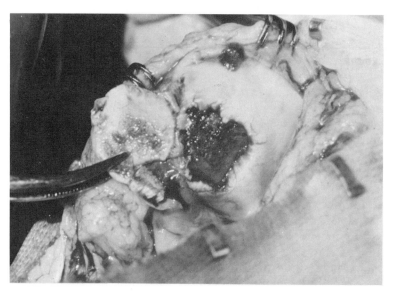

FIGURE 21:43. An osteochondral fracture demonstrated at open arthrotomy. Note the disruption of a large portion of the articular surface.

Each type of trauma produces predictable fracture sites in the involved bones. Exogenous trauma causes fractures in any exposed location such as the medial or lateral aspect of the femoral condyles or the margins of the tibia. These fractures may be large, involving a considerable portion of the articulating surface. Endogenous trauma usually produces smaller lesions in the interior protected areas of the joint, for example, the intercondylar notch region of the medial femoral condyle or the patellofemoral joint. A common area of fracture due to patellar dislocation is the anterolateral aspect of the lateral femoral condyle or medial aspect of the patella. With patellar dislocation, the patella undersurface strikes the lateral femoral condyle, fracturing one or both surfaces. An underlying malalignment of the quadriceps-patella-patellar ligament may be the cause of the acute patellar dislocation.

Pathology

In these fractures an acute fracture line through the subchondral bone produces a fragment consisting of articular cartilage and viable subchondral bone. If the fragment becomes separated, the defect begins to fill in with fibrous tissue, usually within ten days. If the fragment remains in place, the hematoma is invaded by capillaries bringing fibroblasts and other cells involved in bony healing. Just as likely, however, because of inadequate immobilization or the repeated trauma of weight bearing, a fibrous nonunion may develop. In this case, the fracture appears very much like osteochondritis dissecans. This has prompted many authors to hypothesize recently that the osteochondritis lesion is an ununited osteochondral fracture. The bony portion becomes necrotic, the articular cartilage remains viable and the fracture line is filled in with fibrous tissue. The entire piece may later separate and be caught in the joint.

Clinical Presentation

The fracture usually occurs in the adolescent with no pre-existing knee abnormalities. There may be a history of a direct blow to the knee or a violent twisting motion that produced an audible snap or pop. Intra-articular swelling due to blood to the joint occurs within hours. The patient may be unable to bear weight on the extremity due to pain. On aspiration the effusion is bloody. Severe muscle spasm or the fragment displaced as a loose body in the joint may cause the knee to lock in the flexed position. If the fracture is a result of patellar dislocation, an associated tear of the medial retinaculum may produce medial joint line tenderness. This may lead the examiner to diagnose erroneously the condition as a meniscus tear. Ligamentous instability may be associated with osteochondral or chondral fractures. These defects were reported in as many as one fifth of knees with acute anterior cruciate tears. If the patient doesn't present acutely, symptoms may become chronic with vague knee pain and recurrent swelling, the typical picture of osteochondritis dissecans.

The definitive diagnosis depends on visualizing the fragment on roentgenograms or arthroscopically. Since cartilage is not visualized on routine roentgenograms and the bony fragment is usually small, the lesion is commonly missed. Multiple views of the knee may be necessary to rotate the fragment into view where overlap of other bony structures do not obscure it. The usual views are anteroposterior, lateral, right and left obliques, tunnel, and axial patella (sunrise). If the diagnosis remains in doubt, arthroscopy usually defines the true extent of injury and resolves any questions as to the cause of the hemarthrosis in acute injuries.

Treatment

The treatment of osteochondral fractures is usually surgical. If the fracture fragment is very small and on a nonweight-bearing surface, it may be simply excised. Larger fragments and those situated on a weight-bearing surface are anatomically reduced and fixed in place. Afterward, the knee is placed in a cylinder cast and protected from weight bearing. Full weight bearing on the knee is usually not allowed until healing and incorporation of the fracture fragment into the fracture bed. This may require 12 to 16 weeks from the time of surgery. Arthroscopic visualization of the joint surface is sometimes used to determine the extent of healing.

If surgical treatment is delayed past ten days, achieving an anatomic reduction may be difficult because of fibrous tissue ingrowth about the fracture bed. In longstanding lesions it may be impossible to replace the separated fracture fragment. This underscores the urgency of diagnosis and treatment.

The prognosis for the acutely treated lesion is good to excellent. The prognosis for lesions not treated until the chronic phase is reasonably good but not as favorable as acutely treated lesions because of difficulties in restoring the articular surface anatomically. With less than ideal restoration of the joint surface, degenerative changes may occur and the prognosis is poor. Any extensive fracture of the joint surface carries the risk of surface deterioration and future joint arthritis.

FRACTURES ABOUT THE KNEE

Distal Femur Fractures

The supracondylar area extends from the femoral condyles to the junction of the femoral metaphysis and diaphysis. The condylar area is the region from the top of the femoral condyles to the knee joint line (Fig. 21:44). Displacement of fractures in this area can be predicted on the basis of the muscle attachments. Generally, fractures of the distal femur angulate and displace posteriorly. The adductor muscles tend to rotate and shorten the femoral shaft whereas the quadriceps, hamstrings and gastrocnemius contribute to posterior displacement of the condylar fragment.

Severe valgus or varus stress coupled with axial loading or rotational forces produces fractures of the distal femur. While vehicular accidents as in auto racing account for most of

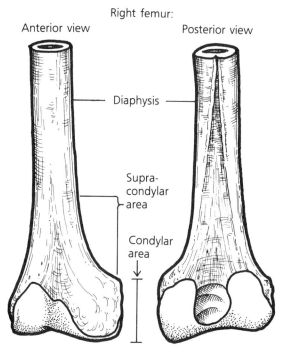

Right femur:

Anterior view   Posterior view

Diaphysis

Supra-
condylar
area

Condylar
area

FIGURE 21:44.   Areas of the femur supracondylar area

these fractures, they may also be produced by a fall on the flexed knee, particularly in the older, osteoporotic, recreational athlete.

Supracondylar Fractures

Supracondylar fractures may be undisplaced, impacted or displaced. Displaced fractures may be transverse or oblique in the orientation of the fracture line, and accompanied by comminution.

History includes major trauma followed immediately by painful swelling and deformity of the distal thigh. Usually there is gross motion and crepitus at the fracture site. Neurovascular enbarrassment associated with this injury is uncommon, but disruption of a major vessel can occur and circulatory status of the lower leg should be carefully evaluated.

Evaluation of this injury requires anteroposterior and lateral x-ray films of the knee as well as anteroposterior and lateral x-ray films of the femur shaft and hip to avoid overlooking serious associated injuries.

Treatment may be closed or surgical. Closed methods entail traction for reduction followed by application of a long leg cast, spica or cast brace. In open treatment traction is followed by operative reduction and fixation with metallic plates and screws or intramedullary rods. After operative treatment, external immobilization by cast or cast brace is usually required. Early knee motion is advised to prevent fibrous ankylosis.

Intercondylar Femur Fractures

Fractures of the femoral metaphysis with extension into the knee joint may be represented as a T or Y fracture, depending on the configuration of the fracture lines, although a variety of fracture configurations may be present. Neer's classification is most widely accepted and is based on displacement and comminution of the supracondylar extension of the fracture line (Fig. 21:45).

In addition to deformity, these fractures are associated with a marked knee effusion and crepitus on passive knee motion. In general, the same mechanism of injury accounts for these injuries as in supracondylar fractures—a blow to the flexed knee as well as varus or valgus combined with rotational forces.

While treatment of these fractures may or may not be operative, the knee intra-articular relationship must be re-established. Surgical intervention is often necessary to achieve this goal. Postoperatively, a cast or cast brace is required, again with a goal of early knee motion.

Femoral Condyle Fractures

Isolated fractures of the femoral condyle are not as common as supracondylar and intercondylar fractures. They are the result of abduction or adduction forces or axial loading. Following injury, crepitus with knee motion and varus or valgus instability may be apparent. A large hemarthrosis develops. While anteroposterior and lateral x-ray films should be obtained to evaluate this injury, oblique views are often necessary to appreciate the full extent of the fracture.

Treatment may be operative or nonoperative. The nondisplaced fracture treated nonsurgically must be carefully observed for any tendency to displace. Open reduction and internal fixation are usually required for displaced or comminuted fractures, again with the goal of early knee motion to prevent fibrous ankylosis.

Proximal Tibia Fractures

Fractures of the proximal tibia may be articular or nonarticular, but loss of knee function is the primary consideration in both. The proximal tibial metaphysis flares from the diaphysis to provide a large, relatively flat surface to articulate with the distal femur. The intercondylar eminence is a nonarticular region between the two tibial condyles to which the anterior cruciate is attached.

Fractures to the tibial condyles are known as "bumper" injuries, but falls from heights and twisting falls also produce these injuries. Forces in vertical compression produce characteristic fractures of a T or Y configuration. Pure varus or valgus forces tend to cause ligament injury whereas, when combined with axial loading forces, they cause various types of fracture configurations. The location and amount of depression of the fracture depends to some extent on the amount of knee flexion at the time of injury. With the knee extended, the compression force is exerted anteriorly. With flexion, the middle or posterior third of the articular surface may be involved.

Undisplaced fractures are those that show less than 4 mm depression or plateau widening. Displaced fractures are compression fractures, split fractures or total plateau fractures.

Compression fractures are divided into two distinct subtypes. In one, the compression is localized to an area roughly shaped to the corresponding femoral condyle. In the second type, compression occurs with splitting-off of a fragment of the metaphysis and articular surface.

These injuries produce acute pain and swelling of the knee. The patient may be aware

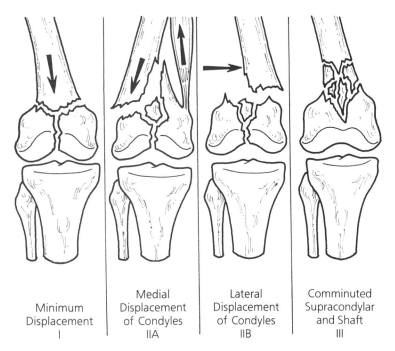

| | | | |
| Minimum Displacement I | Medial Displacement of Condyles IIA | Lateral Displacement of Condyles IIB | Comminuted Supracondylar and Shaft III |

FIGURE 21:45. Neer's classification of fractures

that the knee was deformed at the time of injury. While hemarthrosis is common, sometimes the capsule tears and hemorrhage drains spontaneously into the soft tissues of the knee. Limited motion and pain over the tibial metaphysis is present. Relative varus or valgus instability may be noted with stress testing, which is secondary to the loss in height of the tibial articular surface. Stress x-ray films are often necessary to locate an associated ligamentous injury.

Treatment may be operative or nonoperative, depending on the severity of the fracture. Of paramount importance is restoring the normal articular surface with early knee motion and delayed weight bearing. When the articular surface has been severely depressed, bone grafting may be necessary to maintain the depressed articular surface in a reduced position. Traction is an alternative form of treatment in displaced fractures.

In nondisplaced fractures, plaster immobilization or cast brace immobilization may be

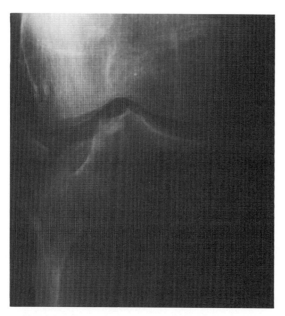

FIGURE 21:46. Compression fracture of the lateral tibial condyle with disruption of the articular surface and severely depressed bone.

employed. Again, weight bearing is delayed but knee motion is encouraged early in the course of treatment. Open reduction usually is necessary, however, with severe depression of the articular surface.

Tibial Spine Fractures

Violent twisting or abduction-adduction injuries may cause fractures of the tibial spine. Avulsion of portions of the intercondylar eminence adjacent to the tibial spine indicates cruciate ligament avulsion. The patient may present with effusion, and often cannot fully extend the knee. Signs of anterior or posterior cruciate ligament insufficiency may be present. Cycling injuries in children commonly cause tibial spine fractures.

Closed treatment is indicated when the avulsed fragment is minimally displaced. If closed reduction cannot be performed, arthrotomy and open reduction with fixation by any number of available methods is performed. Postoperatively, cast immobilization with the knee held in nearly full extension for

five to six weeks is necessary, followed by rehabilitation.

Injuries to the Growth Plate

The seriousness of bony injuries about the knee in growing children cannot be over-emphasized. Not only are these injuries critical in terms of locomotion, but the growth centers about the knee determine approximately 65% of the longitudinal growth of the lower extremity—40% in the distal femoral epiphysis and 25% in the proximal tibial epiphysis.

The growth plate is often the weakest link in the growing child. With angular displacements about the knee, a fracture occurs across the cartilage growth plate, which may injure the cellular component leading to cessation of growth and a short limb. The diagnosis is made by local tenderness about the growth plate region, and varus and valgus stress x-ray views of the knee. With fracture, the growth plate opening can be seen on stress x-ray films.

Because of the stout periosteal layer in the bones of the growing child, joint alignment can usually be obtained by closed means. An anatomical restoration of the growth plate, however, is essential even if surgery is the only means to obtain this. Traditionally, the Salter-Harris classification has been used as a guide for prognosis and treatment (Fig. 21:47). The Type I or shear injury has traditionally been given the best prognosis and Type V or compression injury the worst prognosis for continued growth.

Patellar Fractures

The patella protects the anterior articular surface of the distal femur and increases the force of the quadriceps mechanism by improving the lever arm. Patellar fractures constitute 1% of all skeletal injuries and occur in all ages. The leading causes of injury include falls, direct blows, traffic accidents and falls from heights. Bilateral fractures are uncommon. Ipsilateral fractures (in the same extremity) occur in 15% of patients with patellar fractures.

Patellar fractures are classified into three types: (1) transverse (60% to 75% in frequency), (2) comminuted and stellate (28% to 34% in frequency), and (3) longitudinal (12% to 20% in frequency). Stress fractures, while rare, may occur in the lower patella and result in detachment of the extensor mechanism.

The mechanism of injury and the position of flexion at the time of trauma influences the type of fracture produced. Indirect violence produces a transverse fracture, as does a sudden, forced contraction of the quadriceps when the knee is flexed (eccentric muscle contraction). The patella is literally "pulled apart," fracturing through the plane of tensile stress, which is perpendicular to the muscle pull.

Direct violence is commonly caused by dashboards, but may also occur in any athletic endeavor. These fractures are usually comminuted with or without separation of the fragments. Direct blows may also produce serious ligamentous injuries besides the obvious patellar fracture. Therefore, a thorough physical and roentgenographic examination is necessary to properly evaluate the knee and extremity.

The diagnosis of patellar fractures usually presents little problem. Often an indentation is palpable over the anterior aspect of the knee and the patient is unable to perform a straight leg raise. Roentgenographic diagnosis is usually made in frontal, lateral and axial views. Differential diagnosis includes the bipartite patella, found in 1% to 6% of adolescents. Bipartite patella, often bilateral, occurs in the proximal and lateral aspect of the patella and is nine times more common in men than in women.

The treatment of patellar fractures is based on the nature of the injury and the type of fracture. Nonoperative treatment is recommended for nondisplaced fractures where the extensor mechanism is preserved. A separation of 2 to 3 mm is acceptable, provided the articular surface is without a stepoff. The knee is immobilized in a cylinder plaster cast or knee immobilizer splint for four to six weeks. Then partial weight bearing is followed by rehabilita-

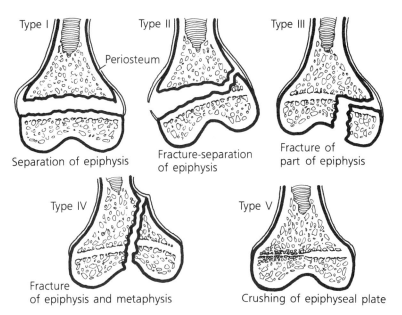

FIGURE 21:47. Salter-Harris classification of fractures

tion. The prognosis is generally excellent for nondisplaced fractures.

Operative treatment is indicated when the fracture fragments are displaced more than 4 mm or with major disruption of the quadriceps extensor mechanism requiring repair. Different surgical treatments are based on the type or severity of fracture. Osteosynthesis, a fixation designed to internally fix and reduce the fracture fragments with wire, screws and pins, is used to obtain bony union. Alternative treatments include partial patellectomy where one large fragment is retained to save patellar function, excising the smaller fragments. The extensor mechanism is repaired as indicated. Total patellectomy is recommended for comminuted fractures when no large fragment can be retained, and also as the last resort.

Rehabilitation is most important after all forms of treatment, operative or nonoperative. Duration of immobilization may vary but muscle strength and power must be regained to return the athlete to the preinjury level of function. Principles of rehabilitation are covered elsewhere. Bone and soft tissue healing require a number of weeks of protection before any strenuous quadriceps exercises are instituted.

MANAGEMENT OF KNEE INJURIES

The proper and appropriate care of the knee begins immediately on injury. Although initially the degree of damage and involvement may not be ascertained in every detail, early evaluation and proper care are necessary for the optimal recovery. In the protocol for knee management, several steps should take place.

1. Determine how the injury occurred, either from the injured athlete or another individual (player, official, etc.) if you did not see it.
2. Determine the area and degree of pain.
3. Determine injury to other areas.
   A. Sensation and circulation in the extremity
   B. Position of the limb
   C. Stability of the knee
   D. Active and passive motion of the joints

The degree of pain and involvement dictates initial care. All of the above information may not be collected immediately. Obviously, if the athlete is down on the field of play and in intense pain and a quick glance indicates an obvious deformity, the course of action is different from when an athlete limps off the field and seeks assistance.

The injured athlete presents in one of several categories.

   I. Injured athlete on the field
   II. Injured athlete who limps off the field
   III. Injured athlete still participating but summons help during the course of competition or practice
   IV. Athlete seen after the game
   V. Next day injury

These categories may in no way indicate severity. The injury seen the next day may be as severe as that seen on the field.

Category I

Pinpoint the problem by asking the injured athlete where the pain is located. In some cases, a severe injury may be apparent and appropriate first-aid steps are then important. The injuries that fall into this category are:

1. Severe ligamentous injury
2. Dislocations (determined by observation)
3. Fractures (determined by observation)
4. Multistructure involvement (determined by observation)

These injuries should be handled as outlined in Chapter 16.

Category II or III

When the athlete comes off the field under his own power, direct him to an area where a thorough examination can be conducted. Collect a complete history. Questions include: ''Where does it hurt? How did it happen? Did you hear anything? What does it feel like?'' The athletic trainer and physician should already be familiar with any history of injury.

In deciding whether immediate return to competition is possible or if a serious injury requires treatment, consider the following:

1. Is there adequate stability?
2. Is there adequate strength?
3. Is there adequate mobility?
4. Is the athlete ready (mentally)?
5. Is added support or taping necessary?

The extent of injury may not be evident immediately, so ice may be applied initially. Later, after the pain has subsided, allow the athlete to move around. Observe for a limp or any inability to use the extremity fully. If the repeat examination reveals no serious injury, permit the athlete to try the knee along the sidelines by light jogging. The trial can progress until the athlete has proven the ability to fully participate without limitation. If there is any question regarding the athlete's condition, refer to a physician.

Injuries treated on the sidelines need to be followed very closely and definitely re-evaluated after the contest or practice. The course of I.C.E. should be followed. Splinting and crutches may even be warranted.

Category IV or V

Serious knee injuries may present after play or the next day. For example, in one study, approximately 15% of those sustaining an anterior cruciate tear after a twisting injury continued to play. After the game or the next day, knee effusion and stiffness brought the athlete to the trainer or physician. Continued participation in sports places the athlete at increased risk for the knee to give way and produce further damage.

The trainer should reinforce the necessity of having every ''knee sprain'' examined. The usual error is to assume the condition is not serious. Continually observe for any limp, stiffness, knee swelling or knee complaints, even those thought to be minor. Additionally, even minor ligament sprains (first degree, no laxity) require vigorous rehabilitation to restore normal muscular strength, endurance and coordination, and prevent more serious injury. Subtle patellofemoral subluxations can produce a gradual weakness and lead to a full giving way episode and serious injury.

Protocol for Management

1. Acute treatment: first 24 hours
   A. I.C.E. (appropriate ice treatment with compression and elevation
   B. Crutches (nonweight bearing)
   C. Pressure wrap (toe to upper two thirds of the thigh)
   D. Splint
2. 24 hours after injury
   A. Appropriate cold therapy
   B. Crutches
   C. Pressure wrap (toe to upper two thirds of the thigh)
   D. Splint
   E. Exercise protocol (refer to section on knee rehabilitation)
   F. Factors that determine when active range of motion is allowed
      1) Absence of laxity or minimal laxity as determined by physician
      2) No effusion
      3) Absence of or minimal pain
      4) Minimal patellar crepitation
3. Early mobilization period to progressive range of motion
   A. Appropriate cold therapy twice a day with active range of motion within pain limits
   B. Patellar mobilization (medial-lateral and proximal-distal)
   C. Crutch walking—progression
      1) Functional range: two crutches
      2) Absence of effusion: one crutch or cane
      3) Absence of pain and limp: discard cane or crutch
      4) Adequate strength (maintain knee extension while weight bearing)
      5) Supportive devices (braces)
   D. Exercise protocol: advance as per section on knee rehabilitation
   E. Taping techniques
      1) Medial or lateral ligament injuries
         a) Anchors (2–3 inch elastic)
         b) Fan (hour glass) (3 inch elastic)
         c) Criss-cross bilaterally (1½ inch cloth, nonstretch)
         d) Spiral (¾ inch elastic)
         e) Slant—for collateral ligament (2 inch elastic)
         f) Covers
      2) Meniscal (medial or lateral)
         a) Anchors
         b) Criss-cross bilaterally
         c) Spiral
         d) Butterfly
         e) Covers
      3) Knee hyperextension
         a) Anchors
         b) Posterior criss-cross
         c) Spiral
         d) Covers
      4) Subluxating patella (taped in internal rotation of the leg)
         a) Anchors
         b) Posterior criss-cross
         c) Butterfly (lateral felt)
         d) Spiral
         e) Covers

5) Anterior cruciate ligament (internally rotated slight flexion)
   a) Anchors
   b) Pes support strips
   c) Criss-cross
   d) Spiral
   e) Cover
6) Triad (medial collateral ligament/anterior collateral ligament meniscal)
   a) Cover
   b) Pes support
   c) Fan (hour glass)
   d) Criss-cross
   e) Spiral
   f) Slant
   g) Butterfly
   h) Covers

REHABILITATION OF THE KNEE

To rehabilitate an injured knee, pain, swelling and the effects of acute injury must first be relieved. Damaged tissue requires time to heal. This is true for both surgically and nonsurgically treated knees. Pain is an important guideline to the extent of healing. Remaining pain is a clear warning of further damage. In the early-injury or postoperative phase, immobilization (splint or cast) and crutches provide the rest necessary for healing and relief of pain.

Every injured or postoperative knee also has some degree of inflammation. Inflammation of the synovial tissues can be secondary to a hemarthrosis. Blood acts as an irritant, causing the synovial tissue to become edematous, and this swelling increases the pain. Decreased swelling and effusion are important signs of improvement. To relieve swelling and inflammation, follow an I.C.E. (ice, compression, elevation) program. Initially use ice for 20 minutes four to eight times per day, placing a towel over the knee and under the surrounding ice bags to avoid burning the skin. Cotton cast padding and Ace wraps provide compression. Rewrap the compressive dressing two to three times per day. Elevation is best done supine with the knee elevated higher than the heart. Aspirin in adequate doses (two tablets four times per day) is commonly the first medication used, but nonsteroidal anti-inflammatory medication may be required. Steroids have too many systemic effects for use in this setting.

After measures to combat pain and inflammation, the next goal is re-educating the knee neuromuscular system. Contraction of muscles in an injured or postoperative knee often causes pain. A reflex response acts to diminish muscle contraction and pain but also causes loss of muscular tone resulting in considerable, rapid atrophy. To minimize this, begin exercises early. Exercise should be pain free. If the exercise evokes pain, then reduce either the repetitions or intensity. Electrical muscle stimulation or transcutaneous nerve stimulation may be required if rehabilitation is delayed or initially painful. Muscle stimulation retards atrophy and produced hypertrophy in some studies. Once neuromuscular re-education and muscle tone are established, pain sometimes diminishes dramatically, especially in disorders of the extensor mechanism and patellofemoral joint.

While specific exercise techniques for strength, power and endurance are discussed below, a word of caution is required. Too vigorous an exercise or improper exercises can damage the knee. The patella surface is most vulnerable. Tremendous loading forces of many times body weight develop between the patella and femur with exercise. Frequently, exercising the quadriceps from 90° to 30° produces pain in the patellofemoral joint. Therefore, initial exercises are often prescribed from 0° to 30° of knee flexion. Carefully follow pain and swelling during the exercise program. Added time for healing is often necessary before any vigorous exercises. After knee surgery, soft tissue must be allowed time to heal before beginning exercises. During immobilization, certain exercises may be done in the cast or splint. Exercise programs must be designed to maintain the patient's interest, as the recovery period is often long and tedious.

After serious ligament injury and surgery, as long as one year's recovery may be necessary. Continued encouragement maintains motivation required for proper rehabilitation and a well-functioning knee.

Besides specific knee exercises, the rest of the lower extremity must not be ignored. Do not focus all the attention on the injured knee only to find later the hip and ankle musculature are weak from disuse, preventing full return to activity or potentially leading to another injury. A comprehensive exercise program should include back, hip, knee and ankle exercises of the injured and uninjured extremities. Upper body exercise programs are also prescribed.

Proper rehabilitation is the key to good results, whether in acute nonsurgical knee injuries, chronic knee conditions or surgically repaired knees. The final functional result is directly related to the therapist and trainer's expertise, interest and ability to motivate the patient.

Rehabilitation Exercises

Although a more complete discussion of the principles of rehabilitation is contained in Chapter 14, this section deals with the specific exercises used to rehabilitate the knee.

Muscular weakness develops in all injured knees. After the relief of pain and recession of inflammation and swelling, the first goal is to regain strength and range of motion. Strength and range of motion are mentioned before power, endurance, speed, agility and coordination because without strength these other functions cannot be obtained (Table 21:6).

In the initial phases of knee rehabilitation, strength building is often started with isometric exercises for several reasons. First, moving the joint through a range of motion may cause pain. Second, isometrics can be done with the leg in a splint or cast. Third, isometrics in full extension put little or no force on the patellofemoral joint, which is important if patellofemoral chondrosis exists. Isometric exercises are started immediately after injury

TABLE 21:6. Rehabilitation Progression

Range of Motion Progression		
1. Active pain-free ROM* with appropriate modality		
2. Patellar mobilization (knee)		
3. Active assistive ROM with PNF†		
4. Resistive assistive ROM		
5. Passive ROM		

Strength Progression		
1. Straight leg raising	8 × 10 to 10 lbs	
2. Short arc knee extensions	8 × 10 to 10 lbs	−30 to 0°
3. Full ROM PRE	4–8 × 10	90° to 0°

*Range of Motion
†Peripheral nerve facilitation

or surgery, and often exercise alone is sufficient to prevent further problems, particularly in the case of patellofemoral disorders. The patient is taught simultaneous contraction of the quadriceps and hamstrings. This develops strength in both muscle groups without joint motion and can be done in any position of immobilized knee flexion.

To teach quadriceps isometrics, the athlete is positioned on a table or bed, lying or sitting, with the knee extended or partially flexed if more comfortable. The athlete places his hand over the quadriceps muscle and palpates the muscle contraction. Usually, the vastus medialis obliquus is the most neglected and atrophied portion of the quadriceps muscle. The athlete specifically palpates the vastus medialis, feeling for a firm, sustained contraction. The "Rule of Tens" is followed: A 20 second contraction, 10 seconds relaxation, repeated ten times each exercise period, done six to ten times daily. If there is pain and reflex inhibition of the muscles, only a poor contraction is obtained.

In isometric exercises, the "shrug" principle is used. As the athlete contracts the muscle, he feels for the tone that is developed. In the middle of the 10 second contraction he may feel the tone diminish, requiring added contraction to regain a firm, hard muscle. He "shrugs" the muscle to increase the tension.

TABLE 21:7.   Rehabilitation Exercise Programs for Common Knee Problems

Diagnosis	Rehabilitation Areas to Stress	Method	Cybex or Orthotron
Chondromalacia patella Subluxating patella S/p‡ surgery for chronic dislocations or chronic irritative processes	1. Strengthening the quads, particularly VMO*, without putting additional stress on patellofemoral surface 2. Achieve or maintain full ROM† 3. General strengthening of hamstrings, ab- & adductors & lower leg musculature	1. Quad sets, straight lifts, lifts, short arcs with progressive resistance 2. ROM & strengthening of hamstrings, ab- & adductors can be done conventionally	Only for strength testing
Anterior cruciate deficient knees, chronic/acute; s/p casting; s/p reconstruction, intra-articular or extra-articular	1. Achieve full ROM 2. Emphasis is placed on strengthening secondary stabilizers to the anterior cruciate	1. Active ROM exercises 2. Hamstring strength aims to equal quad strength of the nonaffected leg, done with programs of isometrics, isotonic with concentric & eccentric contractions; isokinetics 3. Quad strength to be elevated by use of isometrics at 90°, 60°, 30° & full extension; isotonic resistance done only in 90°–45° flexion	1. For strength 2. For hamstring strengthening 3. For quad strengthening 90°–45° only
Medial collateral ligament sprains, chronic/acute, s/p reconstruction; s/p immobilization	1. Special emphasis should be placed on strengthening quads & adductors 2. General ROM 3. General strengthening of hamstrings, adductors & lower leg musculature	1. Achieve or maintain full ROM 2. Quad sets 3. Straight leg lifts with progressive resistance in hip flexion and adduction 4. Isotonics for quads & hamstrings 5. Isokinetics for quads & hamstrings	For testing & workouts

*vastus medialis obliquus muscle
†range of motion
‡status/post

This maintains a near maximal contraction for a full 10 seconds.

Hamstring contractions can be done sitting, standing or lying (prone or supine). The knee is placed in some degree of flexion to obtain a firm hamstring contraction. The therapist or trainer, a fixed object (table, wall, chair or the patient's cast) or simply co-contraction of the quadriceps muscle offers resistance. Other isometric exercises added to the program include hip adductor and adductor and flexion isometrics. Ankle extensor and flexor isometrics may also be done.

Straight leg raises are an important adjunct to isometrics. The patient lies supine on the table. First, he does a maximal isometric quadriceps contraction, then lifts the leg off the table to a height of one to two feet. The athlete "shrugs" the quadriceps during the leg lift to further increase muscle tension. The extremity is held with the knee extended for five seconds, then slowly lowered while the quadriceps shrug is maintained. Full extension (no lag) must be maintained for complete contraction of the quadriceps muscle. If 10 to 15 straight leg raises can be completed with no extensor lag, then weights may be placed at the knee or ankle.

Terminal extensions are another method for early quadriceps rehabilitation. A rolled towel is placed under the knee to give 5° to 10° of knee flexion. The athlete then extends the knee straight and holds to a count of 10. This may also be done with ankle weights. If terminal extension is painful or if the patient cannot lock the knee in extension, eccentric exercises with the leg over the side of the table may be prescribed. With the knee in full extension, a maximum isometric contraction is performed. The athlete gradually allows knee flexion. The trainer may assist the exercise, or ankle weights may be used. Terminal extensions, whether in a concentric or eccentric mode, provide some protection of the patellar surface as the joint is not taken into full flexion.

Lateral step-ups can also be used if terminal extensions are painful. The athlete stands beside a step usually 4 to 6 inches in height (low enough to keep the knee from flexing beyond 20° to 30°). He then steps up sideways and fully extends his knee, progressing to a toe raise. In coming down, the knee is slowly flexed with the body weight over the knee until the opposite foot reaches the ground. This exercises the hip, knee and ankle muscles, using body weight. It is a very effective exercise, yet simple and easy to do, requiring no fancy equipment.

As the situation permits and strength improves the patient can progress to heavier weights and more sophisticated exercise equipment. The previously described exercises may be done at home. However, use of equipment requires trainer supervision. Advancement to the exercise machines begins when the patient is able to do exercises with 10 pounds of ankle weights. The first weight setting on many machines is around 10 pounds and thus the exercise program progresses smoothly. The patellofemoral joint is protected, if required, by blocking the machines to work only in a 0° to 30° extension range for quadriceps exercises. For hamstring exercises no restriction of motion is necessary since the patellofemoral joint is not loaded.

Many techniques are cited for obtaining strength (Table 21:7). Whatever method is used the basic principle remains: the more de-

mand placed on the muscle, the greater the resultant strength. There are many methods for progressively increasing the demand on the muscle, some by daily methods, some weekly. All may be termed progressive resistance exercises (PRE). Suffice it to say that some guidelines and goals must be set for every exercise period to see improvement.

As the PRE program begins to improve strength, attention can be directed to developing power, endurance, speed, agility, flexibility and coordination (Table 21:8). Power is developed by doing the same amount of work faster, or more work at the same speed. This is controlled by putting a limit on the time allowed for one exercise period and requiring the patient to complete his total exercise program in that allotted time. Endurance is gained by exercising the muscle to fatigue with low weights and multiple repetitions. For the knee, this can be done by cycling or by careful use of isokinetics. Too much isokinetic resistance causes thrusting and injurious forces on the patella surface or in healing ligaments. Exercising to fatigue (thigh burn) encourages endurance. Cardiovascular endurance for general body conditioning can be maintained by swimming, or a running program in the swimming pool. Exercise in the pool is an excellent way to provide low forces upon the joint by using the buoyancy of water to maintain balance and also to provide mild resistance to knee motion. Cycling may also be started, as long as the seat of the cycle is raised to a high level, decreasing the amount of flexion at the knee during the pedaling motion. Running activities or individual sports activities are resumed gradually. The running program starts with straight ahead running only. This builds up to figure-of-eight drills and faster type running drills over weeks to months. Speed, agility and coordination are developed by specific skill drills relative to the individual's chosen sport in the latter phases of rehabilitation.

Flexibility is an important aspect of knee rehabilitation. Flexibility exercises are begun early in rehabilitation as the range of motion improves. A good flexibility program includes

TABLE 21:8. Progression of Activity (Endurance)*

Phase I	4 inch step-ups daily	walk 30 min M, W, F	swim 30 min T, Th, Sa	
Phase II	8 inch step-ups daily	rapid walk 30 min M, Th	swim 30 min T, Sa	bike 30 min W, F (when 90° + ROM attained at the knee)
Phase III	12 inch step-ups daily	walk/jog 30 min M, Th	swim 30 min T, Sa	bike 30 min W, F
Phase IV	18 inch step-ups daily	jog 30 min M, W, F	swim 30 min T, Th, Sa	bike 30 min T, Th, Sa	quads PRE at 30 lbs × 10 reps
Phase V	18 inch step-ups daily	full speed sprints 30 min, M, W, F	swim 30 min T, Th, Sa	bike 30 min T, Th, Sa
Phase VI	18 inch step-ups daily	full speed sprints, cutting			quads PRE at 45 lbs × 10 reps
Phase VII	return to competition			

Criteria for Return to Activity After Lower Extremity Injury

Full, pain-free ROM	Running tests without limp
Strength & power equal to uninjured side (80% + may be used in season)	Full speed/straight ahead at preinjury times
	Full speed cutting left & right
Endurance equal to uninjured side	Full speed crossover or carioca
Cardiovascular endurance complete	Able to control any instability
Cerebromuscular rehabilitation complete	No effusion or swelling
	Physician, trainer and athlete agree on return to activity

*In progression of activity, all exercise should be pain-free, without a limp. In patellofemoral problems, eliminate step-ups over 8 inches.

the back, hip, knee and ankle. The safest method is a slow, constant stretching at extremes of motion. Do not use a bouncing technique since it may produce small tears in a tight muscle. It also stimulates firing of the muscle spindles thereby increasing muscle tension. This is the opposite of what is desired, namely, to stretch out the passive element in muscles. Flexibility programs should also be done before and after exercise periods.

Included in the flexibility program are active and passive range of motion. In the early phases of knee rehabilitation, pain and joint stiffness limit the range of motion. Mobilization of the patella is important to achieve complete range of motion. Active range of motion

in which the patient flexes and extends the knee under his own power is the safest. In passive range of motion great care must be taken to avoid manually forcing the knee and causing damage. To perform passive motion, the patient sits on the edge of the table and, with support from his good leg, gradually flexes the knee. This should be done without pain. The trainer may assist passive range of motion, but only with gentle pressure, not pushing. As the range of motion and strength increase and as pain decreases, the PRE program is advanced to exercises performed through a full range of knee motion.

As strength increases and enough time has elapsed for adequate tissue healing, the patient is returned to activity. To aid in making this decision strength and power can be measured isotonically, isokinetically or isometrically (manual muscle test). A strength of 80% to 85% of the uninjured knee is necessary before resuming activity that involves running. Hamstring strength should be 60% of the quadriceps muscles, except in the case of anterior cruciate ligament injuries, when the quadriceps and hamstring strength levels should be equally balanced.

The final stage of rehabilitation is often termed the "return to activity and maintenance stage." There can be no pain, swelling or subjective knee instability. The return to activity is gradual and the athlete must continue to build strength and endurance. Muscles may function adequately for the first 15 minutes or so in practice, then fatigue may set in due to loss of endurance. If the athlete continues to practice, the risk of a repeat injury is markedly increased. Muscle strength and endurance should at least be 80% to 85% of the opposite, normal extremity before any strenuous activity. Skill and running drills and practice situations involving sudden turning or twisting are gradually resumed over weeks to months, depending on the specific knee injury or condition. Agility and proper neuromuscular coordination takes time to build. These qualities must be finely developed, since they ultimately provide dynamic stability to the knee joint. To function athletically or in routine daily activities, knee strength must be maintained. This can be done with exercise periods two to three times per week. Finer skill drills, endurance drills, coordination and agility drills are tailored to the individual.

The Lower Leg

22

ANATOMY

The leg is the lower extremity between the knee and the ankle and includes the tibia, fibula and surrounding soft tissues. The tibia is the second largest bone in the body. It is slightly cup-shaped at its proximal end and is generally cylindrical through most of its shaft (Fig. 22:1). At the distal end it widens to include the ankle mortise. Posteriorly and laterally, it is covered by musculature. Anteriorly, the tibia is subcutaneous through most of its length and is vulnerable to direct impact. It articulates with the distal femur proximally and the talus and fibula distally.

The fibula is a long slender bone lying lateral to the tibia. It forms an arthrodial joint proximally and a syndesmosis distally with the tibia. A nonweight-bearing bone, it serves primarily for muscle attachments. It is also the lateral buttress of the ankle joint. The tibia and fibula are connected by a thick interosseous membrane whose fibers course distally and laterally. This membrane dissipates the forces of weight bearing to the tibia and divides the leg into compartments.

The muscles of the leg are divided into three distinct compartments and separated by thick fascial planes (Fig. 22:2). The anterior compartment contains the anterior tibial, extensor hallucis longus and extensor muscles to the toes, as well as the deep peroneal nerve. The posterior compartment contains the gastrocnemius, soleus, posterior tibial, flexor digitorum longus and flexor hallucis muscles. The peroneal compartment on the lateral aspect of the leg contains the peroneus longus and brevis muscles, which evert the ankle, and the superficial peroneal nerve. The posterior compartment muscles are innervated by the tibial nerve, while the anterior and lateral compartments are innervated by the peroneal nerve.

SOFT TISSUE INJURIES

The anterior aspect of the leg is a common site for direct trauma. When the blow occurs over the anterior lateral aspect of the leg, it may cause an anterior compartment syndrome discussed below. Large hematomas often result and may be painful and difficult to heal. Soft tissue wounds in this area very often are rag-

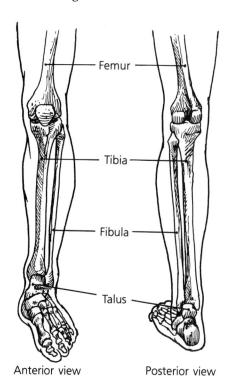

Femur

Tibia

Fibula

Talus

Anterior view   Posterior view

FIGURE 22:1. Leg portion of lower extremity

ged and dirty, usually as a result of cleats or spikes. Because the blood supply to the wound frequently is poor, the wound may be indolent in healing and break down with repeated trauma. Athletes involved in sports where they are likely to injure their shins, e.g., football and soccer, should protect their shins with pads as much as possible.

Treatment for an acute anterior hematoma consists of ice, elevation and compressive dressing. After several days, if the hematoma becomes cystic, it is frequently necessary to open the central portion of the hematoma through a small incision and manually express the old blood clot. This results in more rapid healing and quicker return to activities.

Physical Examination

Most often the overuse syndromes of the leg occur in distance runners. All of these problems result from accumulative impact loading of the lower extremity. The person treating these problems should be familiar with the language of the runner to take an adequate history and physical examination. Up to two thirds of all problems associated with overuse syndromes are related to the training program rather than to abnormal biomechanics. Training errors include excessive mileage, intense workouts, rapid changes in training routines (such as going from cross country to interval workouts), hill running and hard surfaces. An adequate history frequently discloses the cause of the problem and helps in treatment.

Physical examination should include complete evaluation of the lower extremities. A leg length discrepancy should in particular be noted, since this is frequently associated with overuse syndromes, the longer leg usually being injured. Other subtle anatomic abnormalities that may lead to overuse syndromes are femoral anteversion, with excessive internal rotation of the hips and little external rotation; tight hamstrings; genu varum or valgum; excessive Q angles of the patella; patella alta; tibia varum (bow legs); functional shortening

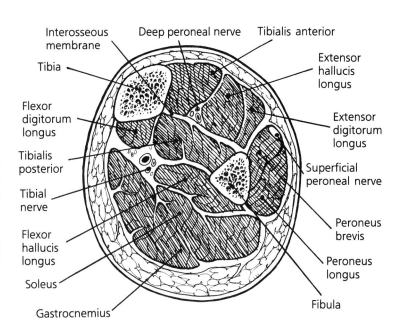

FIGURE 22:2. Three distinct compartments of leg muscles are separated by thick fascial planes.

of the gastronemius-soleus group; and functionally pronated feet.

In examining the runner, note the alignment of the leg to the heel and the heel to the forefoot. Functionally the foot should be positioned so that, with weight bearing, the vertical axis of the heel is parallel to the longitudinal axis of the distal tibia. Likewise, the forefoot should be perpendicular to the vertical axis of the heel. Deviation from normal alignment usually causes compensatory motion through the subtalar joint. These compensatory motions place additional stress on the joints, ligaments and musculotendinous units of the lower extremity resulting in overuse problems.

The most common compensatory movement is excessive and prolonged pronation of the foot during the stance phase of running. This most frequently occurs with mild tibial varum, heel varus and tight gastrocnemius-soleus muscles. Prolonged pronation creates internal tibial torsion, which puts excessive stress on the posterior tibial muscles and the structures around the knee. Treatment may include changing the individual training program, reducing mileage and changing surfaces and/or shoes.

Anatomic abnormalities from abnormal leg to foot alignment usually require a functional orthosis, which is a custom-made arch support. These devices are best fitted by individuals familiar with analysis of leg-heel-forefoot problems, proper casting technique and fabrications. Oral anti-inflammatory drugs, particuarly salicylates, can help treat most of the musculotendinous problems of the leg. Surgery and steroid injections are seldom used.

OVERUSE SYNDROMES

The leg is subject to a number of overuse syndromes, particularly in the jogger and distance runner. The term ''shin splints'' has long been used to describe any sort of leg pain associated with running. This is a wastebasket term that does not identify the specific pathology. If used, it should be reserved for posterior tibial tendonitis or anterior tibial tendonitis.

The overuse syndromes generally present as leg pain without history of a specific injury. They may occur in the novice runner or the well-conditioned athlete. Their common denominator is that they are all associated with exercise. The overuse syndromes include acute muscle cramps; tenosynovitis of the anterior tibial, flexor hallucis longus, posterior tibial or Achilles tendons; periostitis of the tibia; stress fractures of the fibula or tibia; rupture of the Achilles or ''plantaris syndrome'' (tear of the musculotendinous junction of the medial head of the gastrocnemius); or acute anterior or peroneal compartment syndromes.

Muscle Cramps

The simplest and most common overuse syndrome affecting the leg is muscle cramping in the gastrocnemius-soleus group. An acute spasm in the muscle may occur during the late stages of prolonged physical exertion or during the night after a day of strenuous activity. The precise cause of the cramp is unknown. It may be due to electrolyte imbalance or dehydration, or to simple muscle fatigue. Some persons are predisposed to cramps and get them regularly with any physical exertion. Acute cramps are treated with ice packs to numb the muscle, massage and gradual stretching. Preventive measures include a regular stretching program of the gastrocnemius-soleus complex with a slant board and adequate fluid and electrolyte intake during prolonged physical activity.

Anterior Compartment Syndrome

The anterior compartment contains the anterior tibial, extensor hallucis longus and extensor muscles to the foot, as well as the superficial branch of the peroneal nerve and the anterior tibial artery. Because the muscles are encased in a compartment bounded by the tibia and fibula and tough interosseous membrane medially and laterally, and a tough fibrous fascia sheath anteriorly, they are vulnerable to increases in tissue pressure. In the anterior compartment syndrome soft tissue pressure is increased to the point of jeopardizing the viability of the muscles and nerves. The syndrome results most commonly from a direct blow, such as a kick in soccer. It may develop insidiously, however, through minor trauma such as running or simply marching. Classically, the individual sustains a direct blow to the anterior lateral side of the leg resulting in hematoma. The pain progresses and eventually leads to decreased sensation over the superficial peroneal distribution of the foot, and then to total foot drop, with no active eversion or dorsiflexion of toes and foot as the muscles in the compartment become paralyzed. Less frequently, the athlete complains of intermittent claudication after exercise for a period of time, sometimes for several months, before seeking treatment.

The clinical features include a firm, sometimes stony-hard, induration over the anterior compartment of the leg and exquisite tenderness to palpation or to plantar flexion of the ankle. In the late stages, sensation over the dorsum of the foot decreases. In the end stage, there is total foot drop.

When an athlete presents with severe pain and swelling in the anterior compartment area, he must be watched carefully, preferably by someone skilled in managing the problem. If the foot becomes numb, surgical decompression of the leg through fasciotomy of the entire length of the compartment is indicated. This is a true surgical emergency. Once signs of paralysis develop, the muscles involved seldom recover completely. This is one of the few conditions in which watchful observation or continued conservative treatment has no place.

A less common but related condition is the acute peroneal compartment syndrome. This is essentially the same pathologic condition localized to the peroneal musculature on the lateral aspect of the leg. The treatment is the same.

The amount of pressure required to produce a compartmental syndrome depends on a number of factors, including the duration of pressure elevation, the metabolic rate of the tissues, local blood pressure and vascular tone. Functional abnormalities of the nerve are produced within 30 minutes after onset of ischemia, and irreversible loss may occur after 12 to 24 hours. Compartmental syndromes lasting longer than 12 hours are likely to produce chronic functional abnormalities, such as contractures, sensory aberrations and motor weakness. Remember that palpable pulses in the foot are lost late in the syndrome, and occasionally not at all. The patient with palpable pulses can still suffer irreversible tissue damage. It is imperative that the compartmental syndromes be diagnosed as early as possible and fasciotomies performed without undue delay.

The one factor present in any compartment syndrome is increased tissue pressure. The normal tissue pressure is approximately 0 mm of mercury (mm Hg). Ischemia may begin at tissue pressures 10 to 30 mm Hg less than the individual's diastolic pressure.

Posterior Tibial Syndrome

In the posterior tibial syndrome pain occurs along the medial border of the tibia, usually in the distal one third, associated with running. Characteristically, the pain is severe as the individual warms up or begins running, then disappears after a short time, only to recur once activity stops. The condition occurs primarily in the novice runner. When seen in well-conditioned athletes, it is usually secondary to some mechanical abnormality, such as prolonged pronation of the foot during the stance phase of running.

Physical examination reveals a tenderness of the posterior tibial musculature where it attaches along the posterior medial border of the tibia (Fig. 22:3). The tenderness may be confined to a small area in the distal one third of the tibia, or extend through the length of the muscle. Opinions differ regarding the pathology of this condition. Some feel it is actually a periostitis of the tibia caused from pull of the muscles. Others feel it is a pressure phenomenon much like the anterior compartment syn-

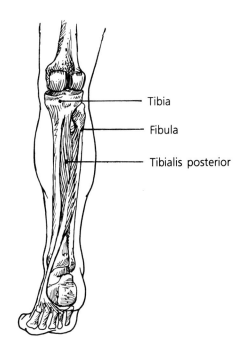

FIGURE 22:3. Posterior tibial musculature

drome where muscles are expanding within a closed compartment.

Differentiating the posterior tibial syndrome from an early stress fracture involving the tibia is sometimes difficult; both may present as pain localized along the posterior medial border of the tibia associated with some bony tenderness. A stress fracture, however, usually leads to some periosteal reaction as it heals, evident on x-rays several weeks after symptoms have begun.

Treatment of the posterior tibial syndrome consists of decreasing the individual's mileage, proper foot alignment and changing surfaces and, possibly, shoes. Anti-inflammatory drugs, such as aspirin in therapeutic doses, usually relieve symptoms. Ice packs or cold water whirlpool to the legs immediately after running and compressive dressings occasionally help. Rehabilitation includes stretching exercises both before and after running, particularly for the gastrocnemius-soleus group, and strengthening of the posterior and anterior tibial muscles through progressive resistance exercise. The posterior tibial syndrome usually subsides with this conservative program as the athlete becomes better conditioned. Any biomechanical abnormalities of foot strike should be corrected with functional orthoses.

Rarely a chronic posterior tibial syndrome is unresponsive to any conservative program, even prolonged rest. Surgical intervention may then be necessary. A fasciotomy of the overlying fascia is performed through a small incision along the medial border of the tibia.

Achilles Tendonitis

Repetitive overextension or overuse of the Achilles tendon, such as jumping in basketball or in distance running, may cause the overlying sheath to become inflamed and thickened. This results in chronic pain and tightness over the Achilles tendon. The condition may be chronic and incapacitating, particularly to the competitive athlete.

Achilles tendonitis usually comes on insidiously from a change in training, such as hill running or increasing mileage too rapidly. The predisposing problem in almost all cases is excessively tight gastrocnemius-soleus muscles, but tibia varus, cavus foot, and heel and forefoot varus deformities may also be predisposing factors. Symptoms include pain both during and after running and with any stretching of the tendon. Examination reveals either diffuse or localized swelling and tenderness to palpation of the tendon. In chronic tendonitis a nodule composed of mucoid degeneration may form inside the tendon. Occasionally motion of the ankle produces crepitus, indicating friction between the tendon and its overlying sheath.

Treatment includes rest until acute inflammation subsides, ice to the affected area and oral nonsteroidal anti-inflammatory drugs. A ½ to ¾ inch heel lift should be inserted into shoes to decrease tension on the tendon. Occasionally orthoses are required to correct biomechanical abnormalities of foot strike, such as with pronated feet. Active stretching and strengthening of the gastrocnemius-soleus muscles begin after acute symptoms subside.

Occasionally the condition persists for a long time and does not respond to conservative measures. The underlying problem in these cases may be a partial tear deep in the Achilles tendon itself, usually as a result of pre-existing degenerative changes within the tendon. Surgery may then be necessary. The overlying tendon sheath, which is usually thickened, fibrotic and constricting the tendon itself, is stripped. If there is evidence of a partial tear, the degenerative area is excised and the tendon repaired. After a postoperative period of rest, the athlete begins gradual stretching exercises. He should also do progressive resistance exercise for the calf muscle, which frequently atrophies after surgery. When the athlete begins running he should use a heel lift for several months, along with well padded running shoes. Patients who have only the Achilles sheath stripped and who show no evidence of any tear within the tendon can usually start running within three to six weeks after surgery. Those with partial tears require longer healing times. Rehabilitation with this injury is therefore slower and more prolonged than in a simple case of tendon sheath excision.

Achilles Tendon Rupture

Acute rupture of the tendon usually occurs 1 or 2 inches above the insertion of the tendon on the calcaneus. The athlete feels a sudden tearing sensation and severe pain, always with sudden loss of function and inability to stand on the toes. Active plantar flexion is weakened, but may still be present because of action in the posterior tibial and flexor hallucis longus muscles. Achilles tendon rupture is disabling and an orthopedist should see the injured athlete as soon as possible.

Physical examination of complete tears reveals swelling and ecchymosis in the posterior aspect of the leg and heel. There is frequently a palpable gap between the tendon ends, and the patient has no active plantar flexion.

A simple test to determine whether the gastrocnemius-soleus complex is intact is the Thompson test (Fig. 22:4). The individual kneels in a chair with his feet hanging free. Squeeze the calf muscle between your fingertips. If there is continuity between the gastrocnemius-soleus muscles and the Achilles tendon, there will be plantar flexion of the foot. Lack of such plantar flexion indicates rupture of the tendon mechanism.

While conservative management of complete Achilles tendon ruptures is sometimes advocated, in the athlete surgical repair produces better results. If an orthopedic surgeon is not readily available, first aid measures are to splint the lower leg and foot in a posterior splint with a compressive dressing with the foot in relaxed plantar flexion.

Partial Achilles tendon ruptures are more difficult to diagnose. The symptoms may be insidious and associated only with activity. A partial rupture should be considered in anybody over the age of 30 with symptoms of chronic Achilles tendonitis. Partial ruptures may be treated conservatively with a long leg cast for three to four weeks followed by a heel lift for several months.

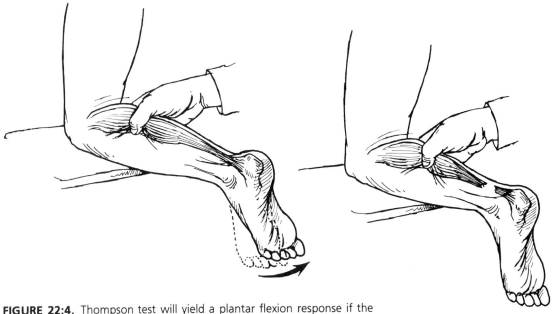

FIGURE 22:4. Thompson test will yield a plantar flexion response if the gastrocnemius-soleus complex is intact. Lack of this response indicates a rupture.

Muscle Strains

The most commonly strained muscle in the leg is the medial head of the gastrocnemius. Most of these cases used to be called the ruptured plantaris syndrome. It is so characteristic in the middle-aged tennis player that in some circles it is called "tennis leg." The symptoms are classic. There is a sudden, painful snapping or tearing sensation in the calf when the plantar flexed foot is suddenly dorsiflexed, usually with the knee in extension. It almost always occurs in active athletes beyond the age of 40. The individual is unable to continue playing, and subsequently marked swelling and ecchymosis of the leg extends down into the ankle and foot. Examination immediately after injury frequently reveals a palpable defect at the musculotendinous junction of the medial head of the gastrocnemius. By the time the athlete has reached a physician, sometimes a day or two later, edema and hematoma may mask this defect.

As in other muscle tears, degrees of injury may vary. Occasionally, swelling is minimal and symptoms subside rapidly. In other cases, swelling is massive and the individual is totally incapacitated for an extended period of time.

Most injuries are first- or second-degree strains and can be managed by elevation of the heel, with gradual active stretching and progressive exercise as tolerated. Some physicians advocate surgical repair of the severe third-degree tear of the muscle or if the individual is unable to sustain his body weight on his tiptoes. Others prefer treatment with plaster with the foot plantar flexed approximately 50° to 60°, and the ankle plantar flexed 15°, for three to four weeks. The muscles should be protected with a heel lift for several months after the patient resumes athletic activities.

Plantaris Muscle Rupture

The small, ribbon-like plantaris muscle originates over the posterior lateral aspect of the knee joint and then curves medially and distally between the two heads of the gastrocnemius to a very small, ribbon-like tendon that inserts along the medial aspect of the calcaneus. It has long been thought the culprit when older people feel pain in calf muscles during strenuous activities. Complete rupture of the plantaris muscle tendon complex has not been documented anatomically, however, and most "plantaris" muscle ruptures are probably tears of the medial head of the gastrocnemius muscle. Occasionally, individuals feel a sharp or tearing pain in the upper midcalf but have little swelling or tenderness. This may be a tear of the plantaris. Since it is a very small muscle with little vascularization, substantial ecchymosis or swelling is unlikely. Treatment consists of symptomatic relief, including crutches, rest, ice, and heel lift. Activities may be resumed as symptoms subside.

Stress Fracture

The tibia and fibula frequently sustain stress fractures as a result of overuse. Stress fractures are most common in distance runners but are also seen in basketball and soccer players. They are not frequent in football.

A stress fracture is a partial or complete disruption of bone produced by rhythmic, repeated, subthreshold stress. Stress fractures do not occur at any particular instant in time but are rather the end product of an adaptive process in which the bone attempts to rapidly remodel itself along the lines of increased stress. A repetitive stress leads to muscle fatigue in the leg. The resulting loss of shock absorbing ability increases stress of the bone and periostitis. The pain produced causes involuntary disuse of the extremity that leads to further muscle atrophy and the process compounds itself. The final result—if stress is not relieved—is fracture of the bone.

Symptoms usually begin with mild discomfort in the lower shaft of the tibia after activity. Simple rest relieves the symptoms. With continued activity, the pain becomes more persistent and lasts from day to day. Ultimately, the pain is severe enough to prohibit activity.

Diagnosis is by clinical examination, which shows localized tenderness to palpation directly over the fracture site. X-ray films frequently are negative early but reveal periosteal reaction or cortical thickening two to four weeks after the onset of symptoms. A bone scan will be positive before x-ray changes and is occasionally needed for diagnosis.

Stress fractures may occur at any level of conditioning, but are more common in women. The usual site is the proximal one third of the tibia. Stress fractures of the fibula occur also, secondary to chronic muscle tension.

Treatment of the tibia stress syndrome or fracture includes rest, changing the training program if indicated and correcting all mechanical abnormalities that may lead to the fracture. The stressful situation, such as running, must be eliminated, but total rest is not necessary. The athlete may continue cardiovascular activities by substituting swimming or cycling. Specific weight training for overall body conditioning and the lower extremity, in particular, should be encouraged within the patient's pain tolerance. It is seldom necessary to keep the patient nonweight bearing or immobilized in plaster. Tibial stress fractures take four to eight weeks to heal, while fibular stress fractures take three to six weeks to heal.

FRACTURES

The tibia and/or fibula may be fractured acutely during collision sports by direct impact, or by twisting or torque forces to the body when the foot is planted. The latter frequently results in long, oblique, spiral fractures of the distal tibia with fracture of the proximal fibula. Tibia fractures are serious injuries to athletes. Deformity, immediate loss of function, pain and motion at the fracture site make the diagnosis easy.

Tibia fractures should be splinted, preferably with an air splint to prevent excessive swelling, and the athlete promptly transported to the nearest medical facility. Fractures of the fibular shaft may occasionally be overlooked, usually passed off as pain from a simple bruise. Fractures of the distal fibula usually require a short leg cast for four to six weeks. Fracture of the midshaft and upper portions of the fibula may be treated with a simple compressive dressing and crutches.

The Ankle

23

The high incidence of ankle injuries accounts for 20% to 25% of all time-loss injuries in every running or jumping sport. The mechanisms of injury and treatment are essentially similar for all sports.

ANATOMY

The ankle joint is formed by three bones: the tibia, fibula and talus. The dome of the talus fits into the mortise formed by the tibia and fibula. The medial and lateral malleoli project downward to articulate with the sides of the talus. The lateral malleolus projects down to the level of the subtalar joint, considerably farther than the medial malleolus, and thus provides greater bony stability for the lateral side of the ankle joint (Fig. 23:1). The ankle joint moves, essentially, in one plane, up and down, about a central axis of rotation. This is associated with a forward and backward movement simultaneously. The talus is wider anteriorly than posteriorly because the lateral wall slopes outward instead of being parallel to the medial wall. The tibial portion of the joint is also wider anteriorly than posteriorly. When the foot is dorsiflexed, the wider anterior portion of the talus is brought into contact with the narrower portion between the malleoli and, therefore, is gripped more tightly. As the ankle goes into plantar flexion, the narrower posterior portion of the talus is brought into contact with the wider anterior portion of the tibia. This permits a small amount of free play in the ankle joint as the wedge effect noted in dorsiflexion is lost. The bony arrangement also helps to promote anterior stability of the ankle joint. As the tibia is driven forward on the plantar-flexed talus, the narrower part of the tibia impinges on the widened anterior portion of the talus, blocking forward dislocation of the tibia on the talus.

The relationship of the tibia, talus and fibula is maintained by three groups of ligaments: the deltoid ligament medially, the lateral collateral ligament and the tibiofibular syndesmosis. The deltoid, the strongest of the three ligaments, is a broad, triangular or delta-shaped band with four parts, as defined by their bony insertions on the navicula, talus and calcaneus. It is functionally divided into a deep and superficial portion. The deep portion attaches to the talus and is horizontal and, therefore, resists lateral displacement of the talus. In coronal sections through the ankle joint, the

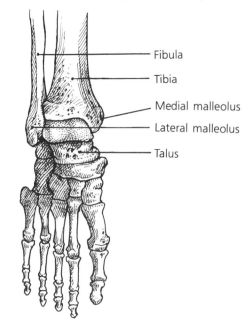

FIGURE 23:1. Bones of the ankle joint

314

vertical position of the superficial portion and the horizontal position of the deep portion are clearly seen. Also, the deep portion is placed posteriorly.

The lateral collateral ligament of the ankle is T-shaped and consists of three distinct parts. The posterior talofibular ligament arises from the posterior portion of the tip of the fibula and runs backward and slightly downward to attach to the lateral tubercle of the posterior process of the talus. This is the strongest of the three ligaments and helps to resist forward dislocation of the leg on the foot. The calcaneofibular ligament is the largest of the three and passes inferiorly in a posterior direction to insert on the lateral surface of the calcaneus. When the foot is in plantar flexion, the calcaneofibular ligament is almost perpendicular to the axis of the fibula. This is extracapsular, but may be associated with the peroneal tendon sheath. On its lateral and dorsal aspects, the calcaneofibular ligament is covered for almost its entire length with the thin inner wall of the tendon sheath. This ligament is completely relaxed when the foot is in a normal standing position. It does not become taut until the calcaneus makes a strong supination movement. The anterior talofibular ligament arises from the anterior border of the lateral malleolus and passes forward and somewhat medially to attach to the neck of the talus. Its direction corresponds to the longitudinal axis of the foot and is taut in all positions of flexion.

The ligaments of the tibiofibular syndesmosis maintain the relationship of the distal tibia and fibula. They consist of the anterior and posterior tibiofibular ligaments and the interosseous membrane. The anterior and posterior tibiofibular ligaments arise respectively from the anterior and posterior caliculi on the lateral side of the tibia. These ligaments actually hold the fibula snug in a groove on the tibia, where the fibula rotates about its vertical axis as well as rises and falls with dorsi- and plantar flexion of the ankle. There is 6° medial rotation of the fibula with dorsiflexion and 6° lateral rotation with plantar flexion. These two ligaments blend into the inter-

osseous membrane 2 to 3 cm above the ankle joint (Fig. 23:2).

Important musculotendinous structures relate to the deltoid and lateral collateral ligaments. Understanding the functions of these muscles is important in preventing ankle injuries as well as rehabilitating the athlete following an ankle injury. The medial stabilizers of the ankle are the tibialis anterior, tibialis posterior, flexor digitorum longus and the flexor hallucis longus. The latter three originate from the posterior compartment of the leg and pass posterior and inferior to the medial malleolus. They are important for plantar flexion and supination of the foot. The posterior tibialis tendon is adjacent to the posterior and middle parts of the deltoid ligament. This explains why this tendon is often trapped between the talus and medial malleolus with severe deltoid ruptures. The tibialis anterior arises in the anterior crural compartment of the leg, passes downward and medially to insert on the first cuneiform and base of the first metatarsal. The lateral stabilizers of the ankle are the peroneal muscles that make up the lateral compartment of the leg. The

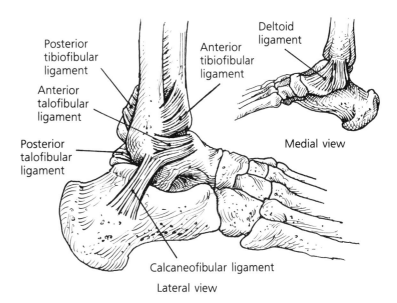

Posterior tibiofibular ligament

Anterior talofibular ligament

Posterior talofibular ligament

Anterior tibiofibular ligament

Deltoid ligament

Medial view

Calcaneofibular ligament

Lateral view

FIGURE 23:2. The anterior and posterior tibiofibular ligaments and the interosseous membrane maintain the relationship of the distal tibia and fibula.

peroneus brevis and longus pass distal and inferior to the lateral malleolus. The brevis inserts on the base of the fifth metatarsal; the longus passes under the cuboid bone in its own groove to insert on the inferior surface of the medial cuneiform and base of the first metatarsal.

As mentioned earlier, the peroneal tendon sheath covers the posterior and lateral portion of the calcaneofibular ligament. When this ligament is ruptured, the overlying inner wall of the peroneal tendon sheath is also torn because it lies adjacent to this ligament. Thus, the peroneal tendon sheath communicates with the ankle joint in this situation. The peroneal tendons are important for pronating and everting the foot. Because of the intricate relationship of these muscles to the stabilizing ligaments of the ankle joint, they are capable of absorbing stress and protecting these ligaments from injury.

MECHANISMS OF INJURY

Injuries to the ankle must be considered in relation to magnitude and direction of forces as applied to the ankle. In sports requiring a cleated shoe, the foot is usually fixed to the ground and the body is rotating and angulating about it. The anatomy and the activity of the running foot are predisposed toward inversion sprains. As mentioned earlier, bony stability is greater laterally than medially, thereby predisposing inversion rather than eversion. Once inversion is initiated, the ankle loses the bony stability of its neutral position. As inversion increases, the medial malleolus may lose its stabilizing function and act as a fulcrum for further inversion. If the everting muscles (peroneals) are not strong enough, the tensile strength of the lateral ligaments may be exceeded, resulting in injury.

The way an athlete uses his ankle may also predispose him to inversion injuries. A cutting or turning maneuver, often the initiating factor in these injuries, involves pushing off to the side from the opposite lead foot. For example, to cut to the left, the direction change

is initiated off the fixed right foot, inverting the ankle and externally rotating and plantar flexing the right foot. Plantar flexion makes the ankle more susceptible to injury because of increased laxity of the joint and the position of the calcaneofibular ligament. As the ankle rotates into more plantar flexion, this ligament goes from a vertical to a horizontal position resulting in less resistance to inversion. The opposite mechanism of injury may occur, although statistically is far less likely. An eversion, external rotation mechanism, can occur when the planted leg receives a lateral blow. This can damage medial structures or rupture the syndesmosis. This same mechanism, however, may result in knee injuries. Another common mechanism of injury is landing on an irregular surface such as another player's foot in basketball or stepping into a hole in a poorly prepared playing field. This usually results in an inversion mechanism.

TYPES OF INJURIES

Since inversion injuries are the most frequent, sprains to the lateral collateral ligament are by far the most common ankle injuries. As a rule, to tear this ligament completely, the fibula must fracture or the anterior tibiofibular ligament must rupture. The same mechanism of inversion and supination can lead to fracture, usually an oblique fracture of the fibular with or without a fracture of the medial malleolus.

The other important mechanism of ankle injury in athletics is pronation and external rotation. This is rarely a pure ligamentous injury, and when it does occur the deltoid and anterior tibiofibular ligaments are torn. Usually, the deltoid ligament rupture is combined with a fracture of the fibula.

CLINICAL EVALUATION

With serious ankle injury, the athlete will say the foot turned under, accompanied by immediate pain and difficulty in bearing weight. Often the injured athlete describes a ''pop'' or ''snap'' or a sensation of giving way.

Initial evaluation reveals localized tenderness over the ligaments involved. Motion may or may not be restricted. The more difficulty the athlete has bearing weight, the more serious his injury. Further participation should be prohibited until a medical evaluation is complete.

At initial evaluation of an acute injury the neurological and vascular function of the extremity must be assessed. Palpate the dorsalis pedis pulse on the dorsum of the foot and the posterior tibial pulse behind the medial malleolus. Evaluation of capillary refill of the toes as well as warmth and color is helpful. Once the neurovascular function is determined to be intact, then transport the athlete to the appropriate facility. If the ankle appears stable, crutches will suffice. However, if there is any question of stability, apply a well padded posterior short leg splint.

Initially a fracture must be differentiated from a sprain. Many fractures about the ankle are obvious, with the exception of the undisplaced spiral fracture of the fibula or the avulsion fracture of the tip of the fibula. Fibular pain with compression or on heel tap often indicates fracture. A fracture of the base of the fifth metatarsal must also be considered. Often careful palpation of these structures helps locate the pathology.

Routine x-ray films of the ankle, including oblique views, can identify fractures. If a fracture of the base of the fifth metatarsal is suspected, then also order x-ray films of the foot.

Sprains must be classified as first-, second- or third-degree before determining treatment and prognosis. A first-degree sprain is a minor ligamentous injury in which the ligament is partially torn and the joint is stable. A second-degree sprain is a more severe injury where the joint remains stable. A third-degree sprain is a ligamentous injury resulting in an unstable joint.

The importance of clinical recognition of the unstable ankle cannot be overemphasized. Physical examination, stress x-rays and arthrography assist in diagnosis. On physical exam, forcefully invert, evert and draw forward the foot to test stability. The most common injury, to the anterior talofibular ligament, results in anterior instability only, demonstrated by a positive anterior drawer test of the ankle (Fig. 23:3). If instability is suspected on clinical exam, repeat stress testing under x-ray. Local anesthesia is needed in acute injuries, as muscle spasm secondary to a painful injury can hide instability. If unsuccessful, a general anesthetic may be necessary. Tilting of the talus within the mortise with supination of the foot is diagnostic of lateral instability. Usually the ankle opens between 5° and 15° on the anteroposterior (AP) view with an isolated tear of the anterior talofibular ligament. However, if the foot is forced forward, the talus will sublux anteriorly (anterior drawer test), as documented on a lateral x-ray film. If, on a straight AP x-ray film, the talus opens 15° to 30° laterally, the diagnosis is rupture of both the anterior talofibular and calcaneofibular ligaments (Fig. 23:4). Gross lateral instability means complete rupture of all three parts of the lateral collateral ligament.

Always suspect an injury to the deltoid ligament with any fracture of the fibula or any pronation mechanism of injury. Again, stress testing can be diagnostic by revealing widening of the medial joint space by x-ray.

Routine plain films including AP, lateral and inversion stress of the ankle are also important. Widening of the distance between the tibia and fibula on the oblique view indicates an injury to the syndesmosis. An avulsion of the very tip of the lateral malleolus is diagnostic of a major injury to the lateral collateral ligament. Osteochondral fractures of the dome of the talus may accompany any injury resulting in instability.

An arthrogram of the ankle offers little information over and above stress x-ray films. It may help localize the specific ligament injured. For instance, if dye escapes from the joint and is seen in the peroneal tendon sheath, there is a tear in the calcaneofibular ligament. Whether this test has true practical value will eventually be determined by further experience and data.

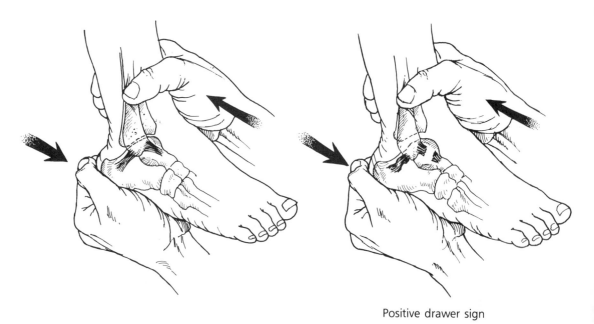

Positive drawer sign

FIGURE 23:3.   Positive anterior drawer test in injury to anterior talo-fibular ligament

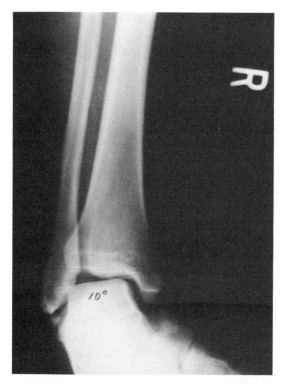 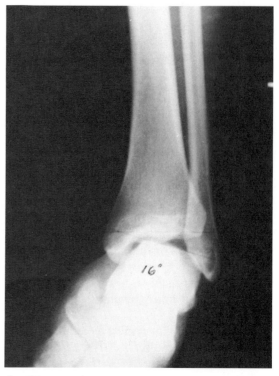

FIGURE 23:4.   Inversion stress film to determine front talar tilts; normal (left) shows 10% talus opening versus abnormal with 16%.

MANAGEMENT PROCEDURES

Once the joint injury has been classified and stability determined, a course of treatment can be outlined and the prognosis established. A first-degree ankle sprain may be treated symptomatically with protective support, non-weight bearing and early rehabilitation. Treatment of second-degree sprains depends on the amount of soft tissue injury and requires various amounts of time for ligament healing, but is basically the same as for a first-degree sprain, only longer. Also, immobilization or splinting is more frequent than with first-degree sprains. The treatment of the unstable third-degree sprain of the lateral collateral ligament is controversial. The choices are a short leg cast for four to six weeks, a cast-brace or a surgical repair. Surgery is considered in displaced intra-articular fractures involving the weight-bearing surface of the joint, or very unstable ankle joints in young competitive athletes. Most authors agree that a torn anterior talofibular ligament with anterior subluxation may be treated conservatively by a cast with the foot at a right angle for four to six weeks or a cast-brace with plantar flexion stop. The literature is confusing concerning treatment of combined tears of the anterior talofibular and calcaneofibular ligaments. This is an ankle sprain that opens 15° to 30° on various stress x-ray films. Acute dislocation of the peroneal tendons is also possible in lateral injuries to the ankle. The mechanism of injury is forceful plantar flexion and valgus of the foot. The groove behind the fibula in which the peroneal tendons slide may be shallow and therefore predisposed to injury. Clinically, the athlete has pain and swelling over the lateral malleolus. The peroneal tendons are usually palpable on the outer aspect of the fibula. Eversion is very painful. Treatment in the athlete frequently requires repair of the torn retinaculum posterior to the fibula along with cast immobilization for six weeks.

To differentiate the spiral fracture and the avulsion fracture of the distal fibula from a sprain is usually possible by careful clinical palpation and localizing the tenderness. An appropriate x-ray film, of course, ultimately confirms the diagnosis.

Severe fracture-dislocations and dislocations of the ankle are usually dramatic events. Fracture-dislocations often occur after a jump, such as in basketball or volleyball. How the athlete lands on his foot determines the type of injury. For instance, landing on an everted foot in plantar flexion can produce an open dislocation of the ankle. The medial malleolus may be exposed through the skin and the foot displaced relative to the lower leg. Immediately remove the shoe and evaluate circulation, sensation and motor function. In an open wound with bone showing, do not attempt closed reduction due to the contamination of the exposed bone. Usually the skin is button-holed around the bone and blocks reduction. Cover this injury with a sterile dressing and apply a well-padded, short leg splint. Transport the patient to the nearest emergency department and notify the team orthopedist immediately. An open wound must be debrided surgically as soon as possible to minimize the chance for infection.

Closed fracture-dislocations of the ankle are usually either bimalleolar fractures or a fibular fracture with a ruptured deltoid ligament (Fig. 23:5). In some instances, these can be severely displaced. As above, the circulation, sensation and motor function of the foot must be assessed immediately. A markedly displaced fracture-dislocation will usually be displaced laterally to the lower leg. This abnormal position can compromise the posterior tibial artery and nerve. In instances of obvious circulatory compromise, flex the knee and apply gentle linear traction to reduce (or replace) the foot on the end of the tibia. However, if the fracture cannot be easily reduced, then splint the ankle in its displaced position, and transport the athlete immediately to an emergency facility. Apply a well-padded, short leg splint (or air splint) before transportation.

Fractures of the ankle are different from sprains in that they all require cast or cast-brace immobilization and may require surgical stabilization. Rehabilitation is more difficult and

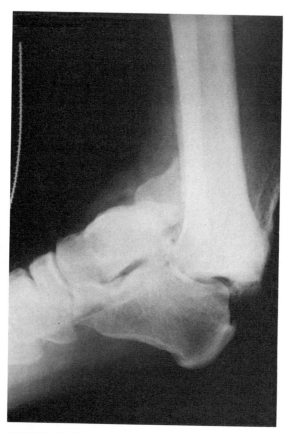

FIGURE 23:5. Radiograph of anterior talar dislocation and distal fibular fracture

prolonged due to the severity of the injury and the muscle atrophy that results from cast immobilization. Rigid internal fixation of these fractures may offer the athlete a shorter period of immobilization and, hence, a faster recovery. The ultimate prognosis in ankle fractures is related to the damage to the articular surface that may not be apparent for some time after the injury.

RECONDITIONING

Rehabilitation of ankle sprains begins almost simultaneously with the onset of treatment. The goal is to obtain a stable, painless, mobile ankle that can undergo the rigors of the athlete's sport. Strengthening of the medial and lateral stabilizers may begin as soon as pain-free exercise is possible. Full weight bearing is not permitted until it can be done without a limp and the athlete has nearly full range of motion without pain. Swimming may begin before weight bearing. Strengthening exercises are initially isometric progressing dynamically as the patient is able to bear weight. Isometric, isotonic, and isokinetic exercises for dorsiflexion, plantar flexion, inversion and eversion exercise the four major muscle groups of the lower leg. Walking is followed by jogging, running, figure-of-eights, and various maneuvers of the sport before return to competition is allowed. Some form of external support, such as taping, an air splint or a cast-brace, is necessary as the athlete with a second- or third-degree sprain returns to running. Taping may be required throughout the remainder of the season to prevent re-injury. Exercises to regain proprioception are also important and can be done on a tilt board or by the athlete's balancing with his eyes closed on the injured leg.

The athlete with recurrent episodes indicating chronic instability should have his ankle taped for all practice sessions and games, and should be on a good ankle conditioning program. If this is not successful, reconstructive surgery should be considered. Rehabilitation following fractures is similar but prolonged relative to the length of immobilization.

The Foot

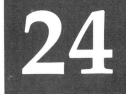

ANATOMY

The bony skeleton of the foot is composed of 26 bones (Fig. 24:1). The talus articulates with the tibia and fibula to make up the ankle joint. Movement at the ankle is basically dorsiflexion and plantar flexion, with some anterior and posterior sliding motion occurring simultaneously. Since the talus is wider in front, the tibiofibular joint spreads with dorsiflexion and narrows with plantar flexion. The inferior surface of the talus articulates with the calcaneus making up the subtalar joint, which contributes greatly to the inversion and eversion foot movements. The head of the talus articulates with the navicular bone on the medial side of the foot and the calcaneus (anterior process) articulates with the cuboid bone on the lateral side of the foot. The combination of movements of these three articulations, talocalcaneal, talonavicular and calcaneocuboid, results in the complex foot movements of eversion and inversion, pronation and supination.

The remaining bones of the foot are the three cuneiforms, five metatarsals and the phalanges, three for each of the lateral four toes and two phalanges for the great toe. The midtarsal joints, navicular-cuneiform and cuneiform-metatarsal, are very stable joints that produce very little movement. The metatarsals and proximal phalanges produce the metatarsophalangeal joints (MP) that are important for push-off, particularly at the first MP joint. The remainder of the toe joints are proximal and distal interphalangeal (IP) joints.

The bones of the foot are arranged structurally to form two arches—the longitudinal arch and the transverse arch. The bones are mortised together to form the architecture of these two arches (Fig. 24:2). The ligaments of the foot provide intrinsic support and the muscles of the leg provide extrinsic support. The longitudinal arch starts at the weight-bearing surface of the calcaneus and ends at the metatarsal heads. It is supported intrinsically by the plantar calcaneonavicular ligament (spring ligament). This ligament supports the head of the talus. The talus is also supported by the plantar fascia, which runs from the calcaneal tuberosity to the phalanges. The plantar fascia acts as a bowstring for the longitudinal arch and supports the muscles on the plantar surface of the foot.

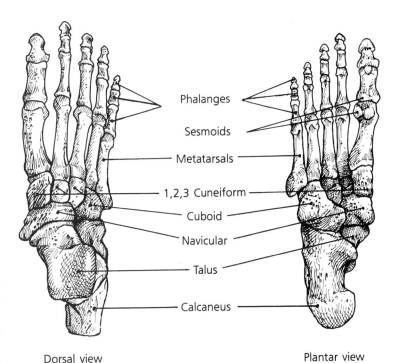

Phalanges

Sesmoids

Metatarsals

1,2,3 Cuneiform

Cuboid

Navicular

Talus

Calcaneus

Dorsal view

Plantar view

FIGURE 24:1. Bony skeleton of the foot

321

The extrinsic support comes from the anterior tibial tendon pulling upon its insertion at the first cuneiform and the posterior tibial tendon and peroneus longus tendon that pass under the foot and create a dynamic sling supporting the longitudinal arch.

The transverse arch is at its highest point, as seen on the frontal plane, at the base of the metatarsals. Its structural support is intrinsic from the mortise effect of the way the bones are put together. There is no transverse arch at the metatarsal heads upon weight bearing, as each of the lateral four metatarsal heads bear one sixth of the body weight and the first metatarsal head (with two sesamoid bones) bears two sixths of the body weight.

The three main muscle groups of the lower leg all insert on the foot, thus controlling the action of the foot. The gastrocnemius soleus, located in the superficial part of the posterior compartment, inserts on the posterior aspect of the calcaneus. The deep portion of the posterior compartment contains three muscles: (1) posterior tibial, (2) flexor digitorum longus, and (3) flexor hallucis longus. The posterior tibial muscle supports the longitudinal arch and inverts the foot. The flexor digitorum longus flexes the lateral four toes and the flexor hallucis longus flexes the great toe.

These three muscles enter the foot through a ligamentous tunnel behind the medial malleolus along with the posterior tibial nerve, artery and vein. The posterior tibial nerve divides into the medial and lateral plantar nerve and supplies sensation to the plantar surface of the foot while innervating the plantar muscles.

The posterior tibial tendon attaches directly on the tuberosity of the navicular bone and indirectly on the plantar surface of the navicular and middle cuneiform bones (see Fig. 24:2). The flexor digitorum longus attaches to the plantar surface of the lateral four toes. The flexor hallucis longus passes between the two sesamoid bones under the first metatarsal head and thus between the two heads of flexor hallucis brevis and inserts on the plantar surface of the distal phalanx of the great toe.

The lateral compartment is composed of two muscles, the peroneus longus and brevis. The longus crosses under the longitudinal arch from lateral to medial and inserts on the plantar surface of the first cuneiform and first metatarsal. The peroneus brevis inserts on the base of the fifth metatarsal. These muscles evert and plantar flex the foot. The anterior compartment consists of (1) the anterior tibialis, which inserts on the medial cuneiform, (2) the extensor digitorum longus and (3) the extensor hallucis longus. This group dorsiflexes the foot and toes. The anterior tibial and extensor hallucis longus muscles are inverters and the extensor digitorum longus is an evertor.

The intrinsic muscles of the foot are primarily related to toe function. There is only one muscle on the dorsum of the foot—the short toe extensor, extensor digitorum brevis. There are 15 small muscles on the plantar surface of the foot arranged in four layers—all related to toe function. They fill in the space between the longitudinal arch and the plantar fascia.

The fat pad is a specialized soft tissue structure designed specifically for weight bearing

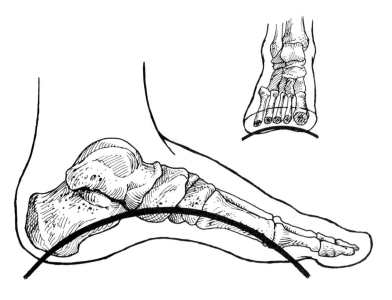

FIGURE 24:2. Longitudinal arch and transverse arch of the foot

and absorbing impact. It consists of specialized fat globules located between the plantar skin and the overlying calcaneus and plantar fascia. These fat globules are contained between vertical fibrous septa. The fatty tissue is packed into multiple fibrous walled compartments that are capable of withstanding the pressure of weight bearing.

BIOMECHANICS

Understanding the normal biomechanics of the running gait and the forces applied to the foot facilitates understanding the mechanism of injury. The normal running gait is divided into a stance, or support, phase and a swing phase (Fig. 24:3). The difference between running and walking is that in the support phase in walking one foot is always on the ground, whereas in running there is an airborne period where neither foot is in contact with the ground. The stance phase begins when the foot strikes the ground. Initial contact is usual-

ly made with the calcaneus, called heel strike. Thus, all the weight-bearing force is absorbed initially by heel contact. The foot then proceeds into midsupport phase. Weight-bearing force passes along the lateral border of the foot to the metatarsal heads. As this occurs, the normal foot is inverted at heel strike and then pronates (rolls inward) as the weight passes from the lateral side of the foot and is spread out along the entire longitudinal arch. This complex series of movements through the subtalar and midtarsal joints absorbs and dissipates the force of heel strike. The foot then progresses from midsupport to toe-off or push-off. The gastrocnemius-soleus muscle group forcefully contracts to assist toe-off as the runner enters the airborne phase (Fig. 24:4).

The trail leg is in swing phase and is just completing follow through as the stance phase leg is in heel strike. The swing phase leg then begins an acceleration phase as the thigh and knee flex and are brought forward. The pelvis rotates around the hip joint of the stance phase

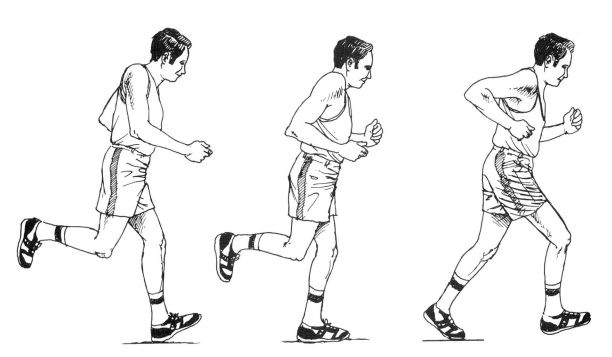

FIGURE 24:3. The three phases of the normal running gait: heel strike, midstance and toe-off

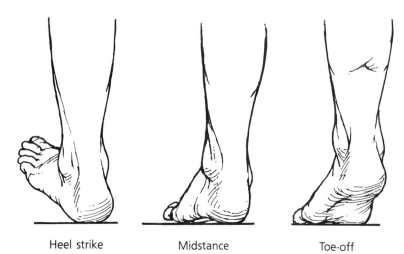

Heel strike   Midstance   Toe-off

FIGURE 24:4. Contraction of gastrocnemius-soleus at toe-off

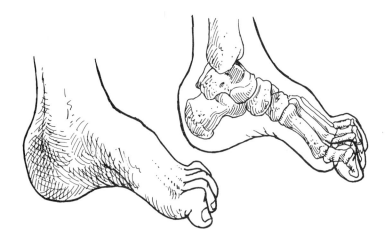

FIGURE 24:5. Cavus foot with elevated longitudinal arch and clawing of the toes

leg. Initially, the pelvis rotates backward (external rotation of the stance phase hip) as the pelvis follows the swing phase leg in follow through. As the swing phase leg comes forward, the pelvis rotates forward with it. Thus in midsupport phase, the center of gravity is directly over the weight-bearing foot and the pelvis is in neutral rotation. The swing phase leg continues forward and begins its deceleration phase as the knee extends and the foot

is preparing for heel strike. At this time, the stance phase leg has completed toe-off and the runner is momentarily airborne.

These complex movements and forces in running explain why some subtle foot deformities and muscle imbalances can cause problems in the foot. The interrelationships between the foot, the knee and the hip in running are extremely complex.

DEFORMITIES

Several foot deformities are sources of potential problems. The cavus foot has an excessively high longitudinal arch. Subtalar motion (inversion and eversion) is frequently restricted, which limits the foot's ability to absorb the forces encountered during heel strike. This deformity may range from just an elevated longitudinal arch to a full blown deformity consisting of a varus heel and clawing of the toes (Fig. 24:5). Athletes with cavus feet frequently complain of plantar fascia pain due to the tripod effect of the deformity and the increased bow-string pull of the fascia. Cavus feet often result in painful callosities on the lateral aspect of the heel, under the metatarsal heads and on the dorsum of the interphalangeal joints if the toes are clawed. An orthosis, a properly placed metatarsal pad, and attention to foot wear may eliminate or prevent symptoms.

The opposite deformity to the cavus foot is the flat foot or pronated foot, in which the longitudinal arch is flattened. The hindfoot may be in valgus. Occasionally, there is an associated accessory navicular bone. In this congenital deformity the ossification center of the navicular tuberosity fails to fuse to the main bone and remains a bony prominence on the medial side of the foot. These are often locally symptomatic and require protection or surgical excision.

Flat feet are classified as flexible or rigid (Fig. 24:6). The flexible flat foot (or pronated foot) is the most common and is usually asymptomatic in the milder forms. Moderate to severe deformities may be symptomatic. Proper attention to foot wear and longitudinal arch supports are helpful. The rigid flat foot is a much more difficult problem and may prohibit such activities as long-distance running. A rigid flat foot is often due to congenital tarsal coalition, although symptoms may be delayed until adolescence or later. The most common tarsal coalitions are talocalcaneal and calcaneonavicular.

Congenital deformities, such as metatarsus varus or valgus, may be present. Metatarsus varus (or adductus) is a deformity of the forefoot in which the forefoot is angulated and rotated medially in relation to the hind foot. Metatarsus valgus (abductus) is the opposite deformity of the forefoot. These deformities may place abnormal stress on the foot, resulting in painful callosities. With these deformities, as with the others, proper foot wear and orthoses may prevent problems. The hindfoot may, also, be in varus (angulated medially) or valgus (angulated laterally). These deformities are usually associated with a cavus (heel varus) or flat foot (heel valgus) deformity.

Deformities of the toes are also common. A Morton's foot is characterized by a short first metatarsal, resulting in an imbalance in the transverse metatarsal arch. This interferes with the normal weight-bearing stresses in the forefoot, placing greater stress on the second metatarsal head, often resulting in pain. This often can be controlled by an orthosis in the shoe. Hallux valgus with or without a bunion, a painful developmental deformity in young athletes, is associated with widening between the first and second metatarsals. Pain may be avoided by proper foot wear. Surgical correction may be indicated in severe cases.

Clawing of the toes is hyperextension of the MP joint and flexion of the IP joints, usually resulting from some subtle muscle imbalance in the foot. Painful callosities often develop on the dorsum of the IP joints from pressure against the shoe and under the metatarsal heads where they press against the sole of the shoe. Proper placement of a metatarsal pad can usually control these symptoms. Hammer toe is a deformity of flexion of the distal IP joint, thus putting pressure on the nail and

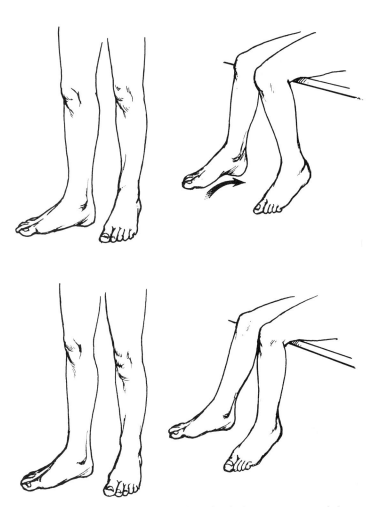

FIGURE 24:6. In a flexible flat foot (top) the transverse arch is present in a nonweight-bearing position. With a rigid flat foot (bottom) there is no change in the flattened longitudinal arch when nonweight-bearing.

end of the toe from contact against the sole of the shoe. These are difficult deformities to control conservatively and may require surgical correction.

A Tailor's bunion is a prominence of the lateral aspect of the fifth metatarsal. Proper foot wear can usually control this deformity.

MECHANISMS AND TYPES OF INJURY

Foot injuries may result from direct trauma during competition or from minor stresses associated with repetitive training. Foot contusions, sprains and fractures are caused frequently by external forces, such as improperly landing from a jump, being stepped on, or striking an object on or near the playing surface. Foot injuries caused by indirect trauma, overuse syndromes, are more difficult to diagnose but equally as disabling as the more obvious traumatic injuries.

Soft Tissue Injuries

A bursa is a soft tissue sac of synovial fluid where tendons slide over bony prominences. External pressure from a poorly fitting shoe may cause inflammation or bursitis, manifested by local pain, swelling and erythema.

The retrocalcaneal bursa, located between the Achilles tendon insertion and the calcaneus and posterior aspect of the talus, is often irritated in athletes. Pain is the presenting symptom and is localized to the soft area just anterior to the Achilles tendon. Pain is usually present with plantar flexion and push-off during gait. The bursitis is often resistant to treatment, which consists of rest from the offending activity, anti-inflammatory medication and occasionally a short leg walking cast for complete rest. At times, a bursitis may develop between the Achilles tendon and the overlying skin. This bursitis is usually related to foot wear and is corrected by shoe modification. With an underlying bony abnormality, such as a bunion, a bursitis may develop over the bony prominence. Again, this is usually due to pressure from the shoe against the abnormal bony prominence. Shoe modification or corrective surgery may be necessary.

A callosity is an area of thickened skin overlying a bony prominence. The presence of a callus usually indicates abnormal pressure between the shoe and the bony protrusion, as seen over the proximal IP joints of claw toes. In this condition, the MP joint is hyperextended, pushing the head of the metatarsal into the sole of the foot. Abnormal pressure can develop under the metatarsal head or at the flexed IP joint of the corresponding toe.

Pain can be often relieved by placing a felt pad in the shoe just proximal to the metatarsal heads, thereby spreading out the pressure and, also, partially correcting the claw toe deformity.

Neuritis, inflammation or irritation of a nerve, can be a troublesome problem for athletes. Morton's neuroma, a common neuritis, is classically characterized by localized pain between the third and fourth metatarsal heads, often radiating into the third and fourth toes, although other interspaces may be involved. The pain is increased by tight shoe wear and is relieved by going barefoot. The medial and lateral plantar nerves converge between the third and fourth toes where the junction becomes enlarged. Tight shoes compress the metatarsal heads against the nerve, producing a painful neuroma. Once the pain starts, it is often difficult to control. Wider shoes with a low heel and a metatarsal pad may help. Surgical excision is often required.

The tarsal tunnel syndrome is another neuritis. The posterior tibial nerve passes through a soft tissue tunnel behind the medial malleolus to enter the foot. The nerve may become inflamed from pronation or direct trauma, swelling and increasing pressure in this area. Pain radiates along the course of the nerve very much like a carpal tunnel syndrome. Patients may demonstrate a decreased conduction time of the posterior tibial nerve. Treatment with rest, anti-inflammatory drugs, shoe correction and occasional local cortisone injections is usually successful. Surgical release of the tarsal tunnel ligament may be required. Neuritis can develop along the course of any of the superficial sensory nerves of the foot, usually the result of pressure from foot wear. Local cortisone injection and modification of foot wear may correct these problems. Care must always be taken not to inject the nerve directly.

The plantar fascia is a dense fibrous band that runs from the calcaneal tuberosity along the plantar surface of the foot and inserts on the plantar surface of the metatarsal heads. This fascia can become irritated from overuse, particularly in running, and may be especially vulnerable in runners with cavus feet. Pain is most severe at the calcaneal tuberosity, but may spread along the course of the fascia. Occasionally, in chronic cases, the fascia calcifies at its insertion on the calcaneal tuberosity, resulting in the so-called heel spur. Treatment is usually conservative: a heel pad, orthosis, local injection with cortisone and rest. In refractory cases, surgical release of the fascia at its insertion may be indicated. The heel pad itself may be injured from direct trauma, the so-called stone bruise. This injury must be differentiated from plantar fasciitis. Rest usually resolves this problem.

Fractures

Stress fractures are fairly common disabling problems for athletes. Fatigue (stress) fractures are related to overuse and often seen in long-distance runners. Although the neck of the second metatarsal is the most common location, stress fractures can occur in any other bone of the foot. Since a negative x-ray film does not rule out a stress fracture, a bone scan may be necessary to make a definitive diagnosis. Fatigue fractures do not require a cast and usually respond to rest from the offending activity.

Direct trauma may cause fractures of any of the bones in the foot. All the bones are vulnerable and the site of the fracture depends on the amount of force and its direction. A fractured phalanx is usually a minor injury, although fracture of the first toe may be more serious. If the injured toe is in good alignment, it can simply be taped to the adjacent toe, taking care not to obstruct circulation. If the phalanx is displaced, the toe must be aligned under local anesthesia and then taped to the adjacent toe. This injury does not cause much lost time. Fractures of the metatarsals and midtarsal bones may require a short leg walking cast. Fractures of the first and fifth metatarsals take longer to heal and may cause more disability. The neck of the talus may be injured by a forceful dorsiflexion injury. Prompt and accurate reduction is mandatory. Since the blood supply to the talus may be lost following the fracture, this injury requires prolonged protection and follow-up. Major fractures of the calcaneus are rare in athletics. However, avulsion fractures at the site of ligamentous and tendinous attachments do occur with inversion injuries, for example, on the anterior process of the calcaneus at the calcaneocuboid joint. Occasionally, the Achilles tendon ruptures at its insertion in the calcaneus, avulsing a bone fragment with it, usually requiring surgical repair.

A very common avulsion fracture in athletics is that of the base of the fifth metatarsal. This injury results from the overpull of the peroneus brevis muscle and fractures the bone at the tendinous insertion. Treatment is usually a short leg walking cast for two to three weeks. Transverse fractures into the proximal shaft are more troublesome and require diligent care. These fractures are often missed when an ankle sprain occurs simultaneously and the concomitant fracture is not suspected.

Sprains may occur in the foot without associated bony injuries. These sprains usually involve the ligaments and/or capsule about the calcaneocuboid joint, the sinus tarsi, midtarsal joints and occasionally the transverse and longitudinal arches. The diagnosis is usually made by finding local tenderness and swelling in the presence of a normal x-ray film. Treatment consists of protected weight bearing and protective strapping.

Dislocation in the foot is most common at the MP joints. Closed reduction and protection for 10 to 14 days is usually sufficient treatment. A more common injury to the MP joint of the great toe is the so-called "turf toe." This is a hyperextension injury with partial tearing of the joint capsule, usually corrected by rest and protective taping. A more severe dislocation is that of the subtalar joint. This dramatic injury may result from a fall from a height (basketball or volleyball) with the foot in inversion. This injury may be open and can seriously impair the blood supply to the foot. Prompt reduction is required to save the foot, usually under a general anesthetic. The usual precautions for open injuries must be followed. Dislocations of the IP joints of the toe also occur and occasionally may be difficult to reduce if the joint capsule is buttonholed by a phalanx.

Avascular necrosis of bone may be seen in adolescents. This should be considered in any adolescent with forefoot pain and is most common in the head of the second metatarsal, Freiberg's disease. Diagnosis is by the x-ray findings of the sclerotic bone corresponding to the area of tenderness. After the pain is controlled by conservative means, the youngster may return to competition.

First Aid

Most acute injuries to the foot require no more than crutches, ice and a compression dressing until a physician can perform a follow-up evaluation. Although these are usually nonemergent injuries, an open dislocation is a real emergency. As the blood supply to the foot may be impaired, this injury must be treated in a hospital as soon as possible. A sterile dressing should be placed over the open wound and splinting applied so as not to impede circulation.

Blisters

Blisters are caused by friction resulting in the separaton of skin layers. Fluid accumulates between the layers. Blisters can be very painful and can become infected.

Avoiding or reducing the friction is the key to preventing blisters. Shoes should be properly fitted and broken in gradually. Multiple pairs of socks, vaseline, Spenco Second Skin and magnesium carbonate-based powders may also help prevent foot blisters. Applying thin adhesive felt (moleskin) over known blister sites prior to their development may also be effective.

If the blister is very large, it may be necessary to drain it. Cleanse the blister and surrounding area with alcohol, soap and water and/or organic iodine. Use a sterile needle or blade to open the blister, allowing it to drain. Do not remove the skin for several days so it can provide natural protection for the sensitive underskin. An antiseptic and/or antibiotic ointment may be applied to the area. Then tape a sterile dressing onto the blister. Check the blister frequently for signs of infection. Should infection occur, the athlete should be seen by a physician, who will probably provide antibiotics and drainage. Hot soaks in warm, soapy water may also be used.

Additional padding and protection of the blister may be necessary for competition. Felt donuts may be used on small blisters to avoid pressure on the blister. Larger blisters may require foot pads that cover a larger area, but avoid the location of the blister. Spenco Second Skin may be applied under the donuts. After the pads have been taped in place, vaseline may be applied to the outside of the taping, over the blister, for more protection from friction.

RECONDITIONING

The rehabilitation of foot injuries must be individualized. In some instances, weight bearing must be avoided, yet early range of motion exercises may be beneficial. This might be the case in midfoot injuries. On the other hand, exercise to strengthen the toes may be possible while a hind foot injury is immobilized in a walking cast. Early motion should be initiated to avoid joint stiffness and muscle atrophy whenever it is not detrimental to the healing process.

Once cast immobilization is discontinued, protected weight bearing is desirable. Swimming is a good early exercise, followed by biking, walking, jogging, and then the activity of the patient's sport. Protective taping may be required for a period following injury. The goal is to regain complete ankle, subtalar, midtarsal and toe motion with normal muscle strength before returning to competition.

Part 7

CARDIORESPIRATORY SYSTEM

The Respiratory System

The primary function of the respiratory system is gas exchange—the addition of oxygen to the venous blood and the removal of carbon dioxide from it. The system is complex and depends on the interaction of multiple anatomic structures. Three areas are important to understanding this system: anatomy, physiology and pathophysiology. The many nonrespiratory functions of the lung and pulmonary circulation—as a reserve for the left ventricle, as an organ of fluid exchange, as a filter to protect the systemic circulation and as a metabolic organ—are not reviewed here.

ANATOMY

The anatomy of the respiratory system may be considered in terms of the communication with the environment via the airways, the primary gas-exchange organ, or lung parenchyma, and the skeletal structures that support these tissues and facilitate air movement in and out of the lungs. The anatomic structures involved in transporting air into the lungs include the nose, mouth, pharynx, larynx, trachea, bronchi and bronchioles (Fig. 25:1). The nose and upper airways humidify the inspired air, bringing it to body temperature, and removing much of the particulate matter contained in the air, besides functioning as an organ of smell. The larynx primarily protects the trachea and lower airways from the inadvertent inhalation of liquids or swallowed particulate matter and secondarily serves as the organ of voice.

The trachea descends from the larynx to the bronchi, where it branches into the two mainstem bronchi, which in turn branch into smaller and smaller conducting airways for approximately 16 generations to the level of the terminal bronchiole (Fig. 25:2). Beyond the terminal bronchiole are an additional seven generations of branching, referred to as the respiratory zone. The air sacs or alveoli are located here and this is where the gas exchange occurs.

The trachea is a cartilaginous and membranous tube. The cartilaginous portion is composed of semicircular ''rings'' that are incomplete posteriorly and are connected by the membranous portion of the trachea composed

25

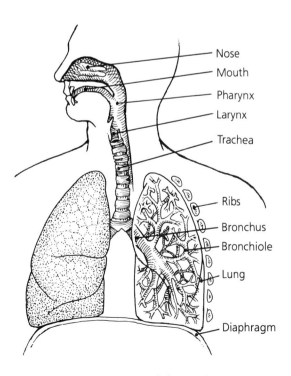

FIGURE 25:1. Anatomy of the respiratory system

331

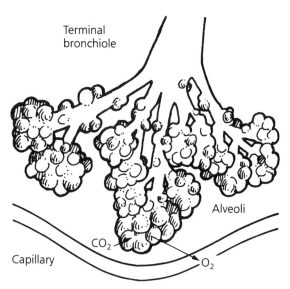

FIGURE 25:2. Terminal bronchiole and alveoli for oxygen and carbon dioxide exchange

of muscle and connective tissue. The semicircular cartilage surrounding the anterior portion of the trachea becomes disk-like in the smaller bronchi and finally disappears at the level of the bronchiole.

The trachea and bronchi are lined by mucosal cells, including columnar ciliated cells, to the level of the terminal bronchiole (the 16th generation of airways). Capillaries and mucus-secreting glands are located in the submucosa. The cilia and mucus have an important protective role in forming what has been referred to as the mucociliary escalator. The approximately 1,000 ml of mucus normally formed every day are swept upward by the ciliary action carrying particulate matter or cellular debris that has been entrapped. The mucus is swallowed when it reaches the pharynx. The walls of the airways also contain certain connective tissues and smooth muscle, which give additional support. Smooth muscle is found in the airway wall as far caudad as the alveolar duct (22nd generation).

The pulmonary parenchyma, or lung itself, is an additional support for conduction airways smaller than 2 mm in diameter. The primary components of this portion of the respiratory system are the alveoli (air sacs), which provide a total volume of about 2,500 ml (as compared with 150 ml in the conduction airways) to the level of the terminal bronchiole. The alveolus contains the interface between the air from the atmosphere and the capillary blood. The most important functional component of the alveolar wall is the capillary. The pulmonary artery from the right ventricle approximately follows the branching of the airways to the level of the alveolus, where it gives rise to the arterioles and in turn to the capillary bed that surrounds the alveolus. Within the walls of the alveoli a fine network of capillary vessels allows a transfer of oxygen from the interalveolar space into the blood, and transfer of carbon dioxide from the blood into the alveolar space. The blood is then returned to the left atrium of the heart via pulmonary veins that run adjacent to the pulmonary arteries (Figs. 25:3A, B).

The musculoskeletal structures surrounding the lung protect and support these structures and make inspiration and expiration possible. The bony ribs of the chest wall articulate with the spinal column posteriorly and sternum anteriorly. On each side, seven vertebrosternal ribs articulate directly with the sternum via their costal cartilages, three vertebrochondral ribs connect indirectly by articulating with the adjacent cartilages, and two ribs are free floating (Fig. 25:4). The ribs are interconnected by intercostal muscles, and a neurovascular bundle that runs along the lower side of the ribs provides the blood supply and nerve innervation to the chest wall. Two tissue layers—the visceral and the parietal pleura—surround each lung and allow for the smooth movement of the lung against the chest wall during inspiratory and expiratory changes. The lungs are separated from the abdominal cavity by the diaphragm, which is a musculomembranous partition through which pass the major vessels (aorta and inferior vena cava) and the esophagus. Other anatomic structures important to respiratory system functioning include the accessory inspiratory muscles, the scalene muscles (which elevate the first two ribs), the

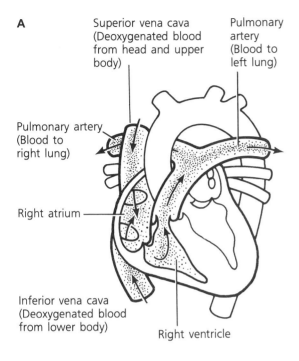

Superior vena cava
(Deoxygenated blood
from head and upper
body)

Pulmonary
artery
(Blood to
left lung)

Pulmonary artery
(Blood to
right lung)

Right atrium

Inferior vena cava
(Deoxygenated blood
from lower body)

Right ventricle

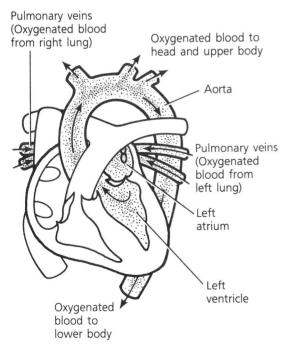

B

Pulmonary veins
(Oxygenated blood
from right lung)

Oxygenated blood to
head and upper body

Aorta

Pulmonary veins
(Oxygenated
blood from
left lung)

Left
atrium

Left
ventricle

Oxygenated
blood to
lower body

FIGURE 25:3. **A** The right-sided, or lower-pressure, pump of the heart circulates blood from the body to the lungs. **B** The left-sided, or higher-pressure, pump of the heart circulates blood from the lungs to the body.

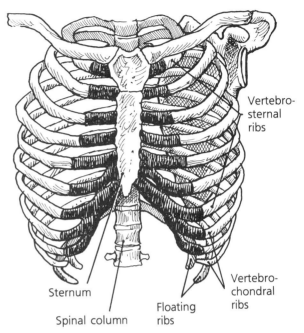

Vertebro-
sternal
ribs

Vertebro-
chondral
ribs

Sternum

Spinal column

Floating
ribs

FIGURE 25:4. Musculoskeletal structures surrounding the lungs

sternomastoid muscles (which raise the sternum) and the primary muscles of expiration in the abdominal wall.

PHYSIOLOGY

The mechanics of how the various anatomic structures of the respiratory system move air from the atmosphere into the lungs and back out again are complex and fascinating. To begin with, consider the volume of air moved into and out of the lung from maximal inspiration to maximal expiration—the vital capacity. Vital capacity is measured by collecting all of the air expired from the point of maximal inspiration to maximal expiration.

Some air remains in the lungs after maximal expiration—residual volume. During normal breathing, the volume of air remaining in the lung at the end of expiration is usually a little greater than the residual volume—functional residual capacity. The amount of air moved in and out of the lungs during normal respiration is the tidal volume and is consid-

Inspiratory reserve volume	Inspiratory capacity	Vital capacity	Total lung volume
Tidal volume			
Expiratory reserve volume	Functional residual capacity		
Residual volume		Residual volume	

FIGURE 25:5. Mechanics of air flow through the respiratory system

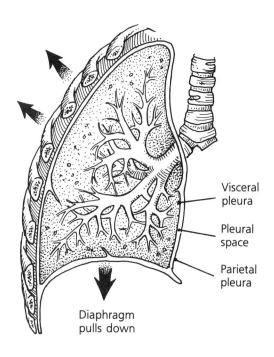

Visceral pleura

Pleural space

Parietal pleura

Diaphragm pulls down

erably less than the vital capacity when the subject is at rest (Fig. 25:5).

At the end of expiration during quiet breathing, a negative pressure in the pleural space between the visceral and the parietal pleura keeps the lung inflated. The natural tendency of the lung to collapse inward and the chest wall to expand outward creates this negative pressure. These properties of the lung and chest become apparent in pneumothorax, or air leak from the atmosphere into the pleural space, when the lung collapses to a volume below residual volume and the chest wall expands outward to a position beyond that seen at total lung capacity. Thus, adjacent surfaces are pulling in opposite directions and are generating a negative pressure in the closed space between them (Fig. 25:6A, B). When the ribs are lifted in a "bucket-handle" type of motion by the intercostal muscles of the scalene and sternomastoid groups and by the downward movement of the contracting diaphragm

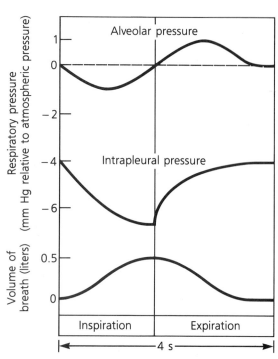

FIGURE 25:6. **A** Negative pressure in pleural space keeps lungs inflated. **B** Alveolar and intrapleural pressure in respiratory cycle

during inspiration, an increasingly negative pressure is generated around and within the lung, resulting in air flow from the atmosphere through the conducting airways into the pulmonary alveoli. When these muscles relax, the lung and chest wall return to their resting positions and air is expired from the lung. During exercise and hyperventilation, expiration is active and is facilitated by the contraction of intercostal and abdominal muscles.

The rapidity and frequency of inspiratory-expiratory efforts thus can be voluntarily manipulated. The characteristics of a curve drawn by measuring the flow rate of the expired air at different lung volumes throughout a forced expiratory maneuver from total lung capacity to residual volume has become a much studied phenomenon among pulmonary physiologists interested in the mechanics of breathing (Fig. 25:7). This measurement is obtained with a spirometer, which provides a timed measurement of the volume of the air expired during the maximal forced expiratory maneuver. From these data, various determinations allow comparison of the pulmonary function of a given subject with predetermined normal values based on the subject's age,

height and sex. Some of these determinations include the volume of the air expired during the first second of the forced vital capacity maneuver, the 1 second forced expiratory volume (FEV_1), the maximal peak expiratory flow (Vmax), the forced expiratory flow from 25% to 75% of the vital capacity (FEF_{25-75}) and the forced vital capacity or lung volume expired during the complete maneuver. In the patient with suspected airway disease, for example, these measurements allow evaluation of pulmonary function as it pertains to the ability to rapidly force the air out of the lungs. The pertinence of this test becomes more apparent with the discussion of respiratory system dysfunction.

The inspiratory and expiratory maneuvers are sometimes described as "in with the good air and out with the bad." Obviously, this is a gross oversimplification, but it warrants some discussion. With inspiration, air (which at sea level contains approximately 20% oxygen) is brought in contact with the alveolocapillary membrane to allow the exchange of gases. Oxygen moves into the blood and carbon dioxide moves out of the blood into the alveolar space, where it is expired into the environment. Most of the oxygen in the blood combines with hemoglobin, though some is dissolved in the blood. Carbon dioxide is carried primarily in the dissolved state, although it may be found in bicarbonate and attached to proteins such as hemoglobin, forming carbamino compounds. The effectiveness of the gas exchange depends to a great extent on the critical matching of ventilation (air in the alveolus) and perfusion (blood in the capillaries surrounding the alveolus) (Fig. 25:8).

Through the process of passive diffusion, oxygen moves from the alveolus into the blood and carbon dioxide moves from the blood into the alveolus. This occurs because the concentration, or partial pressure, of oxygen is higher in the alveolar gas (Fig. 25:9). Other factors that influence the rate of diffusion include the amount of surface area available for diffusion, the thickness of the alveolar capillary membrane through which diffusion occurs, and the

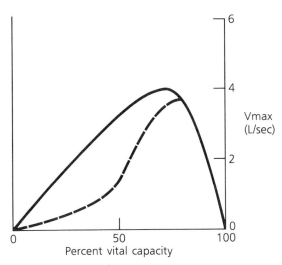

Solid line = normal
Dotted line = smoking teenager

FIGURE 25:7. Expired air volumes measured with spirometry

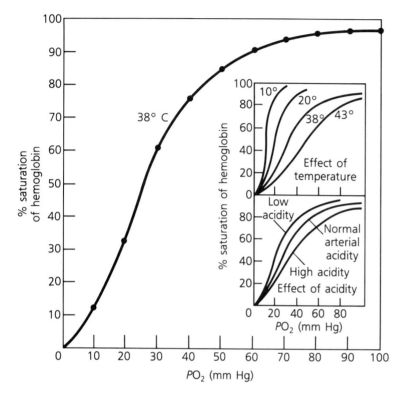

FIGURE 25:8. Hemoglobin–oxygen dissociation curve as affected by temperature and acidity

the range of normal oxygen pressures, whereas the carbon dioxide dissociation curve remains steep in the physiologic range.

If hyperventilation cannot significantly increase the oxygen content of the blood, when exercise increases oxygen demands the cardiac output or the frequency with which a given red blood cell travels from the lung to the heart must increase. Thus, the physiologic requirements of exercise demand a coupling of increased cardiovascular and respiratory activities to meet the gas exchange requirements. With the increased oxygen demands of the muscle, cardiac output or oxygen delivery to the cells must increase; and with the cells' in-

diffusion constant for a given gas. The diffusion constant is proportional to the solubility of the gas in water and is inversely proportional to the square root of its molecular weight. More simply, carbon dioxide diffuses about 20 times more rapidly than oxygen in the lung although it has a similar molecular weight because it is more soluble than oxygen.

In normal persons, hyperventilation significantly reduces the level of carbon dioxide in the blood but does not greatly change the level of oxygen. Physiologically this is a result of the different dissociation curves for oxygen and carbon dioxide. A rapid exchanging of atmospheric and alveolar air allows carbon dioxide to be washed from the blood, reducing the partial pressure of carbon dioxide, but the chemical characteristics of the binding of oxygen with hemoglobin do not allow the oxygen content of the blood to increase significantly. The oxygen dissociation curve becomes flat in

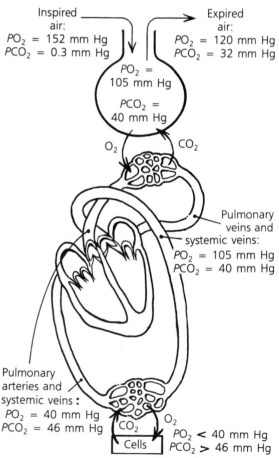

FIGURE 25:9. Process of passive diffusion. Oxygen moves from alveolus into blood and carbon dioxide moves from blood into alveolus.

creased carbon dioxide production in the exercising muscle, alveolar ventilation to remove carbon dioxide from the blood must increase. When delivery of oxygen to the cells is inadequate to meet metabolic demands, lactic acid is produced and released into the bloodstream. The increased acidity stimulates increased alveolar ventilation in an attempt to reduce the acidity of the blood by removing carbon dioxide, which also contributes to overall acidity. The increased production of carbon dioxide by the cell is further aggravated by an increase in carbon dioxide, with the normal buffering processes of the blood, as hydrogen ions combine with bicarbonate ions to form water and more carbon dioxide.

PATHOPHYSIOLOGY

A number of pathologic states interfere with the process of gas exchange. One is exercise induced asthma, precipitated by exercise but similar to other forms of asthma. It is characterized by paroxysmal shortness of breath, cough and a feeling of chest tightness that results primarily from narrowing of the airways by contractions of the smooth muscles in their walls. This is discussed in greater detail in Chapter 44.

Chronic obstructive bronchitis, most commonly associated with long-term cigarette smoking, interferes with gas exchange in much the same manner as asthma but does not consistently have the reversible bronchospasm component (Fig. 25:10A, B). In chronic obstructive bronchitis, the small airways narrow, resulting in an increased resistance to airflow (Fig. 25:10A). On testing with the forced vital capacity maneuver, maximal expiratory flow is reduced predominantly at low lung volumes. This reduction is not episodic and does not significantly improve with bronchodilators. These patients also characteristically have a chronic daily cough that produces an increased amount of bronchial secretions. Thus, with abnormalities in gas exchange, the work of breathing is increased and ventilation and perfusion can become mismatched. Most

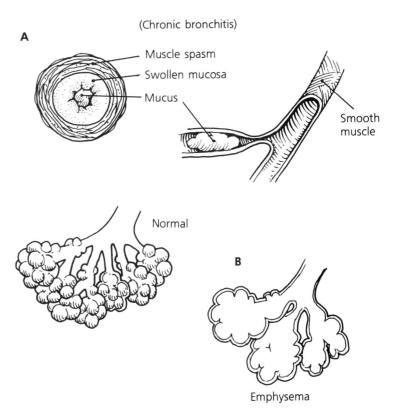

FIGURE 25:10. Narrowing of airways by contraction of smooth muscle in **A** chronic bronchitis compared to normal airway. In emphysema **B** air spaces are over-inflated.

patients with chronic bronchitis also have an emphysema component characterized by an overinflation of the air spaces, resulting in cyst-like deformity in the lung with irreversible destruction of pulmonary tissue (Fig. 25:10B). Mismatching of ventilation and perfusion then results, but the structural support of airways is also lost, with further narrowing and limitation of flow. An inherited form of emphysema, alpha-antitrypsin deficiency, though rare, can be seen in the younger patient who may have never smoked cigarettes. Because of the abnormalities in gas exchange and the increased work of breathing, there may be some exercise limitation. Although the pulmonary component of these diseases is usually irreversible, exercise tolerance may improve with physical conditioning.

RESPIRATORY INFECTIONS

Before considering the anatomic site and different causes of upper and lower respiratory infections, the following generalizations can be made. Symptoms of mild or moderate severity and a few days' duration, such as sore throat, stuffy nose, cough, tiredness and intermittent fever, need not keep an athlete from competing, regardless of cause. Most often these symptoms are caused by viral infections, are self-limited and do not respond to antibiotics. Analgesics, such as aspirin or acetaminophen, may help relieve aches and pains.

Upper respiratory infections involve the throat, tonsils, nose, middle ear, sinuses and/or lymph nodes (glands) in the neck. The common cold viruses cause any or all of the following symptoms: increased nasal congestion and secretions, sore throat, stuffy head and sore, swollen lymph nodes. General symptoms may include tiredness, malaise, headache and intermittent fever. Treatment is symptomatic with nonprescription analgesics and possibly decongestants. Bothersome aching pain localized over the cheeks or about the eyes may indicate a complicating sinus infection. Likewise, earache or a persistent blocked ear may indicate a complicating ear infection. Both of these secondary infections may be caused by bacteria. Logical management includes physician consultation for specific diagnosis and possible antibiotic treatment.

A special word about sore throats. The terms pharyngitis and tonsilitis are used interchangeably. Although most throat infections are viral, a specific diagnosis cannot be made from symptoms or physical examination. Any sore throat that is particularly bothersome, lasts more than a few days, is associated with a persistent fever or with tender, swollen neck lymph nodes, causes pain or restricts opening the mouth should be evaluated for the following possibilities.

1. Streptococcal bacterial infection. This is suspected by symptoms and examination but proven by throat culture. The treatment is antibiotic (penicillin if possible). Athletic

activity can resume when the patient feels better, usually within one to three days.
2. Infectious mononucleosis viral infection. This is suspected by symptoms and examination and proven by a complete blood cell count (CBC) and a blood test for mononucleosis plus a negative throat culture for beta-streptococci. The treatment is symptomatic, plus cortisone in some cases. As the spleen is always involved (and often enlarged) in mononucleosis, the athlete should refrain from athletics until cured and a repeat examination shows a normal spleen. An infected, enlarged spleen is more likely to rupture with trauma. Return to competitive activity usually takes 10 to 14 days.
3. Infection about the tonsils, namely a peritonsillar abscess. This is a bacterial infection suspected by pain and inability to fully open the mouth (trismus). It is diagnosed by examination of the throat. Treatment is close medical supervision plus antibiotics and sometimes drainage of an abscess. The athlete usually misses competition for seven to ten days.
4. Viral throat infection other than mononucleosis. This is suspected by milder symptoms and a "normal" throat examination plus a negative throat culture for beta-streptococci. Blood test results are normal. The treatment is symptomatic and the athlete misses no or minimal competition.

Lower respiratory infections involve the larynx, bronchial tubes and lungs. If a patient coughs, a lower respiratory infection (or allergy) is present. Laryngitis is recognized by hoarseness, a dry, hard cough and some sore throat. Laryngitis, caused by the cold viruses, requires only symptomatic treatment and usually does not limit participation.

The vast majority of lower respiratory infections are viral bronchial infections, i.e., bronchitis or "chest colds." Symptoms include cough aggravated by exercise or lying down. Patients may have an intermittent fever and varying malaise. Whereas an upper respiratory infection (head cold) may last seven to ten days, viral bronchitis often lasts several weeks. The treatment is symptomatic for aches and cough. Symptomatic cough suppression (if needed at night) is often possible with codeine cough medicine, a prescription medicine. Unless bronchitis symptoms are very bothersome or the athlete has a persistent fever, competition is acceptable.

Influenza is a specific viral bronchitis due to influenza viruses A or B. It occurs in epidemics and is often severe, requiring medical consultation for diagnosis or to consider complicating pneumonia.

Pneumonia, an infection of the alveoli, produces coughing, frequently more persistent than with bronchitis, often with fever and malaise. Stethoscopic examination is unreliable but sometimes discloses localized, moist sounds called rales. A chest x-ray film is necessary to diagnose pneumonia. It is frequently difficult to determine whether pneumonia is caused by bacteria, viruses or other virus-like organisms (*Chlamydia*). A physician should decide whether a trial of antibiotics is advisable. The acute phase of most pneumonias lasts seven to ten days, and competition is possible thereafter.

Injuries to the Chest

26

Injuries to the chest are serious because of the likelihood of internal bleeding or direct injury of the heart or lungs. Chest injuries result from automobile accidents, gunshot wounds, stab wounds, falls, blows or compression.

Unless properly treated, a chest injury may be rapidly fatal. Since the body has no capacity to store oxygen, any injury that seriously interferes with the constant replenishment of oxygen through normal breathing must be treated without delay. Specifically, cells in the brain and other parts of the nervous system require a rich supply of oxygen continuously, and may die within minutes if deprived of oxygen. Trainers must be aware of the potential seriousness of chest injuries.

CLASSIFICATION OF CHEST INJURIES

Chest injuries are divided into two categories, open and closed. In open chest injuries the chest wall has been penetrated, as by a knife or a bullet. Open chest injuries may also be associated with severe rib fractures where the broken end of the rib has lacerated the chest wall and the skin. These injuries may be concurrent with contusions or lacerations of the heart, lungs or major blood vessels.

In closed chest injuries, the skin is not broken. However, major damage from fractured ribs or a contusion may exist within the chest. The heart or lungs may be lacerated. Serious closed chest injuries include compression of the chest and severe contusions, such as might result from the blunt trauma of hitting a steering wheel, being struck by a falling object or being buried in a cave-in.

SIGNS OF CHEST INJURIES

The important signs of chest injuries, either open or closed, are:

1. Pain at the site of the injury
2. Pleuritic pain aggravated by or occurring with breathing, localized around the site of a chest injury
3. Dyspnea (difficult or painful respiration)
4. Failure of one or both sides of the chest to expand normally with inspiration
5. Hemoptysis (coughing up blood)
6. Rapid, weak pulse and low blood pressure
7. Cyanosis of the lips, fingertips or fingernails

Any change in the normal breathing pattern is a particularly important sign. An uninjured person breathes from 6 to 20 times a minute without difficulty and without pain, depending on level of physical fitness. The normal rate generally is around 20. Very well trained athletes usually breathe very slowly with large tidal volumes of air. Respiratory rates in excess of 24 per minute are in the range of distress.

Pain in the chest at the site of an obvious fracture or bruise indicates an injury of the chest wall and perhaps lung damage. Pain aggravated by breathing or on inhalation indicates irritation of the pleural surfaces of the lung or the chest wall. Pleural irritation can result from some severe disease processes.

The depth of respiration and difficulty in taking a breath are reliable indicators of respiratory distress. Difficulty in breathing is generally called dyspnea and may result from several causes. In the injured patient, it may arise because the chest cannot expand properly, the patient has lost normal nervous system control of breathing, the airway is obstructed, or the lung itself is being compressed from within the chest by accumulated blood or air.

It is extremely important to observe whether the chest wall fails to expand when the patient inhales. This failure indicates that the muscles of the chest have lost the ability to act appropriately. Such loss of muscular function may result from a direct injury of the chest wall itself, from a severe injury of the nerves controlling the chest wall or from a severe brain injury.

Hemoptysis (coughing up blood) usually indicates that the lung has been lacerated. In such cases, blood enters the bronchial passages within the lungs and is promptly coughed up as the patient tries to clear the passages.

A rapid, weak pulse and low blood pressure are signs of shock. Cyanosis (blue color around the lips, fingernails or fingertips) indicates that blood is being insufficiently oxygenated. This finding in a patient with severe injuries means the patient is unable to bring adequate oxygen to the blood through the lungs. Therefore a chest injury should be suspected. (See Chapter 29 for a more detailed discussion of shock.)

CARE OF CHEST INJURIES

All the various types of chest injuries require almost the same initial care. Emergency medical care is directed to allowing the patient to breathe. The upper airway must be cleared and maintained. Artificial ventilation and supplemental oxygen where necessary must be instituted promptly. The overriding first consideration is to achieve as normal respiration as possible for the patient.

Open chest wounds must be covered. If ribs are broken, the patient should be made comfortable and quiet to minimize the possibility of further damage to the lungs, heart or chest wall. Fractured ribs may be splinted by external supports, usually a sling and swathe (Fig. 26:1). Adhesive taping of the chest wall is

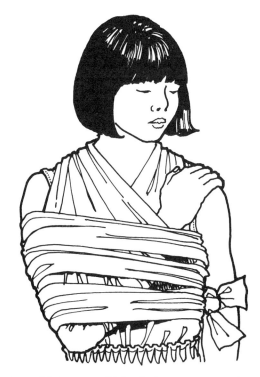

FIGURE 26:1. In multiple rib fractures, a swathe will immobilize injuries.

rarely necessary; further, tape limits the ability of the chest to expand and interferes with proper respiration. Bleeding from the chest wall must be controlled by direct pressure. Embedded or protruding foreign objects, such as knives, should be bandaged in place and left alone. They generally require surgical removal at the hospital.

Vital signs must be observed and recorded. They are the trainer's single means to diagnose and follow the course of internal bleeding. Similarly, the effects of treatment must be observed, since the results frequently show that prompt transport to an emergency care facility is necessary.

Chest wounds usually require expert treatment in a hospital so prompt transportation to an emergency department is of paramount importance. Sometimes the patient is in such extreme circumstances that immediate transportation to the hospital, maintaining adequate oxygen supply and controlling bleeding en route are the only things the trainer should attempt to do.

The following steps should be performed in sequence when handling a patient with a chest injury.

1. Clear and maintain the airway.
2. Use supplemental oxygen and be prepared to give respiratory support with mechanical aids or mouth-to-mouth breathing promptly.
3. Observe and record vital signs.
4. Control all obvious external bleeding.
5. Promptly cover penetrating wounds into the chest cavity.
6. Carefully monitor the effect of treatment and be ready to institute changes, transport rapidly or offer resuscitation promptly. A patient's status may deteriorate very rapidly after a chest injury, or the patient may stabilize and respond to support very well.
7. Transport promptly to the emergency department, and when possible notify the hospital of the type and severity of the injury in advance.

TYPES OF CHEST INJURIES AND EMERGENCY CARE

Rib Fractures

Rib fractures are usually caused by direct blows or compression injuries of the chest. The upper four ribs are rarely fractured, since they are protected by the shoulder girdle (scapula and clavicle). The fifth through the ninth ribs are those commonly fractured. The lower two ribs (11th and 12th) are harder to fracture because they are attached only to the thoracic vertebrae and have greater freedom of movement.

The common finding in all patients with fractured ribs is pain localized at the site of the fracture. Asking the patient to place a finger on the exact area of the pain often determines the location of the injury. There may or may not be a rib deformity, a chest wall contusion or a laceration. Deep breathing, coughing or movement is usually very painful. The patient

generally wants to remain still and may often lean toward the injured side, covering the fractured area with a hand to prevent the chest from moving and to ease local pain.

Simple rib fractures ordinarily are not bound, strapped or taped. If a patient has multiple fractures and is considerably more comfortable with the chest immobilized, the best bandage is a swathe in which the arm is strapped to the chest to limit motion on the injured side (see Fig. 26:1). A swathe of the arm with the forearm in a sling is most effective in immobilizing the chest. Immobilizing both arms may be necessary if the fractures are on both sides. Wide strips of adhesive plaster were often used to immobilize the chest wall in the past. While this lessens the patient's discomfort, the tight bandage of adhesive plaster applied to the skin of the thorax acts as an unyielding corset and hinders whatever expansion the injured chest can achieve. It is better to help the patient to breathe than to try to make him more comfortable by not allowing the chest to expand.

Occasionally, the end of a fractured rib may puncture or lacerate the lung or the skin of the chest wall (Fig. 26:2). In such an instance, some degree of pneumothorax or hemothorax usually occurs (Fig. 26:3). These two conditions are common results of chest injuries and are discussed later in this chapter.

Flail Chest

When three or more ribs are broken, each in two places, the segment of the chest wall lying between the breaks will collapse rather than expand normally with the chest wall on each inhalation. When the patient exhales, this segment protrudes while the rest of the chest wall contracts. The motion of the segment is paradoxical because it is opposite to the normal movement of the chest wall, and is therefore called paradoxical motion. The portion of the chest wall lying between the fractures is called the flail segment (Fig. 26:4). Several terms are used to describe this injury, such as crushed chest or stove-in chest, but the proper one is flail chest. Ordinarily, the paradoxical motion of the flail segment produces considerable pain.

This is a particularly serious injury. Obviously, the lung immediately underneath the flail segment does not expand properly when the patient inhales, and he loses that amount of lung volume. Much more important, however, is that the amount of force exerted on the chest wall needed to multiply fracture a series of ribs and produce a flail chest segment almost always causes severe contusion damage, or bruising, of the lung itself underneath the flail segment. The contusion injury of the lung thus may be far more serious than it appears.

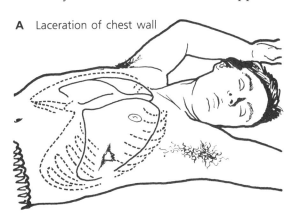

A Laceration of chest wall

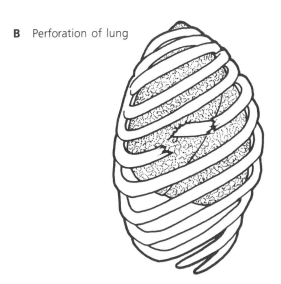

B Perforation of lung

FIGURE 26:2. Fracture of the rib **A** may cause a laceration of the skin or **B** a perforation of the lung.

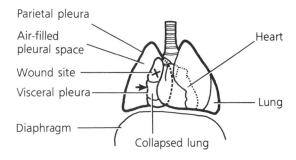

A Pneumothorax

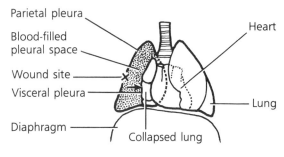

B Hemothorax

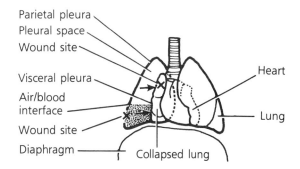

C Hemopneumothorax

FIGURE 26:3. **A** A pneumothorax is a collection of air in the pleural space between the visceral and parietal pleural surfaces. It can result from an opening into the space through the skin or the lung and will collapse the affected lung. **B** A hemothorax is a collection of blood in the pleural space between the visceral and parietal pleural surfaces. It results from bleeding into the chest. **C** A hemothorax may occur alone or in conjunction with a pneumothorax. The latter case is hemopneumothorax.

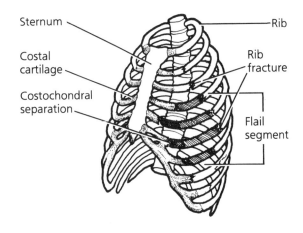

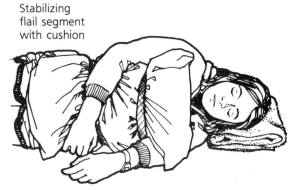

FIGURE 26:4. Flail chest segment (top) and stabilization with cushion

The condition is relatively easy to diagnose through observation. The chest does not rise properly despite the patient's most desperate efforts to inhale deeply. In some patients, signs of lack of oxygen follow rapidly.

In an acute situation, immediately after injury, the major factor limiting adequate respiration is pain on breathing. The patient with a flail chest may breathe more comfortably if positioned with the fractured ribs down or against a bed rail. The patient who has a central flail segment with a fracture of the sternum and fractures in either hemithorax may grasp a pillow to help stabilize the segment when motion causes pain. Occasionally, sandbags may be used, propped against the chest wall to lessen paradoxical motion and pain. If breathing is inadequate, and especial-

ly if cyanosis is present, respiration must be assisted and supplemental oxygen given. Oxygen should be started promptly, since these patients may very soon die without it. The trainer must assist respiration and maintain it until the emergency department is reached. These patients should be transported to the hospital as promptly as possible.

Penetrating Injuries

Stab and gunshot wounds are examples of penetrating chest injuries (Fig. 26:5). They usually produce varying degrees of hemothorax and pneumothorax. Occasionally, they will cause a rib fracture. These injuries frequently create sucking chest wounds that must be made airtight promptly by appropriate dressings (Fig. 26:6).

Penetrating wounds can injure any structure within the thoracic cavity. There is grave

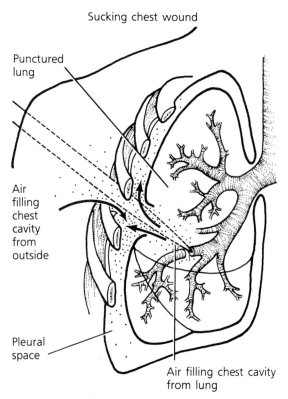

FIGURE 26:5. Sucking chest wound allows free air to leak into chest cavity.

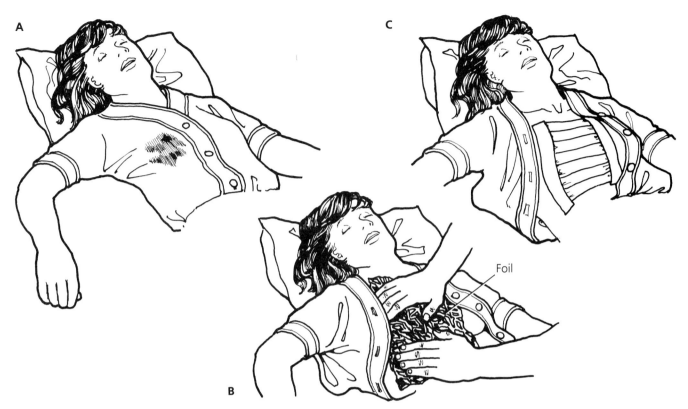

FIGURE 26:6. **A** A sucking chest wound allows free passage of air from the outside to the pleural space. Hemoptysis (coughing up of blood) indicates lung injury. **B** Seal this wound promptly with airtight or impermeable sterile material such as foil. **C** Final bandaging over the seal prevents air from entering the chest through the wound.

danger of a direct laceration or other injury of the heart or the great blood vessels in the chest. Bleeding, which may be massive, is usually into the chest cavity itself, so is rarely visible outside the body. The patient, in addition to having the expected signs of respiratory distress associated with the injury, may be in shock from blood loss and may require artificial ventilation as well as vigorous resuscitation from shock. Prompt transportation to the emergency department is necessary.

When a patient has sustained a penetrating wound of the chest from a gunshot, the chest must be examined carefully for both entrance and exit wounds. This examination will be carried out at the hospital, but evaluation of the patient in the emergency department is much easier if this information is delivered along with the patient.

Compression Injuries

Injuries of the chest can result from sudden circumferential compression of the chest and an accompanying rapid increase in intrathoracic pressure. Multiple rib fractures can occur along with a flail chest. In extreme instances of circumferential compression, the upper part of the body may be cyanotic and edematous, the neck veins distended and the eyes bulging.

Injuries to the Back of the Chest

Injuries to the back of the chest, other than rib fractures, are usually muscle strains or open lacerations. Pain and tenderness locally at the wound site are common. These wounds should be examined for impaled or embedded objects, but such objects should not be removed. Impaled objects may be cut off, if necessary, a few inches from the skin for more comfortable transportation to the emergency department. These patients should always be checked for an injury of the spine (Chapter 32). Observe the patient en route to the emergency department for airway problems. The patient may be more comfortable in a prone position, but the desirability of this posture varies from patient to patient.

An uncommon injury to the back of the chest is a fracture of the scapula, or shoulder blade. This bone is literally buried in a very heavy muscle mass. Accordingly, its fracture indicates that the patient has sustained a particularly severe blow. A bad contusion, hemorrhage or laceration over the shoulder blade should raise the possibility of a scapula fracture. Major injuries to the back of the chest may also cause pulmonary contusion or any of the previously discussed problems within the thorax.

RESULTS OF CHEST INJURIES

The results of chest injuries can be best discussed in a general section because many of the injuries just described have similar results, although the causes may be different. The most common results of chest injuries are considered here.

Pneumothorax

Pneumothorax means the presence of air within the chest cavity in the pleural space, but outside the lung (see Fig. 26:3A). In this condition, the lung has been separated from the chest wall and is said to be collapsed. The volume of the lung is diminished, and so the amount of air that can be inhaled to exchange oxygen and carbon dioxide with the blood is reduced. Hypoxia follows and, as the degree of pneumothorax increases, respiratory distress becomes evident.

Pneumothorax can result from air entering the chest directly through a sucking wound open to the outside. In an intact chest, it can also be caused by air leaking out from a lung lacerated by a fractured rib. In pneumothorax the normal mechanism by which the lung expands, that is, capillary adhesion to the inside of the chest wall, is lost, and the affected, or collapsed, lung cannot expand with inhalation. For patients with an open wound of the chest, the amount of pneumothorax can be minimized by rapid sealing of the hole prior to transportation.

Spontaneous Pneumothorax

Some people have congenitally weak areas on the surface of their lungs. Occasionally, this weak area will rupture, allowing air to leak into the pleural space. Such an event is not usually related to any major trauma and commonly occurs while the patient is sitting quietly. The patient experiences a sudden sharp chest pain and increasing difficulty in breathing. The affected lung undergoes collapse and loses its ability to expand normally. All degrees of this condition exist, from the patient who notices no particular discomfort or difficulty in breathing to the patient who requires emergency transportation to the hospital because of respiratory distress. In the latter instance, the trainer will not be called on to make a diagnosis but must administer respiratory support while transporting the patient promptly to the emergency department.

Tension Pneumothorax

If a spontaneous pneumothorax fails to seal when the lung collapses, a tension pneumothorax may develop (Fig. 26:7). In this condition air continuously leaks out of the lung into the pleural space, expanding the space with every breath the patient takes. Hence, with each breath the affected lung collapses more, until it is completely reduced to a small ball 2 or 3 inches in diameter. At this time, pressure in the affected side of the chest cavity begins to rise, and the collapsed lung is pressed against the heart and the opposite lung. The remaining lung in turn is now compressed. As pressure in the chest cavity rises, it may exceed the normal pressure of blood in veins returning to the heart. Blood can then no longer travel back to the heart to be pumped out. Death can follow rapidly.

Tension pneumothorax is not limited to closed chest injuries. A patient with a fractured rib who has sustained a sucking chest wound (see Sucking Chest Wounds) may also have a severe lung laceration. If the external wound is effectively bandaged and thus sealed and the lung continues to leak, a tension pneumothorax may develop. The condition cannot exist in a patient without an intact or well-sealed chest wall.

The signs of tension pneumothorax are severe, rapidly progressive respiratory distress, a weak pulse, fall in blood pressure, bulging of the tissue in the chest wall between the ribs and above the clavicle, distension of the veins in the neck and cyanosis. The diagnosis is best made by a physician who can immediately relieve the tension in the chest by passing large bore no. 13 or 14 gauge hypodermic needles through the chest wall into the chest cavity. The patient will require ventilatory support, although relief of the tension within the chest often allows normal or near normal respiration to return immediately. For the patient with a bandaged chest wound and a tension pneumothorax, simple release of the dressing is often effective.

It must be emphasized that tension pneumothorax is one of the very few true minute-by-minute emergencies. Prompt treatment can save this patient's life. Some patients with severe tension pneumothorax may die in a very few minutes.

Hemothorax

Hemothorax means the presence of blood in the chest cavity within the pleural space, outside the lung (see Fig. 26:3B). It may occur in open or closed chest injuries and frequently accompanies a pneumothorax. The bleeding may come from lacerated vessels in the chest wall, from lacerated major vessels within the chest cavity itself or, rarely, from a

Tension pneumothorax

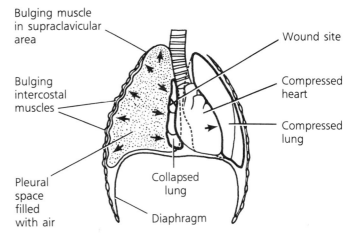

FIGURE 26:7. Air collects in pleural space creating tension pneumothorax.

lacerated lung. If the bleeding in the chest is severe, the patient may show signs of shock from blood loss alone. Shock (Chapter 30) is manifested by pallor, apprehension, a cold, clammy skin, chills, a rapid, weak pulse, fall in blood pressure and thirst.

Hemothorax, like pneumothorax, fills up the chest with something other than the lung. Normal lung expansion cannot occur, and the lung is compressed and loses its volume. Less air can be inhaled, and there may be substantially less blood to carry the reduced amount of oxygen available to the patient. This patient requires immediate ventilatory support, administration of oxygen, and control of obvious bleeding by means of pressure dressings. The patient must then be transported promptly to the emergency department.

Sucking Chest Wounds

In open chest injuries, air may enter the chest cavity through the wound when the patient inhales and the chest expands in the normal respiratory cycle (see Fig. 26:6). Ordinarily, the pressure inside the chest cavity is maintained at somewhat less than atmospheric pressure. Inhalation markedly reduces this pressure. When the chest cavity has been opened, air moves through the wound just as it moves through the nose and mouth during normal respiration. When this happens, the air remains outside the lung in the pleural space, the conditions of a pneumothorax are created and the lung's function is compromised. Air is passed back through the wound to the outside when the patient exhales, and pressure within the thorax rises. Such open chest wounds are called ''sucking chest wounds'' because of a sucking sound at the wound caused by the passage of air through it each time the patient breathes. As an initial emergency step, it is imperative that these wounds be sealed with an airtight dressing (see Fig. 26:6B). Several sterile materials may be used: sterile aluminum foil, vaseline gauze or a folded universal dressing held in place by a pressure dressing. The aim of the dressing is to seal the wound and it must be large enough so that the dressing itself is not sucked into the chest cavity.

Subcutaneous Emphysema

If a lung laceration from a fractured rib has allowed air to escape into the tissues of the chest wall, the trainer will feel a crackling sensation under the fingertips when examining the area of the fracture. The name given to this finding is subcutaneous emphysema. In very severe instances, it can involve the entire chest, neck and face. It indicates that air is being forced out of the lung into the tissues and confirms the presence of fractured ribs and a lacerated lung. This patient should be promptly transported to the hospital for further observation and evaluation.

Pulmonary Contusion

This particular condition is almost uniformly associated with blunt injuries of the chest seen in automobile accidents and severe falls, and has only recently become well recognized. In flail chest, it accounts for the greater part of the severity of the injury, rather than the anatomically disturbed movement of the chest wall itself.

A pulmonary contusion is a bruise of the lung. It behaves in much the same way as bruises of any other tissues in the body. The blood vessels in the lung are injured, and a considerable amount of blood is lost into the lung tissue. Depending on the size of the pulmonary contusion, the patient may or may not be in respiratory distress. Ordinarily, pulmonary contusions do not concern the trainer, as they develop over the first 48 hours of the hospital stay. Some pulmonary contusions are, however, so severe initially that the patient is in respiratory distress almost from the moment the injury occurs. An example is the frail, elderly patient with a chest injury from a bad fall onto the stair railing or the edge of a table or chair. Emergency treatment for these injuries is ventilatory support, including the administration of oxygen. If the pulmonary contusion is associated with several rib fractures, artificial ventilation may be required.

Myocardial Contusion

Blunt injuries of the chest may produce myocardial contusions, which are bruises of the heart muscle itself. Such injuries may not be detectible until fairly sophisticated laboratory and electrocardiographic studies are done. Ordinarily, a severe myocardial contusion disturbs the electrical conduction system that controls the heart rate. In such circumstances the heart is said to be irritable. The signs of such injuries are extra heartbeats, which irregularly interrupt the normal pulse rhythm so the patient has an irregular pulse with occasional pauses and occasional beats coming very close together. The trainer cannot treat this condition but should note the pulse and its character. Early signs of myocardial contusion require prompt transportation of the patient to the emergency department.

Pericardial Tamponade

In pericardial tamponade blood or other fluid is present in the pericardial sac outside the heart, exerting an unusual pressure on the heart itself. It almost always results from gunshot or stab wounds of the heart that have opened one of the heart chambers so that blood leaks out each time the heart beats. The pericardial sac within which the heart lies is a very tough, fibrous membrane and cannot expand suddenly. When blood leaks out of the heart, it is caught within this unyielding sac and, as it accumulates within the pericardial cavity, it compresses the heart so that its chambers can no longer accommodate the blood normally returned to them through the veins. This pressure must be relieved, or death will occur very rapidly.

The signs of the condition are very soft and faint heart tones (hard to hear even with a stethoscope), a weak pulse, blood pressure readings in which the systolic and diastolic pressures come closer and closer together with successive blood pressure readings, and congested and distended veins in the upper part of the body. This patient may require very vigorous emergency respiratory support with ventilatory assistance and oxygen. An emergency operation immediately after arrival at the hospital may be necessary.

Observation of or suspicion of pericardial tamponade is an indication for the trainer to transport that patient to the emergency department as soon as possible. The trainer should, if possible, call ahead to advise the hospital of the type of injury and the patient's status.

Dyspnea

The state of difficult or labored breathing is called dyspnea. It is a serious condition and may be a terrifying one. Dyspnea can be the result of either trauma or disease. Some specific causes are listed here.

1. The flow of air in the trachea and the bronchial tubes may be obstructed, as in many instances of trauma, aspirated vomitus or blood or foreign bodies in the throat or windpipe.

2. Air may not pass easily into or out of the air sacs in the lung, as in patients suffering from asthma or other allergic reactions, because of spasm in the airways themselves. Generally, in this instance it is far easier to inhale than to exhale.

3. A lung may be collapsed and unable to expand, as in spontaneous or traumatic pneumothorax or hemothorax.

4. The air sacs in the lungs themselves may have become inelastic and no longer be responsive to the normal motions of breathing (emphysema).

5. The lungs may be filled with backed-up fluid because the heart muscle has failed and is no longer able to circulate the amount of blood presented to it (pulmonary edema).

Sudden dyspnea may terrify a patient, who may become exhausted simply struggling to breathe. The trainer must approach this patient clearly and calmly. Some persons with dyspnea need only reassurance by a confident professional person to help them relax and breathe more easily. The proper approach to this problem follows these steps.

1. Make certain that the airways are clear of blood, vomitus and other foreign materials.

2. If the patient is unconscious, support the tongue so that it does not obstruct the airway.

3. Have oxygen ready to administer by mask.

4. Assist the conscious patient to find a comfortable position for breathing. This position may be semi-reclining. When dyspnea is the result of cardiac failure, a straight sitting up position may be best.

5. Be prepared to help the patient control vomiting.

6. Try to find out the possible causes of the attack if an injury is not immediately apparent. Causes can include asthma, heart disease, allergy or aspiration of foreign material.

7. Be prepared, once all possible support has been rendered, to transport this patient promptly to the emergency department.

The Hematologic System

27

In the cardiovascular system blood serves many vital functions in the healthy as well as in the diseased person. The primary functions of the blood cells are (1) to distribute oxygen in adequate concentrations to body tissues that require varying levels of oxygen; (2) to maintain hemostasis, especially after an artery or vein has been severed; and (3) to prevent, combat and subdue infections.

Basically, blood can be divided into two phases: the liquid phase (the plasma) and the cellular phase. All of the cellular elements are derived from the bone marrow, which in the adult is primarily found within the central skeletal system—skull, ribs, manubrium, vertebrae and pelvis. In the adult, the distal long bones contain primarily fat in the marrow cavity. In younger people, the long bones have active bone marrow that is replaced by fat with aging.

BLOOD CELLS

Red cells have many functions, but the single most important is delivery of oxygen and return of carbon dioxide. Under normal circumstances, carbon dioxide is released in the lungs as the blood passes through the small capillary beds found in the substance of the lungs. Oxygen from the ambient air crosses in the opposite direction to saturate the hemoglobin contained in the red cells. This material then transports the oxygen to the various tissues and releases it according to the demands of that particular tissue. Brain and myocardium (heart) tissues use much more oxygen than eye, skin and hair tissues. Various diseases and injuries increase oxygen use, especially those conditions associated with fever, infec-

tion or tissue injury such as burns. Persons who have anemia (decreased circulating red cells and hemoglobin) or alterations in their hemoglobin (such as saturation with carbon monoxide displacing oxygen from the normal hemoglobin as in heavy cigarette smokers) will not be able to deliver adequate quantities of oxygen, and therefore certain tissues will suffer. In red cells stored in the blood banks of hospitals or the American Red Cross the capacity for oxygen deliverance during the first 24 hours is greatly reduced, even though the patient's skin may appear to be pink after the transfusion.

There are many different kinds of white cells. Granulocytes (polymorphonuclear leukocytes) can be called to a specific source or site of infection or inflammation to search out and destroy bacteria or foreign substances. These cells can ingest bacteria and destroy it with certain enzymes they contain and rid the body of potentially lethal infections. A large decrease in the number of circulating granulocytes makes a person more susceptible to infections and complications.

Lymphocytes, another form of circulating white blood cell, help fight infections and inflammation in a different way. They respond to various problems by making antibodies that circulate in the plasma, as well as helping other cells remove foreign material, bacteria and viruses from the body. These cells likewise can change into plasma cells (normally not seen circulating in the peripheral blood) that then are directly capable of making antibodies in response to a particular infection. Other white cells, such as basophils, eosinophils and monocytes, have similar but lesser roles in keeping the body free from infections or inflammation. The white cells are one of the many defense mechanisms against infection. Others include the skin, lymphatic system and antibodies.

Platelets are the smallest cellular element in the circulating blood, but their function is still critical to maintaining hemostasis (blood clotting). Too few platelets can lead to bruising and easy bleeding and can aggravate or prolong bleeding when a vessel is injured. Similarly, a person with an extraordinarily high platelet count may have an increased tendency to blood clotting (thrombosis) or, paradoxically, may bleed for unknown reasons.

Many diseases and drugs can affect the normal function and activity of the platelets. For instance, aspirin can interfere with the platelets' stickiness to the vessel walls and, in some persons, can accentuate bleeding abnormalities. Even in some normal persons, bleeding times (one of the many laboratory tests used to evaluate hemostasis) may be prolonged after aspirin ingestion. This effect on the platelets lasts the lifetime of the platelets involved (six to ten days).

BLOOD PLASMA

The plasma or liquid phase of the blood serves numerous functions. Some of the more important are discussed here.

1. Plasma carries wastes and potentially toxic materials from various areas of the body for excretion through the kidneys.
2. Plasma maintains another phase of hemostasis (adequate blood clotting) through a totally different system known as the plasmatic coagulation system. (Patients with so-called classic hemophilia are in this category.) These patients lack a single plasmastic coagulation factor from birth and have a severe bleeding tendency, not only with trauma but also spontaneously into joints, tissues and, rarely, the brain. Acquired defects of coagulation, such as severe liver disease (the organ that makes many of the clotting factors), also can occur.

3. Plasma is the main vehicle for carrying nutrients, including fats, protein and carbohydrates, to and from various organs (especially the liver) for processing and further use in the body's metabolic processes. These nutrients are then stored in tissues for caloric expenditure, that is, energy.
4. Plasma maintains adequate circulation of electrolytes, minerals, nutrients and vitamins. Alterations in their quantities can lead to many different problems, especially in active athletes. Contraction or reduction of the plasma volume, as seen in severe heat exhaustion with dehydration and inadequate fluid replacement, can cause delirium, a rising temperature, confusion, coma and shock. Certain situations give rise to increased amounts of plasma and fluid within the vascular compartment. Excessive swelling in the legs, hands or other tissues may be caused by heart failure, liver failure or an alteration in proteins in the bloodstream that tend to maintain normal water balances within and without the body.
5. Small quantities of oxygen to aid the red cells in oxygen delivery are carried by plasma.

BLOOD PARAMETERS

Hemoglobin Content

Anemia, most commonly due to lack of iron, is seen in women who have heavy menstrual periods and persons bleeding from peptic ulcers or other lesions in the gastrointestinal tract. Occasionally, a person gives blood at his local blood bank every few months and depletes his iron stores without adequate replacement. Over time, this can lead to iron deficiency, especially in the menstruating female. Although there are numerous other reasons for anemia, these are the most commonly encountered in the athlete.

White Blood Cell Count

Alterations in the leukocyte count are much less common, unless the person has a serious disease or a drug-induced low leukocyte count. The normal leukocyte count varies from laboratory to laboratory but usually is between 4,000 and 10,000/cu mm of blood. Persons with bacterial infections may have substantially increased leukocyte counts. Early during the course of a viral illness such as flu, measles, or chickenpox, however, the leukocyte count may decrease to low levels and then return to normal as the disease progresses. This self-limited change is a normal response to a given stimulus. In fact, such alterations may be clues to help identify possible causes of an otherwise unexplained fever and infection.

All athletes should have a screening complete blood cell count (CBC) at the beginning of the school year. A physician should evaluate those with abnormal levels to learn the cause. Proper treatment for either red or white blood cell abnormalities can then be instituted (Table 27:1).

An athlete whose performance has deteriorated or who seems tired or listless may have a blood dyscrasia. If this persists, he should also be referred for medical examination.

Platelet Count

A very low or high platelet count in the blood usually indicates serious disease process and requires extensive evaluation. Excess bruising and bleeding may be the clinical clue. An athlete who bruises too easily should be referred to the team physician for a coagulation evaluation.

Plasma Alterations

In the otherwise healthy person, alterations in the plasmatic (or liquid) phase of the blood usually are not important, as long as adequate hydration and electrolyte balance are maintained. Medication, such as diuretics to remove excessive fluid from the body, can reduce the amount of water in the liquid phase of the blood, sometimes to the point of causing unsteadiness, light-headedness and muscle cramping.

Normal or physiologic plasma alterations can take place, especially with some sports, for example, long-distance running. In addition to certain changes in enzymes and fats in the blood, long-distance runners tend to have lower levels of circulating erythrocytes and hemoglobin than others. These values usually decrease but stay within the normal range. Occasionally patients have a so-called pseudo-anemia when the reduced level of erythrocytes and the increase in plasma volume seen in long-distance runners accounts for the alteration of the hemoglobin, which, in fact, does not signify any particular disease process. Consider these abnormalities with activities that take place over a sustained period and require maximum cardiac output. In runners and other endurance-trained athletes, low or low-normal hemoglobin values are common, seldom reflect true anemia and do not indicate the need for iron, folic acid or vitamin B12 (the building blocks of the bone marrow to produce red cells). In women runners oral iron therapy probably should be given only if blood loss from menstruation seems excessive.

TABLE 27:1. Normal Blood Cell Values*

	Men	Women
Red cell count, cells in millions/mm^3	4.7–6.1	4.2–5.2
Hemoglobin, g%	13.4–17.6	12.0–15.4
Hematocrit, vol%	42–53	38–46
MCV,[†] μm^3	81–96	
MCHC,[‡] g%	30–36	
Total white cell count, cells/mm^3	4–10,000	
Granulocytes		
PMNs,[§] %	38–70	
Eosinophils, %	1–5	
Basophils, %	0–2	
Monocytes, %	1–8	
Lymphocytes, %	15–45	
Platelets, cells/mm^3	200,000–400,000	
Reticulocyte count, %	1–2	

*Slightly variable to labs
[†]Mean corpuscular volume
[‡]Mean corpuscular hemoglobin concentration
[§]Polymorphonuclear leukocytes

The Cardiovascular System

The primary function of the heart is to pump blood at a rate that meets the metabolic needs of the body. The principal metabolic need is oxygen. Hence, the oxygen demands of the tissues of the body, at rest or during exercise, ultimately determine the minute-to-minute cardiac output requirements. The structure and performance of the normal heart are uniquely designed to serve this function.

CARDIAC CYCLE

The cardiac cycle is the electromechanical sequence of events that occurs with one contraction (systole) and relaxation (diastole) of the heart muscles (Fig. 28:1). Knowledge of the physical events of cardiac cycle is fundamental to understanding the heart as a pump.

Each cardiac cycle is initiated by an electrical impulse that propagates over the atria and the ventricles, and results in depolarization and contraction of the individual myocardial cells (Fig. 28:2). Under normal conditions, the impulse originates in the sinoatrial node located in the upper right atrium close to its junction with the superior vena cava. Upon leaving the sinoatrial node, the impulse depolarizes the surrounding atrial muscles, producing atrial contraction, and then travels rapidly via specialized conduction tissue to the left atrium and to the atrioventricular (AV) node. The electrocardiographic correlate of atrial contraction is the P wave.

After traversing the AV node, the impulse proceeds rapidly down the bundle branches to the Purkinje network where the myocardial

28

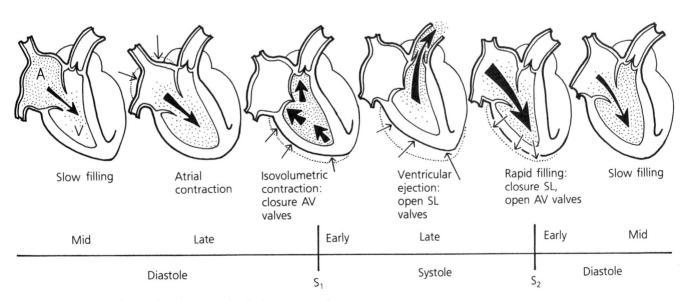

Slow filling	Atrial contraction	Isovolumetric contraction: closure AV valves	Ventricular ejection: open SL valves	Rapid filling: closure SL, open AV valves	Slow filling
Mid	Late	Early	Late	Early	Mid

Diastole — S₁ — Systole — S₂ — Diastole

FIGURE 28:1. Cardiac cycle; electromechanical sequence of events through contraction and relaxation of heart muscles

ATRIAL EXCITATION

Begins   Complete

Sinoatrial node (SA)

Atrioventricular node (AV)

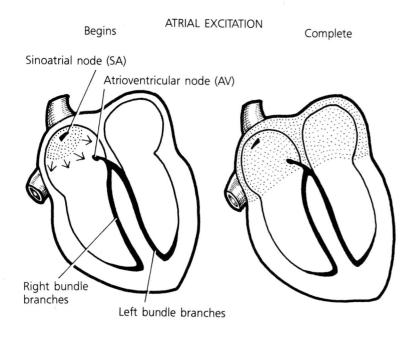

Right bundle
branches

Left bundle branches

VENTRICULAR EXCITATION

Begins   Complete

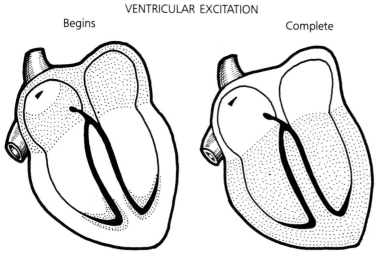

FIGURE 28:2.   Path of electrical impulse that initiates each cardiac cycle

Following the P wave, the atrium contracts, increasing the atrial pressure and propelling blood across the mitral and tricuspid valves. At approximately the peak of the QRS complex, ventricular pressure begins to rapidly rise, initiating ventricular systole. When ventricular pressure exceeds atrial pressure, the AV valves close and may even bulge back into the atrium to some degree. After the closure of the mitral valve and before the opening of the aortic and pulmonary valves, the pressure in the ventricle rises rapidly due to ventricular contraction against its volume of blood.

When the pressure of the ventricle exceeds that of the aorta or pulmonary artery, the semilunar valves open and blood is rapidly ejected out of the heart into these vessels (rapid ejection phase). Ventricular pressure continues to rise briefly, then as the ventricular muscle begins to relax, the pressure begins to fall rapidly. Due to the kinetic energy of the blood, there is still flow across the semilunar valves, even though a pressure gradient no longer exists. Soon vessel pressure exceeds the energy of the outcoming blood, however, and the flow tends to reverse. This causes the semilunar valves to close suddenly, ending the systolic phase, which is followed by a brief rise in aortic and pulmonic pressure (see Fig. 28:4).

When the pressure in the left ventricle drops to a point below the atrial pressure, the mitral valve opens and blood from the atria rushes into the ventricles, initiating the rapid filling phase of the ventricle. Atrial pressure drops rapidly as blood leaves, which reflects this rapid filling phase. As the ventricle accepts this rapid filling, it becomes distended with the in-rushing blood and the pressure begins to rise rapidly. As this occurs, the ventricular and atrial pressures begin to equilibrate and flow into the ventricle is much slower—a slow filling phase. Following this, atrial systole occurs and initiates the cycle again.

CARDIAC OUTPUT

Four major determinants normally regulate the performance of the intact heart. These are in-

cells are activated. Ventricular activation is expressed electrocardiographically by the QRS complex (Fig. 28:3), followed by the T wave that represents ventricular repolarization.

The mechanical events that follow electrical activation of the heart are easily explained by observing the pressure changes that occur in the atria and in the ventricles (Fig. 28:4).

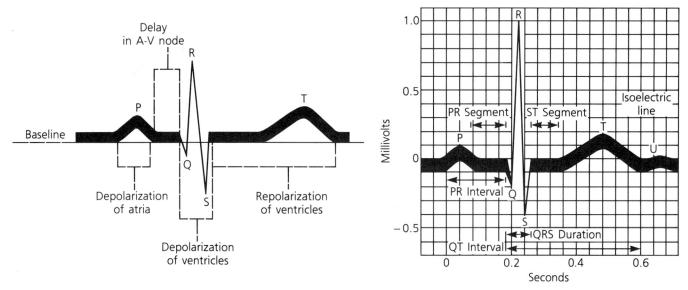

FIGURE 28:3.   The QRS cycle expresses ventricular activation. The T wave represents ventricular repolarization.

tegrated to govern the stroke volume and cardiac output. Stroke volume—the amount of blood ejected per beat—has three determinants—preload, afterload and contractility. Cardiac output—the amount of blood (liters) ejected by the heart per minute—is determined by the frequency of contraction, i.e., heart rate. Thus, cardiac output per se is the stroke volume times the heart rate. Preload is a factor of muscle quality. An elastic distensible ventricle in a young man propels more blood more rapidly than the stiffer, less distensible ventricle in an older man because the stretch in the ventricular muscle fibers from the same volume of blood is greater in the young.

Afterload is simply the impedance of forward flow of blood from the ventricle and relates, therefore, directly to the resistance in the arterial system as manifested by aortic pressure. Left ventricular pressure must exceed aortic pressure before forward flow can occur. Thus, high blood pressure is injurious because it greatly increases the workload of the left ventricle by resisting forward flow. So, too, do obstructing lesions that impede flow out of the left ventricle, such as narrowing of the aortic valves.

Contractility is the most difficult concept to portray, since it cannot be measured directly. Conceptually it refers to the overall capacity of the muscle fibers of the ventricles to shorten and to do useful work. Contractility can be very poor in people with severely diseased or damaged hearts or vigorous with exceptional output in trained athletes.

The final major determinant of cardiac performance is heart rate. It is determined by the firing rate of the sinus node as modulated by the constant flow of neural signals (sympathetic increases rate; parasympathetic decreases rate) from the cardioregulatory centers in the brain, in the chemical (humoral) substances circulating in the blood such as adrenalin and from the thyroid hormones.

These four parameters of cardiac performance—preload (end-diastolic volume or pressure), afterload (aortic pressure), contractile state (inherent power to develop force) and heart rate—not only define the pumping capabilities of the heart, but are also the major determinants of the oxygen needs of the working heart muscle itself (Fig. 28:5). This oxygen demand correlates best in man with the product of the heart rate and blood

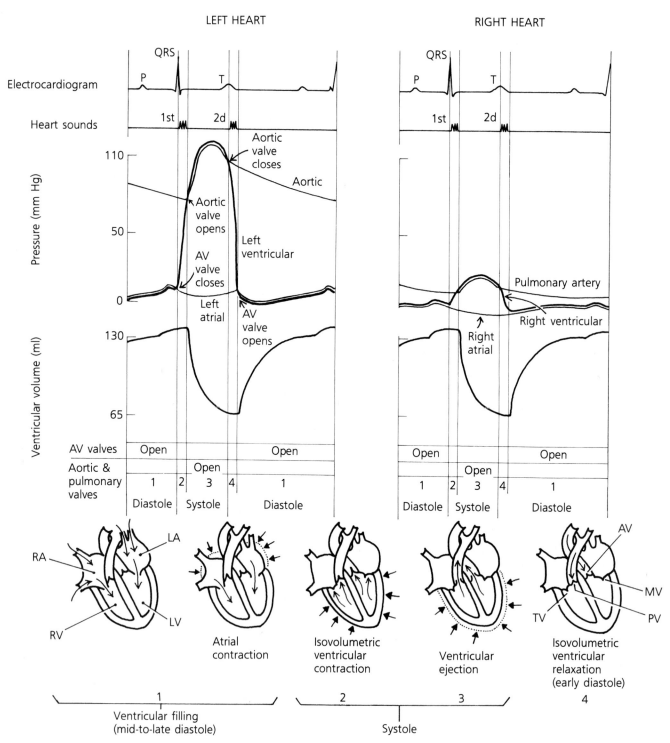

FIGURE 28:4. Atrial and ventricular events in left and right heart corresponding to systole and diastole contractions and relaxations. (AV = aortic valve, MV = mitral valve, PV = pulmonic valve, TV = tricuspid valve)

pressure both at rest and with exercise. More importantly, this oxygen demand generated by the interaction of rate, pressure and activity can only be met by adequate coronary blood flow.

Under resting conditions, the working myocardium uses 8 to 9 mm of oxygen per 100 gm of ventricular tissue, or about 7% of the body's total oxygen requirement. Increase in any of the four parameters of cardiac performance sharply increases this oxygen requirement, which can only be met by increasing flow in the coronary artery. This is because all of the available oxygen presented to the working myocardium is extracted in a single pass. Thus, increased oxygen demands in coronary beds can only be met by increased coronary blood flow. Fortunately, the coronary arterial bed has the capability of increasing flow six-fold or providing for an increased oxygen demand of 500% over base conditions.

From this analysis it is clear that narrowing in one or more of the major coronary arteries can compromise coronary blood flow even at rest, and certainly with exercise. This may result in chest pain or angina due to lack of oxygen available to the working heart muscles. This is simply an imbalance between supply and demand. Complete block of the major coronary vessels results in total lack of oxygen to the functioning myocardial muscle cells and inevitably results in permanent injury—myocardial infarction.

Coronary blood flow is closely regulated by myocardial oxygen demand but also follows certain physical laws of flow inherent in a closed-pipe system such as the circulatory system. These physical principles of flow relate to all blood vessels in the body.

CIRCULATION OF THE BLOOD

Blood flows through vessels because of the pulsatile pumping action of the heart and the pressure differential across the system from the left ventricle (100–110 mm Hg) to the right atrium (5–10 mm Hg). This critical driving force permits adequate flow. Loss of pressure,

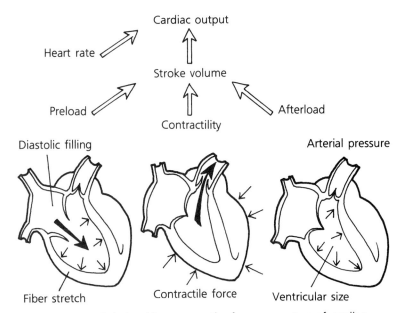

FIGURE 28:5. Relationships among the four parameters of cardiac performance

such as in shock, immediately compromises flow in the critical organs, such as the heart, brain and kidneys, and if prolonged results in death.

Over a century ago, a French physician, Jean Poiseuille, studied continuous flow in small rigid tubes. He carefully delineated the elements that comply with distance and formulated the equations that govern flow in such tubes. His formula, known as Poiseuille's law, indicates that volume flow in a tube is directly proportional to the pressure drop along the length of the tube and to the radius of that tube to the fourth power, and is inversely proportional to the length of the tube and to the viscosity or thickness of the fluid flowing through that tube. Therefore, the geometry of the tube (length and radius) is very important in determining the flow and resistance, and small changes in vessel radius can produce large changes in flow. For example, a 20% increase in radius will produce over a 100% increase in flow (Fig. 28:6).

Poiseuille's law measures internal friction of a fluid. Fluids of high viscosity (i.e., molasses) impede flow to a much greater

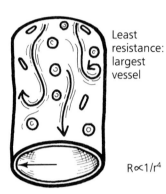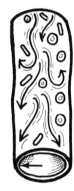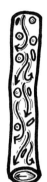

Least resistance: largest vessel

Most resistance: smallest vessel

$R \propto 1/r^4$

FIGURE 28:6. Poiseuille's law of flow through a tube

degree than low viscosity fluids such as water. In man—as hematocrit is the major determinant of viscosity—polycythemic states tend to reduce flow whereas anemia (hemoglobin less than 8 gm) substantially increases blood flow.

The velocity of flow through the circulation is a function of the cross-sectional area of the vessels, such that V1 × A1 = V2 × A2, where V – velocity and A = area. Thus, in the arterial system, where total cross-section area is small, velocities are high. In the capillary system, with its huge total cross-section area, velocity is very slow. In the venous system, which also has a fairly large cross-section area, flows are faster but low compared to those in the arterial system.

In general, sympathetic stimulation increases atrial and ventricular contractility, increases heart rate, and speeds the spread of excitation through the AV node and, slightly, through the ventricles. Vagal stimulation generally has the opposite effect. At any instant, the effect of the nervous system on the heart is a net balance of these two opposing controls, which usually vary reciprocally. The vagal parasympathetic stimulation, generally inhibitory, normally predominates and maintains the usual resting heart rate of about 65 to 75 beats per minute. But during exercise, the sympathetic nervous system becomes dominant.

Neural reflexes, particularly from stretch receptors in the carotid sinus and aorta, form a major intrinsic control mechanism influencing myocardial performance directly and indirectly. Arterial hypotension produces decreased carotid sinus stretch. This triggers the sympathetic nervous system, resulting in increased venous return and thereby increased ventricular end-diastolic fiber length. Simultaneously, carotid sinus hypotension produces arterial vasoconstriction, increasing peripheral vascular resistance and aortic impedance, and thus tends to increase blood pressure. Furthermore, carotid sinus hypotension elicits reflexes that increase atrial and ventricular contractility.

Drugs and Hormones

Myocardial contractility is increased by digitalis, calcium and catecholamines, including norepinephrine, epinephrine, isoproterenol and dopamine. Contractility is also increased by corticosteroids, spironolactone, angiotensin, serotonin, glucagon, some prostaglandins and cardioglobulins. The actions of thyroxine on myocardial contractile functions are complex but, in general, it may be said to enhance cardiac contractility. Myocardial contractility is decreased by hypoxia and by many drugs, including barbiturates, quinidine, propranolol, procainamide and lidocaine. Acidosis also depresses myocardial contractility, particularly if the sympathoadrenal system function is impaired.

EXERCISE AND THE HEART

The mechanisms used to increase cardiac output during exercise vary depending on age, condition, posture and athletic conditioning. In particular, the relative contribution of heart rate and stroke volume is a subject of considerable interest. When in a supine position most normal persons without athletic conditioning appear to increase their cardiac output during mild to moderate exercise mainly by an increase in heart rate rather than an increase in stroke volume. With more extreme exercise, this type of individual increases stroke volume about 10% to 15% in the supine position and

30% to 100% in the upright position, despite a considerably shortened systolic ejection. Normal persons more accustomed to physical exercise show an earlier, more marked increase in stroke volume in both positions, and stroke volume often doubles during upright exercise. Heart rate may increase threefold or even fourfold in trained athletes, whereas stroke volume increases considerably less and can even decline with extreme increases in rate.

The arterial systolic blood pressure often increases 40 mm Hg to 60 mm Hg during moderate or severe exercise, although the mean arterial blood pressure increases much less. The diastolic pressure may increase slightly, decrease slightly or stay the same. Arterial resistance normally decreases considerably during exercise. The combination of vasodilatation of the exercising muscles and the increased activity of the muscles and the abdominal thoracic pump increases the venous return to the heart, further contributing to the increased cardiac output. Exercise also produces a decrease in the volume of blood in venous reservoirs, especially the splenic blood volumes. These shifts make more blood available to the heart, arterial vessels and its exercising muscles. On the other hand, during prolonged exercise, plasma volume may decrease substantially with a resultant increase in hematocrit.

During exercise, there is a major redistribution of the elevated cardiac output. During mild to moderate exercise, coronary blood flow and blood flow to the active skeletal muscle increases and cerebral flow is maintained, whereas renal and splenic flows diminish. During more extreme exercise, these changes are exaggerated and flow to the inactive muscles may decrease. During maximal exercise flow, cerebral flow may also decrease because of hyperventilation and respiratory alkalosis. Skin flow may decrease initially during exercise but then rise during continued exercise to help cool the body.

Physiologically, three kinds of skeletal muscular contractions put demands on the cardiovascular system. The first occurs with iso- metric contraction, such as in a tug of war. The second is dynamic exercise with rhythmical contraction of flexor and extensor muscle groups, such as in walking and jogging. The third is a combination of sustained and dynamic exercise, such as when a person walks rapidly carrying a heavy object. Static exercise to the point of fatigue, such as in a weight lifter, imposes a disproportionate pressure load relative to aerobic requirements on the left ventricle. Dynamic exercise causes a greater acceleration of heart rate, proportional to the greater aerobic requirements. The third type of exercise creates a mixed response. The first and third types of exercise if repeated in rapid sequence can be hazardous, particularly for persons with serious hypertension or coronary vascular disease, because of rapidly developing afterload on the left ventricle. Worse yet for such individuals is that, as cumulative endogenous heart load develops and arterial pressure falls, coronary perfusion may be compromised while demands for peripheral blood flow remain high. Of the three types of exercise, that best suited to develop cardiac fitness is dynamic repetitive exercise such as walking, jogging or swimming.

Currently, in the area of cardiovascular medicine, exercise has a dual role. By increasing the work load of the heart exercise can uncover an imbalance between supply and demand and thus identify coronary artery disease not otherwise suspected in the resting basal state. Safe levels of exercise for middle-aged persons can be established. The other role of exercise, of course, is to achieve cardiovascular fitness. Cardiovascular fitness improves cardiac performance by achieving work loads at less cost. Heart rate and blood pressure response at given work loads are reduced and contractility of the heart and blood supply to the peripheral working muscles are improved. This effect is achieved by exercising for 30 to 40 minutes, three to four times a week, at approximately 75% of the maximal expected oxygen capacity determined primarily by heart rate in the middle-aged in the range of 130 to 145 beats per minute.

CARDIOVASCULAR ENDURANCE

The ability of athletes to reach a high level of performance in most sports partially depends upon the supply of oxygen to the working muscle tissues, especially the heart. This is provided by the cardiovascular system: heart, lungs, arteries, veins and capillaries. As the work load on the muscle tissues increases during athletic activity, the muscles' need for oxygen increases along with a concomitant need to eliminate carbon dioxide.

Cardiovascular endurance is the ability of the cardiovascular system to meet the oxygen-carbon dioxide transport demands of high work loads and maintain efficiency for long periods of time. When the oxygen needs are being met during activity, the athlete is working in aerobic metabolism. If the work load during activity becomes so great that the cardiovascular system is unable to meet the needs of the working muscles, the anaerobic is activated. Performance soon deteriorates and the athlete will eventually have to stop.

Both aerobic and anaerobic metabolism capacities can be increased through training. Aerobic training involves some type of continuous muscular activity with minimal resistance for 20 to 60 minutes. The intensity of the activity should be great enough to increase the heart rate by 70% to 85% of the athlete's maximum. The theoretical maximum heart rate can be roughly calculated by subtracting the athlete's age from 220 and taking 70% of this figure. Thus a 20-year-old athlete would

have a maximum heart rate of 200, and his target heart rate would be 140 beats per minute. Aerobic activities include: running, cycling, cross country skiing, swimming and walking.

Given the trained athlete's greater cardiovascular efficiency, he can exercise at a greater intensity before crossing over into anaerobic metabolism. When the athlete goes into anaerobic metabolism, the muscles will continue contracting for a short period of time, but lactic acid begins to accumulate leading to a deterioration in athletic performance and eventually complete muscle failure. Through training, the athlete can withstand a greater buildup of lactic acid before performance deteriorates.

Anaerobic training should supplement the aerobic training for athletes likely to be involved in short bursts of speed in their sports. The relative emphasis of each type of training depends upon the state of training of the athlete and the physical demands of the sport involved. For instance, a distance runner would concentrate primarily on aerobic training while the sprinter would concentrate primarily on anaerobic training. One type of training, however, carries over to the other, so the sprinter should have some degree of aerobic efficiency and the distance runner some anaerobic training for sprinting near the end of the race. (See Chapter 14 for additional discussion of cardiovascular endurance and anaerobic and aerobic exercise.)

Control of Bleeding

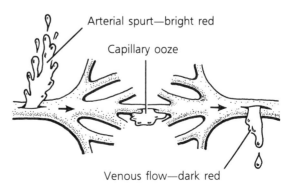

29

Direct pressure on a bleeding point is the most effective way to control hemorrhage. Bleeding and hemorrhage mean the same thing, namely, that blood is escaping from arteries or veins. Bleeding may be external or internal. In either case, it is dangerous. The average adult body has 6 liters of blood. The loss of 1 liter of blood in an adult or 500 ml of blood in a child is very dangerous. In an infant, the loss of even 25 to 30 ml of blood can cause signs of shock. Hemorrhage initially results in weakness and, ultimately, if uncontrolled, in shock and death.

Blood is transported within the circulatory system through blood vessels (Chapter 28). Injury and some diseases disrupt the vessels, resulting in bleeding. Characteristically, blood from an artery spurts and is bright red. Blood from a vein generally comes in a slow and steady flow, and is much darker. Abraded and open, minute capillaries bleed in a continuous, steady ooze (Fig. 29:1). The rapidity of bleeding is very important. The average adult may comfortably lose a pint (500 ml) of blood donated in a blood donor center over 15 or 20 minutes. During the course of the loss of this blood, the body adapts well to its being withdrawn. If larger amounts are lost, especially more suddenly, the patient may show signs and symptoms of shock or permanent vascular changes, or may die.

EXTERNAL BLEEDING

External bleeding is hemorrhage that can be seen coming from a wound. Some examples of external hemorrhage are bleeding from open fractures, bleeding from wounds and nosebleeds. In most instances, bleeding stops naturally in from six to ten minutes because the body has many mechanisms of defense, among which are those that arrest bleeding. If a finger is cut, blood gushes from the lacerated vessels. The vessels react by constricting at the cut ends, which diminishes the hemorrhage. A clot then forms at the cut end, which stops the bleeding as the clot increases in size and plugs the hole. Body tissues and tissue fluid activate the clotting mechanism within blood. Normally, blood within an artery or vein is protected from contact with other body tissues by the vessel wall and does not clot. When blood escapes from an artery or vein and this protection is gone, it clots.

In a severe injury, the damaged blood vessels may be so large that clots cannot physically occlude them. Sometimes only a portion of the vessel wall is torn, and thus the wall cannot retract and constrict. In these cases, bleeding must be stopped by external means. Blood loss may occasionally be so rapid that the patient will bleed to death before normal protective processes can be activated. The

FIGURE 29:1. Abraded capillary loops bleed in a continuous ooze.

trainer must know how to control bleeding. In general, after securing an airway and being certain the patient can breathe, the second matter of immediate concern is the control of hemorrhage.

CONTROLLING BLEEDING

The control of bleeding is often very simple. Local pressure will control almost all instances of external bleeding by stopping the physical flow of blood and permitting normal blood coagulation. External bleeding can be controlled in several ways (Fig. 29:2).

1. With a finger, hand or pressure dressing exert direct pressure over the wound. This method is by far the most effective.
2. Apply pressure on a major artery proximal to the wound to occlude blood flow in that artery. This method may diminish the rate of bleeding but will rarely stop it because of arterial collateral circulation, around the pressure point, to the distal bleeder.
3. Apply a normal splint or air pressure splint.
4. Apply a pneumatic counterpressure device.
5. Apply a tourniquet as a last resort proximal to the wound on an affected extremity.

Local Pressure

Although the initial application of pressure over a wound may be done with a finger or hand, a sterile pressure dressing is preferable. A sterile bandage is made up of gauze pads, with a universal dressing (9 × 36 inches) applied over them at the point where pressure is needed. The actual pressure is maintained by wrapping the wound circumferentially and firmly with sterile, roller, self-adhering bandages. The entire mass of the sterile dressing should be covered above and below the wound by the bandage, stretched sufficiently tight to arrest the hemorrhage. If sterile pads are not immediately available, a handkerchief, a sanitary napkin, a clean cloth or the bare hand can be used to apply pressure. Do not remove a dressing once in place until the pa-

tient is evaluated by the physician in the emergency department. If bleeding continues after the dressing is applied, usually not enough pressure has been used. In such instances, apply more pressure on the wound through the dressing with a hand, tighten the bandage or add additional pads. Any of these methods should stop the bleeding.

Pressure-point Control

When pressure dressings are not available at all, proximal arterial pressure control can sometimes control slow bleeding in an emergency. Pulse points for major arteries were discussed in Chapter 5. Rarely does compression of a major feeding artery proximal to a wound completely arrest hemorrhage from a wound distal to that artery because of the rich supply of collateral arterial vessels around the pressure point. Although proximal arterial pressure should be kept in mind and may occasionally help, often it will not.

Splints

Muscles lacerated by sharp ends of broken bones or vessels lying in the fractured bone create heavy bleeding from injured extremities both externally and internally. So long as the fracture is not controlled, continued laceration and further damage of partially clotted vessels are possible resulting in more bleeding. Often applying a splint to a badly fractured and lacerated extremity (Fig. 29:2) allows prompt control of hemorrhage. In general, injuries are not isolated phenomena. Hemorrhage accompanies nearly all severe injuries, and treating the underlying injury may aid markedly in controlling the hemorrhage. The principles of applying splints are given in Chapter 16.

Tourniquets

A tourniquet to control bleeding is almost never necessary. Tourniquets are not recommended for general use because they sometimes cause more damage to injured extremities than does the injury itself. They crush a

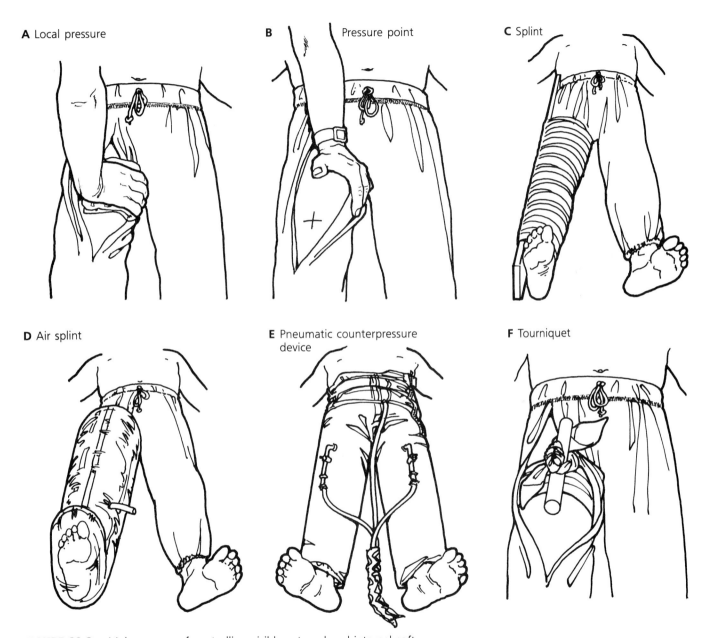

A Local pressure

B Pressure point

C Splint

D Air splint

E Pneumatic counterpressure device

F Tourniquet

FIGURE 29:2. Major means of controlling visible external and internal soft tissue bleeding

considerable amount of tissue beneath them, can cause permanent damage of nerves and blood vessels, and, if left on for any appreciable length of time, can result in the loss of the extremity. Nevertheless, a properly applied tourniquet may save the life of a person bleeding uncontrollably from a major vessel. Specifically, a tourniquet may be called for in a traumatic amputation, either partial or complete, or when local pressure fails to control bleeding. If a tourniquet must be used, apply it correctly (Fig. 29:3).

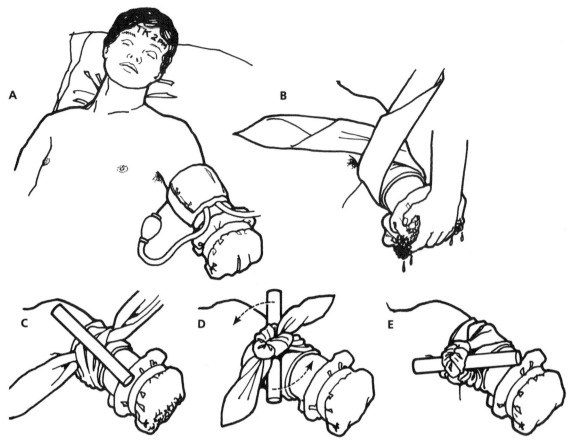

FIGURE 29:3. Proper application of a tourniquet. **A** A sphygmo-manometer cuff can serve. **B–E** Tourniquet application with bandage

1. Fold a triangular bandage to 3 or 4 inches wide and about six or eight layers thick.
2. Wrap this long, 4 inch wide bandage twice around the extremity proximal to the bleeding but as far distal as possible (Fig. 29:3B).
3. Tie one knot in the bandage. Place a stick or metal rod on top of the flat knot and tie the ends of the bandage over the stick in a square knot (Figs. 29:3C, D).
4. Use the stick as a handle to twist the bandage to tighten the tourniquet until the bleeding stops. Once the bleeding has ceased, make no more turns with the stick. Secure the stick or rod in place and make the wrapping neat and smooth (Fig. 29:3E). This technique of using a rod passed through the bandage to achieve pressure is called the Spanish Windlass and is also used to apply traction splints.

When using the tourniquet observe certain precautions.

1. Use as wide a bandage as possible and tighten it securely.

2. Never use wire or any other material that will cut into the skin.
3. Do not loosen the tourniquet until a physician evaluates the patient.
4. Never cover a tourniquet with a bandage. Leave it open and in full view. Always signify that the patient has had a tourniquet applied by writing TK indelibly on the patient's forehead and on any identification tag attached to the patient. Also include the time that the tourniquet was applied on the tag and forehead. In addition, be sure to point out to the medical staff that the patient has a tourniquet.
5. Never place a tourniquet below the knee or elbow because in certain more distal areas in the extremities nerves lie close to the skin and may be injured by compression. Furthermore, bleeding distal to the knee or elbow that requires tourniquet control is rare.
6. If a blood pressure cuff is used, continuously monitor the gauge to be sure that pressure is not being gradually lost.

Shock

30

The term shock has a variety of meanings, physiological and otherwise. It is used to denote any amount of electric current received by a person. Some refer to a sudden hemorrhage or clot in the brain as a shock or, more commonly, a stroke. Generally, in medicine shock means the cardiovascular system is in a state of collapse.

The cardiovascular system circulates blood to all the cells, bringing them oxygen and food and removing waste products. The brain, the spinal cord, the peripheral nervous system and the heart require a constant flow of blood to live. Any suspension of blood flow for more than a very few minutes, especially in the nervous system, and their component cells die.

The cardiovascular system consists of two parts: a container and its contents. The container is the heart and its system of blood vessels, arteries, veins, innumerable small arterioles, venules and capillaries. These tubes extend to every cell in the body. Within this container is the blood.

The arteries and the arterial ends of the capillaries have distinct muscular walls—they can open and close as directed. The fine capillaries that pass between individual cells and link the arterioles to the venules can also open or close. The opening or closing of these vessels is entirely automatic and is under the control of the autonomic nervous system (sympathetic and parasympathetic). Stimuli that cause the opening or closing of these vessels include fright, heat, cold, an organ's need for oxygen or an organ's need to dispose of waste. In a normal person never are all the vessels fully opened or fully closed.

Normally there is just enough blood in the container to fill the system absolutely full. In an average adult, this amount is 6 liters. If the heart pumps 6 liters a minute through a system that can hold just 6 liters, every part of the system receives a regular supply of blood every minute. The condition in which this system fails to provide sufficient circulation to every part of the body is called shock.

Perfusion means the circulation of blood within an organ. An organ is perfused if blood enters it through the arteries and leaves it through the veins. Thus, blood must pass through the capillaries, give up nutrients and oxygen and pick up waste. Perfusion of the whole body by blood keeps the component cells of the body healthy. In states of shock, the perfusion of organs and tissues fails.

Certain organs of the body are more susceptible than others to lack of adequate perfusions. The brain, the spinal cord and peripheral nervous system cannot lose perfusion for more than 4 to 6 minutes without permanent damage of their cells. Damage in the kidney results after inadequate perfusion for 30 to 45 minutes. The heart requires constant perfusion or it will not function properly. Skeletal muscle can be permanently damaged if it loses perfusion for 2 hours. The gastrointestinal tract can survive with impaired perfusion for a number of hours but no part of the body can exist without adequate perfusion for an indefinite period. Permanent injury results when the organ system most sensitive to the lack of adequate perfusion is damaged—the central and peripheral nervous system.

The concept of perfusion is the unifying element in shock. While there are several separate causes for shock, they induce shock in only three ways. Whatever the cause of shock,

365

deficient perfusion in organs and tissues causes them to start to die.

Shock is a relative loss of intravascular oxygen-carrying mass. There are three major causes of shock.

1. The heart can be damaged so that it fails to perform properly as a pump.
2. Blood can be lost so that the volume of fluid within the vascular container is insufficient.
3. The blood vessels constituting the container can dilate so that the blood within them, even though of normal volume, is still insufficient to fill the system and provide efficient circulation.

In all instances, the results of shock are exactly the same. There is insufficient perfusion of blood through the tissues of the body to provide adequate food and oxygen and to carry away waste. All normal bodily processes are affected and vital functions slow down. If the conditions causing shock are not promptly arrested and reversed, death soon follows.

Shock is a certain precursor of death unless it is treated and reversed. One does not see shock itself, however, but a falling blood pressure, a rising pulse, a pale, ashen, cold, clammy skin, poor urinary flow, agitation and air hunger. These signs herald imminent, severe cardiovascular collapse.

Shock is likely in many clinical situations: massive bleeding, internal or external; multiple severe fractures; an acute abdomen; spinal injuries and generalized sepsis.

TYPES AND CAUSES OF SHOCK

Shock may accompany many different emergency situations. Ordinarily, they can all be related to one of the three major causes. Common types of shock are:

1. Hemorrhagic (blood loss)
2. Respiratory (inadequate oxygen supply)
3. Neurogenic (loss of vascular control by the nervous system)
4. Psychogenic (the common faint)
5. Cardiogenic (inadequate functioning of the heart)
6. Septic (severe infection and blood vessel damage)
7. Anaphylactic (allergic reaction)
8. Metabolic (loss of body fluid)

Hemorrhagic Shock

Shock following trauma is commonly due to blood loss. External bleeding may accompany severe lacerations or fractures. Internal bleeding follows rupture of the liver, the spleen or the great vessels within the abdomen or chest. Hemorrhagic shock is also seen with severe burns and extremely severe contusions or fractures. There may be no visible hemorrhage but a considerable amount of intravascular fluid (plasma or blood) is lost into the muscular tissues. Burns in particular produce extensive and alarming losses of plasma (the colorless part of the blood) and other body fluids into the burned tissues.

In crush injuries damaged blood vessels may also leak both blood and plasma into the injured tissues. If the patient is dehydrated (loss of body water) before injury, the state of shock is aggravated. This particular situation was commonly seen in personnel wounded in military actions in the tropics. In this environment they were constantly exposed to the sun and sweated heavily. In all the instances enumerated, the common factor is insufficient blood within the vascular container to provide adequate circulation to all organs of the body. This whole range of conditions is called hemorrhagic shock, or sometimes hypovolemic shock (''hypo'' meaning ''small'' and ''volemic'' meaning ''volume'').

Respiratory Shock

A sucking chest wound, a flail chest, an obstructed airway or a pneumothorax all may result in an inability to breathe adequately, so that an insufficient amount of oxygen is inspired. This condition may produce respiratory shock. If the patient has a broken neck with a spinal cord injury, the chest muscles may be paralyzed. Able to breathe only with the diaphragm, the patient may not be able to inspire adequately to take in enough oxygen.

Inadequate breathing can produce shock as rapidly as hemorrhage. In this instance, shock is produced because the amount of oxygen in the blood is insufficient. The volume of blood, the volume of the vascular container and the action of the heart are all normal, but the supply of oxygen carried in the blood is not. Without oxygen, the organs in the body cannot survive and their functions gradually deteriorate.

Neurogenic Shock

Paralysis of the autonomic nerves after spinal cord injuries may cause neurogenic shock. In this condition, the muscles of the blood vessels are essentially deprived of nerve supply and thus relax, causing general dilation of the cardiovascular system. Normally the muscles in these blood vessels, under the control of the autonomic nervous system, are in some degree of constriction. When the controlling nervous system is injured by spinal or neck trauma, vessels are released from its effect. Under no control at all, the vessels dilate widely. The available 6 liters of blood can then no longer fill the vascular system, which has become a much larger container. The entire system fails, perfusion of all organs becomes inadequate and shock ensues.

Psychogenic Shock

Psychogenic shock, or the common faint, is a sudden reaction of the nervous system that allows momentary vascular dilation. The result is a temporary reduction of blood supply to the brain because blood momentarily pools in the dilated vessels in other parts of the body. With this sudden sharply reduced blood supply, the brain ceases to function, and fainting ensues. Fear, bad news, sometimes good news, the sight of an injury or blood, the prospect of medical treatment, severe pain or anxiety are among the many precipitating causes of this condition. A person who is not feeling well, is tired or worried, or even obliged to stand quietly in a stuffy room may be more susceptible to fainting. Once the person has collapsed and become supine, circulation in the brain is restored and the episode passes promptly. In this type of shock, the major concern is any injury sustained during the fainting spell, such as when striking the head.

Cardiogenic Shock

Cardiogenic shock is shock caused by inadequate functioning of the heart. Circulation of blood throughout the vascular bed requires the constant action of a normal and vigorous heart muscle. Many types of disease cause the destruction or inflammation of this muscle. Within certain limits, the heart can adapt to these injuries, but with too much muscular impairment, as following some heart attacks, the heart no longer functions well. Shock from cardiac origin develops when the heart muscle can no longer impart sufficient pressure and force to circulate blood to all organs.

Septic Shock

In some patients with severe bacterial infections, the bacteria liberate toxins (poisons) into the blood stream and produce a state of shock called septic shock. In this condition the small vessels of the vascular system are dilated and plasma is lost through injured vessel walls. The toxins formed by the bacteria directly attack small blood vessel walls, rendering them leaky so that blood and plasma are lost from the capillaries into the tissues. The muscular elements of the walls of arterioles are damaged and no longer contract on direct stimulation.

This type of shock presents a rather complex problem. The volume of fluid is insufficient because much of the blood has leaked out of the vascular system into the tissues, while at the same time there is a larger than normal blood vessel bed to contain the smaller than normal volume of intravascular blood. This type of shock is almost always seen as a complication of prolonged hospitalization for serious illness, injury or surgery.

Anaphylactic Shock

Anaphylactic shock occurs when a person is sensitized to some substance by previous contact and reacts violently to another dose or contact. It is the most severe form of allergic reaction. Substances that most often cause allergic reactions in sensitized persons may be grouped as follows.

1. Injections of sera such as tetanus antitoxin or drugs such as penicillin
2. Ingestion of fish, shellfish or berries, medications or drugs such as oral penicillin can cause slower but equally severe reactions
3. Stings of the bee, wasp, yellow jacket or hornet can cause very rapid and severe, generalized anaphylactic reactions.
4. Inhalation of dusts, pollens or materials may similarly cause rapid and severe reactions

Anaphylactic shock is a very special and complex kind of allergic reaction. It is occasionally seen, however, and the trainer should know its signs and immediate treatment.

Metabolic Shock

In severe, untreated illnesses, such as diabetes, a state of shock may occur occasionally because of profound fluid loss from vomiting, diarrhea, excess urination or severe disturbance of the body fluid and acid-base balance. Patients who develop shock in the course of this type of chronic disease are desperately ill and may have reached the end stage of their disease. The trainer may be called to transport such a patient who has been neglected. During transportation, this patient requires all supportive measures available.

SIGNS AND SYMPTOMS OF SHOCK

Certain signs and symptoms are common to all types of shock. Anaphylactic shock presents some very special signs, which are discussed separately for added emphasis. The common indications of shock are:

1. Restlessness and anxiety, which may precede all other signs
2. Weak and rapid pulse
3. Cold and wet skin (commonly described as clammy)
4. Profuse sweating
5. Pale face perhaps later becoming cyanotic (blue) around the mouth
6. Shallow, labored, rapid or possibly irregular or gasping respirations, especially with chest injury
7. Dull or lusterless eyes, with dilated pupils
8. Thirst
9. Nausea or vomiting
10. Gradually and steadily falling blood pressure. A systolic blood pressure of only 90 to 100 mm Hg may be normal, but assume that shock is developing in any injured adult whose blood pressure is 100 mm Hg or less.
11. In rapidly developing shock, loss of consciousness

Anaphylactic reactions occur in minutes or even seconds following contact with the substances to which the patient is allergic. Disturbances in the skin, respiratory system and circulation are obvious. The major signs of an anaphylactic reaction are:

1. Skin—flushing, itching or burning sensation, especially of the face and upper chest. Hives may spread over large areas of the body. Edema (swelling), especially of the face and tongue, may occur. A specific swelling of the lips may be seen. Cyanosis may become rapidly visible about the lips.
2. Respiratory system—a tightness or pain in the chest with an irritating and persistent cough. Wheezing and difficulty in breathing develop. Fluid is lost into the bronchi, and the patient tries to cough it up. The smaller bronchi constrict and the passage of air is increasingly difficult. Therefore wheezing results, especially on expiration.

3. Circulatory system—a perceptible drop in blood pressure, a weak or imperceptible pulse, pallor and dizziness. Faintness and even coma may follow.

CARE AND TREATMENT OF SHOCK

A patient who exhibits any of the foregoing signs or symptoms should be treated vigorously for shock immediately. Recognizing the probable cause of shock allows treatment to be adjusted accordingly. However, many specific principles of initial treatment apply to all patients in shock.

1. Secure and maintain a clear airway and give oxygen as needed. Do this first, before doing anything else.
2. Control all obvious bleeding by gentle, firm compression.
3. Elevate the lower extremities about 12 inches, unless injury makes this maneuver inadvisable or impossible.
4. Splint fractures. This lessens bleeding, pain and discomfort, which further aggravate shock.
5. Avoid rough and excessive handling.
6. Prevent the loss of body heat by putting blankets under and over the patient. Do not load the patient with covers or attempt to warm the patient.
7. In general, keep an injured patient supine. However, remember that some patients in shock after a severe heart attack or with lung disease cannot breathe as well supine as sitting up or in a semi-reclining position. With such a patient, use the most comfortable position.
8. Record accurately the patient's initial pulse, blood pressure and other vital signs, and maintain a record of them at five minute intervals until arrival at the emergency department.
9. Do not give the patient anything to eat or drink.
10. Plan to use a pneumatic counterpressure device when appropriate. For patients in

shock from injuries of the pelvis, hips or femurs, or from intra-abdominal bleeding, the pneumatic counterpressure device may force blood from the lower extremities and abdomen back to the head.

It is important to check the patient's breathing. Lack of oxygen rapidly causes shock. Inadequate ventilation may be either the primary cause or a contributing factor in shock. An easily removed obstruction of the throat may be found. Establish and maintain an open airway, and be sure that breathing is adequate. Give oxygen to all patients in shock. A few assisted breaths by a ventilatory apparatus with added oxygen usually raises the patient's blood oxygen to an acceptable level.

An oxygen-adding device can provide oxygen on demand to a patient (conscious or unconscious) having difficulty breathing. Disposable plastic masks, with or without a breathing bag, may be used to administer the oxygen. Unless oxygen is humidified, limit inhalation to avoid drying the mouth, nasal passages and throat. If the respiratory muscles do not function after the airway is cleared, assisted ventilation by either a ventilatory apparatus or a mouth-to-mouth technique may be lifesaving. In some instances all available knowledge of artificial breathing and cardiac compression is needed to save the patient.

Control all obvious bleeding with sterile gauze compresses placed over the bleeding sites and bandaged with direct pressure applied. Bandaging minimizes the loss of blood. Sufficient pressure must be applied to stop any bleeding. The use of tourniquets is a last resort (see Chapter 29).

Elevating the lower extremities allows the blood in the legs to return to the heart more readily. It is a simple way, after a severe hemorrhage, of supplying as much blood to the heart as possible. Do not elevate fractured legs unless they are well splinted. Elevation may aggravate any unsplinted fracture and cause more soft-tissue damage.

Splint fractures although splinting at this point is not a definitive treatment. Splinting minimizes the amount of damage that the broken ends of bone can do to adjacent soft tissue and, thus, limits hemorrhage around the fracture site. In general, splinting makes moving the patient much easier and makes him much more comfortable. Some soft tissue injuries may be handled best by splinting and occasionally by air splints for compression.

Avoid rough or excessive handling of the patient. An attendant should ride with the patient to offer reassurance and keep him quiet. Transportation should be carried out at a safe speed.

Prevent the loss of body heat, but do not add more heat. It is better that the patient be slightly cool than too warm. External heat, such as hot water bottles or heating pads, may be harmful and should only be used in cold weather to prevent chilling. Observe all precautions concerning the use of external heat because it is easy to burn a semiconscious patient.

Do not give any liquids to the patient in shock, especially if the patient is vomiting, has an obvious abdominal injury or is unable to swallow. Nothing should be given orally until a physician has seen the patient in the emergency department. Never give alcoholic drinks to treat shock. Other stimulants such as ammonia or coffee have little or no value. The intense thirst that frequently accompanies shock may be allayed by allowing the patient to chew or suck on a moist sponge.

Recently, a pneumatic counterpressure device (pneumatic trousers or air-pressure pants) has been proposed to treat hypovolemic shock. It is effective in some specific instances:

1. To control severe bleeding into tissues from a fractured pelvis or fractures of the hips or femurs
2. To control severe intra-abdominal bleeding
3. To stabilize fractures of the pelvis, hips or femurs
4. To apply when blood pressure is below 100 mm Hg (systolic) and a bleeding source is not evident

The device takes account of the fact that the greatest volume of blood, at any one time, is in the capillary circulation. Compressing the abdomen and lower extremities forces much of the blood centrally to nourish vital organs and also aids in local control of bleeding and fractures. The few contraindications to the use of a pneumatic counterpressure device include pregnancy, pulmonary edema from myocardial damage and the need for the device to be worn for over two hours.

Major complications of a pneumatic counterpressure device have arisen because deflation was too rapid or unsupervised. Although the trainer will not ordinarily participate in this phase of treatment, he must, however, inform emergency department personnel of the patient's blood pressure when the device was applied and the results observed after its application. The device is removed in the emergency department or operating room after gradual deflation and with appropriate intravenous solutions. Figure 30:1 illustrates application of the pneumatic counterpressure device.

TREATMENT FOR SHOCK

Hemorrhagic Shock

The emergency treatment of hemorrhagic shock begins with control of obvious bleeding after the patient can breathe properly. Failure to apply pressure to obvious bleeding wounds, failure to splint fractures and rough handling allows continued bleeding.

Elevate the lower extremities a maximum of 12 inches by raising the legs from the hips, keeping the knees straight. This maneuver increases the blood flow returning to the heart and combats shock. A litter may be placed with the patient's head lowered if moving the legs is contraindicated. In this position the entire weight of the abdominal organs falls on the diaphragm and may make breathing difficult, thus requiring assisted ventilation.

Blood passed from the mouth or rectum means internal hemorrhage. Nothing can be done locally to control this bleeding. Give

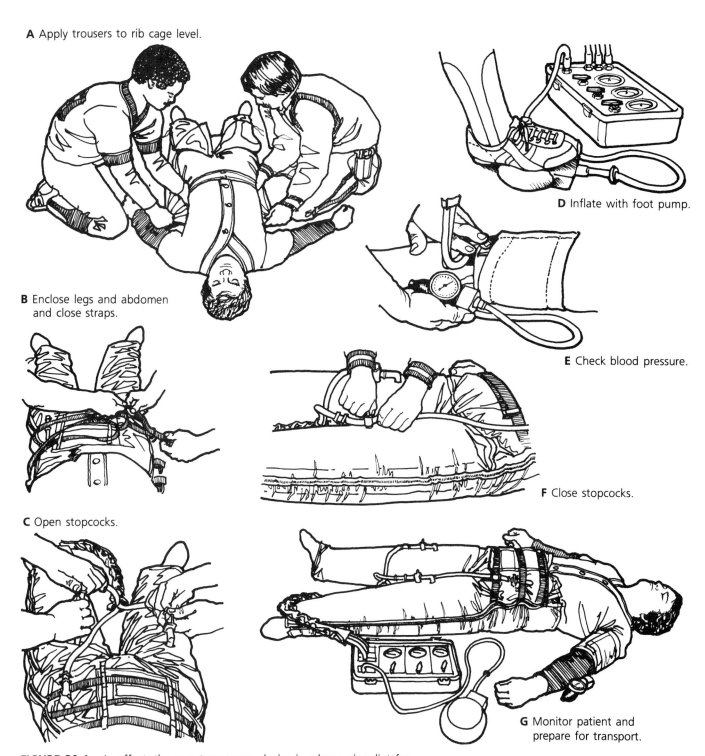

A Apply trousers to rib cage level.

B Enclose legs and abdomen and close straps.

C Open stopcocks.

D Inflate with foot pump.

E Check blood pressure.

F Close stopcocks.

G Monitor patient and prepare for transport.

FIGURE 30:1. In effect, the counterpressure device is a large air splint for the lower half of the body. It can provide stability for severe pelvic, hip and femoral fractures and effectively combat shock from any cause. A team using this method of shock control should be very familiar with its application.

general support, insure that the patient does not aspirate any vomitus and institute all the general methods for treating shock. In instances of hemorrhage about the pelvis, hips or femurs, or intra-abdominally, the pneumatic counterpressure device may be very effective.

Ventilator support should be part of this treatment and may include assisted ventilation and supplemental oxygen while the patient is transported to the hospital. Take this patient as promptly as possible to the emergency department for definitive care.

Respiratory Shock

Proper management of respiratory shock involves, first, securing and maintaining an airway. Clear the mouth and the throat down to the larynx of mucus, vomitus, foreign material or anything else obstructing the passage. Administer artificial ventilation, using ventilatory aids or mouth-to-mouth resuscitation and supplemental oxygen. These patients generally have severe medical emergencies and must be treated as rapidly as patients with obviously severe chest injuries. Prompt transportation to the emergency department is mandatory.

Neurogenic Shock

Shock accompanying severe spinal cord injuries or arising from a neurogenic cause is best treated by a combination of all supportive measures. This patient will probably require extended hospitalization. Emergency treatment should be directed at obtaining and maintaining a proper airway and conserving body heat with blankets. The patient may not be losing blood, but the vascular capacity may have become considerably larger than the volume of blood it contains. In this instance, a pneumatic counterpressure device may also be very useful. Provide supplemental oxygen so that the blood may carry a greater than normal concentration. Keep the patient as warm as possible, since normal body control of temperature is lost with such an injury. Prompt transportation to the hospital is mandatory,

since this patient may require specialized care to survive.

Psychogenic Shock

Usually a common fainting spell passes very quickly. If the patient has fallen, be alert for any injuries. These might include fractures of the long bones or of any bones that may have been struck, most particularly fractures of the skull, or cerebral concussions or contusions. As soon as the person falls and becomes supine, the blood supply to the brain improves and consciousness usually returns quickly. If the person does not awake or is confused after such an attack, suspect a head injury. Transport the person to the emergency department promptly and record initial observations and the length of time the patient was unconscious.

Cardiogenic Shock

The patient in shock as a result of a heart attack does not require a blood transfusion, intravenous fluid, elevation of the legs or a pneumatic counterpressure device. In this case, shock is due to the inability of the heart to handle the blood volume already present. If chronic lung disease is associated with this condition, as it frequently is, oxygenation of the blood passing through the lungs is normally poor, and the states of cardiogenic shock and hypoxia aggravate each other. This patient is often able to breathe better in a sitting position and this should be permitted.

Usually these patients do not have injuries but have had and may still have chest pain. Often the pulse is irregular and may be weak. The blood pressure is low. Cyanosis is frequently seen about the lips and under the fingernails. They may very well be anxious and occasionally may vomit.

These patients should be placed in the position in which they can breathe most easily, be given oxygen and assisted ventilation when necessary and transported promptly to the emergency department. Reassure them and maintain a calm demeanor.

Septic Shock

Septic shock requires complex hospital management. If this condition is suspected, transport the patient to the hospital as promptly as possible while giving all the general support available, including oxygen. Ventilatory support may be necessary. Septic shock does not ordinarily concern the trainer, as it usually occurs during a long hospitalization and in the course of prolonged and debilitating illness. If occasionally faced with this condition, remember that the presence of uncontrolled infection may produce shock.

Anaphylactic Shock

The only really effective treatment for acute allergic reactions is immediate subcutaneous, intramuscular or intravenous injection of medication to combat the agent causing the reaction. In general the injection of 0.5 to 1.0 ml of 1:1000 epinephrine alleviates the immediate signs of these reactions. Often patients are aware of their specific sensitivities and may have kits with epinephrine to combat the reactions. Assist the patient in administering epinephrine and be ready to repeat the injection as the signs and symptoms recur or worsen. Frequently, specific counteragents for the compound causing the reaction can be given, usually by a physician at a medical facility. Try to discover or identify what caused the reaction—drugs, insect bites or food—and how it was received, whether by mouth, by inhalation or by injection (needle or insect sting).

The severity of such reactions varies greatly. The symptoms may range from mild itching and burning of the skin to a generalized edema, profound coma and death. Because the severity of any reaction cannot be predicted, prompt transportation to a medical facility is important. Supportive measures must be carried out en route.

Metabolic Shock

Metabolic shock is usually the result of long-term illness associated with loss of fluid through vomiting, diarrhea or urination. With inadequate food and fluid intake to cover the loss of body water, the patient may have literally dried up. Transport this patient to the hospital as promptly as possible, again giving all the support necessary, including oxygen during transport. Try to ascertain the presence of any contributory illness, such as diabetes or severe enteritis.

Basic Life Support

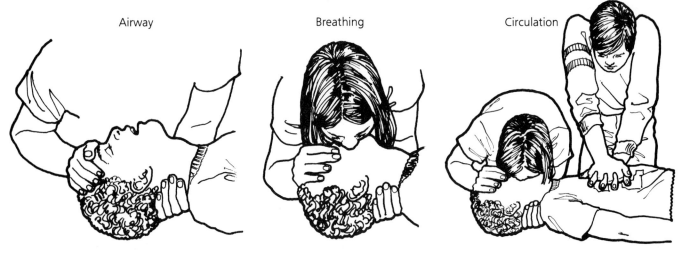

Basic life support is an emergency life-saving procedure that consists of recognizing and correcting failure of the respiratory or cardiovascular system. Oxygen, present in the atmosphere in a concentration of about 21%, is essential for the life of all cells. The brain starts to die if deprived of oxygen for as little as four minutes. To deliver oxygen from the atmosphere to the brain cells, two actions are necessary—breathing and circulation. Any profound disturbance of the airway, breathing or the circulation can promptly produce brain death.

ABC OF CPR

Basic life support includes the ABC steps of cardiopulmonary resuscitation (CPR) (Fig. 31:1):

A—Airway obstruction
B—Breathing (respiratory arrest)
C—Circulatory or Cardiac (heart) arrest

Basic life support requires no instruments or supplies, and the correct application of the steps of CPR can maintain life until the patient recovers sufficiently to be transported to a hospital or until advanced life support can be delivered.

Basic life support is not the same as advanced life support. The latter uses equipment, cardiac monitoring, defibrillation, an intravenous line and the infusion of appropriate drugs.

Basic life support demands a maximal sense of urgency. The outstanding advantage of CPR is that it permits the earliest possible treatment of airway obstruction, respiratory arrest or cardiac arrest by properly trained persons. Ideally, only seconds should intervene between recognizing the need and starting the treatment. The inadequacy or absence of breathing or circulation must be determined immediately.

Airway   Breathing   Circulation

FIGURE 31:1. The ABC steps of cardiopulmonary resuscitation—Airway, Breathing, Circulation

If breathing alone is inadequate or absent, either opening the airway or artificial ventilation is all that is necessary. If circulation is also absent, artificial circulation must be instituted in combination with the artificial ventilation. If breathing stops before the heart stops, enough oxygen will be available in the lungs to maintain life for several minutes. But if heart arrest occurs first, delivery of oxygen to the brain ceases immediately. Brain damage is possible if the brain is deprived of oxygen for four to six minutes. Beyond six minutes without oxygen, brain damage is very likely (Fig. 31:2). Speed is essential in determining the need for and beginning the procedures of basic life support.

Beginning and Terminating Basic Life Support

CPR is most effective when started immediately after cardiac arrest. If there is any question of how long the arrest has lasted, give the patient the benefit of the doubt and start resuscitation at once. However, CPR is not indicated for a patient known to be in the terminal stages of an incurable condition.

When resuscitation is indicated and begun in the absence of a physician, continue until one of the following events occurs.

1. Effective, spontaneous circulation and ventilation are restored.
2. Resuscitation efforts are transferred to another responsible person who continues basic life support.
3. A physician assumes responsibility.
4. The trainer is exhausted and unable to continue resuscitation efforts.

Unconsciousness

Check an unconscious patient carefully to determine which steps of basic life support are needed. Unconsciousness is established by observing the patient's responses to verbal or painful stimuli. In addition, to exclude a head injury as the cause of unconsciousness and to determine the possibility of spinal injuries,

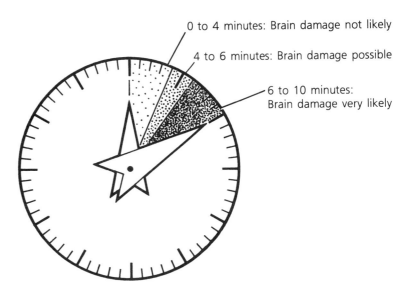

FIGURE 31:2. If the brain is deprived of O_2 for four to six minutes, brain damage is likely. After six minutes brain damage is extremely likely.

while checking breathing and circulation ask witnesses if the patient had a fall or look for evidence of an accident or fall. Without evidence of such injuries, start life support without concern for spinal damage. Conversely, if spinal injury is suspected, take care to protect the spinal cord. Unconscious states and spinal and head injuries are each treated in separate chapters in this text.

Positioning the Patient

For CPR to be effective, the patient must be horizontal, supine (lying face up) and on a firm surface. Even when flawlessly performed, external chest compression produces no blood flow to the brain if the body is vertical. Airway management and artificial ventilation are done more easily when the patient is supine.

It is therefore imperative to place the unconscious patient in a supine position as quickly as possible when he is found in a vertical position. Also, if the patient is lying crumpled up or face down, repositioning is necessary. Considerable caution must be taken, particularly if a neck or back injury is suspected. The patient must be rolled as a single unit of head, neck and back. Elevating the lower extremities about 12 inches while keeping the rest of the body horizontal may promote venous blood return and assist artificial circulation if external chest compression is required.

Kneel by the patient, not in bodily contact, and sufficiently far away so that when the patient is rolled, he does not end up in your lap. Rapidly straighten the patient's legs and move the nearer arm above the head (Fig. 31:3A), then place one hand behind the back of the patient's head and neck and the other hand on the distant shoulder (Fig. 31:3B). Then turn the patient toward yourself by pulling on the shoulder, and control the head and neck so that they turn with the rest of the torso as a

unit (Fig. 31:3C). In this way, the head and neck remain in the same vertical plane as the back, preventing aggravation of any spinal injury. When the patient is flat on his back, bring the patient's arm back to his side (Fig. 31:3D). Now airway, breathing and circulation can be assessed and treated.

ARTIFICIAL VENTILATION

Respiratory inadequacy may result from an obstruction of the airway or from respiratory failure. An obstructed airway is sometimes difficult to recognize until the initial steps of air-

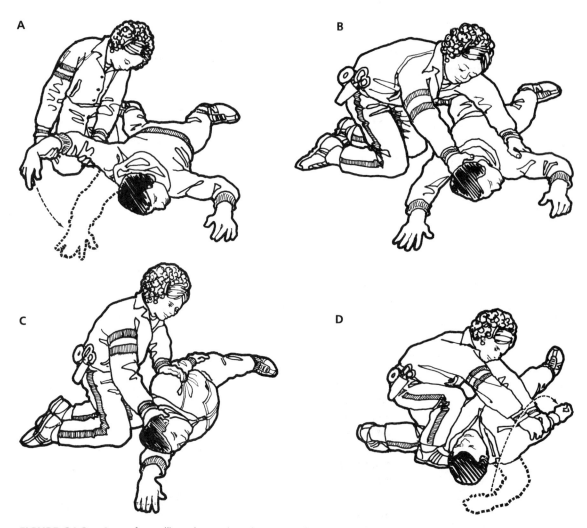

FIGURE 31:3. Steps for rolling the patient into a supine position

way management have been attempted. At other times, a partially obstructed airway can be recognized by labored breathing, by excessive respiratory efforts involving the accessory muscles of respiration, and by retraction of the intercostal, supraclavicular and suprasternal spaces. Respiratory failure or arrest is characterized by minimal or absent respiratory efforts, failure of the chest or upper abdomen to move, and no detectible air movement through the nose or mouth.

Opening the airway and restoring breathing are the basic steps of artificial ventilation. The steps can be performed quickly under almost any circumstances, without equipment, and without help from another person. These steps constitute emergency medical care for airway obstruction, respiratory failure or respiratory arrest.

Opening the Airway

Immediate opening of the airway is the most important factor in successful artificial ventilation. The airway may be blocked by the patient's own tongue or by foreign material in the mouth or throat.

Head-Tilt Maneuver

With loss of consciousness, muscles relax. An unconscious patient's tongue can fall back into the pharynx, blocking it and obstructing the upper airway (Fig. 31:4).

The obstruction caused by the tongue is relieved easily and quickly by tilting the patient's head backward as far as possible—the head-tilt maneuver (Fig. 31:5). Sometimes this simple maneuver is all that is required for the patient to resume breathing spontaneously. For the head tilt to be performed, the patient must be lying on his back. Kneeling close to the patient, place a hand on the patient's forehead and apply firm backward pressure with the palm. This moves the patient's head as far backward as possible. Use the other hand to perform either a neck-lift or a chin-lift. The head-tilt is the initial and most important step in opening the airway.

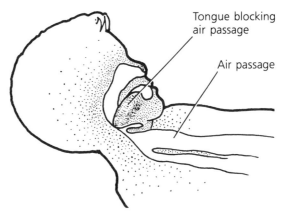

FIGURE 31:4. When the neck is in flexion (chin down on chest), the tongue falls back into the throat and obstructs the airway.

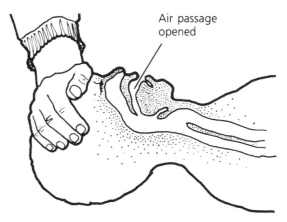

FIGURE 31:5. The head-tilt maneuver. Open the airway by extending the neck with firm pressure applied to the forehead.

Head Tilt-Neck Lift

Having achieved head tilt by placing one hand on the forehead and applying backward pressure, place the other hand beneath the neck and lift and/or support it upward (Fig. 31:6). Excess force in performing this maneuver may cause cervical spine injury. Since the specific movement used is extension of the head at the junction with the neck rather than hyperextension of the cervical vertebrae, place the hand lifting the neck close to the back

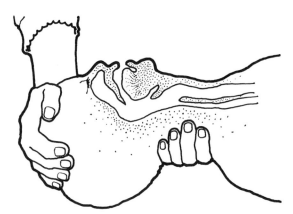

FIGURE 31:6. The head tilt-neck lift, further opening the airway

of the head to lessen extension of the cervical spine. Always be gentle but firm when lifting the neck.

Head Tilt-Chin Lift

In the conscious patient making spontaneous respiratory effort, chin-lift combined with head-tilt is highly effective in opening the airway when used initially. In addition, head tilt-chin lift may open the airway in some persons in whom head tilt-neck lift is not effective. For this reason, be familiar with the chin-lift technique so you can perform it as well as the neck-lift. The lower jaw may be supported by lifting the chin. Place the tips of the fingers of one

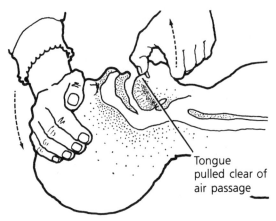

Tongue pulled clear of air passage

FIGURE 31:7. Head tilt-chin lift technique. While tilting the head backward with one hand, lift the chin forward with the fingers of the other.

hand under the lower jaw on the bony part near the chin, bringing the chin forward, supporting the jaw and helping to tilt the head back (Fig. 31:7). Do not compress the soft tissues under the chin, which might obstruct the airway. Continue to press on the patient's forehead with the other hand to tilt the head back. Lift the chin so the teeth are nearly brought together, but avoid closing the mouth completely. The thumb is used rarely when lifting the chin and then only to depress the lower lip slightly so the mouth will remain open. If the patient has loose dentures, they can be held in position with this maneuver, making obstruction by the lips less likely. If artificial ventilation is needed, the mouth-to-mouth seal is easier when the dentures are in place. If dentures cannot be managed in place, they should be removed.

In summary, either the head tilt-neck lift or the head tilt-chin lift can be used to open the airway. While the traditional head tilt-neck lift is effective, the chin lift may be needed if the neck lift does not restore airway patency. From field experiences trainers will be able to identify the usefulness of both methods.

The neck should not be hyperextended in patients who have suffered an actual or suspected injury to the cervical spine, as it may cause permanent paralysis. The possibility of a cervical spine injury must be considered at all times, especially in those patients who have suffered a fall or been involved in an accident.

Jaw-Thrust Maneuver

The methods described above are effective for most patients. If not, an additional forward movement of the lower jaw—the jaw-thrust—may be required. In this triple maneuver place the fingers behind the angle of the patient's lower jaw, and then:

1. Forcefully bring the jaw forward.
2. Tilt the head backward.
3. Use the thumb to pull the patient's lower lip down, which allows breathing through the mouth as well as the nose (Fig. 31:8).

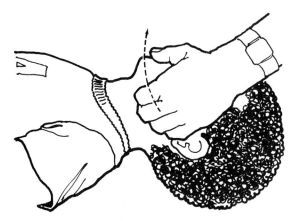

FIGURE 31:8. In the jaw-thrust maneuver, place your fingers behind the angle of the patient's jaw and forcefully bring it forward.

The jaw-thrust is best performed with the trainer kneeling by the patient's head.

If a cervical spine injury is suspected, this triple maneuver can be modified by keeping the head in a neutral position, thrusting the jaw forward and opening the mouth as described. This may permit opening the airway without need to move the head from a neutral position.

Once the airway has been opened, the patient may or may not start to breathe again. To assess whether breathing has returned, place your ear about 1 inch above the patient's nose and mouth (Fig. 31:9). If you can feel and hear movement of air and can see the patient's chest and abdomen move, breathing has returned. Feeling and hearing are far more important than seeing. With airway obstruction, there may be no air movement, even though the chest and abdomen rise and fall with the patient's attempts to breathe. Also, observing chest and abdominal movement is difficult in a fully clothed patient. Finally, the chest may not move even with normal breathing in patients who have chronic obstructive pulmonary disease.

Restoring Breathing

No equipment is required to give effective artificial ventilation. It should never be delayed while obtaining or applying devices for ventilatory assistance. Artificial ventilation, whether mouth-to-mouth, mouth-to-nose or mouth-to-stoma, should deliver at least 12 breaths per minute in the adult.

Mouth-to-Mouth

If the patient does not promptly resume adequate breathing after the airway is opened, start artificial ventilation. The exhaled air used in artificial ventilation contains about 16% oxygen. This is sufficient to sustain the patient's life.

In mouth-to-mouth ventilation, place one hand under the patient's neck and, with the other hand, pinch the patient's nostrils together, using the thumb and index finger. At the same time, with the heel of the hand, continue to exert pressure on the forehead to maintain the backward tilt of the head (Fig. 31:10A). Alternatively, use the head tilt-chin lift technique for keeping the airway open during mouth-to-mouth ventilation. Open the mouth wide, take a deep breath, make a tight seal around the patient's mouth and exhale

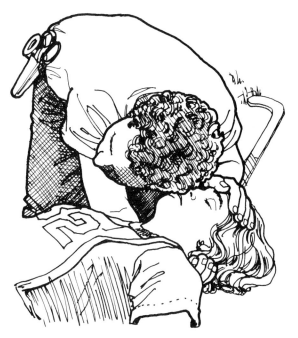

FIGURE 31:9. Respiration is determined by feeling, hearing and seeing.

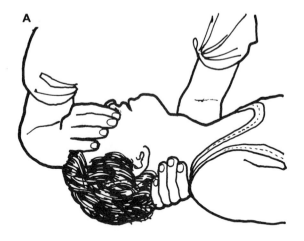

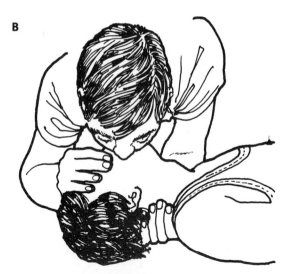

FIGURE 31:10. Mouth-to-mouth ventilation is achieved, **A** by sealing off the patient's nose, and **B** by encircling the patient's open mouth and exhaling deeply into it.

(Fig. 31:10B). Then remove your mouth and allow the patient to exhale passively, turning slightly to watch the patient's chest fall. The first four breaths must be given in rapid succession without waiting for the patient's lungs to deflate completely between breaths. This succession of breaths helps to re-expand the collapsed lungs.

Adequate ventilation is insured if, on every breath, you:

1. See the chest rise and fall
2. Feel the resistance of the lungs as they expand
3. Hear and feel the air escape during exhalation

If the head tilt-chin lift technique is used, the thumb of the hand lifting the chin can be used to depress the lower lip, thus keeping the mouth open during mouth-to-mouth ventilation. When using the jaw-thrust for mouth-to-mouth ventilation, move to the patient's side, keep the patient's mouth open with both thumbs, and seal the nose by placing a cheek against the nostrils.

Mouth-to-Nose

In some cases, mouth-to-nose ventilation is more effective than mouth-to-mouth ventilation. It is recommended when it is impossible to open the patient's mouth; when it is impossible to ventilate the patient through the mouth because of severe facial injuries; when a tight seal around the mouth of a patient without teeth is difficult; or when, for some other reason, the nasal route is preferred.

For the mouth-to-nose technique, keep the patient's head tilted back with one hand on the

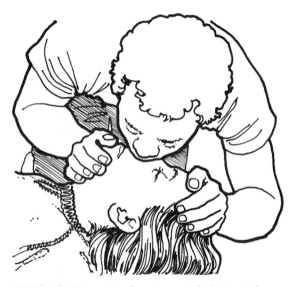

FIGURE 31:11. Mouth-to-nose technique, sealing the lips by lifting lower jaw

forehead and use the other hand to lift the patient's lower jaw (Fig. 31:11). This maneuver seals the lips. Then take a deep breath, seal your lips around the patient's nose and blow in until you feel the lungs expand. Remove your mouth and allow the patient to exhale passively. Watch the chest fall when the patient exhales. It may be necessary to open the patient's mouth or separate the lips to allow air to escape during exhalation because the soft palate may block the nasopharynx and prevent air from exiting through the nose. When using the jaw-thrust for mouth-to-nose ventilation, use your cheek to seal the patient's mouth and do not use thumbs to retract the lower lip.

Mouth-to-Stoma

Direct mouth-to-stoma ventilation may be used for patients who have had a laryngectomy. These patients have a permanent stoma (opening) in the neck, which connects the trachea directly to the skin. It may be seen as an opening at the center, in front and at the base of the neck. Many of these patients have other openings in the neck, according to the type of operation done and reconstruction attempted. However, any opening other than the main, midline tracheal stoma should be ignored. In general, any other neck opening lies on one side or the other but not in the midline.

Neither head-tilt nor jaw-thrust maneuvers are required for mouth-to-stoma ventilation. If the patient has a tube in the stoma, blow into the tube. When blowing into a stoma, it should be standard practice to seal the patient's mouth and nose with a hand to prevent air leaking up the trachea.

Gastric Distention

Artificial ventilation frequently causes distention of the stomach. This occurs most often in children, but it is also common in adults. It is usually caused by excessive pressures used for ventilation or an obstructed airway. Slight gastric distention may be disregarded, but marked inflation of the stomach is dangerous because it promotes regurgitation and re-

duces lung volume by elevating the diaphragm. Promptly relieve gastric distention that interferes with adequate ventilation. Frequently, exerting moderate pressure on the patient's abdomen between the umbilicus and the rib cage with the flat of the hand is effective. To prevent aspiration of gastric contents during this maneuver, turn the patient's head and shoulder to one side and keep a suction device ready for immediate use.

AIRWAY OBSTRUCTION

Upper airway obstruction can cause unconsciousness and cardiopulmonary arrest, or it can be the result of the arrest itself. Either event can be fatal. Sudden airway obstruction by a foreign body in an adult usually occurs during eating. In a child it occurs during eating or at play (sucking small objects).

Other causes of airway obstruction include the unconscious patient who suffers airway obstruction because the tongue falls back into the pharynx, blocking it and obstructing the upper airway. Gastric contents can be regurgitated into the pharynx during cardiopulmonary arrest or CPR and thereby block the airway. Also, in head and facial injuries, blood clots, tooth and bone fragments and loose tissue may obstruct the upper airway, particularly if the patient is unconscious.

Recognition of Foreign Body Obstruction

Early recognition of airway obstruction is crucial to successful management. Learn to differentiate between primary airway obstruction and other conditions resulting in respiratory failure or arrest, such as fainting, stroke or heart attack. Upper airway obstruction may present in two ways: the patient may be conscious when discovered but become unconscious, or the patient may be unconscious when discovered.

Conscious Patient

Sudden upper airway obstruction usually occurs when a person who is eating or has just finished eating is suddenly unable to speak or cough, grasps his throat, appears cyanotic or shows exaggerated breathing efforts. Air movement is either absent or not detectable. Initially the patient remains conscious, but if the obstruction is not removed within a few minutes, the oxygen in the lungs is used up because the obstructed airway prevents the entry of air into the lungs. Unconsciousness and death follow.

Unconscious Patient

When a patient is discovered unconscious, the cause is initially unknown. The unconsciousness may have been caused by airway obstruction or cardiopulmonary arrest. Any patient found unconscious must be managed as a patient with cardiopulmonary arrest, and the obstructed airway should be dealt with only as it becomes apparent during the correct sequence of resuscitative maneuvers.

Relieving Upper Airway Obstruction

Three manual maneuvers are recommended for relieving foreign body obstruction: back blows, manual thrusts and finger sweeps.

Back Blows

Deliver a series of four sharp back blows in rapid succession with the hand over the patient's spine between the scapulae. Apply the technique whether the patient is sitting, standing or lying down.

With the patient sitting or standing:

1. Stay at the side of and slightly behind the patient.
2. Deliver sharp blows with the hand to the patient's spine between the scapulae.
3. Place the other hand in front of the patient's chest for support.

With the patient lying down:

1. Kneel down and roll the patient so that the patient's chest rests against your knees.
2. Deliver sharp blows with the hand to the patient's spine between the scapulae.

Manual Thrusts

Deliver a rapid series of up to four thrusts to the upper abdomen (abdominal thrust) or lower chest (chest thrust). To perform an abdominal thrust with the patient sitting or standing (Fig. 31:12):

1. Stand behind the patient, with arms wrapped about the patient's waist.
2. Grasp one fist with the other hand and place the thumb side of the fist against the patient's abdomen between the xiphoid and umbilicus.
3. Press your fist into the patient's abdomen with a quick upward thrust. Repeat this three more times.

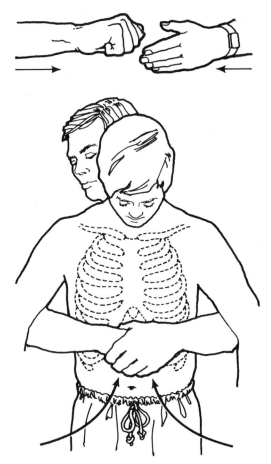

FIGURE 31:12. Proper positioning of the hands for applying abdominal thrusts in the erect adult

For the abdominal thrust with the patient lying down, modify the technique as follows (Fig. 31:13):

1. Positioning the patient supine, kneel close to the patient's hips or straddle either the hips or one leg of the patient.
2. Place the heel of one hand against the patient's abdomen between the xiphoid and umbilicus, and place the second hand on top of the first.
3. Press the hand into the patient's abdomen with a quick upward thrust and repeat the thrust as above if necessary.

In advanced pregnancy or gross obesity when it is impossible to encircle the abdomen fully, an alternative technique, the chest thrust, can be applied (Fig. 31:14).

With the patient sitting or standing:

1. Wrap your hands under the patient's arms to encircle the lower chest.
2. Grasp one fist with the other hand, with the thumb side of the fist on the lower sternum but clear of the xiphoid process.
3. Press the fist into the patient's chest with a quick backward thrust. Deliver up to four thrusts if necessary.

With the patient lying down:

1. Position the patient supine and kneel close to the side of the patient's body.
2. Place your hands on the sternum in exactly the same manner as for external chest compression and apply compressions as would be performed for CPR. Apply four downward thrusts.

Back Blows Plus Manual Thrusts

Back blows produce an instantaneous increase in pressure in the respiratory passages, which may partially or completely dislodge a foreign body. Manual thrusts produce a lower, although more sustained, increase in pressure in the respiratory passages and may further assist in dislodging the foreign body. Combining these two techniques appears to be more effective in clearing upper airway obstruction

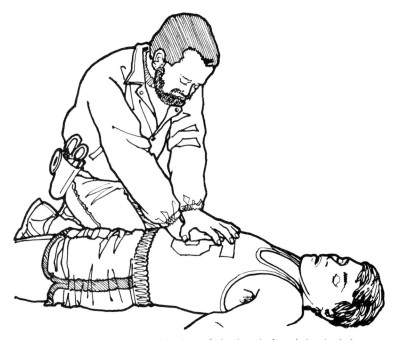

FIGURE 31:13. Proper positioning of the hands for abdominal thrusts in the supine patient

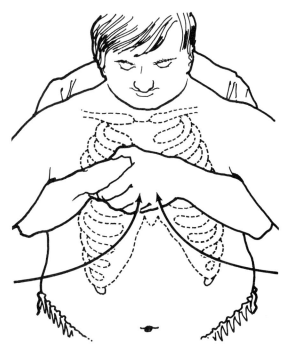

FIGURE 31:14. Proper technique of the chest thrust in the erect patient

than either used singly. Whether one sequence is more effective than another is not clear, however, and thus either back blows followed by thrusts or thrusts followed by back blows can be used.

Manual Removal of Foreign Body

If the foreign body causing the airway obstruction appears in the mouth or may be in the mouth, remove it cautiously with the fingers. Back blows and manual thrusts may dislodge the foreign body but not expel it because the unconscious patient's jaw muscles relax. Use either a cross-finger technique or a tongue-jaw lift to probe the mouth with a finger.

In the cross-finger technique (Fig. 31:15):

1. Cross the thumb under the index finger.
2. Brace the thumb and index finger against the patient's lower and upper teeth, respectively.
3. Push the fingers apart to force the patient's jaw open.

For the tongue-jaw lift:

1. Keep the head in the neutral position.
2. Open the patient's mouth by grasping both the tongue and lower jaw between the thumb and fingers and lifting them forward. This action pulls the tongue away from the back of the throat and away from the foreign body that may be lodged there.

For the finger probe:

1. Hold the patient's mouth open with either the cross-finger or tongue-jaw lift technique.
2. Use the index finger of the other hand to sweep down the inside of the patient's cheek to the base of the tongue.
3. Use the index finger as a hook to try to dislodge the impacted foreign body up into the mouth.
4. When the foreign body comes within reach, grasp and remove it.

Take care with finger probes not to push the dislodged foreign body back into the airway.

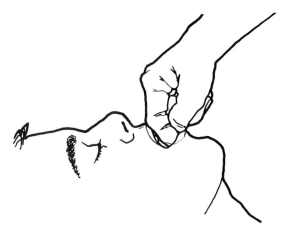

FIGURE 31:15. Cross-finger technique

ARTIFICIAL CIRCULATION

A disturbance of the regular rhythm of the heart may prevent adequate cardiac contraction, resulting in failure to generate blood flow and produce a pulse. The absence of a strong, palpable central pulse, such as the carotid pulse in the neck, indicates no blood flow and hence cardiac arrest.

After determining unconsciousness, turning the patient if necessary, opening the airway and giving four quick breaths, assess the status of the patient's circulation by checking for a palpable pulse in a large artery. The carotid is such an artery; it is close to the heart, large in diameter and palpable in the neck. It is found most easily by locating the larynx at the front of the neck and then sliding two fingers toward either side of the neck. The carotid pulse is felt in the groove between the larynx and the sternocleidomastoid muscle with the pulp of the index and long fingers (Fig. 31:16). Light pressure is sufficient. Avoid excessive pressure because it can obstruct the circulation, dislodge blood clots or produce marked cardiac slowing.

Leave the hand on the forehead in position to maintain backward head tilt, but it is not necessary to continue to pinch off the nostrils. Use the hand previously placed beneath the neck for locating the carotid pulse.

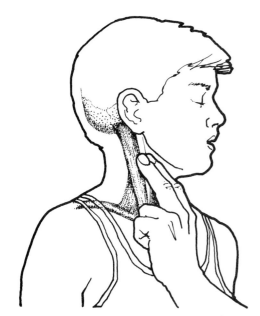

FIGURE 31:16. The carotid pulse is felt in the groove between the larynx and the sternocleidomastoid muscle.

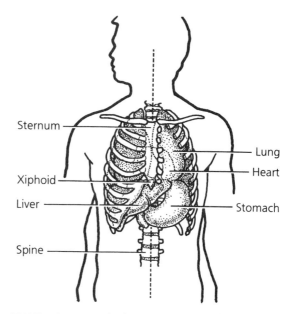

FIGURE 31:17. Rhythmic pressure on the lower half of the sternum will provide compression of the heart, provided the spine is on a flat, solid surface.

If the pulse is present but breathing is absent, ventilate the patient once every five seconds until adequate breathing resumes. If the pulse is absent, start external chest compression, which adds artificial circulation to the already initiated artificial ventilation.

External Chest Compression

The heart lies slightly to the left of the chest midline between the sternum and the spine (Fig. 31:17). Rhythmic pressure and relaxation applied to the lower half of the sternum compresses the heart and produces artificial circulation. In a patient with cardiac arrest, the carotid artery flow resulting from external chest compression is only about one quarter to one third of normal. **External chest compression must always be accompanied by artificial ventilation.** The patient must be on a firm, flat surface—the ground, the floor or a spine board on an ambulance litter. If in bed, place the patient on the floor rather than looking for some type of support and delaying cardiac compression.

Kneel close to the patient's side, with one knee at the level of the head and the other at the level of the upper chest, and place the heel of one hand on the lower half of the sternum. Take great care not to place the hand on the xiphoid process, which extends downward over the upper abdomen, or beside the sternum into the ribs (Fig. 31:18). To correctly posi-

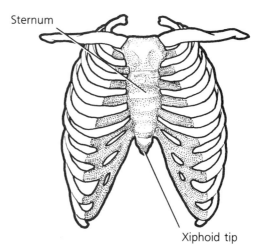

FIGURE 31:18. The xiphoid process

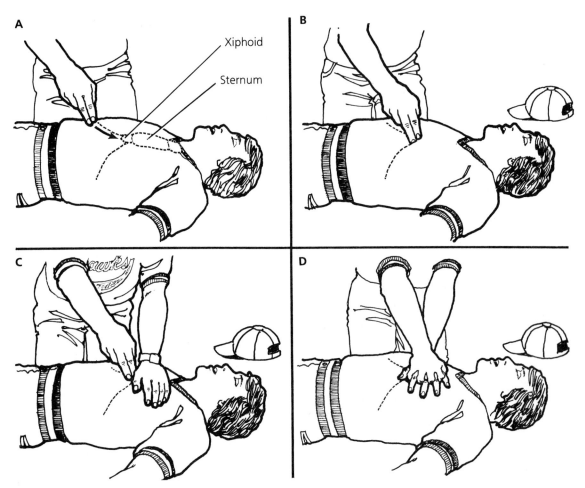

FIGURE 31:19. Steps to position the hands correctly to perform CPR. See text for complete description.

tion the hands, slide the index and long fingers of the hand nearer the patient's feet along the edge of the rib cage until the fingers reach the notch in the center chest (Fig. 31:19A). Push the long finger as high as possible into the notch, and lay the index finger on the lower portion of the sternum with the two fingers touching (Fig. 31:19B).

Then place the heel of the other hand on the lower half of the sternum (Fig. 31:19C) so that it touches the index finger of the first hand. Remove the first hand from the notch in the center of the rib cage and place it over and parallel to the hand now resting on the patient's lower sternum (Fig. 31:19D). **Only the heel of one hand is in contact with the lower half of the sternum.**

The technique may be improved or made more comfortable for the trainer by interlocking the fingers of the lower hand with the fingers of the upper and pulling them slightly away from the chest wall. Pressure is exerted vertically downward through both arms to depress the adult sternum 1½ to 2 inches. A rocking motion allows pressure to be delivered vertically downward from the shoulder while keeping the arms straight (Fig. 31:20).

Vertical pressure downward produces a compression, which should be immediately followed by a period of relaxation. The time

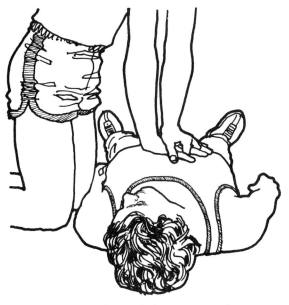

FIGURE 31:20. External chest compression

diac compression is not interrupted, blood pressure never falls to zero.

If a second person becomes available after single-person CPR is in progress, the recommended procedure for entry of the second person is as follows. Without stopping CPR, the original person lets the new person know that everything is ready for switch to two-person CPR. The new person should check the patient's pulse to make sure that the patient's condition has been correctly diagnosed. The new person should then kneel down on the side of the patient opposite the original person, in position for artificial ventilation, fingers in position to feel the carotid pulse. If compressions are adequate, a pulse should be present.

spent in the compression phase is a crucial factor in determining blood flow. At least 50% of the compression-relaxation cycle should be spent in compression. Short, jabbing compressions are ineffective in producing blood flow. Do not remove the heel of the hand from the chest during relaxation, but completely release the pressure on the sternum so that it can return to its normal resting position between compressions. Compression and relaxation must be rhythmic. Do not jab downward or allow the hands to bounce or come away from the patient's chest (Fig. 31:21).

RESUSCITATION

With two-person CPR, the compression rate should be 60 per minute, with a single breath given after each fifth compression (ratio 5:1). The person delivering the compression can count: "one thousand one, one thousand two, one thousand three," etc., as approximately one second is required to say this phrase. Two persons can provide more effective CPR than one because ventilation can be delivered without any pause in compression and, since car-

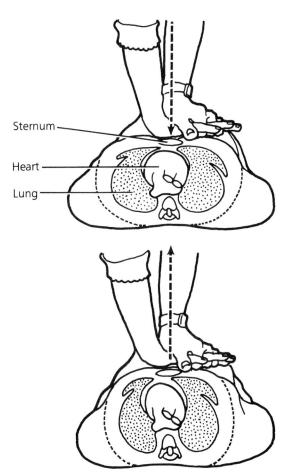

FIGURE 31:21. Compression and relaxation should be rhythmic and of equal duration.

If no pulse is felt, the compressor's technique should be evaluated. The new person should call out, after feeling a pulse with each compression, "Stop compression." Compression should be stopped for 5 seconds so that the new person can check for a spontaneous pulse. If none is found, two-person CPR is begun. The new person should deliver a breath immediately after confirming pulselessness. This entire process, from the moment the new person arrives to the point when a breath is delivered, should be done as quickly as possible to insure that CPR continues effectively. As soon as this breath is delivered, the original person changes to the two-person rate. Artificial ventilation is then interposed during the upstroke of each fifth cardiac compression.

Two-person CPR is performed with the resuscitators on opposite sides of the patient (Fig. 31:22). They can then switch positions when necessary without major interruption in

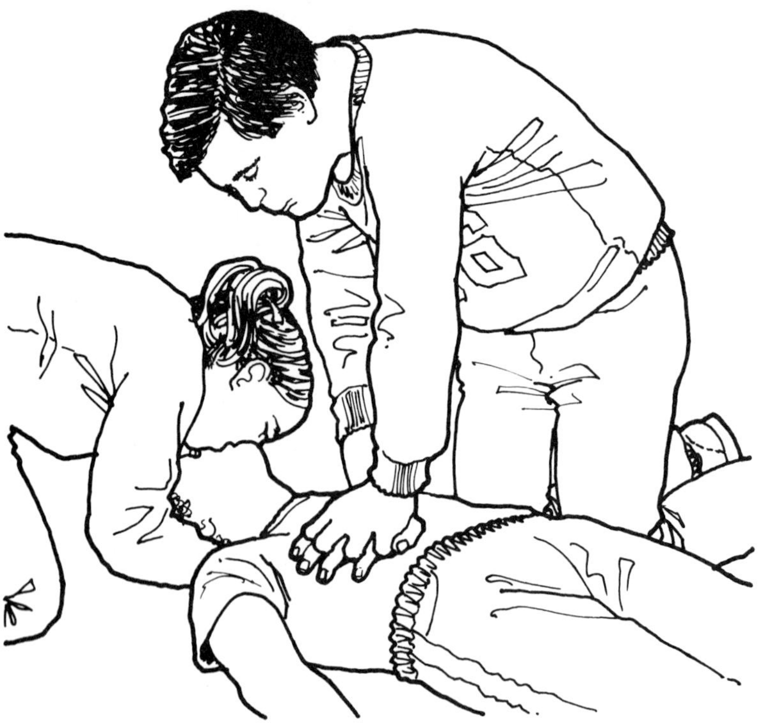

FIGURE 31:22. With two-person CPR, one is on each side of the patient.

the 5:1 sequence. To switch, the person who is providing ventilation, after giving a breath, moves into position for compressions. The person performing compression, after the fifth compression, moves to the patient's head and checks the pulse for 5 seconds but no longer. If no pulse is felt, the person at the head ventilates the patient and says, "continue CPR."

When performing CPR on a litter in an ambulance, both persons must perform from the same side of the patient. They switch positions using the following technique. The ventilator rapidly moves behind the compressor and assumes the role of compressor. The original compressor moves to the head of the patient to continue ventilation.

Because of the interruptions for ventilation, one-person CPR must be carried out at the faster rate of 80 compressions per minute to achieve an actual compression rate of 60 per minute. After 15 compressions, deliver two ventilations (ratio 15:2). The 15 compressions are delivered in 10 to 11 seconds, followed by two full, rapid ventilations (with minimal exhalation time) delivered in four to five seconds.

Effectiveness of CPR

Check the reaction of the pupils to light periodically during CPR. Pupils that constrict when exposed to light indicate adequate oxygenation and blood flow to the brain. If the pupils remain widely dilated and do not react to light, serious brain damage may be imminent or may have occurred (see Fig. 5:3). Dilated but reactive pupils are a less ominous sign. However, it must be emphasized that normal pupillary reactions may be altered in the elderly and frequently are altered in any individual by the administration of drugs.

Palpate the carotid pulse periodically during CPR to check the effectiveness of external cardiac compression or the return of a spontaneous effective heartbeat. Palpate the carotid artery after the first minute of CPR and every few minutes thereafter. The person ventilating should check pupils and pulse, particularly just before the change of trainers.

CPR Interruption

Do not interrupt CPR for more than 5 seconds for any reason, except when a patient must be moved up or down a stairway, where it may be difficult to continue effective resuscitation. Under these circumstances, perform CPR at the head or foot of the stairs, then interrupt at a given signal and move quickly to the next level, and resume effective CPR. These interruptions should not exceed 15 seconds each. Do not move the patient to a more convenient site until stable and ready for transportation or until arrangements have been made for uninterrupted CPR during movement.

Without the addition of monitoring, an intravenous line, drugs and defibrillation (advanced life support), basic life support will rarely be sufficient for patient survival, regardless of how well it is performed. If advanced life-support modalities cannot be brought to the scene, the patient must be moved promptly to the hospital. It is good practice to choose a stable, competent person from those at the scene (preferably a third trainer or a law enforcement officer) to drive, so that the two original resuscitators can continue CPR while the ambulance proceeds to the hospital.

Basic Life Support in Infants and Children

The basic principles of CPR are the same whether the patient is an infant, child or adult. The underlying causes of emergencies in infants and children may be different and techniques must be varied due to size of the patient. In most instances, cardiopulmonary arrest in infants and children begins with respiratory arrest with secondary cardiac arrest resulting from hypoxia. Therefore, major attention must be directed to the airway and ventilation. In many cases, restoration of an open airway and adequate ventilation of the lungs is all that is needed for resuscitation. Some of the major crises that commonly necessitate resuscitation in infants and children include aspiration of foreign bodies into the airway, e.g., peanuts, candy and small toys; poisonings and drug overdose; near drowning; and sudden infant death syndrome. For the purposes of CPR, anyone under 1 year of age is considered an infant. A child is between the ages of 1 and 8 years. Above 8 years, techniques used for adults can generally be applied. These definitions are guidelines only, recognizing the variations among infants and children in size relative to age.

Part 8

NERVOUS SYSTEM

Injuries of the Head and Spine

The skull and spine form a unit to protect the central nervous system, composed of the brain and spinal cord (Fig. 32:1). The central nervous system coordinates nerve messages from receptors on the surface of the body, in muscles, tendons and ligaments, as well as in the visceral organs of the thorax and abdomen and numerous other sites. Reflex arcs function involuntarily but the voluntary responses of the muscles in propelling the musculoskeletal system are the important ones in athletics. While most injuries sustained in sports do not result in catastrophic and irreversible damage, the potential for injury to the brain and spinal cord is of utmost concern for those who care for the athlete.

32

ANATOMY OF THE HEAD

The scalp serves as a protective coating for the bony structure. Because of its mobility, it allows for some transmission of forces struck over the skull.

The scalp consists of four layers: hair, skin, subcutaneous connective tissue and pericranium. The scalp has a healthy blood supply and scalp and face lacerations often bleed profusely. This bleeding can be controlled by applying a pressure bandage until the lacerations can be treated. Hematoma formation between the scalp and skull often needs roentgenographic evaluation to diagnosis any associated underlying skull fracture. Accumulation of this hematoma can be reduced by ice and pressure techniques. If there is a question of an underlying skull fracture, pressure should be used judiciously.

Skull

The skull is a natural helmet. Its hard outer shell protects the soft brain inside a fluid-filled cushion. The bones of the skull are united by sutures and synchondroses (Fig. 32:2). The bones of the skull composing the cranial cavity are the frontal, parietal, occipital, sphenoid, ethmoid and temporal. Of these, only the parietal and temporal are paired. The bones of the

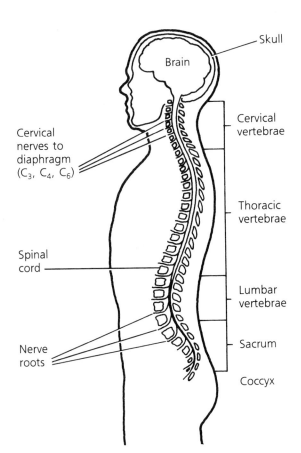

FIGURE 32:1. Lateral view of the spine

393

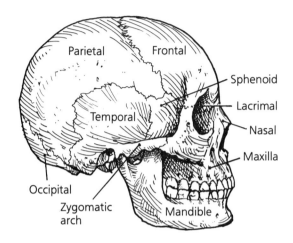

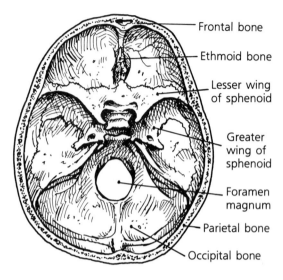

FIGURE 32:3. Interior of the base of the skull

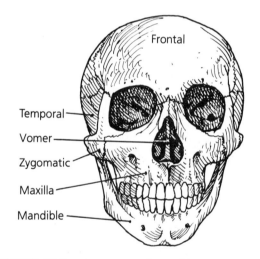

FIGURE 32:2. Anteroposterior and lateral views of the bones of the skull

face and nasal cavities are the maxilla, zygomatic, palatine, nasal, lacrimal, inferior nasal concha, vomer and mandible. Of these, only the vomer and mandible are unpaired.

The foramen magnum is the large aperture at the base of the skull through which the medulla and spinal cord pass and enter into the bony spinal canal in the neck (Fig. 32:3). The bones of the adult skull are constructed of firm outer and inner layers, or tables, and interspersed between these layers is softer bone containing blood channels. Some of

these larger vascular pathways are visible on skull x-ray films.

Whenever an athlete suffers a severe blow to the head, a skull fracture should be suspected. While the incidence of these fractures is low, those that do occur are potentially serious. Skull fractures are classed as linear, nondepressed or depressed but may be difficult to determine clinically (Fig. 32:4). Even a depressed skull fracture may be confused clinically with a deep scalp hematoma. Therefore, x-ray evaluation is crucial to detection and management. In evaluating and observing athletes who have sustained skull fractures, always consider associated brain injury.

Brain

The brain and spinal cord are surrounded and protected by layers of non-nervous tissue, collectively termed the meninges (Fig. 32:5). These layers, from without inward, are the dura mater, arachnoid and pia mater. The dura mater is a tough, fibrous membrane. Within the skull the dura mater lies immediately internal to the bone and contains venous channels, or sinuses, that carry blood from the brain to the veins in the neck. The dura mater covering the spinal cord is separated from the bone by an interval, the epidural space, that contains fat and many small veins.

The arachnoid, so called because it resembles a spider web, is a thin, cellular membrane. It is separated from the dura mater by a space of capillary thinness, the subdural space. The arachnoid is very closely connected by a meshwork of connective tissue strands to the innermost meningeal layer, the pia mater. The pia mater is a loose tissue that covers the brain and sheaths blood vessels as they enter the brain. The space between the arachnoid and the pia mater is the subarachnoid space that contains the cerebral spinal fluid. The arachnoid and pia mater are more widely separated from each other around the spinal cord than over the brain.

Cerebral Spinal Fluid

The ventricles of the brain contain a vascular choroid plexus from which an almost protein-free cerebral spinal fluid is formed. This fluid circulates through the ventricles, enters the subarachnoid space and eventually filters back into the venous system (Fig. 32:6). Cerebral spinal fluid serves to minimize dam-

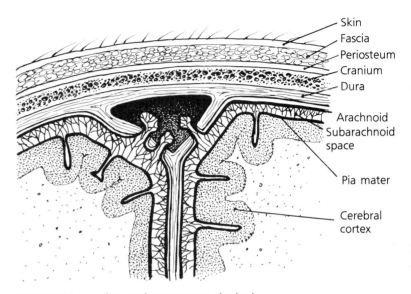

FIGURE 32:5. The meninges protect the brain.

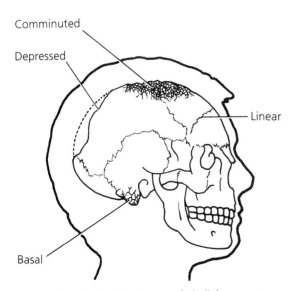

FIGURE 32:4. Various types of skull fractures

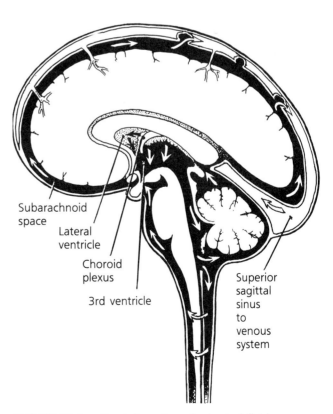

FIGURE 32:6. Circulation of cerebral spinal fluid

age to the brain and spinal cord by protecting them from blows to the head and neck.

Pressure of the cerebral spinal fluid is usually between 100 and 200 millimeters of water (mm H₂O). This is the fluid removed during a lumbar puncture. Certain anesthetics as well as contrast radiographic material for determining the positions of masses, tumors, ruptured discs and displaced fracture fragments can be administered into the space occupied by the fluid.

The cerebral branches of the vertebral and internal carotid arteries supply blood to the brain (Fig. 32:7). The middle meningeal branch of the maxillary artery mainly supplies the meninges. Vertebral arteries and segmental arteries supply the spinal cord and spinal roots. A number of small branches along the course of the nerves supply the peripheral nerves.

The brain is a large mass of nervous tissue distinguished by the folds or convolutions of much of its surface. The bulk of the brain is formed by two convoluted cerebral hemispheres. The diencephalon lies between the hemispheres and forms the upper part of what

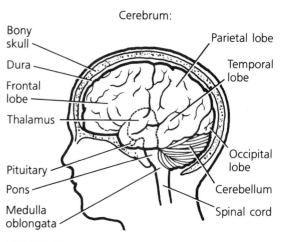

FIGURE 32:8.   Cross section of head

is generally called the brain stem, or unpaired stalk or stem, that descends from the base of the brain.

The brain has four lobes—frontal, parietal, occipital and temporal—plus the brain stem that connects the cerebral hemispheres with the spinal cord at the foramen magnum (Fig. 32:8). The cerebellum is a fissured mass of grey matter that occupies the posterior cranium and is attached to the brain stem by three pairs of peduncles.

The cortex, the outer part of the hemisphere, is only a few millimeters in thickness and is composed of grey matter, in contrast to the interior of the brain, which is composed partly of white matter. Grey matter is largely bodies of nerve cells whereas white matter is largely the processes or fibers of the nerve cells. The interior of the cerebral hemispheres, including the diencephalon, contains not only white matter but well demarcated masses of grey matter, known collectively as a basal ganglia. The cortex of the cerebellum, like that of the cerebral hemisphere, is composed mainly of white matter but also contains nerve cell nuclei, or grey matter. The brain stem, by contrast, contains nuclei in diffuse masses of grey matter in its interior.

The highest mental and behavioral activities of man are a function of the cerebral hemi-

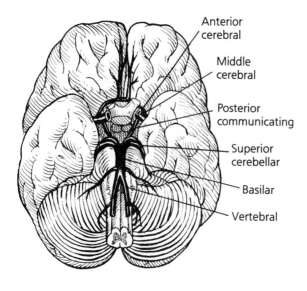

FIGURE 32:7.   Arterial circulation of the brain

sphere, in particular the cerebral cortex. The cerebral cortex is also concerned with speech, motor and sensory functions. The brain stem, which contains the centers for the cranial nerves and those concerned with respiration and circulation and other visceral activities, also connects with the cerebellum. The cerebellum, important to the automatic regulation of movement and posture, functions closely with the cerebral cortex and the brain stem.

Cranial Nerves

The 12 pairs of cranial nerves are special nerves associated with the brain (Fig. 32:9). The fibers in the cranial nerves are of two main, functional types, some composed primarily of sensory fibers and some primarily of motor fibers.

Cranial Nerve I: olfactory—smell
Cranial Nerve II: optic—vision
Cranial Nerves III, IV, & VI: oculomotor, trochlear and abducent—motor nerves controlling the movement of the eye
Cranial Nerve V: trigeminal—sensation of the head, face and movement of the jaw
Cranial Nerve VII: facial—special sensory, motor and autonomic nervous components that allow taste, facial movements and secretion of tears and saliva
Cranial Nerve VIII: acoustic—the cochlear and vestibular parts are important in hearing and equilibrium, respectively
Cranial Nerve IX: glossopharyngeal—sensory and motor components dealing with taste, sensation in the pharynx and movement of the pharynx; autonomic function in secretion of saliva and sensory components in visceral reflexes
Cranial Nerve X: vagus—controls taste, sensation to the pharynx, larynx and tracheobronchial tree; important in movements of the pharynx and larynx, secretions of the thoracic and abdominal viscera and visceral reflexes
Cranial Nerve XI: spinal accessory—motor nerve concerned with movements of the pharynx, larynx, head and shoulders

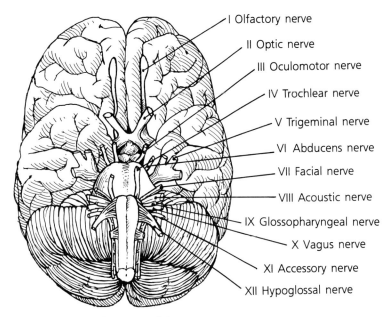

I Olfactory nerve
II Optic nerve
III Oculomotor nerve
IV Trochlear nerve
V Trigeminal nerve
VI Abducens nerve
VII Facial nerve
VIII Acoustic nerve
IX Glossopharyngeal nerve
X Vagus nerve
XI Accessory nerve
XII Hypoglossal nerve

FIGURE 32:9. The 12 cranial nerves

Cranial Nerve XII: hypoglossal—primarily a motor nerve concerned with the movements of the tongue.

Generations of medical students have learned these nerves with the mnemonic "On Old Olympus' Towering Tops, A Finn And Greek Viewed Some Hops."

INJURY TO THE BRAIN

Cerebral concussion is a basic insult to the brain itself and can be classified into three degrees of severity (Table 32:1). These distinctions are important in determining treatment and prognosis.

First-Degree Concussion

A first-degree concussion is the mildest, involving no loss of consciousness. The force of impact causes transient aberration in the electrophysiology of the brain substance, creating slight mental confusion. Memory loss, dizziness and tinnitus may occur, but there is no loss of coordination. Because of the rapid recovery rate, it is important to remember that

TABLE 32:1.   Three Levels of Cerebral Concussion

Level	Consciousness	Memory Loss	Dizziness	Tinnitus	Loss of Coordination	Recovery Time
I	No loss	May occur	May occur	May occur	No	Rapid
II	Momentary loss 10 seconds–5 minutes	Transient confusion; mild retrograde amnesia	Moderate	Moderate	May occur	Varies
III	Prolonged loss	Severe	Severe	Severe	Marked	Prolonged beyond 5 minutes

an individual may suffer a minor concussion without loss of consciousness.

Second-Degree Concussion

With a second-degree concussion there is momentary loss of consciousness. This may last from seconds up to 5 minutes and can be associated with transient confusion, moderate dizziness, tinnitus, unsteadiness and prolonged, mild retrograde amnesia. There is a wide range of findings between first-degree concussions and third-degree concussions. Second-degree concussions demand careful clinical observation and skilled judgment, especially as to a decision to return to play at a later date.

Third-Degree Concussion

Third-degree concussions are more severe and result in prolonged loss of consciousness. Neuromuscular coordination is markedly compromised with severe mental confusion, tinnitus, dizziness and retrograde amnesia. The recovery period is also prolonged beyond 5 minutes.

The question of return to competition after concussion is very individual, and conservatism seems the wisest course in almost all cases. There may be rare exceptions following a mild concussion, however, when experienced personnel in attendance to constantly monitor and re-evaluate the athlete's status allow him to return to competition. Symptoms of concussion may be associated with more serious and progressive underlying brain injury. The athlete who sustains repeated concussions requires special evaluation before returning to a sport with the potential for further brain injury. Most team physicians follow the "1-2-3 Rule": One concussion and you are out of the game; two concussions and you are out for the season; three concussions and you should no longer play.

Cerebral Contusion

The brain substance may suffer a contusion when an object impacts with the skull or vice versa. This "bruising" causes internal bleeding from injured vessels with concomitant loss of consciousness. This may be associated with partial paralysis or hemiplegia, one-sided pupil dilatation, or altered vital signs and may last for prolonged periods of time. Progressive swelling may produce further danger to brain tissue not injured in the original trauma. Even with severe contusions, however, eventual recovery without the necessity of intracranial surgery is the rule. The prognosis is often determined by the supportive care delivered from the moment of injury, including adequate ventilation and CPR, proper transport techniques and prompt expert evaluation.

Cerebral Hematoma

Finally, there is the cerebral hematoma. The skull fits the brain like a custom-made helmet, leaving little room for lesions like blood clots that occupy space. Blood clots are of two types, epidural and subdural, depending on whether they are outside or inside the dura (Fig. 32:10).

An epidural hematoma in the athlete most commonly results from a severe blow to the head producing a skull fracture in the temporoparietal region. The middle meningeal artery may be severed, producing an epidural hematoma. Thus, there may be a hiatus of 10 to 20 minutes or longer before the injured athlete's neurologic status begins to deteriorate progressively. Immediate surgery may be required to decompress the hematoma and to control the bleeding artery.

The mechanism of the subdural hematoma is more complex. The force of a blow to the skull thrusts the brain against the point of impact. The subdural vessels on the opposite side of the brain are torn, resulting in venous bleeding. As bleeding is low pressure with slow clot formation, symptoms may not become evident until hours, days or even weeks later, when the clot may absorb fluid and expand. Prolonged observation and monitoring are advised in an athlete suffering loss of consciousness or altered mental status, as associated bleeding may contribute to subsequent deterioration. Surgical intervention may be necessary to evacuate the hematoma and decompress the brain.

Unit		Time
I Vital signs	Blood pressure Pulse Respiration Temperature	
II Conscious and	Oriented Disoriented Restless Combative	
III Speech	Clear Rambling Garbled None	
IV Will awaken to	Name Shaking Light pain Strong pain	
V Nonverbal reaction to pain	Appropriate Inappropriate "Decerebrate" None	
VI Pupils	Size on right Size on left Reacts on right Reacts on left	
VII Ability to move	Right arm Left arm Right leg Left leg	

TABLE 32:2.   Neural Watch Chart

INITIAL ASSESSMENT

Head trauma in an athletic situation requires immediate assessment for appropriate emergency action (Table 32:2). Rarely do athletes sustain such serious head injuries that require immediate evacuation to the nearest medical facility and then constant monitoring and observation. The athlete is initially evaluated at the site of injury. Observe his respiratory and cardiac status. Determine the level of consciousness by simple questions directed toward orientation and observe the appropriate response of the athlete. Evaluate recent

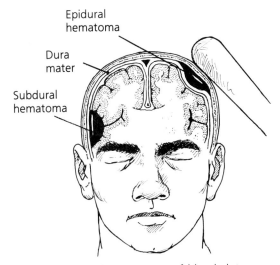

FIGURE 32:10.   The two types of blood clots are epidural and subdural.

memory and assess the voluntary response of muscle control of all extremities. Briefly evaluate the appropriateness of response to pain and establish whether the athlete has sensation in the extremities.

The player who is conscious or who was momentarily unconscious is transported to the sidelines or locker room for further evaluation after the initial on-site evaluation. If the athlete is unconscious, moving and positioning should be done carefully, assuming possible associated cervical injury. It is not necessary to remove the helmet unless in some way it compromises maintenance of adequate ventilation. Often an adequate airway can be maintained by removing only face masks or straps (Fig. 32:11A). Move the unconscious player with care, avoiding motion of the neck by gentle, firm support, and transport on a backboard (Fig. 32:11B–F).

Examination on the Sidelines

Once the athlete is in an area where a more detailed examination can be carried out and is conscious, remove the helmet. Obtain a more complete history of exactly what happened, noting how the athlete recalls his injury. Ask further questions to determine the athlete's mental status. Examine motor functions in detail including evaluation of strength, reflexes and sensory and pain response. It is essential that the trainer document and record the initial findings and subsequent monitoring of the head-injured athlete. It is difficult to make specific recommendations on return to competition. Important factors to consider are:

1. History of head trauma
2. Observation and monitoring by experienced personnel during recovery
3. Determination of recovery and potential for further neurologic deterioration

After head trauma, the athlete should return to competition with great caution. Most athletes who are unconscious for a period of time require extensive evaluation and monitoring. Even though the majority recover without

any permanent neurological deficit or need for surgery, major head trauma potentially threatens life. Following head injury, the athlete should not return to competition that day, and must be free of headaches for 24 hours before he resumes training. Recurrent head injuries are commonly seen and may be avoided by assuring complete recovery from the initial episode. A physician should see any athlete who was unconscious or has headaches.

ARTICULATED VERTEBRAL COLUMN

The vertebral column consists of 24 moveable vertebrae, the sacrum and the coccyx (Fig. 32:12). The vertebral column with its muscles and joints represents an axis of the body capable of rigidity and flexibility. The head pivots on it and the upper limbs are attached to it. The vertebral column completely surrounds and encases the spinal cord and partly shields the thoracic and abdominal viscera. It transmits the weight of the rest of the body to the lower limbs and to the ground when a person is standing, supports the weight for locomotion and protects the spinal cord and the roots of the spinal nerves. The vertebral column is flexible because it is composed of many slightly moveable parts—the vertebrae. Its stability depends largely upon ligaments and muscles. Some stability, however, is provided by the form of the column and the constituent parts. The vertebrae become progressively larger from the skull to the sacrum and then become progressively smaller. The length of the vertebral column amounts to about two-fifths of the total height of the body.

Curves of the Vertebral Column

The cervical, thoracic, lumbar and sacral portions of the vertebral column all have characteristic curves. Abnormal curves are called curvatures. Accentuation of the normal curve is called lordosis in the lumbar spine and kyphosis in the thoracic spine (Fig. 32:13).

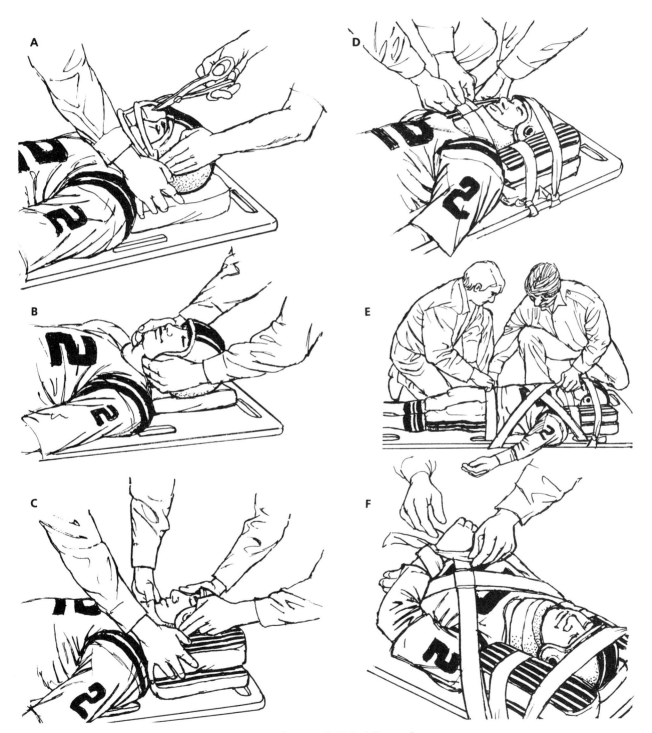

FIGURE 32:11. **A** Cutters can be used to remove face mask. **B** Stabilize and apply traction as needed. **C–F** To secure the patient to the spine board, place sandbags next to the head **C**, secure the head and sandbags to the board **D**, secure limbs and trunk to board **E** and tie wrists loosely together **F**.

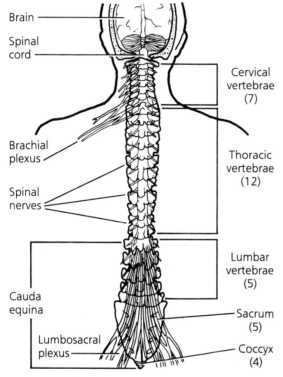

FIGURE 32:12. The vertebral column

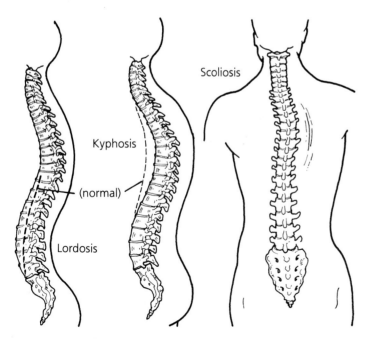

FIGURE 32:13. Abnormal curves of the lumbar and thoracic spines, called curvatures

These curvatures may be associated with underlying developmental problems in the young athlete. While there is normally kyphosis in the thoracic area and lordosis in the lumbar area, these terms more commonly refer to exaggeration of the normal curve resulting from a pathological condition.

Lateral curvature of the spine, to the left or right, is termed scoliosis, and may be accompanied by major rib cage deformity and postural changes. These become permanent if not treated soon enough. Scoliosis commonly starts in the preadolescent and increases during adolescence, especially in the female.

Movement between the vertebrae is the least in regions where the intervertebral discs are the thinnest—in the thoracic and pelvic cavities. In these areas the column is concave. The intervertebral disc is a fibrocartilaginous disc whose peripheral part is composed of concentric layers of fibers called the anulus fibrosis (Fig. 32:14). The center of the disc is filled with a gelatinous pulp, the nucleus pulposus, which acts as a cushion and a shock absorber.

Vertebral Bodies

The typical vertebra consists of a body, vertebral arch and several processes for muscular and articular connections (Fig. 32:15). Each vertebra has three relatively short processes (two transverse and one spinous), and the 12 thoracic vertebrae are connected with ribs. The body of the vertebra gives strength and supports weight. It is separated from the bodies of the vertebrae above and below by the intervertebral disc. Posterior to the body is the vertebral arch which, with the posterior surface of the body, forms the walls of the spinal canal. These walls enclose and protect the spinal cord. The vertebral arch is composed of right and left pedicles and right and left laminae. Superior and inferior articular processes on each side (superior and inferior articular facets, respectively) form the small joints of the posterior elements. The lower edge of each pedicle has a deep notch, while the upper edge of each pedicle has a shallow

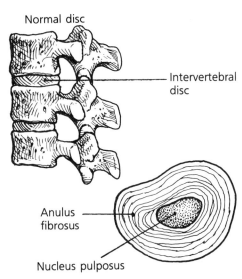

FIGURE 32:14. Normal disc and intervertebral spacing of spinal cord

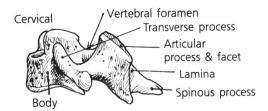

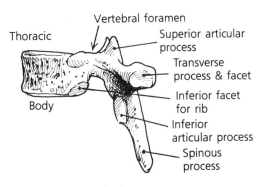

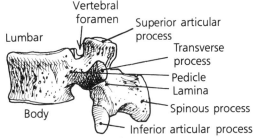

FIGURE 32:15. Anatomy of vertebrae

notch. Two adjacent notches together with the intervening body and the intervertebral disc form the intervertebral foramina that transmits the spinal nerve and its vessels.

The seven cervical vertebrae are between the skull and the thorax. They are characterized by the presence of a foramina that transmits a vertebral artery in each transverse process. The first cervical vertebra, the atlas, is ring shaped and the skull rests on it. The second cervical vertebra, the axis, forms a pivot around which the atlas can rotate, carrying with it the skull. The atlas and axis are the two specialized cervical vertebrae (Fig. 32:16). The third to sixth cervical vertebrae have small, broad bodies with large triangular vertebral foramina and are similar in shape. The seventh cervical vertebra is characterized by a long spine that gives attachment to a strong cord, the ligamentum nuchae, that also attaches the skull.

The 12 thoracic vertebrae bear the ribs and form the posterior point of the chest wall.

The five lumbar vertebrae are between the thorax and sacrum and are distinguished by their large size and the absence of costal facets and foramina transversarium. The sacrum consists of five vertebrae that are fused in the adult

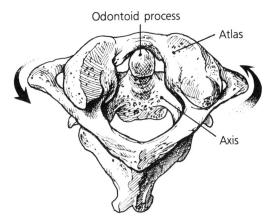

FIGURE 32:16. The axis forms a pivot for the atlas to rotate the skull.

into wedge-shaped bone that forms the back of the pelvis. Below the sacrum, the coccyx lies slightly above and behind the anus. Like the sacrum, it resembles a wedge and usually consists of four segments.

Spinal Cord

The spinal cord is a continuation of the central nervous system to provide pathways to and from the brain. It is widest in the mid-cervical region, narrows in the thoracic area, and ends in the upper lumbar area in the L1-2 intervertebral space (Fig. 32:17). From this point down, the nerves continue as the cauda equina through the lower lumbar and sacral areas. Attached to the spinal cord on each side is a series of pairs of nerves and spinal roots, termed the dorsal and ventral according to their position. Generally, 31 pairs comprise 8 cervical, 12 thoracic, 5 lumbar, 5 sacral and 1 coccygeal.

Many of the cells of the spinal cord, as well as the brain stem, are concerned with reflexes. A reflex may be defined as a fairly fixed pattern of response or behavior similar for any given stimulus. The reflex pathway consists of sensory fibers bringing impulses into the spinal cord. These sensory fibers connect with motor cells and impulses reaching back to the muscle cells by way of the nerves innervating them (Fig. 32:18).

Autonomic Nervous System

The autonomic nervous system is the portion of the nervous system that mainly regulates the activity of the cardiac muscle, the smooth muscle and the glands. The autonomic nervous system has two parts: the sympathetic system and the parasympathetic system. The sympathetic, or thoracolumbar, part of the autonomic system comprises fibers that come from the length of the spinal cord. The para-

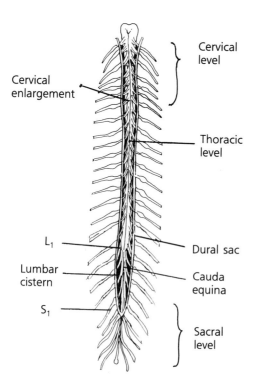

FIGURE 32:17. The spinal cord at the cervical, thoracic, lumbar and sacral levels

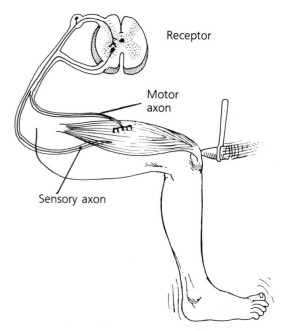

FIGURE 32:18. Reflex arc through sensory arc receptor and motor axon

sympathetic, or craniosacral, part of the autonomic system comprises fibers that come from the brain stem and the sacral portion of the spinal cord. The autonomic system is important to keeping the internal environment of the body constant by maintaining temperature, fluid balance and the ionic composition of the blood. There are many specific functions in the parasympathetic and sympathetic systems and they are particularly important to the athlete's "fight-or-flight" response to stress.

NECK: SOFT TISSUE INJURY

The esophagus lies in front of the vertebral bodies and behind the trachea and larynx. The carotid arteries that carry blood to the brain are on each side of the trachea and are easily palpable just under the sternocleidomastoid muscles. The muscle and ligaments that control the motion of the neck can be grouped into the posterior group attached to the lamina, extending from the skull to the shoulders, and the anterior group, consisting of a deep group of muscles that attach to the skull, vertebral bodies and the upper ribs. The most superficial and largest anterior muscle is the sternocleidomastoid, which arises from the clavicle and sternum below and attaches to the base of the skull at the mastoid process above (Fig. 32:19).

A cervical strain is an injury to the musculotendinous unit that may or may not be associated with a ligamentous sprain. Cervical sprains and strains are common in athletic events. They can occur at the extremes of motion, such as hyperflexion, hyperextension or excessive rotation, or in association with violent muscle contraction. Cervical sprains and strains associated with muscle spasms, limited motion, painful motion or radiating pain, numbness or tingling into the upper or lower extremities require further evaluation, including roentgenographic studies. These studies should ascertain the stability of the cervical spine and may require flexion-extension views, cinematography or traction studies.

Acute cervical intervertebral disc herniation may be associated with restricted cervical mo-

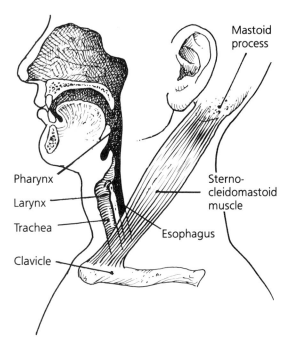

FIGURE 32:19. Soft tissue structures of the neck

tion, cervical pain, radiating pain, numbness and tingling. Routine roentgenograms, although usually not helpful in making this diagnosis, should be obtained. The neurologic examination is the basis of diagnosis. After appropriate evaluation and conservative measures including bed rest and traction have failed, a myelogram or CT scan may be necessary to confirm the diagnosis, to plan further treatment and to give a more accurate prognosis. Repeated injury or even a single episode of injury to the intervertebral disc in the cervical spine may be associated with degenerative changes at the involved level. These can even occur in young athletes and on cervical roentgenograms appear as narrowing of the space occupied by the intervertebral disc with osteophyte formation at the vertebral margins. These chronic changes are most often seen in the disc spaces of the lower cervical spine and may become associated with symptoms related to the impingement of the neural elements as they exit the spinal canal.

One of the most common cervical injuries seen in athletics, especially football, is forced

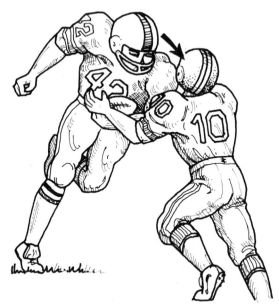

FIGURE 32:20. Forced lateral deviation of the neck, commonly called a "stinger" or "burner"

lateral deviation of the neck (Fig. 32:20). This injury is often associated with pain, numbness or tingling into the upper extremity and is commonly called a "stinger" or "burner."

The neck may not only be driven laterally, but may have associated rotation or anterior and posterior motion. This displacement may be associated with a stretch injury to the nerve trunks of the upper portion of the brachial plexus. These nerves may be stretched and, on rare instances, completely pulled away from the spinal cord. A complete pull-off, or avulsion, results in permanent paralysis of the muscles innervated by those specific nerves. These uncommon nerve avulsions can be demonstrated by special techniques of cervical myelography.

In general, however, most injuries to the upper brachial plexus are brief, transient episodes of paresthesia and pain extending into the upper extremities. The initial cause is usually a stretch of the neural elements on the opposite side to which the head is driven. Symptoms are commonly pain extending out into the shoulder and down the extremity, accompanied by weakness. The athlete usually describes a burning sensation and says that his arm "has gone numb." This injury most frequently involves areas innervated by the fifth and sixth cervical roots and may result in weakness of the deltoid and biceps muscles and depression of the biceps reflex. The pain is usually transient, lasting only a few minutes. Those athletes with muscle weakness associated with their paresthesia require a decision on returning to competition. When the symptoms pass, the athlete typically wishes to resume competition. If the initial episode is severe or recurrent, neurologic changes may develop. Initially these may involve pronation and supination of the forearm but with more marked involvement prolonged weakness of the deltoid and biceps muscle may develop.

In football, wearing a collar restricting the extremes of cervical motion may offer some degree of protection. This collar needs to fit well on the shoulder pads and provide an effective block beneath the helmet. Off-season strengthening of cervical musculature and improved blocking and tackling techniques may be beneficial.

Blunt trauma to the front of the neck can be associated with injury to the larynx and trachea with acute airway obstruction. This can become a medical emergency and may require tracheotomy.

CERVICAL SPINE FRACTURES

Cervical spine fractures can only be diagnosed and confirmed by roentgenographic evaluation. On the field consider the possibility in any athlete sustaining a cervical injury with persistent pain or symptoms following injury, with or without neurologic impairment. Fractures are often accompanied by instability of the cervical spine and injury to the spinal cord and nerve roots. Even if the neural elements were not injured at the time of the fracture, injudicious movement of the head and neck in an unstable spine can cause permanent spinal cord or nerve root injury. A subluxation or dislocation of the cervical spine means normal anatomical alignment may be lost with associated ligament, tendon, muscle, disc, bone and neural element injuries. The varying degrees of injuries may result in paralysis and even sudden death. Mechanisms of injury of the cervical spine are complex and usually represent a combination of forces rather than one single mechanism. These include flexion and extension in the anteroposterior plane, lateral flexion, rotation and compressive axial loading of the vertebral column. The most common devastating fracture dislocations of the cervical spine in athletic participation occur with flexion and compression loading.

The first cervical vertebra is atypical, composed primarily of a large ring in which there is usually more than adequate room for the spinal cord. This extra room often allows the spinal cord to escape injury in fractures, causing only minor displacement. A bursting fracture of this ring of C-1 (the so-called Jefferson fracture) occurs when the condyles of the occiput are driven down against the ring of the atlas, splitting this fragile bone (Fig. 32:21). The danger in this injury is that it may be difficult to detect clinically, and may be overlooked on roentgenographic examination unless special views are taken that demonstrate widening in this ring. Even without neurologic damage, the clinical picture of paraspinacervical muscle spasms associated with pain and resistance to rotation on examination should alert the trainer to the possibility of this injury. It is important to suspect the fracture, stabilize the neck and eliminate any further contact until adequate evaluation.

Fractures and dislocations of the atlantoaxial joint mean an alteration in the alignment between the first two cervical vertebrae. The odontoid process of the second cervical vertebra may rupture the transverse ligament of the first cervical vertebra, allowing the atlas to slide forward on the second cervical vertebra encroaching on the space occupied by the spinal cord. Fractures of the odontoid process may also occur and, like all injuries in this area, can only be evaluated with specific roentgenographic views. The hangman's fracture is a fracture of the pedicles of C-2 (Fig. 32:22).

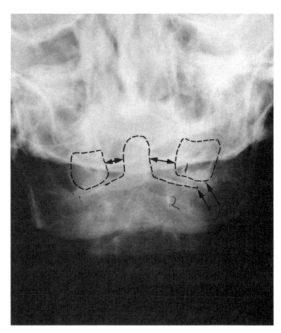

FIGURE 32:21. Odontoid view showing a burst fracture of the ring of C_1 (Jefferson fracture). This fracture can be inferred by noting the subtle displacement of the left C_1 lateral mass.

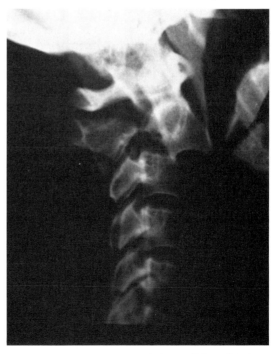

FIGURE 32:22. Fracture of the pedicles of C-2, the so-called hangman's fracture

Damage to the upper cervical spinal cord is a life-threatening injury because the centers that control respiration are located in this area. Fractures and dislocations of the lower cervical spine, associated with spinal cord injuries in athletes, are most commonly observed at the fourth, fifth and sixth cervical levels. Like fracture dislocations of the cervical spine anywhere, these injuries may be associated with varying degrees of damage to the neural elements and can cause transient, partial or complete paralysis.

The brachial plexus exits from the lower portion of the cervical spine, and the degree of involvement of the upper extremity following a spinal cord injury is determined by which level sustains the damage. This potential for neurologic damage makes care of the injured cervical spine critical.

UPPER BACK AND THORACIC SPINE INJURIES

Although lacking the dramatic impact of a "broken neck" or the frequency of low back injury, disorders and injuries of the thoracic spine merit careful attention. The nature of injuries in this area differs because of the stability offered by the rib cage. The special consideration in this area is that the muscles can be divided into two functional groups—those that join the shoulder mechanism to the back, and those that power movement between individual vertebrae and ribs.

Fractures of the bony elements of the upper back also vary in severity and degree of involvement of adjacent neural elements. The traditional concepts of bony injury of the spine have been fractures of the vertebrae or ribs resulting from a single, forceful impact. The potential for spinal injury, however, resulting from recurrent microtrauma from repetitive flexing or extending of the spine is becoming increasingly apparent. The young athlete, particularly during the adolescent growth spurt, appears to be especially subject to recurrent microtraumatic injuries that produce stress fractures.

Posterior rib fractures are usually caused by a direct blow. Because they bleed and swell, they can be easily confused with a muscle contusion. Direct tenderness at the site of the injury can be misleading, but pain referred to the site of injury from pressure over an uninvolved portion of the same rib may indicate a fractured rib. Sometimes, of course, only an x-ray can differentiate between fracture and contusion. This differentiation is important because a fractured rib can puncture the pleura lining of the chest cavity, or even the lung itself. If this occurs, air leaks into this potential space and collapses the lung.

Dorsal spine fractures can result from either direct or indirect force. Fracture from a direct blow is extremely rare, usually the result of vertical loading of the spine or a rotational force. These fractures generally occur at the lower levels of the dorsal spine, or at the thoracolumbar junction, where forces tend to concentrate because of the change of the spinal curves from the thoracic kyphosis to the lumbar lordosis. The stabilizing structures of the spine at this point, including the posterior joints and ligaments, also appear to be weaker than the structures above and below.

Spinal fractures are classed as stable or unstable, depending on the risk of injury to the spinal cord or nerve roots from movement at the time of injury or during the period shortly after the injury. The vertebral body compression, or wedge fracture, is the most common and is almost always stable in the dorsal spine. Another fracture, the Chance or slice fracture, is frequently unstable. Often special x-ray techniques are necessary to differentiate these fractures.

Despite the fact that most fractures of the thoracic spine occurring in sports are stable, any athlete suspected of having a spinal fracture must be treated as a spinal emergency and appropriate evacuation and transport techniques used until definitive assessment.

Musculotendinous Injuries

Contusions of the upper back muscles are fairly common in contact sports. Because of the double function of these muscles, both back motion and shoulder motion can be affected. As with any contusion of large muscle groups, immediate ICE management helps minimize disability. On occasion, particularly if the shoulder girdle muscles are involved, a sling on the involved side can improve comfort. Musculotendinous strains in this area can result from either excessive extrinsic stretch of the back muscles, such as from twisting, or from a sustained overloading contraction of the muscles.

Upper back sprains can be difficult to distinguish from a musculotendinous strain, particularly when a sprain is followed by extensive reflex protective muscle spasm of the dorsal muscles. Usually, however, no anatomic area of muscle tenderness can be palpated with a sprain, although "trigger points" of increased sensitivity can sometimes be identified. In addition, with a sprain the athlete may strongly resist lateral or rotational motion. Upper back sprains may show dramatic improvement in 24 to 48 hours, while a true muscle tendon strain of the dorsal musculature may take three to four weeks or more to resolve.

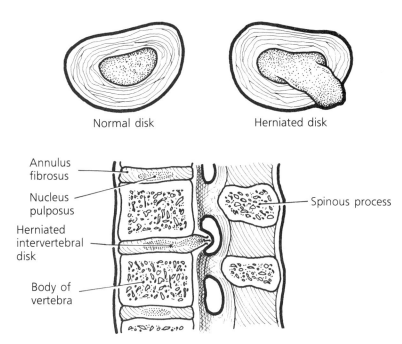

FIGURE 32:23. Normal and herniated intervertebral discs

LUMBAR SPINE

Serious disabling injuries to the low back are unusual in athletes. Contusions of the muscles, sprains and strains and even subtle fractures of the lumbar vertebrae ordinarily heal with no persistent disability. If low back pain and disability persist, the underlying cause must be identified. Most acute low back pain in athletes is self-limited and resolves within two to three weeks. Persistent symptoms indicate more established and chronic problems needing careful diagnosis and management.

Symptomatic Lumbar Disc

A young athlete with low back pain associated with radiating pain into the lower extremities, especially when the pain is associated with sciatica, may have a herniated disc (Fig. 32:23). The differential diagnosis of lesions

mimicking a herniated lumbar disc in an athlete includes neoplasms, bony compromise of the nerve root canal or foramina and other rare conditions irritating the neural elements more distal to the spinal column.

A posterior or lateral disc herniation pressing against the adjacent neural elements may be very incapacitating. Young athletes may successfully return to competition with or without disc surgery. Once a young athlete has had a prolonged irritation of the neural elements, however, he may have great difficulty returning to his previous performance level or tolerance for activity and may have to select other sports or a less demanding position in the same sport.

Pars Interarticularis: Spondylolysis and Spondylolisthesis

Chronic pain confined to the lumbar spine may be caused by segmental instability associated with lumbar pars interarticularis defects. These defects may be associated with spon-

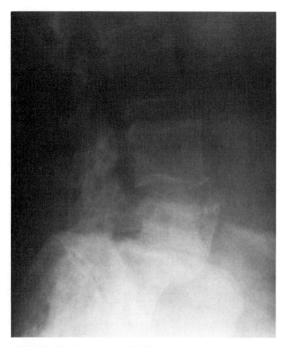

FIGURE 32:24. Spondylolisthesis, forward sub-luxation of the lower lumbar vertebrae (in this case L5 on S1), may cause chronic leg and back pain.

dylolysis, a dissolution of a vertebra, and spondylolisthesis—vertebral slippage (Fig. 32:24). Vertebral slippage in the lower lumbar spine, commonly seen at the L5–S1 level, occurs most often between the ages of 9 and 13 in athletic women. A more vertical sacrum with hamstring tightness and loss of flexibility are signs of a possible spondylolisthesis.

Lumbar Spine Fracture

Transverse processes or spinous processes fractures, either from direct blows or violent muscle contraction, occur occasionally in the athlete and may lead to periods of disability. Subtle fractures of the vertebral bodies other than the more obvious compression fractures can also be seen and be disabling.

Compression fractures of the lumbar vertebrae are most frequently seen at L1 due to the mechanical vulnerability of the thoraco-lumbar junction. These fractures are usually caused by vertical loading and flexion. Frac-

ture dislocations of the lumbar spine with or without neural injury are rare in athletic participation. The spinal cord ends at L2. Therefore, fractures or dislocations of the lumbar spine below this point may injure the roots but not the cord.

At the present time, no protective athletic equipment is adequate to prevent trauma to the spinal vertebral column or the spinal cord. The helmet protects the head, but does nothing to protect the cervical, thoracic or lumbar spine from potential injuries. Technique and chance protect the spine.

The incidence of spinal injuries can be reduced primarily by minimizing exposure to risks. Those caring for sports injuries to the head and spine share the responsibility of keeping the risks to a minimum. Yet even with the greatest care, spinal injuries will occur, and collision sports have a higher incidence of potentially devastating head and spine injuries.

EMERGENCY CARE AND TRANSPORTATION

Basic principles must be observed to adequately protect someone with a head or spine injury from damage to the brain or spinal cord, producing paralysis or even death. When a person with a head injury is unconscious, the forces that caused cerebral injury may have been sufficient to damage the cervical spine. Therefore, every traumatic episode resulting in an unconscious athlete may have an associated injury to the cervical spine, with neurological damage possible until proven otherwise. All such injuries should be treated as neck injuries until ruled out by subsequent examination.

Paralysis does not have to be present for an athlete to have a severely injured head or spine. If the athlete complains of numbness or tingling, buzzing sensations, radiating pain or inability to move a body part, take extreme care and consider the possibility of a neurologic injury. Immobilize the athlete with potential spinal injuries to prevent further damage and increased neurologic deficits during transportation. A person with a fracture that results in instability to the spine may be rendered para- or quadriplegic by injudicious movement.

Initially, of course, the basic considerations of airway and cardiopulmonary functions are paramount. An injured person may have to be moved promptly in order to maintain adequate breathing or initiate resuscitation. In spite of a spinal injury, it is of little value to protect the spine while neglecting vital functions although every possible care should be taken within reason.

Immobilization and splinting should be accomplished without twisting or bending the spine in any direction. However, if the victim's head is in a position that obstructs the airway, gentle traction on the head followed by positioning into normal alignment is necessary. Opening the airway of the victim with a suspected neck fracture may often be done by the chin-lift method or by the jaw-forward technique. Do not overextend or overflex the neck while performing CPR on such a victim. Do not try to straighten the deformity simply to make splinting easier or more convenient. Straighten only to establish an airway; otherwise, it is better to splint the neck or back in the position of deformity. Because people with spinal cord injuries have neurogenic shock, and because the chest muscles may become paralyzed, insure that an adequate airway is maintained during transportation.

Before making any attempt to move the victim, generally assess the situation. A simple series of steps for checking signs of spinal fracture and dislocation in a conscious patient is to ASK, LOOK, FEEL and ASK others at the scene what happened. Ask a conscious patient several questions to aid in evaluating the seriousness of the injury: Is there pain in the neck or back? Is there numbness or tingling? Then ask the patient to voluntarily move, one by one, the hands, feet, arms and legs. If the person cannot perform these simple motions, avoid moving him until adequate immobilization and transportation can be arranged, unless absolutely necessary for other lifesaving reasons, i.e., cardiac or respiratory distress. The importance of stabilizing the neck to prevent secondary mechanical bony or vascular damage to the spinal cord cannot be overemphasized. A stabilization board must be available either at the athletic site or from the emergency transportation vehicle.

Apply only gentle traction to a cervical injury prior to roentgenographic evaluation. Immobilization to prevent motion should always be the initial treatment. This can be done by sandbagging on either side of the head, or by protecting the spine with a cervical immobilizer applied judiciously.

Do not flex the neck when lifting the patient onto a board. At least three people are required to move a patient with cervical spine injury with adequate care. However, in a dire emergency, if the unconscious person is in an extremely precarious position, a lone rescuer may grasp the person by the armpits, with the head cradled flat against the rescuer's forearm, and drag the patient backward along the body's longitudinal axis.

Diving injuries may be associated with unstable fractures of the cervical spine. In removing an unconscious diving accident victim from the water, remember that such an injury could be aggravated by hyperextension or hyperflexion of the cervical spine. Splint such injuries properly before moving the victim from the water unless there are enough persons available to protect the head and neck from bending.

Facial Injuries

33

Facial injuries are commonly associated with head injuries. Soft tissue injuries to the head and face are treated identically to soft tissue injuries elsewhere. Bleeding can easily be controlled by direct pressure.

EYE

The eye is most commonly injured by a foreign body. Carefully remove the offending object, preferably by gentle, mild irrigation. On occasion, removal of the foreign body requires inversion of the upper lid (Fig. 33:1). The foreign body may have caused a corneal abrasion, which often requires further evaluation using a fluorescein solution instilled into the eye. The cornea is inspected carefully, using special lighting. If small corneal abrasions are detected, antibiotic ointment can be applied and an eye patch worn for a period of time. Larger abrasions, penetrating injuries or contusions or lacerations of the globe itself require immediate medical care, and the athlete should be evacuated immediately to the nearest appropriate facility. A direct blow may cause detachment of the retina.

Hyphema is a serious eye injury, characterized by bleeding within the eye caused by trauma. This can be diagnosed by examining the pupil with a small flashlight. In hyphema a red discoloration is seen. Comparison with the normal eye helps in making the diagnosis. This injury calls for complete rest of the eye and consultation with an ophthalmologist.

Another frequent injury is the eyelid contusion or "black eye." Early ice application may help limit swelling. Disability is limited to one to two days with rapid absorption of the swelling. Lid laceration, particularly in the region of the tear ducts, may require special suturing techniques necessitating referral.

With fracture of the bones surrounding the eye, the globe itself may actually descend into the maxillary sinus resulting in diplopia and occasionally even enophthalmos. X-ray films in the frontal and oblique projections and

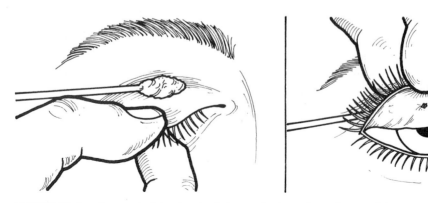

FIGURE 33:1. Removal of foreign body in eye by inversion of upper lid. Holding the lid and stick in place with one hand, use sterile cotton swab to lift out foreign body.

Waters's view make the diagnosis definitive. Treatment for orbital fracture includes open reduction and possibly internal fixation.

Fractures of the medial wall of the orbit may violate the ethmoid sinus. This may result in puffiness around the nose and eye, which increases markedly after blowing the nose. The athlete must be cautioned against this, and appropriate antibiotics instituted.

FACIAL BONE FRACTURES

Facial bone fractures are often overlooked in evaluating the athlete with head trauma. Fractures may be masked by the severe swelling often associated with facial contusions or abrasions, as well as the inadequacy of conventional roentgenograms in demonstrating subtle fractures. Reduction is much easier in the initial hours following the injury than later. Special roentgenographic views should be obtained early on to obviate the need for technically difficult and unsatisfactory late reconstructive procedures.

A common by-product of impact injuries, facial fractures may result in severe deformities and bleeding, both of which may cause airway obstruction. Emergency care is directed at maintaining an airway and controlling hemorrhage. Bleeding can often be controlled by direct pressure. Check for bleeding sites inside the mouth and lacerations of the tongue. Blood draining into the throat may cause vomiting and airway obstruction.

Depression of the zygomatic arch is of only cosmetic importance when occurring as an isolated injury (Fig. 33:2). Zygomatic arch fractures can usually be easily reduced surgically and may not require internal fixation.

Fractures of the maxilla and mandible may not be obvious if undisplaced. Maxillary fractures can be treated by wiring the teeth or the bony fragments if no upper teeth are present. Maxillary and mandibular fractures should be suspected with any irregularity in occlusion of the teeth. Roentgenograms confirm the fracture and reduction can often be accomplished by wiring the teeth. One crucial precaution

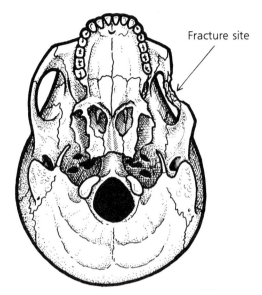

Fracture site

FIGURE 33:2. Compression fracture of the zygomatic arch

with bilateral or comminuted mandibular fractures is to secure the airway by drawing the tongue forward. Tracheostomy is needed in only the most severe cases.

Nasal Fractures

Nasal fractures are the most common facial bone fractures. They are usually recognized by palpation of the bony structures of the nose. Bleeding is frequent and may be controlled with an ice pack over the nose, pinching the nostrils when tolerable or packing the nostrils with gauze. Hemorrhage around the septal cartilage may result in late pressure necrosis. Nasal fractures with septal deviation often require special treatment to prevent later problems with nasal breathing. Fractures involving the nasal cartilage as well as the bone may require packing and external and internal fixation with wires and a splint. Nasal fractures associated with fractures in the cribriform plate may result in leakage of spinal fluid from the nose. This serious problem requires antibiotics and rest. The clear fluid should be tested for sugar content to be sure it is spinal fluid. These fractures are difficult to see on x-ray films. A simple nasal fracture may mean only several days' disability if a nose guard is worn.

TEETH INJURIES

The teeth themselves may be loosened, chipped or completely fractured. Chipped teeth can be capped to prevent devitalization. Even loosened teeth, when still viable, can be preserved by wiring them to adjacent teeth. When teeth are injured by facial trauma, associated maxillary or mandibular fractures must be suspected. On the field, palpate the gingiva and underlying bony structures directly. Barring secondary infection or retained root fragments, rapid recovery can generally be expected following trauma isolated to the teeth. Encourage athletes who have already suffered injuries to the teeth to wear mouth protection.

MOUTH LACERATIONS

Aside from injuries to the teeth, the most common injury to the mouth is contusion or laceration of the lip. Proper repair of lip lacerations requires exact alignment of the vermilion border, the junction of the mucous membrane and skin. Through and through lacerations of the lip may bleed profusely and require special suturing techniques. When loss of lip substance is excessive, referral to a plastic surgeon for immediate reconstructive flaps is advised. The only other mucous membrane lacerations of serious consequence are those involving the opening of the submaxillary or parotid duct. In these cases, the duct must be identified and cannulized with a small plastic catheter, and the repair done around this catheter.

Lacerations of the tongue usually result from forcible contact with the teeth. They may require careful suturing to minimize scar formation. A badly scarred tongue is apt to be sensitive and uncomfortable and may interfere with proper speech patterns. The undersurface of the tongue should be examined to determine the full extent of any lacerations. All mouth lacerations should be monitored and require special attention to mouth hygiene. The period of disability for mouth injuries is usually brief. Most mouth injuries are preventable though the use of properly fitted mouth guards, which should be mandatory.

EAR

Foreign bodies are less common in the ear than the eye and usually more innocuous. Occasionally water may be retained in the ear canal after swimming or bathing, but most foreign bodies in the ear are easily removed with the aid of a speculum. The tympanic membrane itself may rupture as a result of a blow to the head or from pressure changes or infection. Barring complications following a tympanic membrane rupture, the disability is usually minor, but referral to an otorhinolaryngologist is suggested for further evaluation. Basilar skull fractures may be associated with bleeding behind the tympanic membrane or from the auditory canal and, in certain extensive skull fractures, spinal fluid may even be found in the auditory canal. Examination of the ear and the external auditory canal after head injury is an appropriate part of the examination.

Contusions to the external ear may cause considerable extravasated blood around the ear cartilage, necessitating aspiration to avoid pressure and permanent cartilage damage ("cauliflower ear"). With severe lacerations, every bit of viable cartilage should be preserved. The ear has a remarkable ability to survive, and resuturing is usually attempted even if circulation seems minimal. Missing pieces of both the ear and nose may be restored later if found and maintained properly.

Part 9

GASTROINTESTINAL AND GENITOURINARY SYSTEMS

The Abdomen and Digestive System

ABDOMINAL CAVITY

The two major body cavities are the thorax and the abdomen. The abdomen is inferior to the thorax. The superior boundary of the abdomen is the diaphragm. The interior boundary is at the level of an imaginary plane between the pubis and the sacrum. The anterior and posterior boundaries are the musculoskeletal body walls (Fig. 34:1). Immediately beneath the inferior plane lies the pelvic cavity, the lowermost part of the abdomen, surrounded by the bony pelvic ring.

The abdominal cavity contains the liver, gallbladder and bile ducts, spleen, stomach and intestines (Fig. 34:2). Immediately behind the peritoneum and between it and the major back muscles and spine lie the kidneys with their drainage tubes (the ureters), the adrenal glands, the pancreas and much of the duo-denum. In this same plane, between the peritoneum and the spine, lie the aorta and the inferior vena cava, supplying blood to the whole lower half of the body. Many nerves and lymph glands accompany these large vessels. The organs and vessels are supported against the body wall by the peritoneum and are termed retroperitoneal (Figs. 34:3A, B).

In the pelvic cavity lie the rectum, the urinary bladder and, in the female, the internal reproductive organs. Strictly speaking, the urinary bladder is outside the cavity, as it lies between the pubic bone in front and the pelvic peritoneum behind it. It is, however, a pelvic organ and is frequently injured when the pelvis is fractured.

Both cavities, abdominal and pelvic, are lined by a smooth, glistening, thin, transparent layer of tissue called the peritoneum.

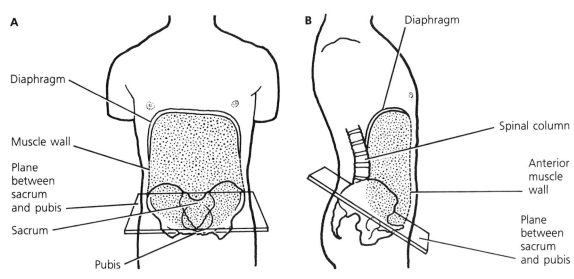

FIGURE 34:1. Boundaries of the abdominal cavity with imaginary plane

417

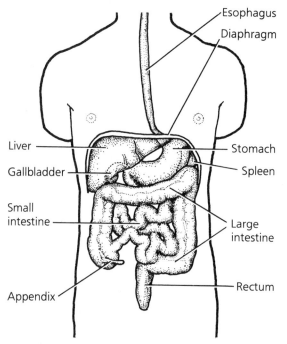

FIGURE 34:2.   Major intra-abdominal organs

Except where organs lie immediately beneath it, the peritoneum lies directly over the muscles of the body wall that serve to protect the organs within. Peritoneum is reflected from the body wall to cover the organs within the abdomen, so that wherever two surfaces are in contact, the surfaces are peritoneal. When peritoneum covers organs, it is called serosa (see Fig. 34:3B).

Nearly all the organs within the abdomen are suspended from the body walls by sheets of tissue called mesentery, very delicate tissue formed by peritoneum. As peritoneum that lines the body cavity is reflected to cover the organs, it forms the mesentery. Mesentery carries blood vessels and nerves to all the organs. Mesenteric attachments allow the organs to shift position with regard to one another because they hang fairly freely. The continuous muscular activity of the bowel requires an easily movable organ, and the mesenteric attachment provides mobility (see Fig. 34:3B).

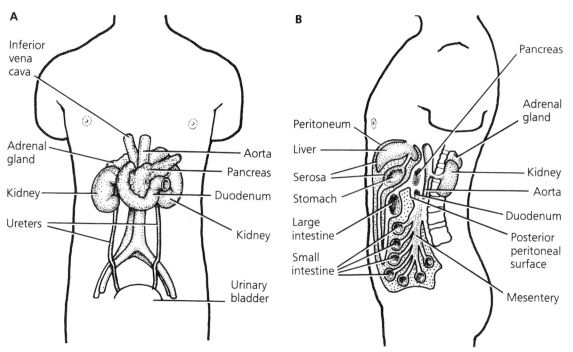

FIGURE 34:3.   **A** Major retroperitoneal organs seen in frontal view.
B Relationship of retroperitoneal organs in side view

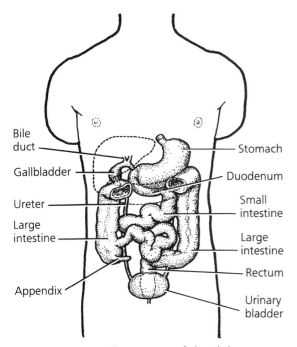

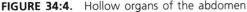

FIGURE 34:4.   Hollow organs of the abdomen

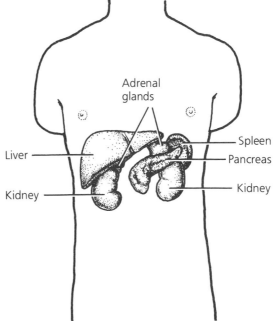

FIGURE 34:5.   Solid organs of the abdomen

Peritoneum, like all other tissues, has a nerve supply. The peritoneum lining the abdominal wall has the same ability to perceive sensation as the skin of the wall itself because it is directly supplied by the same somatic nerves that innervate the skin. The peritoneum forming mesentery and serosa perceives only one sensation—stretch or pressure—and is innervated by the autonomic, not the somatic, nervous system. This system cannot localize pain and can only perceive tension. The visceral innervation gives rise to the phenomenon of referred pain.

In general, these organs—abdominal, retroperitoneal and pelvic—are regarded as hollow or solid. Hollow organs are tubes through which materials pass. For example, the stomach and intestines conduct food through the body, and the ureters and bladder conduct and store urine until expelled. Solid organs are solid masses of tissue where much of the chemical work of the body takes place. The stomach, duodenum, small intestine, large intestine (colon), rectum, appendix, gallbladder,

bile ducts, urinary bladder and ureters are the hollow organs (Fig. 34:4). The liver, spleen, pancreas, kidneys and adrenal glands are the solid organs of this region (Fig. 34:5).

Injuries within the abdomen can involve either hollow or solid organs. In general, hollow organs discharge their contents into the abdominal cavity or adjacent tissue when they are lacerated, while solid organs tend to bleed copiously. Spilled contents usually cause an intense, painful inflammatory reaction—peritonitis. Bleeding from solid organs may be rapidly fatal and frequently causes shock. Mesentery supporting hollow organs can be lacerated. In such instances, bleeding from the torn mesentery can be severe, and the organ that is torn away loses its blood supply.

Bony landmarks in the abdomen include the pubic symphysis, the costal arch, the iliac crests and the anterior superior iliac spines. The major soft tissue landmark is the umbilicus, which overlies the fourth lumbar vertebra, or the junction of the fourth and fifth vertebrae in some patients. For ease of description, the abdomen is arbitrarily divided into quadrants by two perpendicular lines intersecting at the umbilicus (see Fig. 4:6 for visual representation of quadrants).

On the right, the liver lies very well protected by the eighth through twelfth ribs. Normally it is entirely under the costal arch and not palpable. Similarly, on the left, the stomach and the spleen are protected by the lowermost ribs, and only a very small portion of the stomach is not covered by bone and cartilage. The aorta and vena cava divide to form the common iliac arteries and veins at the level of the fourth lumbar vertebra or underneath the umbilicus. The pubic symphysis lies immediately anterior to the bladder and forms the anteriormost potion of the bony ring that surrounds and protects the organs within the pelvic cavity.

DIGESTIVE SYSTEM

The digestive system is composed of the gastrointestinal tract (stomach and intestines), mouth, salivary glands, pharynx, esophagus, liver, gallbladder, pancreas, rectum and anus. It transcends the boundaries of the abdomen and the thorax (Fig. 34:6). The system processes food to nourish the individual cells of the body. The process of digestion begins in the mouth.

Digestion of liquid and solid food, from the time it is taken into the mouth until essential compounds are extracted and delivered by the circulatory system to nourish all the cells of the body, is a complicated chemical process. In succession, different secretions are added by the salivary glands, stomach, liver, pancreas and small intestine to convert food into basic sugars, fatty acids and amino acids.

These products are then carried in the venous blood from the intestine to the liver. In the liver these basic products of digestion are further changed to simpler materials that nourish individual tissues and cells. The products are then pumped in the blood through the heart and arteries to the capillaries, where they pass through the capillary walls and the cell walls to feed the body's cells. Digestion within the small bowel produces many poisonous chemical compounds. They cannot be passed safely into the general circulation until the liver has transformed them. The fact that all the blood leaving the intestine must first pass through the liver protects the body as a whole against such compounds.

Mouth

The mouth consists of the lips, cheeks, gums, teeth and tongue. A mucous membrane lines the mouth. Hard and soft palates form the roof of the mouth (see Fig. 34:6). The hard palate is a bony plate lying anteriorly, while the soft palate is a fold of mucous membrane

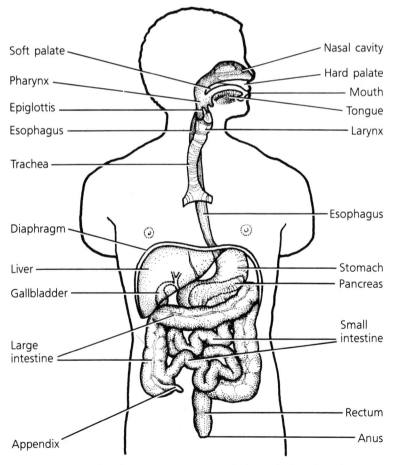

Soft palate
Pharynx
Epiglottis
Esophagus
Trachea
Diaphragm
Liver
Gallbladder
Large intestine
Appendix

Nasal cavity
Hard palate
Mouth
Tongue
Larynx
Esophagus
Stomach
Pancreas
Small intestine
Rectum
Anus

FIGURE 34:6. The digestive system extends from the head to the anus.

and muscle that extends posteriorly into the throat. It is adapted to hold food that is being chewed within the mouth and to initiate swallowing.

Salivary Glands

Three paired salivary glands are located on each side of the lower jaw just under the tongue, on each side of the lower jaw just below the angle of the mandible, and on each cheek in the tissue just in front of the ears. They produce nearly 1.5 liters of saliva daily to keep the mouth and pharynx normally moist. Saliva is poured into the mouth through salivary ducts and is approximately 98% water. The remaining 2% is mucus, salts and organic compounds. Mucus serves as a binder for chewed food and as a lubricant within the mouth.

Digestive enzymes actually accomplish the chemical conversion of food within the gastro-intestinal tract, breaking it down from starch, fat and protein to simple sugar, fatty acids and amino acids. There is only one digestive enzyme, ptyalin, in saliva. Ptyalin initiates the digestion of starch, converting it to a simple sugar. Otherwise, in the mouth, food is converted into a soft mush mixed with mucus and saliva and easily swallowed.

Pharynx

The pharynx, or throat, is a tubular structure about 5 inches long, extending vertically from the back of the mouth to the esophagus and trachea. The trachea, or windpipe, lies just in front of the esophagus. It is connected with the pharynx by the larynx, or voice box. The larynx is covered by a leaf-shaped valve called the epiglottis. An automatic movement of the pharynx permits the epiglottis to close over the larynx when swallowing so that liquids and solids are moved into the esophagus and away from the trachea.

Esophagus

The esophagus is a collapsible tube about 10 inches long. It extends from the end of the pharynx to the stomach, and lies just anterior to the spinal column in the chest. Contractions of the muscle in the esophagus propel food through it toward the stomach. Liquids pass with very little assistance. Semisolid foods seldom take more than 10 seconds to pass through the esophagus to the stomach.

Stomach

The stomach, an abdominal hollow organ, is located in the upper left portion of the abdominal cavity largely protected by the lower left ribs. Muscular movement and gastric juice, which contains much mucus, convert ingested food to a thoroughly mixed, semisolid mass. The major function of the stomach is to receive food in large, intermittent quantities, store it and provide for its movement into the small bowel in regular small amounts. Approximately 1.5 liters of gastric juice are produced each day and pass into the first division of the small intestine, the duodenum, with the ingested food.

In 1 to 3 hours, the semisolid food mass is entirely propelled into the duodenum by muscular contractions. Poisoning or any reaction to trauma may paralyze gastric muscular action and cause the retention of food in the stomach. In these instances, only vomiting or a stomach tube can empty this organ.

Only one digestive enzyme, pepsin, is produced in the stomach. This agent initiates the digestion of protein.

Pancreas

The pancreas, a flat, solid organ, lies below and behind the liver and stomach and behind the peritoneum on the spine and muscles of the back. It is oriented transversely in the upper abdomen. It is firmly fixed in position, deep within the abdomen, and is not easily damaged. It contains two kinds of glands.

One kind secretes nearly 2 liters of pancreatic juice daily. This juice contains many enzymes that digest of fat, starch and protein. It flows directly into the duodenum through the pancreatic ducts. This secretion is very important in the digestion of food.

The other kind of gland, called the islets of Langerhans, does not connect to any duct but secretes its products into the bloodstream across the capillaries. These islets produce a hormone, insulin, that regulates the amount of sugar in blood, and secrete several other regulatory hormones.

Liver

The liver is a large, solid organ that takes up most of the area immediately beneath the diaphragm on the right side. It is largely protected by the lower right ribs and the costal arch. It is the largest solid organ in the abdomen and consequently the one most often injured. It is a vital organ with several functions. Poisonous substances produced by digestion are brought to it by the blood and rendered harmless. Factors necessary for blood clotting and for producing normal plasma are formed here. The liver makes between 0.5 and 1.0 liter of bile daily to function in the normal digestion of fat. The liver is the principal organ for storing sugar for immediate use by the body. It also produces many of the factors that aid in regulating immune responses.

Essentially, the liver is a large mass of blood vessels and cells packed tightly together. For this reason, it is very fragile and easily injured. Blood flow in the liver is very high, since all of the blood that is pumped from the gastrointestinal tract passes through the liver before it returns to the heart. In addition, the liver receives a generous arterial blood supply of its own.

Biliary System

The liver is connected to the intestine by a duct system consisting of the gallbladder and the bile ducts, properly considered hollow organs. The gallbladder is a reservoir for bile received from the liver. It discharges the bile into the duodenum through the common bile duct. The presence of fat, food or acid peptic juice in the duodenum triggers a contraction of the gallbladder so that it can empty. It usually contains 2 to 3 ounces of bile. The liver is connected directly to the duodenum by the bile ducts, while the gallbladder is a pouch connected to the side of the common bile duct. Stones can form in the gallbladder and can pass into the common bile duct to obstruct it. Injuries of the gallbladder and bile ducts are not common, since these organs are fairly small and well protected.

Small Intestine

The small intestine, the major abdominal hollow organ, is so named because of its diameter in comparison to the large intestine and stomach. It includes the duodenum, jejunum and ileum.

The duodenum, about 12 inches long, passes from the stomach to the jejunum. Most "stomach ulcers" are really ulcers of the duodenum. Most of this organ lies behind the peritoneum and closely curls around the head of the pancreas (see Fig. 34:3). The duodenum is thus well protected and is rarely injured. However, duodenum injuries do occur, particularly from a steering wheel impact against the abdomen. Such injuries are very serious because they are difficult to treat and are usually associated with pancreatic damage. The duodenum is the part of the bowel into which secretions from the pancreas and liver empty to take part in digestion.

The jejunum and ileum together measure more than 20 feet on the average and, with the duodenum, make up the small bowel. The jejunum is the first half and the ileum the second half. The small intestine empties into the large intestine through the iliocecal valve between the ileum and cecum, the first part of the large bowel. This valve allows passage of bowel contents in only one direction—into the colon. The junction of small and large bowel is normally in the right lower quadrant of the abdominal cavity.

The small intestine lies entirely free within the abdomen, supported by its mesentery, which is attached to the back wall of the body.

Arteries from the aorta to the intestine and veins carrying blood to the liver lie in this supporting tissue. These vessels may be damaged in abdominal injury. Within the small intestine are the bile, pancreatic juice and small bowel secretions. Some 3 liters of small bowel juice containing mucus and potent enzymes are secreted daily.

Bile, produced by the liver and stored in the gallbladder, is emptied as needed into the duodenum. It is greenish-black in color but, through changes during digestion, it gives feces their typical brown color. Its major digestive function lies in emulsifying and digesting fat. Pancreatic and small bowel juice each contain the powerful chemical enzymes that carry out the final processes of digestion of protein, fat and carbohydrate. Within the small bowel, food is digested (broken down to its basic chemical constituents). The products of digestion—water, ingested vitamins and minerals—are then absorbed primarily in the terminal ileum for transportation to the liver.

Large Intestine

The large intestine, another major hollow organ, is about 5 feet long. It encircles the outer border of the abdomen around the small bowel. It lies partly behind the peritoneum (both ascending and descending portions) and partly on a mesentery, hanging free like the small bowel. It is most susceptible to injury at those areas where it changes from a fixed to a freely movable organ. The major function of the colon, which it shares with the very end of the small bowel, is to absorb the final 5% to 10% of water remaining in the fluid fecal stream to form solid stool, which is stored in the rectum and passed out of the body through the anus.

Appendix

The appendix is a small tube that opens into the cecum in the lower right quadrant of the abdomen. It is closed at the other end and is 3 or 4 inches long. It may easily become ob-structed and, as a result, inflamed. Appendicitis, the term for this inflammation, is one of the major causes of severe abdominal distress.

The appendix is a vestigial organ and has no major function in the human being. In early life it may play a role in developing normal immune response. It does not have any role in the usual processes of digestion.

Rectum and Anus

The lowermost end of the colon is the rectum. It is a large hollow organ adapted to store quantities of feces until expelled. It lies in the hollow of the sacrum within the pelvic cavity. At its terminal end is the anal canal, lined by normal skin and approximately 2 inches long. The rectum and anus are supplied with a complex series of circular muscles, called sphincters, that control the escape of liquids, gases and solids from the digestive tract. In general, the most distal anal sphincter, voluntarily controlled, can prevent or permit the escape of gas and some liquid. True rectal control is given by a broad shelf of muscle called the levator ani, which forms the entire pelvic floor.

Sensation within the rectum and anus is very specialized. The rectum is adapted to expand and, at a critical point, to expel its contents. Some rectal tumors fill up the organ and trigger this expelling reflex but cannot, in turn, be expelled. The resulting urge to defecate, which cannot be satisfied, is called tenesmus. Within the short terminal anal canal, sensation is exactly like that of the skin. Ulceration, irritations and lacerations are as painful as on a finger or toe. Because the anus is so richly supplied with nerves, an irritation here may result in profound systemic reactions.

Peristalsis

There are two layers of involuntary or smooth muscle throughout the wall of the entire intestinal tract from esophagus to rectum. Involuntary muscle is so called because it continues to contract rhythmically regardless of conscious will. It is also called smooth muscle from its microscopic appearance. Involuntary

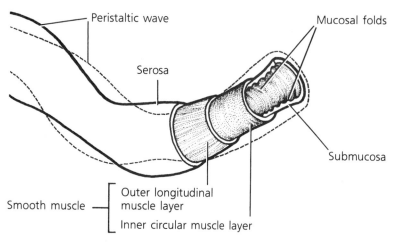

FIGURE 34:7. Smooth muscle layers or individual fibers allow tubular organs (intestine, blood vessels, or bronchi) to contract or dilate producing a peristaltic wave of intestinal contraction.

muscle handles the work of all the internal organs except the heart. Blood vessels constrict or dilate in response to heat or cold, work load or rest, fright or a number of other stimuli. Smooth muscle fibers in the vessel walls perform this action. We can exert no conscious control over it. The bronchi and bronchioles (air passages in the lung) dilate or constrict in response to cold or inhaled irritants because of involuntary muscle action in their walls.

In the gastrointestinal tract are two layers of smooth muscle, one oriented around the bowel and one longitudinally. Peristalsis, a coordinated wavelike contraction of this involuntary muscle, starts at the stomach and proceeds to the anus, propelling food through the digestive tract (Fig. 34:7). Swallowing initiates peristalsis in the esophagus. In the gastrointestinal tract, it is initiated by gastric distension. Once started, a wave passes through the entire system. When peristaltic waves are especially strong or when they are interrupted by an obstruction so that the contents cannot be propelled along, the contraction causes a painful cramp, called colic. Normal peristalsis is responsible for the bowel sounds heard when listening to the abdomen with a stethoscope. They represent the passage of gas and fluid through a narrow hollow organ.

Involuntary muscles are constantly responding to changes in their immediate surroundings, although the person does not consciously perceive many of the specific stimuli. These stimuli and their muscular surroundings keep us automatically in balance and maintain much of the body's routine work.

Spleen

The spleen, a major solid organ, is smaller than the liver. It, too, is filled with large blood vessels and is even more fragile. It lies in the left upper quadrant of the abdomen just beneath the diaphragm and immediately beneath the 9th to 11th ribs. It is fixed in position by three major ligaments that attach it to the kidney, colon and diaphragm, and it is well protected. It is adjacent to the lateral border of the stomach (which receives a considerable portion of its blood supply from the spleen) and the tail of the pancreas. Injuries to the spleen frequently mean damage of these nearby organs.

Blunt injuries can easily tear the supporting ligaments from the spleen, and bleeding from the lacerated organ may be very severe, controllable only by its removal. Injuries that fracture the 8th through 12th ribs on the left side are also likely to lacerate the spleen. Penetrating injuries of the stomach, spleen or pancreas must always be investigated for associated injuries to any of the other organs lying closely adjacent to them.

The spleen is not required for life, nor is it associated with the digestive tract. The function of the organ lies in the normal production and destruction of blood cells. When it is injured, the liver and bone marrow can assume its function.

The Acute Abdomen

35

In medicine the term acute abdomen indicates an abdominal pathology causing acute irritation or inflammation of the peritoneum and, consequently, severe pain. All penetrating abdominal wounds and all blunt injuries severe enough to damage abdominal organs result in the signs of an acute abdomen—abdominal tenderness, distention and pain. This chapter examines the development of these signs without preceding injury.

The term abdominal catastrophe is occasionally used to denote the most severe form of acute abdomen. Neither term, acute abdomen or abdominal catastrophe, is exact and neither refers to a disease of any specific organ. Both mean that severe abdominal pathology is causing peritonitis, usually sudden in onset. Since many diseases in many different organs result in the same signs and complaints of pain and tenderness in the abdomen, they can all be considered under these terms. A skilled practitioner often has difficulty determining the exact cause of acute abdomen. The trainer should recognize such an abdominal condition, but need not know the exact cause.

Conditions giving rise to acute abdominal signs are frequently sudden in onset and rapidly progressive. They may quickly result in death. The overriding principle of emergency care in these conditions is to correct life-threatening problems and transport the patient to a hospital without delay. Such conditions may require emergency surgery which must not be delayed.

ACUTE ABDOMEN SIGNS

The signs of an acute abdomen arise from irritation or inflammation of the peritoneum—peritonitis. The patient complains of abdominal pain and tenderness when the abdomen is palpated or moved. The degree of pain and tenderness usually reflects the severity of the inflammation.

The sensory nervous supply of the peritoneum is rich and twofold. The parietal peritoneum (lining of the wall of the abdomen) receives its innervation from the sensory nerves of the lower intercostal and lumbar segments that supply the trunk. It perceives sensations similar to those felt by the skin: irritation, heavy touch, stretch, pressure and temperature change. The nerves of the parietal peritoneum can localize an irritating point with little difficulty.

The visceral peritoneum (serosa or mesentery) is supplied by the sympathetic chain and vagus nerves, the autonomic nervous system. Visceral sensory nerves are less able to localize pain. The type of pain perceived is limited to that arising from activation of stretch receptors, caused by distention or forceful contraction within organs. This type of activation is usually interpreted as colic, a severe, intermittent, cramping pain.

The autonomic peritoneal innervation gives rise to the phenomenon of referred pain. An irritated peritoneal surface over an organ may cause pain on a distant surface of the body linked to the same area of the spinal cord as the irritated organ. For example, acute cholecystitis (inflammation of the gallbladder) may cause pain in the right shoulder, since the sympathetic nerves serving the gallbladder arise in the same area as the somatic nerves innervating the skin of the shoulder. There is no shoulder problem, but each set of nerves is activated (Fig. 35:1).

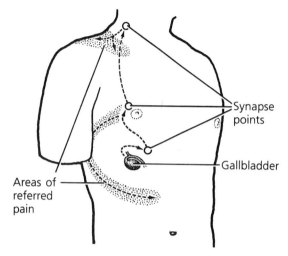

FIGURE 35:1. Nervous pathways causing referred pain in acute cholecystitis

diverticulitis, cholecystitis or pelvic inflammatory disease, may have substantial temperature elevations. Table 35:1 lists the common signs and symptoms of acute abdomen.

TABLE 35:1. The Acute Abdomen: Signs and Symptoms

 1. No evident abdominal injury
 2. Abdominal pain, local or diffuse
 3. Abdominal tenderness, local or diffuse
 4. A quiet patient who does not want to move because it hurts
 5. A patient who is breathing rapidly and not deeply because a deep breath hurts
 6. Rapid pulse (tachycardia)
 7. Low blood pressure
 8. A tense, often distended, abdomen
 9. Referred (distant) pain
10. Fever

Peritonitis always causes ileus—paralysis of normal intestinal peristalsis. Abdominal distention from retained gas and feces in these patients is common. In the presence of such paralysis, nothing that is eaten will be passed out of the stomach or through the bowel. Vomiting is the only way the stomach can empty itself, and it usually does so. Normally, muscular activity in the bowel is continuous as long as the patient is active. As soon as irritation causes a disturbance in the bowel action, distention develops proximal to the area of disturbance.

In peritonitis body fluid is always lost into the abdomen. This loss decreases the volume of the circulating blood (hypovolemia) and may eventually cause shock. Depending on the stage of the development of peritonitis, the patient may have normal vital signs or may have a very rapid pulse and low blood pressure. If peritonitis is associated with hemorrhage, the signs of shock are much more acute.

Depending on the cause of the acute abdomen, fever may be evident. The usual patient with acute appendicitis, aged 12 to 20, does not have fever until the appendix has perforated and an abscess is forming. On the other hand, patients with other acute diseases,

Degrees of pain and tenderness vary. Pain may be sharply localized or diffuse. When localized, it gives a clue to the cause. Tenderness may be minimal, or it may be so great that the patient will not allow the abdomen to be touched but "guards" it with the muscles so that the abdominal wall is absolutely rigid. The position of the patient is an important clue. In some diseases, patients can obtain comfort only by lying in one position. The patient with appendicitis may draw up the right knee. The patient with pancreatitis may lie curled up on the right side. Each position tends to relax muscles adjacent to the inflamed organ and lessen pain.

Severe peritonitis may make breathing painful. Pulse and blood pressure may be greatly changed or not altered at all, but usually reflect the severity of the process and its duration. Distention can easily be gauged by looking at the patient's abdomen. Distention is apparent within a few hours after intestinal muscular activity has ceased.

Examination of the abdomen may be done quickly, using the steps listed in Table 35:2, and yields much information. Do not prolong

TABLE 35:2.   The Acute Abdomen: Examination

1. Determine whether the patient is restless or quiet, whether motion causes pain, or whether any characteristic position, distention, or abnormality is present
2. Feel the abdomen gently to see whether it is tense (guarded) or soft
3. Determine whether the patient can relax the abdominal wall on command
4. Determine whether the abdomen is tender when touched

this examination, as the physician will do it in much more detail at the hospital. Carry out all abdominal palpation very gently. Occasionally an organ within the abdomen will be greatly enlarged and very fragile. Rough palpation can rupture aneurysms of the aorta or lacerate an enlarged spleen.

CAUSES OF ABDOMINAL DISEASE

The solid and hollow organs in the abdominal cavity making up the gastrointestinal and genitourinary systems are wholly covered with peritoneum, which lines the inside of the cavity and the outside of the organs. The entire cavity normally contains a very small amount of peritoneal fluid bathing the organs. Any condition that allows pus, blood, feces, urine, gastric juice, intestinal contents, amniotic fluid, dead or severely inflamed tissue to lie within or adjacent to this cavity can give rise to the signs of an acute abdomen.

Among the common diseases that produce these signs are acute appendicitis, perforated peptic ulcer, cholecystitis and diverticulitis—an inflammation of pockets along the distal colon. The list of diseases that can produce an acute abdomen is long, however, and includes nearly every abdominal problem. Rarely, and most often in children, a primary infection of the peritoneum occurs. This infection can also give rise to the signs of acute abdominal inflammation. Table 35:3 lists some common emergency problems and the location of the direct and referred pain produced.

Since the peritoneum is richly supplied with nerves sensitive to the presence of inflammation, disease or inflammation of the organs that lie behind or beneath it in the pelvic cavity can produce all the signs of peritonitis that accompany actual inflammation within the cavity itself. Pancreatitis can produce a severe inflammation difficult to distinguish from a perforated ulcer. Kidney stones causing ureteral colic are frequently associated with paralysis of bowel action. One of the very common causes of an acute abdomen in women is pelvic inflammatory disease, a venereal infection usually involving the fallopian tubes and surrounding tissue. It is one of the major diseases that must be distinguished from appendicitis in women. Infections of the upper and lower urinary tracts, kidney and ureter, or bladder and urethra, respectively, may also cause peritoneal irritation.

The aorta lies immediately behind the peritoneum on the spinal column. In older people it often develops weak areas that swell and are called aneurysms. Aneurysms are rarely associated with symptoms because they develop slowly. If this weak area ruptures, however, massive hemorrhage may occur, and some of the signs of an acute peritoneal irritation arise, along with severe back pain, because the peritoneum is rapidly stripped away from the body wall. In such instances, peritoneal signs are accompanied by profound shock.

CARE OF THE ACUTE ABDOMEN PATIENT

Acute abdomen signs justify a working diagnosis of an abdominal surgical emergency. Transport the patient to the emergency department without delay.

These patients often vomit as the emergency frequently develops just after the patient has eaten a large meal or has drunk heavily. The patient's throat and airway must be cleared of vomited material and kept clear.

The administration of oxygen may be necessary. Usually the exchange of air in the lungs

TABLE 35:3. Acute Abdomen: Direct and Referred Pain

Disease	Localization of Pain
Appendicitis	Around navel (referred); right lower quadrant (direct)
Cholecystitis	Right shoulder (referred); right upper quadrant (direct)
Duodenal ulcer	Upper midabdomen (direct) or upper back (direct)
Diverticulitis	Left lower quadrant
Perforated peptic ulcer	Generalized
Aortic aneurysm (ruptured)	Back and right lower quadrant
Cystitis (bladder inflammation)	Lower midabdomen (retropubic)
Pancreatitis	Upper back or upper abdomen
Pyelonephritis (R or L)	Right or left angles between last rib and lumbar vertebrae (back)
Kidney stones	Either right or left sides, radiating to genitalia
Pelvic inflammation (gonorrhea)	Both lower quadrants

or the airway is not blocked. Pain makes breathing physically difficult, however, and supplemental oxygen can compensate for a small respiratory volume.

Under no circumstances should a patient with acute abdominal signs be given anything to eat or drink. Ingestion of food or fluid can only aggravate many of the symptoms. Also, if emergency surgery is required, food in the stomach makes the procedure much more dangerous. In the presence of peritoneal irritation and intestinal paralysis, food does not pass out of the stomach and only increases distention and consequent vomiting.

No matter how distressed the patient is, do not give any medication for the pain or any sedatives. The examining physician must know exactly where the pain is and how much it hurts. Medication frequently masks these findings and may delay an ultimate diagnosis until it is too late to effect proper treatment.

Do not try to diagnose the patient's disease, but listen to the description of the location of pain and tenderness and the severity of symptoms. Record the patient's description of how the process started and the vital signs as soon as possible so the physician will have this information. Shock is common in these patients. It must be recognized early, for its presence makes prompt transport to the hospital even more imperative. Make the patient as comfortable as possible, conserve body heat with blankets and transport the patient gently and promptly to the emergency department.

Injuries of the Abdomen

36

Abdominal injuries may be closed or open, and they may involve hollow or solid organs. In closed injuries the abdomen is damaged by a severe blow but the skin remains intact, such as hitting a steering wheel or the dashboard of a car, or being tackled in football. In open injuries a foreign body has entered the abdomen, opening the peritoneum-lined cavity to the outside. Stab or gunshot wounds are open injuries.

Some penetrating injuries may only lacerate the abdominal wall itself. Whether the abdominal cavity is penetrated may not be clear. If the injury is a gunshot or stab wound, always assume that the bullet or knife has entered the abdominal cavity and give emergency care accordingly. The only certain way to determine if organs have been injured is through exploratory surgery. Emergency medical care for penetrating abdominal wounds is based on the assumption that penetration has occurred and one or several organs have been injured.

The abdomen contains both hollow and solid organs, any of which may be injured. The hollow organs usually contain a stream of food that is being digested. When these organs are ruptured or lacerated their contents spill into the peritoneal cavity. Digested or undigested food, the bowel contents, gastric juice or other digestive enzymes cause an intense inflammatory reaction—peritonitis. This reaction produces prompt and severe abdominal tenderness, muscular rigidity and intense pain. Bowel movement is paralyzed and the abdomen becomes distended.

Injuries of the solid organs usually cause severe hemorrhage due to their rich blood supply. Blood within the peritoneal cavity is not very irritating. The first signs of these injuries may be changes in pulse and blood pressure together with other signs indicating shock, such as an ashen, pale color and cold, clammy skin.

Either closed or open abdominal injuries may involve the aorta, inferior vena cava, or any other large blood vessels. The hemorrhage may be severe and fatal.

EVALUATING THE INJURED ABDOMEN

Abdominal injuries may be very easy to perceive or quite subtle. In general, the overriding complaint of a patient with abdominal injury is pain. Blunt injury may leave bruises as clues to the nature of the wounding agent. Patients with penetrating injuries generally have obvious abdominal wounds, through which bowel or fat may be protruding. In addition to pain, patients frequently feel nauseated and may want to vomit. In general, when peritonitis is developing because of irritation of the peritoneal surface, patients prefer to lie still because it hurts to move.

The signs of an abdominal injury are generally more definite. (A clinical sign, as opposed to a symptom, is a finding that can be elicited by the examiner. Tenderness when the abdomen is palpated is a sign, while pain within the abdomen, of which the patient complains, is a symptom.) Abdominal tenderness, and specifically, localized abdominal tenderness, is a very important clinical sign. Difficulty in moving because of abdominal pain is another. Obvious wounds, of both entry and exit, are excellent clues for injuries, as are bruises. Altered vital signs such as low blood pressure, a rapid pulse and rapid, shallow respirations are also important.

The method of evaluating an abdominal injury is the same for blunt and penetrating trauma. Permit the patient to lie supine, as comfortably as possible, with knees slightly flexed and supported. Remove or loosen clothes. Rapidly assess the patient's condition by simple inspection. First, record vital signs, especially pulse, blood pressure and rate of respiration. Many abdominal emergencies, aside from those that cause severe bleeding, can cause a rapid pulse and low blood pressure. It is absolutely necessary that a record of vital signs be made as early as possible and that they be recorded from time to time thereafter to help the physician evaluate the progress and severity of the problem.

At first inspection, note how the patient is lying. The patient with severe abdominal disease or injury who prefers to lie still usually lies with the legs drawn up. Rapid, shallow breaths limit movement of the abdominal contents. A patient with acute pancreatitis or a ruptured appendix may lie on the right side with the legs drawn up. Motion of the body or the abdominal organs irritates the inflamed peritoneum and causes additional pain, which the patient instinctively tries to avoid.

In evaluating abdominal injuries, perceive important clinical signs and symptoms (Table 36:1) and be aware of their significance.

Penetrating objects such as knives should be noted, stabilized and left alone after sup-portive bandaging. Bruises help determine the cause and severity of any blunt injury. The location of bruises or wounds is a clue to the organs that may be injured underneath. With severe lacerations of the abdominal wall, inner organs may protrude through the wound. This is called evisceration.

The patient may say where the abdomen hurts, feel nauseated or vomit. A patient with abdominal injuries may have a stomach full of food or drink. If vomiting occurs, especially in a patient who is comatose or nearly so, the throat must be kept clear of vomitus so that it is not aspirated into the lungs. Turn the patient's head to one side, and try to keep it lower than the chest. Note material vomited: undigested food, blood, mucus or bile.

The initial evaluation should determine the type of injury, blunt or penetrating, its possible extent and the presence of shock. The patient should be transported promptly to the hospital.

Blunt Abdominal Wounds

Blunt abdominal wounds may cause severe bruises of the abdominal wall. Within the abdomen, the liver and spleen may be lacerated. The intestine may be ruptured. Supporting mesenteries may be torn, and their vessels injured. The kidneys may be ruptured or torn from their arteries and veins. The bladder may be ruptured, especially in a patient who has been drinking heavily and whose bladder may have been full and distended. These patients may have severe intra-abdominal hemorrhage as well as peritoneal irritation and inflammation from the ruptured hollow organs.

Place the patient supine in a comfortable position with the head turned to one side. Clear the mouth and throat of vomitus. Note signs of shock: pallor, cold sweat, a rapid, thready pulse or low blood pressure. Institute all appropriate measures to combat shock. Assist respiration by clearing the airway, and use oxygen when needed. Transport the patient promptly and gently to the emergency department.

TABLE 36:1. Abdominal Injuries: Blunt or Penetrating

Signs	Symptoms
1. Bruises	1. Pain (abdominal)
2. Lacerations or stab wounds	2. Pain (referred)
3. Lowered blood pressure	3. Nausea
4. Elevated pulse	4. Anxiety
5. Rapid, shallow aspirations	5. Desire not to be moved
6. Ashen color	
7. Local or diffuse abdominal tenderness	
8. Distention	
9. Shock	
10. Vomiting	

Penetrating Abdominal Injuries

In the penetrating abdominal wound, it may be very difficult to determine without surgery if an object has penetrated the abdomen and, if it has, what organs it injured. Assume major damage even if no obvious signs are present immediately, since such signs often develop slowly. In these injuries, hollow organs are usually lacerated, discharging their contents into the abdominal cavity with resulting inflammation. If major blood vessels are cut or if major solid organs are lacerated, hemorrhage may be rapid and severe.

Initial steps in the care of these patients have already been outlined elsewhere. Note the areas of the abdomen penetrated including exit wounds. Leave a penetrating instrument in place and bandage it so that external bleeding is controlled and the instrument is stable. Control other obvious external bleeding with pressure. Protect the patient from aspirating vomitus and maintain the airway. Provide respiratory support and oxygen when needed. Make the patient as comfortable as possible, and transport him promptly and gently to the emergency department.

The Genitourinary System

37

The urinary and genital systems are commonly discussed together because their various organs and passages develop from the same embryologic beginnings and they thus share many structures. The urinary system controls the discharge of certain waste materials filtered from the blood. The genital system controls the reproductive processes. In the urinary system, the kidneys are solid organs, while the bladder and ureters are hollow organs (Fig. 37:1). The female genitalia, uterus, ovaries and fallopian tubes, are contained entirely within the pelvis (Fig. 37:2). The male genitalia, except for the prostate gland and seminal vesicles, are outside the abdomen (Fig. 37:3).

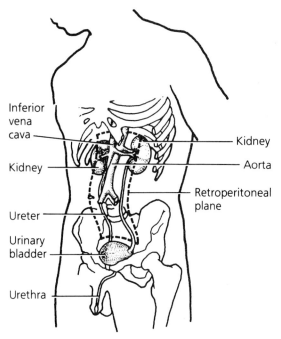

FIGURE 37:1. The urinary system lies outside the peritoneal cavity.

URINARY SYSTEM

Kidneys

The body's two kidneys lie on the posterior muscular wall of the abdomen behind the peritoneum. These vital organs rid the blood of toxic waste products and control its balance of water and salt. If the kidneys are destroyed or, for any reason, no longer function adequately, uremia occurs. Waste accumulates within the bloodstream, the balance of salt and water is disturbed, and death may result.

Nearly 20% of the output of blood from the heart each minute passes through the kidneys. Large vessels attach the kidneys directly to the aorta and the inferior vena cava. Blood flow in the kidneys is high. Waste products and water are constantly filtered from the blood to form urine. The kidneys continuously concentrate this filtered urine by reabsorbing the water as it is passed through a system of specialized tubes within them. These tubes finally unite to form the renal pelvis, a cone-shaped collecting area that connects the ureter and the kidney. Normally, each kidney drains its urine into one ureter, through which the urine passes to the bladder.

Ureters

Each kidney is usually drained by one ureter, although anomalies exist. The ureter passes from the kidney along the surface of the posterior wall to drain into the urinary bladder. The ureters are small (diameter 0.5 cm), hollow, muscular tubes. Peristalsis in these tubes moves the urine to the bladder. Injuries of the ureters are rare because they are small and well protected.

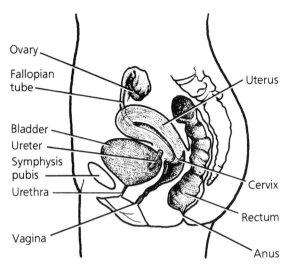

FIGURE 37:2. The female genital system is entirely contained within the pelvis.

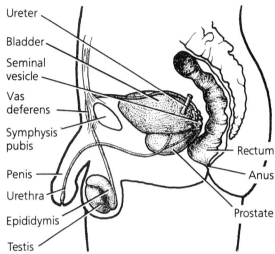

FIGURE 37:3. The male genital system is outside the abdomen, except for the prostate gland and seminal vesicles.

Urinary Bladder and Urethra

The urinary bladder is situated immediately behind the pubic symphysis in the pelvis. It is covered by peritoneum and hence lies outside the abdominal cavity and in front of it. The ureters enter posteriorly at its base. It empties to the outside of the body through the urethra. In men, the urethra passes from the anterior base of the bladder into the penis (see Fig. 37:3). In women, the urethra opens at the front of the vagina (see Fig. 37:2).

The bladder is formed of smooth muscle with a specialized lining membrane. Smooth muscle reacts to automatic stimuli transmitted by the autonomic nervous system. Urination is largely an autonomic function that can, however, be controlled voluntarily. Ordinarily, bladder contraction and the stimulus to void are the automatic results of stimulation of the bladder at a certain critical point of fullness. This is another regulatory function of smooth muscle. Sensory cells then send messages to the brain, notifying it that the bladder is ready to empty, and the bladder contracts, forcing urine through the urethra to the outside of the body. The normal adult forms 1.5 to 2.0 liters of concentrated urine every day. This waste is extracted and concentrated from the 1,500 liters of blood circulated through the kidneys daily.

GENITAL SYSTEM

Genitalia

The genitalia include the male and female reproductive organs and the male urethra. The male and female reproductive organs have certain similarities and, of course, basic differences. They produce sperm and egg cells, appropriate hormones, make possible sexual intercourse and, ultimately, reproduction.

Male Reproductive System and Organs

The male reproductive system includes the testicles, vasa deferens, seminal vesicles, prostate gland, urethra and penis (see Fig. 37:3). Each testicle contains specialized cells and ducts. Certain cells produce male hormones and others develop sperm. The hormones are absorbed directly into the blood from the testicles. The vasa deferens travel from the testicles up beneath the skin of the abdominal wall for a short distance. They then pass through an opening into the abdominal cavity and down into the prostate gland to meet the urethra. The seminal vesicles are small storage sacs for sperm and seminal fluid. These vesicles also empty into the urethra at the prostate. Semen (seminal fluid) contains sperm cells carried up each vas from a testis to be mixed with fluid from the seminal vesicles and prostate gland.

The prostate gland is a small gland that surrounds the urethra where it emerges from the urinary bladder. Fluids from the prostate gland and from the seminal vesicles come together during intercourse. During the act of intercourse, special mechanisms in the nervous system prevent the passage of urine into the urethra. Only seminal fluid, prostatic fluid and sperm pass from the penis into the vagina during ejaculation.

The penis has a special type of tissue called erectile tissue. This tissue is largely vascular and, when filled with blood, distends the penis into a state of erection. As the vessels fill under pressure from the circulatory system, the penis becomes a rigid organ that can enter the vagina. Certain spinal injuries, some diseases and drugs cause a permanent and painful erection called priapism.

Female Reproductive System and Organs

The female reproductive organs include the ovaries, fallopian tubes, uterus and vagina (see Fig. 37:2). The ovaries, like the testicles, produce sex hormones and specialized cells for reproduction. The female sex hormones are absorbed directly into the blood. A specialized cell, called an ovum, is produced with regularity during the adult female's reproductive years. The ovaries release a mature egg, or ovum, approximately once every 28 days. This egg travels through the fallopian tubes to the uterus.

The fallopian tubes connect with the uterus and carry the ovum to the cavity of the uterus. The uterus is a pear-shaped, hollow organ with muscular walls. A narrow opening from the uterus to the vagina is called the cervix.

The vagina is a muscular, distensible tube connecting the uterus with the vulva—the external female genitalia. The vagina receives the male penis during intercourse, when semen and sperm are deposited in it. The sperm may pass into the uterus and fertilize an egg, causing pregnancy. Should the pregnancy come to completion, at the end of nine months the baby will pass through the vagina and be born. The vagina also channels the menstrual flow from the uterus out of the body.

Menstrual Cycle

The menstrual period is the end of the monthly female reproductive cycle. A woman has monthly periods of menstruation from the start of the first menstrual period at about age 12 until menopause at about age 50. Each month the endometrium (lining of the uterus) is stimulated by the female sex hormones to form a special bed. This bed is prepared so that, if a sperm and ovum unite making a fertilized egg, the uterus is ready to receive it and provide a place for it to grow. Approximately 15 days after a menstrual period ceases, one ovary produces an egg. This egg travels into the uterus through the fallopian tubes.

If a sperm is able to travel from the vagina through the cervix to fertilize the egg, either in the uterus or in the fallopian tubes, the fertilized egg settles in the uterus and begins to grow in the lining there.

If the egg is not fertilized, there is a menstrual period. During the period, the uterus sheds its recently formed special lining, a very thin layer of cells and blood. The lining, in the form of the menstrual flow, passes out of the uterus into the vagina and out of the body. The flow lasts about five days. After it ceases the uterus begins to prepare a new lining as a bed to receive a new egg, and the cycle is repeated.

GENITOURINARY INJURIES

Kidney

The rare injury of the kidney may result from blunt or penetrating trauma. The intensity of a blow required to damage the kidney is such that the injury is almost always associated with fractured ribs or other severely injured intra-abdominal organs. The kidneys are so well-protected that a penetrating wound nearly always involves other organs as well as the kidney or its vessels.

A history or physical evidence of an abrasion, laceration, bleeding into the tissues or a penetrating wound in the region of the lower rib cage, the flank or the upper abdomen should make the trainer suspect accompanying kidney damage. The patient with fractures on either side of the lower rib cage or of the lower thoracic or upper lumbar vertebrae is also a likely candidate for a kidney injury (Fig. 37:4). Force sufficient to fracture these ribs or vertebrae is strong enough that associated soft tissue damage is inevitable.

Except for signs of severe injury on the skin, such as bruises, evidence of kidney damage is not manifest on external examination. Shock may be seen early when the injury is associated with major blood loss. Since the function of the kidney is to form urine, an injury produces blood in the urine—hematuria. Thus, any urine passed by the patient while under observation should be measured and saved for analysis at the hospital. A small amount of blood will not turn the urine red and can only be confirmed on microscopic examination.

A patient with suspected kidney damage should be placed at total rest. Monitor vital signs carefully until arrival at the emergency department. Shock or associated severe injuries may be present. The patient should be transported promptly.

Urinary Bladder

Injury of the urinary bladder, either blunt or penetrating, is usually a rupture. Urine is spilled into the surrounding tissue. Any urine that passes through the urethra is likely to be bloody. Blunt injuries of the lower abdomen or pelvis frequently cause an explosive rupture of the urinary bladder, particularly when it is full and distended. In fractures of the pelvis, the urinary bladder is often torn by the sharp, bony fragments of the pelvis (Fig. 37:5). Sudden deceleration, especially with a full bladder in the male, can literally shear it off the urethra (see Fig. 37:3). Penetrating wounds of the lower midabdomen or perineum (the pelvic floor and associated structures occupying the pelvic outliet) can directly involve the blad-

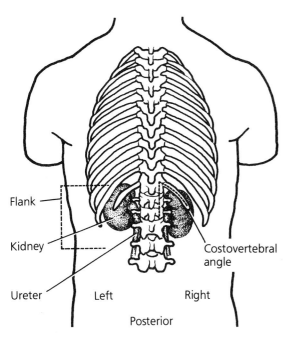

FIGURE 37:4. Posterior view shows proximity of lower ribs to kidneys.

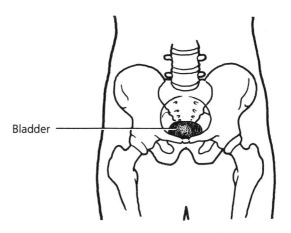

FIGURE 37:5. Frontal view shows proximity of urinary bladder to bony pelvic ring.

der. A history of any of the above types of injury, evidence on physical examination of trauma in the lower abdomen, pelvis or perineum or blood at the urethral opening all point to a bladder injury. Final documentation of the presence and severity of a bladder injury depends on x-ray studies. Save a specimen of any urine passed by a patient with suspected bladder injury for analysis at the hospital.

Male Genitalia

Injuries of the external male genitalia include all types of soft tissue wounds: avulsions, lacerations, abrasions, penetrations and contusions. Although rarely life-threatening, they are extremely painful and generally a source of great concern to the patient.

Direct blows on the scrotum and its contents can rupture a testis or cause a substantial accumulation of blood about the testes. Application of an ice pack to the scrotal-perineal area is desirable while the patient is being transported.

In treating injuries involving the male external genitalia a few general rules apply to several specific instances. The trainer should be able to differentiate between the contusion of the testicle, epididymitis and torsion of the testicle. Certainly this latter diagnosis must be considered in any acute problem involving this organ system, as early recognition and treatment are important.

Other conditions that may disable the athlete are hydroceles and varicoceles diagnosed by increasing fluid in the sac or increased venous pattern as in the case of the varicocele. A urologist should see patients who have this problem to institute appropriate treatment. Frequently only an appropriate athletic supporter is necessary to prevent the possibility of contusion in a swollen organ.

Hernias are usually ruled out during a pre-season examination or cared for at that time. However, an athlete may suffer acute herniation during his training program. Hernias produce pain, frequently into the testicles and groin. Palpation of the inguinal canal and the protrusion of the hernial sac when the athlete coughs yields the diagnosis. Treatment is generally surgical. The team physician can advise whether surgery is necessary immediately or can be postponed until the season is finished.

The absence of a testicle indicates an undescended testicle or one with a short spermatic cord tending to protract up into the abdomen and should be mentioned to the team physician. Frequently the testicle can be moved down into the scrotal sac. If this is impossible then surgery may be advised to try to preserve an organ that may otherwise deteriorate. The question of allowing an athlete with an undescended testicle to participate in sports is still open to question. The athlete and his parents should discuss with the team physician the possible consequences of further injury to the remaining testicle.

Protective devices are extremely beneficial and are mandatory in certain sports. For example, the catcher in baseball certainly should wear an aluminum cup, and the same is true for a hockey goaltender, as the hard missiles can cause severe damage to unprotected external genitalia. Athletic supporters are frequently worn for comfort in other sports, particularly in running sports, although many athletes prefer not to wear them.

Female Genitalia

The uterus, ovaries and fallopian tubes are subject to the same kinds of injuries as any other internal organ. However, they are rarely damaged because they are small and well-protected by the pelvis (see Fig. 37:2). Unlike the bladder, they do not lie adjacent to the bony pelvis and most often are not injured when it is fractured.

The external female genitalia include the vulva, the clitoris and the major and minor labia (lips) at the entrance of the vagina. The female urethra enters the anterior vagina.

Injuries of the external female genitalia can include all types of soft tissue damage. These genital parts have a rich nerve supply, and injuries are very painful. Lacerations, abrasions and avulsions should be treated with moist compresses, local pressure to control bleeding and a diaper-type bandage to hold dressings in place. Major bleeding will require control in the operating room. Under no circumstances should dressings or packs be placed in the vagina.

In general, although these injuries are painful, they probably are not life-threatening in most cases. Bleeding may be copious, but it can usually be controlled by local ice and compression. The priority for transportation to the emergency department is dictated by associated injuries, amount of hemorrhage and the presence of shock.

Common Gastrointestinal and Genitourinary Complaints

38

The trainer will often have to deal with complaints indicating gastrointestinal (GI) and genitourinary (GU) disease. Frequently these complaints interfere with the person's normal daily habits. In some cases, emergency help and transportation to the emergency department may be advisable.

Within the GI system, emergency complaints not associated with injuries or an acute abdomen include dysphagia (difficulty in swallowing), vomiting, hematemesis (vomiting of blood), diarrhea, melena (dark, black stools indicative of blood), hematochezia (bright red blood in the stool) and jaundice. Within the GU system, complaints are dysuria (painful or burning urination), hematuria (blood in the urine), frequency, incontinence, urethral discharge or renal colic.

GASTROINTESTINAL SYSTEM

Dysphagia

Dysphagia is the sensation of difficulty in swallowing. Obstructing lesions in the esophagus range from swallowed foreign bodies to carcinoma. In general, the patient complains of a sensation of food sticking under the breastbone or at the back of the throat. In many instances, the dysphagia slowly progresses, starting with chunks of meat and becoming more severe, so that only liquids or very soft gruel can be swallowed. Many people ignore dysphagia until it becomes very severe. A drink of water at meals eases difficult swallowing and people tend to forget about the problem until the next meal, since this condition does not cause pain.

Dysphagia usually represents long-standing disease and professional help should be obtained promptly. It is not an emergency condition, but is associated with a number of very serious ailments.

Vomiting

Vomiting, one of the most common gastrointestinal complaints, results from a multitude of causes. Any situation causing peritonitis, an acute abdomen, and subsequent paralytic ileus can reduce peristalsis in the GI tract so that vomiting is the only way the stomach can empty. Any disease or situation causing a specific inflammation of the lining of the GI tract, especially the stomach, will also cause vomiting. Gastroenteritis, of viral or bacterial origin, is a very common cause as is the ingestion of irritating agents, most commonly seen in the athlete who has indulged very heavily in alcohol, which stimulates gastric juice as well as irritates gastric mucosa. Food poisoning often causes vomiting as the stomach attempts to rid itself of the noxious agent, as does the excessive use of an irritant drug such as aspirin. Any mechanical obstruction to the passage of material through the GI tract will also cause vomiting. Vomiting, the response of the stomach to a stimulus such as irritation, infection or obstruction, should be distinguished from regurgitation, the result of overfilling or overdistention with air and fluid. The "burp" is an example of regurgitation.

Vomiting is always serious, since the trainer does not know its cause, which may be much more serious than gastroenteritis or too much whiskey. Rarely, however, is vomiting an emergency in itself, unless neglected for several days during which the patient has not eaten or drunk enough to replace that lost in the vomitus. In such situations, the patient may actually be in shock because of the amount of fluid and salt lost from his body. This particular state is termed metabolic shock (see Chapter 30).

Care of the vomiting patient is usually straightforward unless the patient is drunk. The alert patient, vomiting as a result of an illness, is rarely if ever in danger of aspiration, since all the reflexes guarding the airway are active. The somnolent or semiconscious drunken patient may vomit in bed or when supine and frequently does aspirate. In this patient, clearing and protecting the airway are of paramount importance. The vomiting patient who is in shock is a genuine emergency patient. After protecting the airway and providing other support, transport the patient promptly to the emergency department.

Vomiting as a consequence of injury is discussed in chapters dealing with specific trauma. In these patients, anticipate vomiting and protect the airway.

Hematemesis

Vomiting of blood is particularly disturbing for the patient. In general, it is associated with problems arising in the esophagus or the stomach. Hematemesis can produce ''coffee ground'' vomitus in small quantities or large quantities of bright red blood.

Probably the most common disease in the United States associated with hematemesis is peptic ulcer in the stomach. Peptic ulcers in the duodenum that bleed usually do not produce hematemesis because the pylorus, the muscle that separates the stomach from the duodenum, prevents the blood from returning into the stomach. In these instances, the blood tends to pass distally down the GI tract and

out with the feces, rather than up and out as vomitus. Ulcers in the stomach, however, and lesions in the esophagus produce hematemesis. Coffee ground vomitus is so called because the material produced looks exactly like coffee grounds suspended in the clear mucus and liquid of normal gastric juice. This event indicates a very slow rate of gastric bleeding. Small quantities of blood are ingested in the stomach and turned dark brown by hydrochloric acid. A very briskly bleeding ulcer may produce large quantities of bright red blood. Some rapidly bleeding duodenal ulcers also cause hematemesis. Whatever the type, hematemesis is a reason for prompt transport to the emergency department. Estimate and record the amount of blood vomited and collect a sample to take to the hospital with the patient.

Another very common cause of upper GI bleeding is esophageal varices. In this situation, a result of long-standing alcohol abuse, cirrhosis of the liver causes blood flow from the GI tract which normally goes to be shunted around the liver instead of through it. Because of the shunting, huge collateral veins (varices) develop in the esophagus. They are distended, very thin, and contain blood at three or four times the normal pressure for this type of vessel. Bleeding from esophageal varices is copious, bright red, and may be rapidly fatal. Ordinarily, the person with esophageal variceal bleeding has a long history of alcohol abuse, may be on a drinking binge and generally has blood in the vomitus from the first moment of vomiting on. There is little or no pain associated with variceal bleeding, but the extent of the hemorrhage makes the emergency nature of the situation obvious. Prompt transport to the emergency department is mandatory, and treatment en route may be required for hypovolemic shock as well as protection of the airway.

Another fairly common cause of GI bleeding is gastritis—inflammation of the lining of the stomach. This complex disease has a number of causes. Specific agents in everyday use, such as aspirin, alcohol and a number of related compounds, can irritate the gastric mucosa to the extent that diffuse gastritis and hemorrhage develop. Stress can also cause gastric bleeding. Some medications, such as cortisone, are also associated with this type of bleeding. Hemorrhage is often copious, and vital signs may be unstable. The patient usually has vague, indefinite epigastric and left upper quadrant pain. Again, prompt transport with treatment for shock and airway protection is needed.

Very rarely, forceful or prolonged vomiting will completely rupture the stomach or esophagus. The patient suddenly has excruciatingly severe left chest pain and left upper quadrant abdominal pain in association with the vomiting. By the time the trainer sees this patient, the patient will usually be in shock and desperately ill. Transport the patient immediately, using all measures to combat hypovolemic shock and provide respiratory support.

Diarrhea

Just as vomiting has many causes, so does diarrhea, abnormally frequent and liquid bowel movements. Anxiety, gastroenteritis (the common flu), severe infections with bacteria, such as typhoid fever, or parasitic infestation with an amoeba can all cause diarrhea. Inflammatory processes in the bowel of unknown causes, including ulcerative colitis, granulomatous colitis or enteritis, can also result in diarrhea. In the elderly, one of the most common causes of diarrhea is a partial obstruction of the bowel by fecal impaction. Only liquid material can pass beyond the impacted feces, and this liquid material produces the diarrhea.

Very rarely does diarrhea cause an acute problem. If it has been present for several days and if the patient has been unable to take sufficient food or fluid to balance the amount lost, then obvious evidence of dehydration and electrolyte imbalance or starvation may be present. This patient, just like the neglected vomiter, may have unstable vital signs and be in metabolic shock. The trainer will not see this type of patient very frequently. Remember, however, that uncontrolled diarrhea or vomiting over several days or weeks may result in a desperately ill individual. Ordinarily, the patient with diarrhea necessitating an emergency call should be transported to the hospital to assess the cause of the problem. It is not generally, however, a first priority emergency.

Melena

The term melena is derived from a Greek term meaning black. Melena is the passage of a dark black stool, very tarry or sticky in consistency. It has a characteristic, particularly foul odor. The black color is due to blood in the stool that has been digested within the GI tract. In general, melena is associated with slow, continuous GI bleeding in the upper GI tract, such as with peptic ulcer in the duodenum or ulceration within the small bowel or proximal large bowel.

Melena is not an emergency unless it has been ignored for many weeks and the patient exhibits signs of hypovolemic shock. It is, however, a cause for grave concern, and the bleeding source must be identified as expeditiously as possible. Some medications, such as bismuth and iron-containing compounds, impart the same dark black color to the stool. In general, however, the trainer will not be required to make this differential diagnosis.

Hematochezia

The passage of bright red blood in the stool is called hematochezia. This also has several causes ranging from colonic and rectal carcinoma to hemorrhoids and anal fissures. Bright red blood in the stool is not ordinarily an emergency and, except in a very few obvious instances, bleeding is not massive. It is, however, distinctly abnormal and requires immediate diagnosis of the cause. Faced with hematochezia or melena as major complaints, be sure vital signs are stable and transfer the patient to the emergency department for examination and diagnosis as expeditiously as possible. A recorded estimate of the volume of bloody stool passed is helpful to the evaluating physician.

Jaundice

Jaundice is derived from a French word meaning ''yellow,'' and implies a yellow color of the skin. Many diseases cause jaundice, almost all from some malfunction of the liver or the biliary tract. To form bile within its cells, the liver uses the products of the destruction of worn-out red blood cells. The bile is secreted through the common bile duct into the duodenum, where it plays an essential role in digesting fat in the GI tract. A considerable portion of the excreted bile is reabsorbed in the GI tract and returned to the liver.

Any disease that overloads the liver with red cell destruction products causes jaundice, as does any disease that interferes with the function of the normal liver cell so that bile cannot be made or excreted properly. Any situation in which the outflow of bile from the liver to the GI tract is blocked also causes jaundice.

Ordinarily, jaundice is not an emergency, but the patient should be transported to the hospital for immediate medical attention. Jaundice is most readily detected by looking at portions of the body that are normally white, the sclera of the eye or the conjunctiva. In Caucasians jaundice is easily detected. In pigmented individuals, jaundice may be evident only by examining normally pale areas, such as the undersurface of the tongue, the conjunctiva, the scleral surfaces of the eyes, or the palms of the hands.

Colic

The term colic implies a characteristic intraabdominal pain associated with obstruction of largely muscular hollow tubes. The pain is intermittent, rises sharply to an excruciating peak and relents suddenly as the muscle relaxes. Colic can accompany obstruction of the GI tract by tumors, polyps, foreign bodies or adhesions. When a urinary stone is obstructing a ureter, there is a characteristic radiation of pain from the flank and into the genitalia. Colic is a very common complaint in children. It is caused by active peristalsis in the GI tract when a wave of contraction catches up with the immediately preceding wave, subjecting the segment of bowel between the two waves to extreme tension. In the adult colic often accompanies the viral flu syndrome and diarrhea and again is associated with extreme hyperperistaltic activity of the GI tract. Frequently the patient describes colic as a cramp or a gas pain.

The trainer should be familiar with the term colic and be able to recognize this type of pain when described. It is a very distressing complaint for the patient, and its cause must be assessed by a physician. Thus the patient should be seen by a physician, but the situation is usually not urgent.

GENITOURINARY SYSTEM

Dysuria

Dysuria is the sensation of pain, burning or itching on urination. It generally indicates an inflammatory process or infection within the lower urinary tract (external urethral opening, urethra and bladder). Urinary tract infections are found much more frequently in women than in men. It is a symptomatic indication of a problem that should be treated, although it is not an emergency. When an athlete's major complaint is dysuria, he should be seen by a physician for diagnosis and treatment.

Hematuria

The passage of blood in the urine is called hematuria. Occasionally it is gross and visible to the naked eye. Much more frequently, blood in the urine can be identified only on microscopic examination of urinary sediment. The causes of hematuria include tumors within the urinary tract, stones causing abrasions and bleeding from the kidney or the ureters and trauma. The trainer is concerned only with hematuria that the athlete notices. An athlete with this problem should be promptly seen by a physician for the appropriate diagnostic workup. Except following injury, hematuria is not an emergency. Hematuria easily seen by the unaided eye points to a very serious problem within the urinary tract needing prompt diagnosis. Hematuria associated with trauma is discussed in Chapter 37. Bring any urine voided by the patient with urinary complaints to the physician. Hemastix testing of voided specimens may be helpful.

Urinary Frequency

The term urinary frequency means an abnormally high number of voiding episodes during a 24 hour period. Frequency is associated with dysuria and bladder infections. Commonly very small quantities of urine are passed at very frequent intervals. Generally, this urine smells unusually bad. In the aging male, the prostate gland surrounding the upper portion of the urethra, adjacent to the bladder, can enlarge and encroach on the urethral passage partially obstructing it. A sign of this obstruction is urinary frequency, persisting not only during the day but throughout the night, requiring the patient to get up to void. The necessary passage of urine at night is called nocturia and is also regarded as a sign of lower urinary tract obstruction.

Frequency is not an emergency and is seen in association with a number of problems of the lower urinary tract. The trainer should recognize this condition and realize it indicates an underlying disorder.

Incontinence

The uncontrolled passage of urine or feces and soiling of clothing is incontinence. While not an emergency it occurs in association with many emergency conditions. Patients are frequently incontinent during epileptic seizures, but this does not indicate major urinary or bowel disease. The patient with a severe spinal injury resulting in paraplegia loses control of both urinary and fecal discharge. Ordinarily, incontinence in this patient is an obligatory

overflow from a distended bladder that can no longer contract in a coordinated fashion or respond to the stimulus of being full. Episodic incontinence is frequently associated with unconsciousness or semiconsciousness, as in an alcoholic binge. The older patient may be incontinent as a result of generalized senile degeneration. When incontinence is sudden, unexpected and not associated with any obvious cause, it may signal a serious underlying disorder in the lower urinary tract. For this reason, do not ignore its occurrence but do not ordinarily consider it an emergency.

Urethral Discharge

The most common indication of venereal infection in the man is a penile urethral discharge. In women, these infections result in an intrapelvic inflammation about the fallopian tubes and the ovaries—pelvic inflammatory disease. The discharge may be thin and serous, or it may be grossly purulent. Any material passed out of the male urethra, other than urine or semen, is abnormal and requires medical attention. Venereal disease is extremely common in the United States today, and the athlete whose only complaint is unexplained urethral discharge may consult the trainer.

The situation is not an emergency but the cause of the discharge should be treated immediately. These diseases can become chronic and can have devastating later effects for the individual.

Renal Colic

A fairly common problem is a renal stone, usually formed from a combination of calcium and oxalate crystals. Once formed, virtually no agent is able to dissolve this complex. Much less common, but next in frequency, are renal stones formed of uric acid in patients with gout. While the stones are in the kidney, they are asymptomatic or may produce hematuria, only apparent on microscopic examination of the urine. If a stone passes from the kidney into the ureter, it can quickly obstruct the very small caliber tube. Urine is formed continuously in the kidney, and each kidney passes approximately 1 liter into the bladder every day. Since there is no reservoir capacity for urine above the bladder and since the volume within the ureters and the collecting system of the kidney is very small, it is absolutely necessary that this liter of urine pass constantly into the bladder without impediment. When a stone obstructs a ureter, a characteristic colicky pain ensues as the muscular ureter tries to overcome the obstruction by vigorous peristalsis proximal to the stone. The pain is an excruciatingly sharp colic in the flank on either side of the back. As the stone progresses down the ureter, the pain may radiate down to either side of the external genitalia in both men and women. Renal colic is one of the most severe forms of pain and requires vigorous measures for immediate relief.

The patient suffering from renal colic may give a typical history of the type of pain and its location and radiation. This patient is generally restless, forever seeking a position of some comfort, getting up or lying down. This situation is not life threatening but is urgent because the patient demands and requires relief. Transport this patient promptly to the emergency department. Ordinarily no major measures for support of other body systems are necessary. Collect any urine discharged for analysis at the hospital.

Part 10

MEDICAL EMERGENCIES

Acute Chest Pain

39

CARDIAC FUNCTION

The myocardium (heart muscle) must have a continuous supply of oxygen to carry out its pumping function. The coronary arteries carry oxygen and nutrients to the myocardium. When the heart must increase its work, as during periods of physical exertion or stress, the myocardium requires more oxygen and therefore more blood flow. In the normal heart, the coronary arteries dilate, which easily increases blood flow. Atherosclerosis (thickening of the arterial walls caused by fatty deposits) within these arteries interferes with their ability to dilate and carry additional blood. Indeed, atherosclerosis can cause complete occlusion of a coronary artery and thus can reduce the amount of oxygen available to the myocardium. Acute myocardial infarction (death of heart muscle) and angina pectoris (chest pain, generally considered to mean only the pain of too little oxygen for the heart) are both conditions arising from a reduced oxygen supply. Each represents a different degree of coronary arteriosclerosis.

The coronary arteries originate at the base of the aorta, just above the aortic valve. The right coronary artery supplies the right ventricle and, in most people, the underside of the left ventricle. The left coronary artery divides into the left anterior descending and the left circumflex arteries, both supplying the left ventricle (Fig. 39:1).

Atherosclerosis, which can occur in any artery of the body, begins with a deposit of cholesterol laid down just beneath the endothelium (inner cell layer) of an artery. Deposits may be apparent as early as age 18. As a person ages, more of this fatty material is de-

posited, narrowing the lumen (the inside diameter) of the artery. The deposits grow until they finally disrupt the endothelial covering and cause thrombosis or scarring of the artery. Calcium deposited within the scar further narrows the artery.

By a person's 40s or 50s, coronary artery damage may be so extensive as to limit any increase in blood flow to the heart at times of peak activity, such as running or exercising. Therefore, during these periods the oxygen supply to the heart can no longer meet the heart's requirements.

In the United States, the peak incidence of heart disease lies in the decades between 40 and 70, but heart attack and angina may occur any time from the teens to the 90s. In a

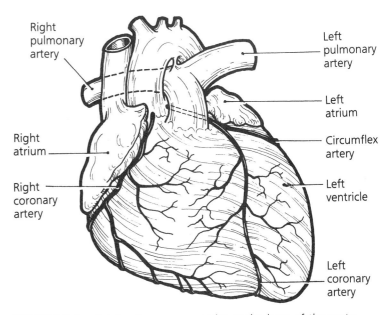

FIGURE 39:1. Origin of coronary arteries at the base of the aorta. Note division of left coronary artery.

28-year-old with chest pain the possibility of a heart attack cannot be excluded.

ANGINA PECTORIS

If the heart has too little oxygen for its needs for more than several seconds, severe pain occurs. This pain is called angina pectoris. Since the occurrence of angina pectoris indicates coronary artery disease, it is important to understand the pain and to recognize it.

Since angina pectoris occurs when the need of the heart for oxygen exceeds its supply, it generally occurs at times when the heart is working hard, during periods of physical or emotional stress. The key characteristic of angina pectoris is pain that comes on with exertion and is relieved by rest. The pain is felt substernally, can radiate to the jaw, arms (especially the left arm) or epigastrium (the upper middle region of the abdomen). It is a pressure or a squeezing sensation, ''like someone standing on my chest.'' It usually lasts from three to eight minutes, rarely longer than ten, and may be associated with shortness of breath, nausea and sweating. The pain is relieved promptly when the oxygen supply of the heart equals or exceeds the demand, as when the stress diminishes or ceases. Occasionally, discomfort or pain is noted not in the chest but only at the point of referral (jaw, left arm or epigastrium). In such instances, the patient may call it ''indigestion'' or it may be confused with gallbladder disease. By no means is physical exertion the only cause of angina. Emotional stress, a large meal or common anxiety may all trigger an attack.

Angina pectoris is treated with nitroglycerin in the form of a small white tablet, one-half the size of aspirin, placed under the tongue. Nitroglycerin works in seconds to relax vascular smooth muscle, dilating coronary vessels and increasing blood flow and oxygen supply to the heart muscle, thus relieving the pain of angina pectoris. It also relaxes and dilates the vessels in the brain and meninges, sometimes causing a severe headache, and it can be used to relax smooth muscle in the gastrointestinal tract. Although angina pectoris is painful, it does not mean death of the myocardium, and it does not lead to the death of the patient or to permanent damage of the heart. Angina pectoris is an indicator that coronary artery disease exists.

MYOCARDIAL INFARCTION

If the narrowing of the coronary artery by atherosclerosis is severe enough, or if a blood clot forms at this point, the oxygen supply in the area of the heart served by that vessel can be so diminished that the myocardium dies. This condition is an acute myocardial infarction (AMI).

Myocardial infarction occurs predominantly in the left ventricle, the thick walled chamber that produces the higher systemic blood pressure. It requires a greater blood supply and much more oxygen than does the lower pressure right ventricle. The left ventricle suffers most from a lack of oxygen. A myocardial infarction has serious consequences:

1. Sudden death from an arrhythmia (unorganized, ineffective beating of the heart)
2. Congestive heart failure
3. Shock

Sudden Death

Approximately 40% of all patients who suffer a myocardial infarction die before they reach the hospital. These deaths occur because of abnormalities of the heart rhythm (arrhythmias), which prevent any effective pumping action of the heart. The chance of an arrhythmia occurring after AMI is greatest within the first hour after the event. It diminishes to a very small risk after three to five hours. Arrhythmias range from irregular heart beats to completely disorganized quivering (fibrillation) or asystole (absence of any beat at all). In either case, the heart is said to be in cardiac arrest. This situation requires cardiopulmonary resuscitation (CPR).

Congestive Heart Failure

The heart fails when the muscle is so damaged by the infarction that it can no longer pump enough blood for the needs of the body. This can occur any time after an infarction, but it is usually manifest between the third and seventh days after the heart attack. These patients may develop pulmonary edema (fluid in the lungs) with frothy pink sputum. They consequently may have difficulty breathing. There may also be evidence of generalized swelling in the body (edema).

Cardiogenic shock is an early complication of an infarction, within 24 hours of the event. It means that the heart has been so damaged that it is unable to sustain a normal systemic blood pressure.

Clinical Presentation of AMI

AMI may have the following signs.

1. Sudden onset of weakness, nausea and sweating without a clear cause
2. Chest pain
3. Sudden arrhythmia accompanied by syncope (fainting)
4. Pulmonary edema
5. Sudden death

Unfortunately, the first sign of coronary heart disease may be sudden death—40% of all patients with AMI may never reach the hospital. Fifty percent of these people will have had no previous knowledge of any heart disease, while in the other 50% coronary artery disease will have been diagnosed. Sudden death from AMI, caused by an arrhythmia, is usually a result of cardiac arrest from ventricular fibrillation. Only beginning CPR promptly can save such a patient. Ventricular asystole, the lack of any heartbeat, may also cause sudden death, but the incidence is hard to determine, since many dangerous ventricular arrhythmias rapidly end in asystole if no treatment is given.

The chance of sudden death is extremely high at the instant of the infarction—this moment is the most dangerous time for the patient. Rapid institution of basic life support mechanisms has successfully resuscitated many patients with cardiac arrest.

Most patients with AMI who do not die at the onset of the infarct develop chest pain. Classically, the pain is:

1. Substernal in location
2. Squeezing in character, or felt as a heaviness or pressure
3. Longer lasting than 30 minutes
4. Not related to exertion, and not relieved by rest or nitroglycerin
5. Perceived as radiating to the jaw, the left arm, to both arms or to the epigastrium

The pain of AMI differs from that of angina pectoris in two ways. It lasts longer than that of angina pectoris. Whereas anginal pain usually lasts no longer than three to ten minutes, AMI pain lasts 30 minutes to hours. Unlike that of angina pectoris, AMI pain is not related to exertion or mental or emotional stress. It is not relieved by rest or by nitroglycerin. AMI pain may come on at any time, waking the person from sleep or while he is sitting reading quietly. Table 39:1 compares findings and treatment of angina with AMI.

About 90% of patients with AMI develop some sort of cardiac arrhythmia, usually extra beats arising in the damaged ventricle. These extra beats, called ventricular premature contractions, may group together and produce a serious disturbance called ventricular tachycardia. If ventricular tachycardia persists, it can become ventricular fibrillation, the totally ineffective quavering that is cardiac arrest. Some patients with AMI may not feel pain but may notice the irregularity of the heartbeat. The episodes of ventricular arrhythmia may cause syncope. Therefore, AMI must be suspected in any patient who develops sudden syncope, especially with any chest pain or discomfort prior to or after the faint.

The sudden onset of left ventricular failure, causing pulmonary edema and difficult breathing, may be the first sign of AMI, and it should be treated as such. If the infarction causes enough damage, the heart can no longer pump

TABLE 39:1. Angina versus Acute Myocardial Infarction

Condition	Common Precipitants	Duration	Frequent Manifestations (Singular or in Combination)	Treatment
Angina	Physical stress Emotional stress Large meals	3-10 min	Substernal pain Epigastric pain-radiating pain to jaw or arms Pressure in chest Shortness of breath Nausea Sweating	1. Rest 2. Nitroglycerin 3. Medical follow-up
Acute Myocardial Infarction	Not necessarily related to stress; may occur at rest	Longer than 30 minutes	Substernal pain Crushing chest pain Heaviness in chest Irregularity of heartbeat Radiation of pain to jaw, arms, epigastrium Feeling faint or lightheaded Shortness of breath or air hunger	1. Reassurance 2. Monitor vital signs 3. Send to ED as soon as possible. Alert hospital of patient's status and estimated time of arrival

blood effectively. Since myocardial infarction usually occurs in the left ventricle, that ventricle does not efficiently pump out the blood coming from the lungs. However, the right ventricle continues to function, pumping blood into the lungs. Pressure within the lung capillaries rises, and fluid pours out from the blood vessels into the pulmonary alveoli. The lungs literally fill with fluid, and the patient feels the sensation of drowning, cannot breathe enough to get oxygen from the air and has a marked feeling of shortness of breath. At times, the fluid in the alveoli may actually come out of the mouth and nose as pink foam. If such a patient has no history of shortness of breath or heart failure, and if the pulmonary edema is sudden in onset, the episode must be treated as one of AMI. Emergency medical treatment for the pulmonary edema should be started at the same time. It usually includes positioning with the head up and giving supplemental oxygen.

Because the left ventricular muscle is damaged by AMI, the amount of blood pumped per minute falls. The occasional patient who does not have pain or an arrhythmia may sud-denly feel weak and be unable to stand or walk. This extreme weakness is probably a result of the fall in cardiac output. Assume such persons are having an AMI and treat them as such.

Physical Findings of AMI

The physical findings of AMI are variable. Generally, the pulse rate is increased as a normal response to stress, fear or the actual injury of the myocardium. Since arrhythmias are the rule rather than the exception, an irregularity of the pulse may be noted. In some cases of AMI, bradycardia (an abnormal slowing of the pulse) develops rather than tachycardia (an abnormally rapid pulse). Blood pressure falls as a result of diminished cardiac output and diminished capability of the ventricle to pump. Respirations are normal unless pulmonary edema occurs, which produces rapid, shallow respirations. The patient appears very frightened and is often in a cold sweat. The patient may feel nauseated and may vomit. The skin is often ashen as a result of poor cardiac output and circulation.

One of the unexplained aspects of AMI is the fact that many patients have an almost overwhelming feeling of impending doom. In this mental state, they are convinced, almost resigned, that they are about to die.

Approach to the Patient

In the conscious patient with suspected heart disease or infarct, the following steps are appropriate.

Reassure the patient. Act professionally, be calm, and speak to the patient in a voice that is neither too loud nor too soft. Tell the patient that trained people are present to provide care, and that he will shortly be taken to the hospital. Remember, all patients are frightened. Some may act carefree, and some may be demanding, but all are frightened. The professional attitude of the trainer is the single most important factor in gaining the patient's co-operation. Patient agitation and anxiety is directly related to an increased number and frequency of paroxysmal ventricular extrasystoles (irregular, extra beats). This arrhythmia may rapidly lead to totally disorganized ventricular activity, fibrillation and death. Thus, apart from providing reassurance and comfort, the calmness and poise of the trainer may materially contribute to preventing a fatal worsening of the patient's condition. Alert the nearest hospital and its emergency department as to the status of the patient and the estimated time of arrival.

Shortness of Breath

40

Dyspnea is defined as the sensation of shortness of breath. It may be accompanied by distinct signs of labored or difficult breathing. Difficult breathing or dyspnea may result from a variety of medical or traumatic causes. Chapter 25 discusses the traumatic causes while this chapter is limited to dyspnea for nontraumatic causes.

PULMONARY PHYSIOLOGY

The major function of the lungs is to provide oxygen to the blood and to take carbon dioxide from the blood to be expelled in the expired, or breathed out, air. To carry out this exchange

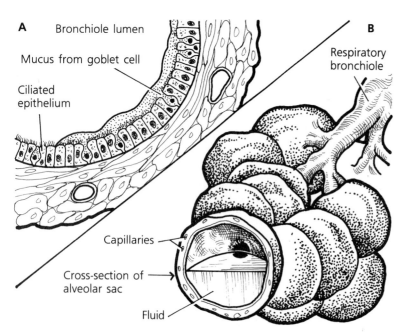

FIGURE 40:1. **A** Cross-section of bronchial wall obstructed by mucus leading to long-term damage if obstruction persists. **B** Dilated bronchiole with fluid preventing exchange of O_2 and CO_2

A
Bronchiole lumen
Mucus from goblet cell
Ciliated epithelium
B
Respiratory bronchiole
Capillaries
Cross-section of alveolar sac
Fluid

of oxygen and carbon dioxide properly, the flow of inspired air (air breathed in) and expired air to and from the pulmonary alveoli (air sacs) must not be impaired. The alveoli are microscopic, thin-walled sacs lying close against the pulmonary arteries and veins through which oxygen and carbon dioxide exchange between the air in the sacs and the blood in the pulmonary vessels easily takes place. In most disorders of the lung, however, the pulmonary vessels are physically separated from the air sacs by fluid or infection. Major air passages are increasingly obstructed by spasm or mucus, or the air sacs are damaged and cannot transport gases well across their own walls (Fig. 40:1). All of these conditions prevent the proper exchange of oxygen and carbon dioxide. Abnormalities of the pulmonary blood vessels themselves may interfere with blood flow and thus hinder transfer of oxygen and carbon dioxide. The first and second mechanisms are those usually seen in athletes.

Too little oxygen entering the blood for any reason harms the body. An excessive level of carbon dioxide may also have an adverse effect. The stimulus that causes a person to breathe is the level of carbon dioxide in the arterial blood. If the carbon dioxide in the blood drops below its normal level, one automatically breathes less deeply and at a lower rate per minute. By decreasing the carbon dioxide expired, this response allows the amount of carbon dioxide in the blood to rise to normal. On the other hand, should carbon dioxide build up in the arterial blood, one breathes more deeply and rapidly, "blowing off" carbon dioxide. The arterial level of carbon dioxide is controlled breath by breath and is regulated so that it varies little in the normal, healthy person. A low level of oxygen in the blood also impels one to breathe, although the stimulus of falling oxygen is not as strong as that of rising carbon dioxide.

DYSPNEA IN SPORTS

Medical problems where dyspnea, or evidence of breathing difficulty, is present include:

1. Acute pulmonary edema
2. Obstruction of the airway by aspiration of vomitus or a foreign object
3. Asthma, exercise-induced asthma or allergic reactions
4. Dyspnea without lung abnormalities (hyperventilation)

Acute Pulmonary Edema

Acute pulmonary edema is usually a concomitant of acute myocardial damage or incompetency, when the heart muscle has been so damaged it cannot circulate the blood properly. In this case, the left side of the heart cannot remove blood and fluid from the lung as fast as the right side delivers it (Fig. 40:2). Fluid collects within the alveoli and the lung tissue itself. This accumulation of fluid is called pulmonary edema. It interferes physically with the exchange of carbon dioxide and oxygen, and the patient may experience dyspnea. In very severe instances, a frothy pink sputum is apparent in nose and mouth. This may occur in high altitude activities such as skiing or mountain climbing. In athletes on salicylate anti-inflammatory therapy, overdose may also produce pulmonary edema.

Obstruction

The airway may be obstructed in semiconscious and unconscious persons as a result of the position of the head, obstruction by the tongue or aspiration of vomitus. Proper opening of the airway by neck extension may solve the problem, but this may be done only after a head or neck injury has been ruled out. If

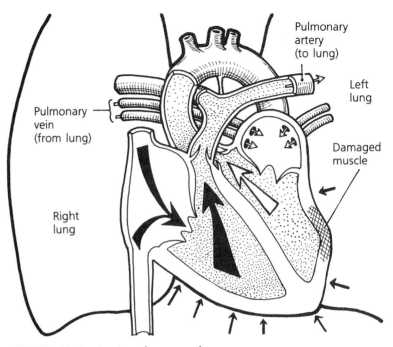

FIGURE 40:2. Acute pulmonary edema

simple opening of the airway does not correct the breathing problem, search for an upper airway obstruction. Foreign body upper airway obstruction must be considered as a first diagnosis in any dyspneic athlete. (Review the techniques of relieving upper airway obstruction—breaths, blows, thrusts, probes—in Chapter 31.) In sports obstruction occurs most often following head injury and should be considered in every unconscious player. In addition, large tonsils and adenoids may be a potential cause of airway obstruction in the adolescent. Chewing gum, tobacco, mouth piece or other material in the mouth during athletic activity may cause obstruction (Table 40:1).

Asthma and Allergic Reactions

Bronchial asthma may occur at any age. The disease is caused by an acute spasm of the airways, which produces a characteristic wheezing as the patient attempts to breathe out. Often, the spasm results from inhalation, ingestion or injection of some agent to which the

TABLE 40:1.   Airway Obstruction

Conscious Athlete	Unconscious Athlete
1. If athlete is breathing or coughing, leave alone but continue to watch.	1. Head tilt if no neck injury is suspected
2. If no air is going in and out of lungs, administer A. 4 Back blows B. 4 Abdominal thrusts	2. No response—try to ventilate
	3. No success—reposition head and try to ventilate again
3. Repeat until A. Athlete can breath on his own B. Athlete becomes unconscious	4. Roll away from you and administer 4 back blows
	5. If unsuccessful, follow with 4 abdominal thrusts
	6. Quick sweep of the mouth
	7. If unsuccessful, repeat steps 1–6 until A. There is no longer obstruction B. Qualified help arrives. A tracheotomy may follow if obstruction continues

patient has become sensitized (allergic). Usually no abnormality in the level of blood gases, oxygen and carbon dioxide occurs, and many athletes have normal lung function between attacks. An allergic response to a bee sting or to substances such as a medication may produce an acute asthmatic attack. At its most severe, this allergic reaction can produce anaphylactic shock (see Chapters 30 and 51). In athletics, preparticipation evaluation should identify the susceptible individual and a record of medication dosage and frequency kept. Exercise-induced asthma (EIA) is probably the most common form of asthma in the athlete with no history of breathing difficulties. Exercise in a cold, dry environment is the usual predisposing factor. This results in heat and fluid loss from the airway and produces bronchospasm and wheezing respiration. Athletes working in humidified warm environments (swimmers and wrestlers) rarely have this problem. There is no evidence that any permanent or long-term problems result from

EIA, nor does this disorder result in chronic asthma (see Chapter 44).

Dyspnea Without Lung Abnormalities

Hyperventilation is overbreathing to the extent that arterial carbon dioxide is abnormally lowered. When overbreathing blows off too much carbon dioxide, the blood pH (a measure of blood acidity) is raised above normal and alkalosis, the cause of many of the symptoms associated with overbreathing, develops. Hyperventilation is a common response to psychological stress, almost as common a reaction as headache or stomach upset. The symptoms can be produced by breathing as deeply and as rapidly as possible for 3 to 5 minutes. However, an athlete often will not realize that he has been hyperventilating.

Anerobic exercise may result in a feeling of air hunger, most commonly in interval training or workouts involving hill climbs. It is probably due to mild metabolic acidosis and muscle fatigue, and is often accompanied by an aching pain in the lower chest or upper abdomen.

Dyspnea associated with fainting during exercise is a cardinal warning sign. Stop all further exercise and refer the athlete to a physician for a careful cardiopulmonary evaluation.

TREATMENT OF DYSPNEA

Acute Pulmonary Edema

For the pulmonary problem, the athlete requires supplemental oxygen, clearing of the copious secretions from the airway and prompt transport to an emergency department. Transport from high altitudes and restriction of activity reduces the demands on the heart and relieves the problem.

Obstruction

The first step is to clear the upper airway. Supplemental oxygen and prompt transport to an emergency department are indicated, especially if one encounters difficulty in clearing the air passage. Tongue forceps and bolt cutter (to remove facial protection) may be necessary to adequately assess and maintain the airway.

Asthma and Allergic Reactions

The asthmatic athlete may be in respiratory distress, and wheezing on expiration heard without a stethoscope. The outflow of air is greatly restricted, causing the person literally to labor to push out each breath. Sternocleido-mastoid retraction may be seen, and is an important sign that the athlete with severe wheezing is beginning to tire. The effort to breathe out is tiring and frightening.

The history of asthma is episodic attacks of shortness of breath, with completely normal breathing between episodes. Chest pain is rarely present. The pulse rate is normal, and the blood pressure may be slightly elevated as a consequence of tension and anxiety or medication that may have been taken to alleviate the attack. The respiratory rate is also increased.

A trainer or physician should have a good initial history available on each athlete. An athlete with respiratory distress secondary to a bee sting may have symptoms masquerading as a mechanical obstruction. Response to bee or wasp stings may rapidly progress to anaphylactic shock. Thus, a history of preceding events is crucial. Reassure the patient and give oxygen. Allow the person to sit, as breathing is much easier in this position.

Many athletes with asthma or known sensitivities have medications to take when an attack occurs. The patient with full-blown anaphylactic shock may be unconscious and require assisted respiration as well as supple-

mental oxygen. Kits are now available for the subcutaneous or intramuscular injection of .5 ml of 1:1,000 epinephrine. Epinephrine may rapidly reverse an anaphylactic reaction.

The treatment of exercise-induced asthma is to breathe warm moist air, as in a shower room. Commercially available inhalers (such as Albuterol) may be used to reduce wheezing for up to six hours. Such an inhaler used prior to participation prevents the wheezing associated with this problem. Teenagers tend to have fewer problems as they get older, and this problem does not appear to be associated with chronic asthma.

Hyperventilation

The hyperventilating patient may feel he cannot get enough air into the chest, despite the fact that a larger quantity than usual is being exchanged. Dizziness and feeling faint are common. Often the person feels a numbness or tingling of the hands and feet, which he may also describe as "being cold." Fainting or sticking, stabbing chest pains that increase with respiration may occur. Vital signs reveal rapid breathing and a high pulse rate (tachycardia) with normal blood pressure.

Assess the athlete's status and obtain a history. The presence or absence of chest pain, cardiac problems, the coughing of blood and diabetes may be easily noted. In the absence of any of these causes for hyperventilation, the best treatment is kindness and reassurance.

To build up the blood carbon dioxide, ask the patient to breathe into a paper bag. Rebreathing expired breath raises the arterial carbon dioxide. Do not worry about oxygen. The patient receives sufficient oxygen because expired breath is not exclusively carbon dioxide.

Sudden Loss of Consciousness

41

In caring for the unconscious athlete, provide needed life support initially, then move the patient to an appropriate facility for evaluation and treatment. Steps in emergency medical care are similar, regardless of the cause of the unconscious state. The trainer is in an excellent position to accumulate and retrieve data concerning the cause of the patient's problem.

Many clinical problems result in unconsciousness. Table 41:1 lists most of the common problems causing unconsciousness, as well as their pathophysiology and emergency medical management.

EMERGENCY CARE

In general, emergency medical treatment follows a consistent pattern for every unconscious patient.

1. Secure and maintain an airway.
2. Institute cardiopulmonary resuscitation (CPR) when necessary.
3. Observe and record vital signs.
4. Observe the incident, record history when available and note any items that might serve as evidence regarding the cause of the unconscious state.
5. Attempt to define the specific cause of unconsciousness.

For every unconscious patient, maintain an open airway and provide respiratory support when necessary. A supine, unconscious patient is in danger of aspiration of vomitus or other oral contents and suffocation from an obstructed airway. If neck injury has been ruled out and the airway opened, place the patient on one side, with head lower than the feet and be sure to keep the airway open. Transport the patient to the emergency department in this position continuing to monitor respiration (Fig. 41:1).

When the unconscious patient has sustained a cardiopulmonary arrest, start CPR. Many runners with arrhythmias or acute myocardial infarctions have been saved by CPR immediately after the attack.

Obtain a history regarding previous episodes of unconsciousness, epilepsy, any known medical illness, details of drug use and the possibility of a drug overdose. Preparticipation evaluation should provide valuable historical information.

Record vital signs and note and describe any injury. Note whether the pupils of the eyes are constricted or widely dilated. Transport the patient promptly to the emergency department.

CAUSES OF UNCONSCIOUSNESS

After resuscitation the trainer's first consideration is to find the cause of unconsciousness so that prompt emergency medical treatment can reverse the condition as soon as possible. In general, the unconscious state can be assigned to diseases, injuries, emotions, environmental causes or injected or ingested poisonous agents.

Diseases

Common diseases that may produce unconsciousness are diabetes (see Chapter 43), arteriosclerosis involving the coronary vessels of the heart or disorders of the cerebral vessels in the brain.

TABLE 41:1.   Causes of Unconsciousness in the Athlete

Category	Problem	Cause	Pathophysiology	Management
General	Loss of consciousness	Injury or disease	Shock, head injury, other injuries, diabetes, arteriosclerosis	Need for CPR, triage
Diseases	Diabetic coma	Hyperglycemia and acidosis	Inadequate use of sugar, acidosis	Complex treatment for acidosis
	Insulin shock	Hypoglycemia	Excess insulin	Sugar
	Myocardial infarct	Damaged myocardium	Insufficient cardiac output	O_2, CPR, transport
	Stroke	Damaged brain	Loss of arterial supply to brain or hemorrhage within brain	Support, gentle transport
Injury	Hemorrhagic shock	Bleeding	Hypovolemia	Control external bleeding, recognize internal bleeding, CPR, transport
	Respiratory shock	Insufficient O_2	Paralysis, chest damage, airway obstruction	Clear airway, supplemental O_2, CPR, transport
	Anaphylactic shock	Acute contact with agent to which patient is sensitive	Allergic reaction	Intramuscular epinephrine, support, CPR, transport
	Cerebral contusion, concussion or hematoma	Blunt head injury	Bleeding into or around brain, concussive effect	Airway, supplemental O_2, CPR, careful monitoring, transport
Emotions	Psychogenic shock	Emotional reaction	Sudden drop in cerebral blood flow	Place supine, make comfortable, observe for injuries
Environment	Heatstroke	Excessive heat, inability to sweat	Brain damage from heat	Immediate cooling, support, CPR, transport
	Electric shock	Contact with electric current	Cardiac abnormalities, fibrillation	CPR, transport; do not treat until current controlled
	Systemic hypothermia	Prolonged exposure to cold	Diminished cerebral function, cardiac arrhythmias	CPR, rapid transport, warming at hospital
	Drowning	O_2, CO_2, breath holding, H_2O	Cerebral damage	CPR, transport
	Air embolism	Intravascular air	Obstruction to arterial blood flow by nitrogen bubbles	CPR, recompression
	Decompression sickness ("bends")	Intravascular nitrogen	Obstruction to arterial blood flow by nitrogen bubbles	CPR, recompression
Injected or ingested agents	Alcohol	Excess intake	Cerebral depression	Support, CPR, transport
	Drugs	Excess intake	Cerebral depression	Support, CPR, transport (bring drug)
	Plant poisons	Contact, ingestion	Direct cerebral or other toxic effect	Support, recognition, CPR, identify plant, local wound care, transport
	Animal poisons	Contact, ingestion, injection	Direct cerebral or other toxic effect	Recognition, support, CPR, identify agent, local wound care, transport
Neurological	Epilepsy	Brain injury, scar, genetic predisposition, disease	Excitable focus of motor activity in brain	Support, protect patient, transport in status epilepticus

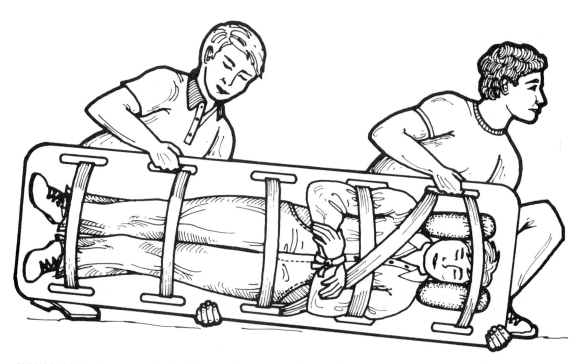

FIGURE 41:1.   Proper method of transporting unconscious athlete to sidelines

Arteriosclerosis

Atherosclerotic blood vessel disease can attack every artery in the body. When it damages arterial vessels supplying the heart with subsequent occlusion, a heart attack may follow. Loss of consciousness may be sudden because of acute disordered beating of the damaged heart. In this situation, CPR may be lifesaving. The many presentations of heart attacks are discussed in Chapter 31.

Stroke

Normal brain function requires a continuous supply of oxygen and glucose and, therefore, a continuous blood flow. Interruption of flow in a cerebral artery for more than six minutes usually causes irreversible damage in the area of the brain supplied by that artery. Since specific areas of the brain correspond to specific functions of the body, the results of damage in the brain depend on the area of the brain destroyed.

A stroke (cerebrovascular accident, or CVA) is the term given to the set of symptoms and signs caused by any interruption of blood flow that lasts long enough to damage the brain. A number of events can interrupt cerebral flow.

1. Clot formation (thrombus) at the site of damage within an arterial wall can occlude a cerebral artery. This is usually the result of atherosclerotic vascular disease.

2. An artery can rupture and bleed into the brain. The bleeding may cause spasm of the leaking artery and further lessen blood flow within the vessel. Brain damage may result directly from the hemorrhage into the tissue or from the impaired circulation. Generally, bleeding comes from a weakened, bulging area of an intracerebral vessel—an aneurysm. These arterial lesions are common causes of strokes in younger patients. Aneurysms can be congenital or acquired. Occasionally, a stroke is associated with hypertension alone, in which case the

bleeding is not caused by a weakened, damaged vessel but by too great an intraluminal arterial pressure.

3. A blood clot formed elsewhere, usually within the heart, may travel to a cerebral vessel as an embolus (clot or plug) and obstruct it.

An embolism in a cerebral vessel occurs most often in individuals with heart disease. Valvular damage is frequently the cause of the clot, which forms within the heart itself and breaks loose to pass to the brain, but any heart disease that causes an abnormal rhythm, usually atrial fibrillation, may also be the cause.

The three different events that can interrupt blood flow to the brain cause three distinct clinical pictures. Clotting of a cerebral artery causes a lessening of body function, generally without pain or seizures. An arterial rupture is frequently accompanied by a sudden, severe headache with rapid loss of consciousness. A cerebral embolism may also occur suddenly with a convulsion, paralysis or the abrupt loss of consciousness.

Strokes may produce the following effects:

1. Paralysis of extremities, unilateral or bilateral
2. Diminished consciousness, varying from coma to confusion to dizziness
3. Difficulty with speech or vision
4. Convulsions (although many individuals have epilepsy or experience convulsions from other causes without any damage of the brain)
5. Headache alone

The initial care of a patient with a stroke should include careful observation of vital signs, respiration, pulse and blood pressure. Is respiration regular or irregular? Some patients with stroke exhibit certain characteristic hesitancies in their breathing patterns. Others may have very rapid, but not labored, respiration. Judge whether the frequency of breathing is sufficient, or whether supportive respiratory is required.

Take a pulse both at the wrist and the throat. Early in the course of a stroke observing whether both carotid pulses (one on each side of the neck) are present is helpful. Absence of a carotid pulse may indicate a thrombosis of that vessel. When palpating the pulse, note its rhythm. An irregularity may indicate underlying heart disease and therefore suggest an embolic cause for the stroke.

Take the blood pressure. A very high blood pressure associated with a slow pulse is often a sign of marked swelling of the brain. Immediate care by a physician is necessary for this patient to promptly control blood pressure and cerebral swelling.

Administer oxygen only if the patient is having breathing difficulty or cyanosis. When lifting and transporting the patient, always protect paralyzed arms and legs from further injury.

Do not give anything by mouth, as the throat may be paralyzed. If a patient is semiconscious or comatose and choking on saliva, position him on one side, preferably with the paralyzed side down, during transport. This position frees the patient's useful extremities. Take care, however, to adequately cushion the paralyzed side although ordinarily it is not injured during routine transport. Clear the airway by suction, and give oxygen when needed. Transportation to the emergency department must be as gentle but as prompt as possible.

Injury

Many injuries result in loss of consciousness. All injuries that cause excessive blood loss may precipitate hypovolemic shock. In this situation, insufficient blood is left in the vascular system to circulate so perfusion of both the brain and heart is inadequate. Loss of consciousness from hypovolemic shock, associated with obvious external or suspected internal bleeding, is an end-stage situation in the picture of shock. This patient is critically ill and requires the promptest possible transport to a source of medical care.

Similarly, unconsciousness due to lack of sufficient oxygen for whatever reason is a very serious situation in which the trainer's primary responsibility is to provide an adequate airway and supplemental oxygen as soon as possible. These situations, hypovolemic and respiratory shock, along with several other causes of shock, are discussed in Chapter 30.

Most important in dealing with the person with a head injury is to observe the initial state of consciousness and any subsequent changes. A changing state of consciousness in a person with a head injury and consequent direct damage within the brain may require very rapid transport to the emergency department and an immediate operation to correct the condition. This situation is discussed in Chapter 32.

Emotions

The common faint or psychogenic shock is an emotional reaction that results in a transient, sudden general dilatation of the blood vessels without increased cardiac output. Momentarily, blood supply for the brain is inadequate, impairing its function. In general, consciousness is restored very promptly when the patient lies down. Be alert for injuries sustained if the patient falls during a fainting episode.

Environment

Among environmental causes for loss of consciousness are heat, cold, electricity, water and exposure to gases under extreme pressure. Generally, heatstroke or systemic hypothermia is easily diagnosed by virtue of the circumstances and body temperature.

Many pieces of equipment in the training room can produce electric shock. With a patient who has sustained electric shock, the trainer must first think of self-protection. The electric current must be controlled before any treatment is given to the patient. The patient may have a cardiopulmonary arrest as a result of the shock and require CPR as an initial step. Prevention by adequate grounding of equipment is a necessity.

In general, drowning patients require basic life support and prompt transport to the nearest emergency department.

Patients with suspected air embolism or decompression sickness from a diving accident may require treatment in a recompression chamber. These patients may need support up to and including CPR and prompt transport to the emergency department, where the recompression treatment may be arranged.

Injected or Ingested Agents

All manner of agents may be injected or ingested. Some are very toxic in minute amounts. Others, such as alcohol, are used routinely by a large portion of the population and to great excess by some.

The medical treatment for all toxic overdoses, whether of alcohol, drugs or other agents, is to support the patient until the drug is cleared or metabolized by the body. In some cases, treatment may include a specific antagonist, such as sugar for insulin. In most overdose situations, respiratory function is lowered. Take great care to insure that the airway is open and that artificial respiration is given if necessary.

If blood pressure falls, elevate the patient's legs slightly. Note the response of the pupils to light. Widely dilated pupils are characteristic of overdoses of such drugs as barbiturates, whereas constricted pupils accompany narcotic use such as Demerol or heroin.

EPILEPSY

Epilepsy is a common condition usually easily controlled by medication. When uncontrolled, it is manifested by seizures. The seizures take a variety of forms, from simply ''blacking out'' for a few seconds to severe convulsions. Epilepsy can be caused by an old brain injury with a scar, acute head trauma, a brain tumor, a cerebral embolus acutely blocking blood flow within a cerebral vessel, infection, birth injury or a genetic predisposition. The seizures are caused by an abnormal focus of activity within the brain that produces severe motor responses or changes in consciousness. Most seizures involve altered states of consciousness lasting for a variable period of time and are followed by a period of unconsciousness. Patients with uncontrolled epilepsy and recurrent seizures can frequently be identified by medical identification tags or by close questioning of family members.

Not all seizures are due to epilepsy. Many other serious illnesses can cause seizures. It is especially important to determine the cause in the patient with no history of previous seizures. This may require an extensive medical workup in the hospital.

Seizures are generally classified according to the degree and location of electrical activity in the brain. Seizure episodes are classified in two categories, generalized seizures and partial seizures, either simple or complex.

A generalized seizure (convulsive or tonic-clonic seizure) involves most of the brain. Contraction of the jaw muscles leads to biting the tongue or lips. Loss of bowel or bladder control is common. Partial seizures involve less extensive areas of the brain. The seizure activity may be limited to one or more extremities or one side of the body (simple partial seizures), or the consciousness may be clouded and the patient may display automatic behavior such as chewing, fumbling with clothes, walking aimlessly, muttering or unresponsiveness. These seizures are called complex partial seizures.

Management

To manage a convulsive or tonic-clonic seizure, keep the patient from injury during the attack, and assure an open airway and proper respiration during the unconscious state. Protect the patient's head, arms and legs but do not rigidly restrain them. If the patient's teeth are not clenched, place a padded tongue blade between the molars to prevent biting of his tongue, cheek or lip. Do not place anything between the front teeth. Never place fingers

Epileptic Management Chart

1. Protect from injury during seizure.
2. Remove others from scene—the patient should not have undue stress during this episode.
3. If mouth is open, insert padded tongue blade.
4. Allow sleep for recovery.
5. If status epilepticus or first seizure, seek medical help.

between the teeth. Never allow the padded tongue blade or anything else to migrate into the pharynx, further obstructing the airway.

Contractions of all chest muscles may make the patient appear to have an airway obstruction and to become cyanotic. Normal respiration during the attack rarely presents a problem unless several convulsions follow one another in quick succession. The airway can be best kept open by putting the patient on one side so that gravity aids in keeping the tongue out of the pharynx, and vomited material is not aspirated as easily.

Following the period of excessive muscular activity, the patient is lethargic, perhaps disoriented, and only partially conscious. Normal respirations almost always follow. However, clear the airway and maintain it adequately until the patient is fully awake.

In the patient who has frequent, recurrent epileptic seizures, medical assistance following the seizure and subsequent transportation to the emergency department is usually not necessary. At most, the patient usually needs only to sleep to completely recover. Seek medical assistance for these patients only when seizures last ten minutes or more, or when a second seizure follows immediately upon the first. This state of continuous seizures, in which the person does not fully recover consciousness between seizures, is called status epilepticus.

Any patient without a history of previous seizures should be transported to the hospital for a thorough medical evaluation. Since most seizure patients take some type of medication, take all his medications to the hospital.

In managing partial seizures, the same general rules apply as for convulsive seizures. A complex partial seizure may be mistaken for intoxication, drug abuse or other medical condition causing abnormal behavior. A cardinal rule in handling a patient with aberrant behavior is not to physically restrain the patient unless essential for safety. These patients may react violently to restraint, although not aware of their actions. During the seizure, which may last 15 minutes or longer, the patient is confused but is usually amenable to suggestions and comments made in a pleasant and friendly manner. It is thus possible to control the person for the duration of the seizure. Stay with the patient, provide reassurance and observe him carefully until the abnormal behavior ceases. A thorough medical evaluation in the hospital may be needed to diagnose this type of seizure disorder accurately.

Part 11

SPECIAL
MEDICAL
CONSIDERATIONS

Women Athletes

In the last several years, greater numbers of women have become athletic competitors. Trainers used to dealing only with men in the training room now must cope with women. Anatomic and physiologic differences make each sex unique in athletics. Physiological factors influence the participation and performance of women athletes. Data on injury rates in women show specific injuries are seen more frequently in women than in men. Correct conditioning and rehabilitation techniques can decrease these injury rates. Women, in addition, may have special medical problems, such as amenorrhea and iron deficiency.

ANATOMIC AND PHYSIOLOGIC SEX DIFFERENCES

The anatomic and physiologic differences explain the uniqueness of each sex in athletics. Despite the data on the "typical" man and "typical" woman, the spectrum of these differences overlaps so that in reality these differences are not so definitive as they may seem in the following discussion. Neither do these differences define male and female sports dominions, although, without a doubt, the "typical" woman has a greater chance of surpassing a man in some areas because of these differences, as does the man in other areas. Yet training diminishes the absolute genetic advantages and disadvantages of each sex. Therefore, these differences are explained not to catalog the abilities of each sex but rather to have those who work with the conditioning, treating and rehabilitation of athletes recognize the inherent genetic strengths and weaknesses of each athlete, and so maximize the performance of each.

In general, women have smaller bones and correspondingly smaller areas of articular surfaces. Men have longer legs, comprising 56% of their height as compared to 51% in the woman. The man's heavier, larger, more rugged structure gives him a mechanical and structural advantage in athletic activities. His longer bones act as greater levers, producing more forces in sports requiring striking, hitting and kicking. The woman has narrower shoulders, a wider pelvis and greater valgus angulation at the knees than does the man. In women the greater varus of the hips and valgus of the knee are sometimes blamed for the increased number of overuse syndromes seen about the hip and knee, especially in the unconditioned state (Fig. 42:1). Because of their

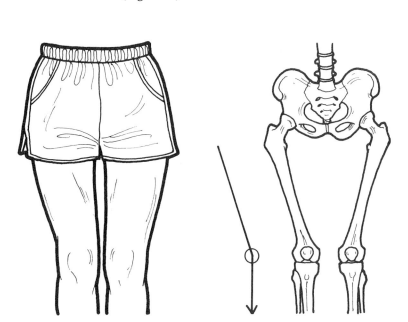

FIGURE 42:1. Wider female pelvis can result in genu valgum.

465

wider pelvises and shorter lower extremities, women have a lower center of gravity, 56.1% of their height compared to 56.7% in men. This gives women a distinct advantage in balance sports such as gymnastics. The man must widen his stance to obtain the same degree of balance as the woman. Hence, events like the balance beam, one of the four major events of women's gymnastic competition, are not events in male gymnastic competition.

For the same body weight, women have smaller hearts, lower diastolic and systolic blood pressures, and smaller lungs and thoracic cavities than equally trained men. This decreases their effectiveness in both anerobic (burst) and aerobic (endurance) activities. Aerobic capacity depends upon one's genetic ability to maximally consume oxygen. Training can and does enhance maximal oxygen consumption, but the baseline is genetically determined. Maximum oxygen consumption (VO_2 max) reflects the body's ability to maximally extract and use oxygen for aerobic metabolism. VO_2 max measures the lung's ability to extract oxygen, the heart's ability to deliver the oxygen to the muscle, and the muscle's ability to assimilate oxygen in energy pathways maximally. Because of her smaller heart, stroke volume and lung and muscle mass, a woman with the same weight and conditioned state as a man has a lower baseline VO_2 max upon which to build her aerobic capacity. Each of these parameters has a continuum for each sex. Indeed, some women on the upper spectrum of the VO_2 max capacity have a greater genetic baseline than some men on the lower end of the masculine profile.

Normal college women are approximately 25% fat per body weight, whereas normal college men are about 15% fat per body weight. In studies analyzing body fat in conditioned athletes, there is great variability among athletes participating in different sports. For track athletes, the average conditioned woman is about 10% to 15% body fat while the conditioned man is generally less than 7%.

As noted above, the woman has less muscle mass per body weight (23%) than an equally trained male (40%). Therefore, it is more difficult for her to achieve the same power and speed as an equally trained man of the same body weight. The woman's greater percentage of fat per body weight also hinders power and speed.

The woman's increased percentage of body fat per body weight is a disadvantage even when matched with a man of equal muscle mass, since the woman must use the same muscle mass to "energize" her extra body fat. If a man performs in a weighted vest equal to a woman's excess body fat, his VO_2 max is lowered to her range. Women athletes have been compared with race horses carrying a heavier handicap. Their extra load of fat reduces their work capacity and stamina. But fat does insulate and give buoyancy—an advantage for swimmers, especially in natural water. Women hold the records for swimming the English Channel, with the best one way time of 7 hours, 40 minutes set by Peggy Bean in 1978 and the best double crossing time of 39 hours, 14 minutes set by Cynthia Nichols in 1979. Fat may also provide energy when glycogen is depleted. Women may be able to convert to fatty acid metabolism more readily than their male counterparts, an advantage in marathons and ultra marathons.

It used to be thought that women were more prone to heat exhaustion than men, and that they needed higher core body temperatures before increasing their sudorific (sweating) response. However, recent evidence demonstrates that equally trained and conditioned men and women are equal in their thermal regulation.

Basic metabolic rate is lower in women and, therefore, for the same amount of activity, the female needs fewer calories. This is important to keep in mind when planning training tables and pregame meals for female athletes. Women need a nutritionally balanced meal, yet with fewer total calories than do men. This fact, although it seems so obvious, can be easily overlooked. In fact, when women first entered the military academies, the diet of the cadets was not altered. The women gained weight eating the high-calorie foods (gravy, potatoes, sauces, etc.) provided for the male cadets to insure them of adequate calorie intake to maintain their base body weights during this time of intense physical effort. The academies learned that they had to provide nutritional meals with fewer total calories—lean meats, fewer sauces, more fruits and vegetables—for their female cadets.

Coordination and dexterity are difficult parameters to measure, but are probably equal between the sexes.

The foregoing anatomic and physiologic comparisons apply to hormonally mature men and women. The prepubertal female best approximates her male counterpart in strength, aerobic power, oxygen pulse, heart size and weight. Puberty in the man is a time of maturation of fitness, but in the woman it is a period of great alteration of physical characteristics and abilities, making her no longer equal to men in size or strength. The woman must adjust timing and performance techniques to accommodate her increase in weight and height without the help of a parallel increase in muscle mass. Recall the prepubertal Nadia Comaneci of the 1976 Olympics, the darling, talented gymnast who won everyone's heart and performed outstandingly (Fig. 42:2). Four years later, puberty had taken its toll. Her percentage of body fat had increased, curves had replaced her previously straight lines, and her center of gravity had obviously changed. It took her several years to readjust her gymnastic timing to her new body.

PSYCHOLOGICAL ADJUSTMENT

Puberty is only one of the many psychological adjustments the female athlete must make. Since ancient Greek times, independence, fortitude, aggressiveness, achievement, and the desire to win or conquer have been classified as masculine or ''nonfeminine'' qualities. Yet, these are the important characteristics in the successful athlete. The winning male athlete has proven his masculinity, whereas the winning female athlete often finds she must justify

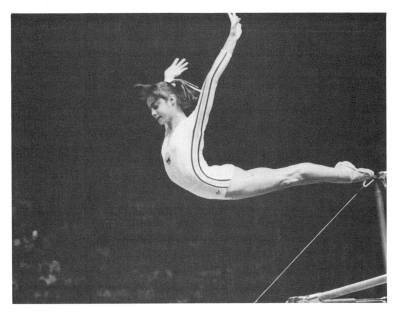

FIGURE 42:2. Nadia Comaneci scoring a perfect 10 at the 1976 Olympic women's gymnastic competition

her femininity. This attitude is slowly changing, but it will be years before the prejudices arbitrarily qualifying masculinity and femininity disappear. The athletic female may face depression because she feels that she is not living up to the image expectations of her sex. Those involved in the care of the female athlete must be aware that these feelings can develop, and must help the athlete cope with them. Trainers must be attuned to the psychological as well as the physiological needs of their athletes. The athlete often confides his or her fears and frustrations to the trainer. Injury can be precipitated by lack of confidence or athletes may appear for sick call for many minor ''hurts.'' Physically, they are fine, but are reaching out for psychological reassurance. The trainer must be sensitive to this need, recognize it and respond to it.

CONDITIONING AND REHABILITATION

Prior to the 1980s, authorities blocked women's participation in long-distance running events because they felt women were not physically strong enough to sustain such an activity and would physically harm themselves. The performance of the first women to run the 800 meter race only reinforced this idea. The majority of the participants, untrained and uncoached, tried to sprint the entire distance, and many collapsed along the way.

Lack of conditioning may also be responsible for early reports of more injuries in female athletes compared with men. Similarly, studies of the first female cadets admitted to the military academies found women had an increase in minor injuries and a greater time loss from duty. The early conclusion from these studies (unfairly drawn) was that women were physiologically inferior to men. In reality, these studies merely reflected that women entering the military academy had not, during their high school years, been subjected to physical training programs as rigorous as those of the men. After several months at the academy, the number of minor injuries and days lost from duty decreased significantly for women. Recently, several studies have demonstrated greater differences in the number and types of injuries sustained by women in different sports than by men and women in the same sport. Just as in male athletes, most injuries seen in women's sports are sprains, strains and contusions, especially of the lower extremities. Injury studies done on women athletes show that conditioning programs, including properly structured weight training programs, are as important for women as they are for men. Conditioning increases endurance, strength and flexibility and, therefore, decreases the number of injuries.

Weight training will not produce musclebound females, a common myth. A woman can increase her strength by 44% without any significant increase in muscle mass. Muscle size is hormonally regulated. Within a sex, the secretion of testosterone, androgen and estrogen, the sex hormones, varies considerably and accounts for the marked variations in terms of muscularity and general morphology among men and women. Some female athletes are indeed muscular and would be so whether they participated in sports or not.

COMMON ORTHOPEDIC PROBLEMS

Some orthopedic problems seen more commonly in female athletes than in male athletes that present challenging treatment problems include retropatella pain, shoulder pain, spondylolysis, scoliosis, stress fractures and bunions.

Women commonly complain of retropatellar pain, or pain behind the kneecap. Pain may develop from direct trauma to the patella or from repetitive knee flexion-extension activities. Decreasing retropatella pain is frequently difficult for the physician and therapist. Hamstring stretching and quadriceps strengthening exercises are the basis of any therapy program. As in most acute inflammatory processes, icing following activity may be helpful. Physicians may also prescribe various braces, shoe orthoses or oral anti-inflammatory medications. Muscle-stimulating units to enhance the strength of the vastus medialis obliquus have also had some success. Eliminate stair climbing and deep squats from the athlete's conditioning program.

Shoulder pain in women, particularly in swimmers and softball players, is usually due to either impingement or subluxation. The woman with shoulder subluxation complains of pain in the anterior region of her shoulder when her shoulder is placed in external rotation, abduction and extension (Fig. 42:3). In this position, the humeral head subluxes against the anterior shoulder capsule, stretching the capsular tissue and thereby causing pain in this area. With impingement because of a weak rotator cuff, the humerus is elevated superiorly in the glenoid with deltoid contraction as seen with overhead motions such as throwing, tennis serves and the swim crawl. This pinches the tissue, tendons and bursa, between the acromion and the upwardly migrated humeral head, causing inflammation and pain, with resultant tendonitis and bursitis. A downward pressure on the acromion while elevating the humerus in a forward-flexed manner reduces the pain. Both shoulder impingement and shoulder subluxation can be managed by strengthening programs for the rotator cuff and shoulder muscles. Rubber tubing provides an excellent way to perform exercises in a pseudo isokinetic fashion.

Low back pain in female athletes may be associated with defects in the posterior elements of the spine, a condition called spondylolysis (Fig. 42:4). This defect occurs with four times greater frequency in the female gymnast than in the normal population. The team physician should determine whether this defect is an acute stress fracture or a chronic injury. If an acute stress fracture, prolonged rest is recommended. In cases of chronic spondylolysis, rest during the acute phase with gradual return to activity is usually prescribed. Anti-inflammatories, muscle relaxants, ice massage and other physical therapy modalities may be helpful. A regular exercise program for abdominal and back muscles should be instituted.

The greater incidence of stress fractures in female athletes probably represents a lack of conditioning and proper training techniques rather than a true predisposition to injury. Stress fractures occur when the rate of bone breakdown from activity (a normal process) is greater than the rate of bone formation (repair). Slow and sensible conditioning for her sport is necessary to give her bone time to increase in cortical thickness to meet the mechanical demands. The pain of a stress fracture is typically restricted to a specific area, worse with activity, and may often be relieved with rest. Initially, radiographs may not demonstrate the area of fracture, since many stress fractures are ''microfractures'' of bone. X-ray films become positive at about two weeks, when healing with increased bony reaction around the microfracture site occurs. A bone scan is more sensitive than routine radiographs and is positive in the early phases of bone healing, before enough bone is laid down to be detected on plain radiographs.

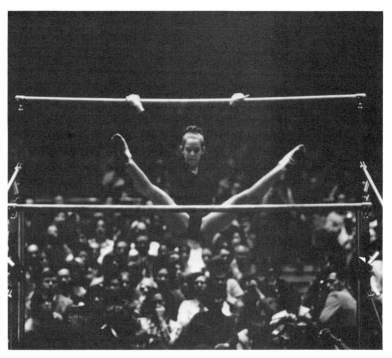

FIGURE 42:3.   Reverse eagle on uneven bars places the shoulder in external rotation, abduction and extension.

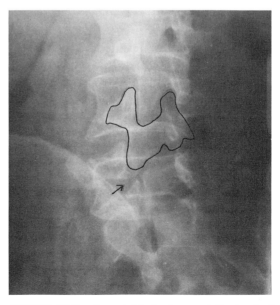

FIGURE 42:4.   Spondylolysis shown at the level of L_3. Note the Scotty dog configuration at L_4 and L_3. The disruption at the dog's neck in L_5 is spondylolysis.

Perhaps because of shoe styles, bunions of the big toes (inflammation of the bursa over the medial side of the metatarsal phalangeal joint of the great toe) are more common in women than in men. The inflamed bursa is generally associated with a deformity of the toe at this level, and bony hypertrophy of the metatarsal head often underlies the inflamed bursa. All conservative modalities should be used to treat bunions, since surgery may alter foot mechanics and precipitate other problems for the athlete. Shoe alterations, orthoses and protective pads, as well as taping, are often successful in diminishing symptoms.

COMMON MEDICAL PROBLEMS

Common medical problems unique to women include amenorrhea, dysmenorrhea, vaginitis and iron deficiency with or without anemia. Because a woman can lose up to 1.2 to 2 mg of iron per day during menstruation, menstruating females have a higher incidence of iron deficiency than the general population. The mineral iron, present in the hemoglobin molecules within red blood cells, is necessary for oxygen transport. A normal iron level, then, is especially important in athletics where maximal oxygen-carrying capacity is needed for maximal energy output. Iron may also participate as a catalyst in removing the lactate formed during aerobic exercise. Women who are iron deficient but not anemic have increased lactate levels with submaximal exercises when compared with women with normal levels of iron. Strenuous exercise during early conditioning programs has also been reported to lower plasma iron levels in both sexes, perhaps because of increased destruction of red cells with vigorous activity, but the exact cause is not known. Therefore, iron supplementation in women is advised unless sufficient quantities are part of the athlete's diet. The recommended daily allowance of iron for women after the beginning of menstruation increases from 10 mg per day to 18 mg per day. Only 10% of all ingested iron is absorbed through the gut. Foods high in iron include

liver, oysters, beef, turkey, dried apricots and prune juice. Ferrous sulphate, taken as a 300 mg tablet each day, may be used to supplement dietary iron sources. A multivitamin plus iron generally has only 12 mg of iron, but may be used instead of ferrous sulphate as an iron supplement for the athletic woman. "Mega doses" of iron are not helpful because one cannot make blood "iron rich" and thereby improve oxygen-carrying capacity. In fact, iron overdose can be toxic.

Normal ovulation and menstruation depend upon proper hormonal secretion by the hypothalamus, the pituitary and the ovaries. A delicate balance of positive and negative feedback channels exists within this system. Basically, the hypothalamus, located at the base of the brain, secretes releasing and inhibiting factors that act on the pituitary to cause it to release pituitary hormones—follicular-stimulating hormone (FSH) and luteinizing hormone (LH). These hormones travel to the ovaries, where they promote the development of ovarian follicles and the production of estrogen and progesterone—the ovarian hormones. Ovarian follicles have two basic stages: a follicular stage prior to ovulation and a luteal phase that follows ovulation. FSH causes follicles within the ovary to mature and produce estrogen. This increased estrogen causes the pituitary to respond by producing a surge of LH. This surge of LH combined with the FSH produced by the pituitary acts on the ovary to stimulate ovulation in the ovarian follicle that is most mature at this time. Following ovulation, the follicle that produced the ovum involutes, forming the corpus luteum that secretes progesterone, as well as estrogen, beginning the luteal, or second, phase of the monthly menstrual cycle. The normal menstrual cycle is 28 days, with a range of 25 to 32 days. The length of the follicular and luteal phases of the cycle are equal, approximately 14 days each.

Secondary amenorrhea is the cessation of normal menstrual periods in a previously menstruating female. This is not uncommon in women athletes and has been related to physical and emotional stresses as well as to the low percentage of body fat in conditioned athletes with high energy demands. There is also a high incidence of secondary amenorrhea in women cadets in the military academies during their first few months of training. Stress or increased energy demands may play a major role in causing secondary amenorrhea and, in fact, may be more important than a low percentage of body fat. This stress-related secondary amenorrhea is thought to be due to the absence of the LH surge necessary for proper ovulation and menstruation. Those who argue that the athlete's secondary amenorrhea is due to a low percentage of body fat suggest that the pituitary realizes that the body lacks sufficient fat to support pregnancy and therefore ''turns off'' the pituitary axis. This hypoestrogenic amenorrhea is commonly seen in anorexia nervosa, a psychological disturbance resulting in the lack of food intake.

Much is still to be learned regarding secondary amenorrhea in the female athlete. It seems fairly certain that this secondary amenorrhea is reversible and does not result in long-term fertility problems. Basically, if the athlete cuts down slightly in her training or gains a little weight, normal menstrual cycles return. Since an athlete with secondary amenorrhea may begin a normal cycle at any time (implying that she is then ovulating normally), she can becoming pregnant then. Athletes with secondary amenorrhea should be advised of this, since many feel that the lack of regular periods protects against pregnancy. Because secondary amenorrhea is relatively common in female athletes, most gynecologists feel that evaluation is necessary only if the amenorrhea persists for longer than one year.

Dysmenorrhea, or painful menstruation, is far less common in athletic women than in nonathletic women. The pain appears to be caused by the release of prostaglandins (another hormonal type substance) by the lining of the uterus. Prostaglandin inhibitors, such as ibuprofen, aspirin and naproxen, may help control dysmenorrhea.

Vaginitis is common in women and typically results in a pruritic discharge. Yeast and Trichomonas infections are the two most frequent causes of vaginitis. A physician should examine athletes with vaginal discharge so that the correct diagnosis can be made from a smear of the discharged fluid. Vaginal suppositories for yeast infections and oral medication for Trichomonas infections are extremely effective in controlling this problem.

Various contraceptive devices, birth control pills, intrauterine devices, diaphragms, foams, spermicidal jellies and suppositories are of concern to female athletes. Some find that oral contraceptives cause increased water retention and a feeling of premenstrual sluggishness. For others, intrauterine devices cause heavy menstrual flow and pelvic pain that can influence performance. Diaphragms, if worn during training episodes, have been reported to cause cramping and abdominal pain. No means of contraception seems universally acceptable. On the other hand, there is certainly no specific contraindication to the use of any type of contraception for any particular athlete. However, all women should be warned not to use birth control pills to alter the normal menstrual cycle prior to competition merely because a woman feels she performs best at certain times in her cycle. A study done in the 1972 Olympics found gold medalists in all phases of their menstrual cycles. For the sake of complete information, it should be stated that menstruation is no contraindication to athletic performance, even aquatic sports.

While there was much initial discussion regarding protective equipment for the external female genitalia, injuries to these areas are extremely rare. Protective pelvic girdles and protective bras with molded plastic cups are no longer marketed. Sport bras with few if any metal fasteners and broad straps designed not to slide off easily, or cut into, the shoulder are available. For maximal comfort, these bras are generally made of a light-weight material that ''breathes'' and is easy to launder. However, bras manufactured as sport bras are expensive, and a conventional bra style may have all of the characteristics of a sport bra but be less expensive.

It is a myth that the breast needs maximal support during exercise to prevent the elastic fibers in breast tissue from stretching irreparably, causing sagging breasts in later years. The amount of breast support needed during exercise depends on the individual preference and should be determined by comfort rather than by any arbitrary standard. Some women prefer very supportive bras, and others prefer to wear no bra, a preference not always determined by breast size. The type of sport does not seem to influence the degree of support preferred by the athlete. Surveys indicate that women generally want the same type of bra for all sports.

Nipple chafing and excoriation occurs in both men and women, especially in women who wear no bras. Long-distance runners are particularly susceptible to nipple irritation from shirts rubbing over the nipple area. Vaseline smeared on the nipples, with or without bandage coverage, may decrease symptoms.

The Diabetic Athlete

Carbohydrates are important sources of energy in the diet. Following ingestion, carbohydrates are digested to monosaccharides and absorbed in the duodenum and jejunum. Once carbohydrates are absorbed, the blood glucose rises and then gradually returns to normal.

Insulin, a blood glucose-lowering hormone, is produced by the beta cells of the islets of Langerhans of the pancreas. Several hormones raise blood glucose levels: epinephrine secreted by the adrenal medulla, glucocorticoids secreted by the adrenal cortex, glucogen secreted by the alpha cells of the islets of Langerhans and growth hormone secreted by the anterior pituitary. These systems act as regulators of blood glucose levels. Unfortunately, in diabetes, these regulators may fail, causing severe imbalances.

Several etiologies of diabetes are postulated.

1. Abnormal beta cell function or number
2. Environmental factors altering beta cell function
3. Abnormal glucogen secretion
4. Abnormal insulin activity

Depending on its course, diabetes is managed by diet, physical activity and hypoglycemic agents. A careful balance of these is particularly important to the diabetic. In some cases, diet and exercise alone can control diabetes. In other cases, insulin must be supplemented to assist in regulation.

THE INSULIN-DEPENDENT DIABETIC ATHLETE

The insulin-dependent diabetic athlete must try to balance insulin intake with physical activity and food intake to maintain stable glucose concentrations in the blood. Without this control, blood glucose use is markedly affected.

Acute exercise reduces the blood glucose level in insulin-treated diabetics, and there is enhanced sensitivity to insulin after physical training. In short-term exercise, glucose uptake increases sevenfold to twentyfold. With more prolonged exercise, free fatty acids provide the energy needs to muscle, minimizing the fall in blood glucose. Exercise may accelerate insulin absorption from the injection site, leading to increased insulin levels in the blood. The diabetic can then deplete glycogen stores by strenuous exercise over several days but, following this, must have several days of reduced exercise to replenish glycogen stores. Supplemental carbohydrate feeding during competition may be used to avoid carbohydrate depletion and insulin reaction.

A diabetic participating in running sports should use sugar in a dilute solution to avoid hypoglycemia and heat exhaustion. He may also have a meal before competition similar to that of a nondiabetic athlete. He should refrain from exercise at the time of peak insulin effect, however, or should consume a carbohydrate snack about 30 minutes before exercising. In other words, the insulin dosage is not altered but the food intake is increased.

Imbalance in insulin and blood sugar can produce several complications. The athletic trainer should be extremely familiar with their signs and treatment.

The waste products from the body's use of fat to meet normal energy requirements markedly increase the acidity of the blood. If the loss of fluid (from the high level of sugar in the blood and increased urinary frequency)

43

and the increase of acidity are severe enough, diabetic coma (diabetic ketoacidosis) occurs. The very high sugar level in the blood does not directly cause coma. Rather the presence of acid waste products in the blood and the loss of fluid cause the coma.

Coma commonly develops when a diabetic patient who is untreated or who fails to take prescribed insulin undergoes some sort of stress, such as an infection. The patient may then be found comatose with the following physical signs.

1. Air hunger, manifested by rapid and deep sighing respirations (Kussmaul respiration)
2. Dehydration, or excessive loss of body water, manifested by a dry, warm skin and sunken eyes
3. A sweet or fruity (acetone) odor on the breath, caused by the acid in the blood
4. A rapid, weak pulse
5. A normal or slightly low blood pressure
6. Varying degrees of unresponsiveness

Insulin Shock (Hypoglycemia)

Insulin shock may result when too much insulin is given or when the patient takes a regular dose of insulin but does not eat enough food or exercises excessively. Sugar is then rapidly driven out of the blood and into the cells. This means that insufficient sugar is available in the blood for use by the brain. Since the brain requires a constant supply of glucose just as it requires a constant supply of oxygen, unconsciousness and permanent brain damage can occur quickly if blood sugar remains low.

Insufficient sugar in the blood (hypoglycemia) is associated with the following signs and symptoms.

1. Normal respiration
2. Pale, moist skin
3. Dizziness, headache
4. Full, rapid pulse
5. Normal blood pressure
6. Fainting, seizures, coma

DIAGNOSIS AND TREATMENT

An inexperienced person, even one who knows the patient has diabetes, may have difficulty distinguishing between the signs of diabetic coma and insulin shock. In either case, a patient who has not yet become comatose may feel sick or be semiconscious. This patient can frequently reveal the exact cause of the illness. In taking care of an ill diabetic patient, ask the patient or the family these two questions:

1. Have you eaten today?
2. Have you taken your insulin today?

If the patient has eaten but has not taken insulin, the problem is probably diabetic coma. If the patient has taken insulin but has not eaten, the problem is probably insulin shock. A diabetic patient will usually know what is the matter, so listen carefully.

If the patient is unconscious, try to decide on the basis of the signs and symptoms just discussed whether the problem is diabetic coma or insulin shock. The primary visible difference is in the patient's breathing: deep, sighing respiration in diabetic coma and normal respiration in insulin shock. A diabetic patient who is unconscious and having seizures is more likely to be in insulin shock. Care for these conditions includes these steps.

1. The patient in diabetic coma (too much blood sugar) needs insulin and possibly other medications. Promptly transport this patient to the hospital for proper medical care.
2. The patient in insulin shock (low blood sugar) needs sugar. The administration of any sugar solution may promptly reverse insulin shock.

When undecided, give sugar to any diabetic patient with the symptoms described, even though the final diagnosis may be diabetic coma. This is because untreated insulin shock resulting in unconsciousness can quickly cause brain damage or death. The patient in insulin shock is in a far more critical condition and is far more likely to have brain damage than the patient in diabetic coma. Thus, giving sugar to a patient in insulin shock may save the patient's life or prevent brain damage. The patient in insulin shock will respond to the giving of sugar within 1 to 2 minutes and must be transported to a hospital as soon as possible. Whether hospitalization is required is then the physician's decision.

Give the conscious patient sugar cubes, granulated sugar, candy or any fruit juice (sweetened with additional sugar if available) to reverse an insulin reaction. The unconscious patient must be given intravenous glucose at the emergency department. The trainer is not responsible for starting an intravenous solution, but for promptly transporting the patient so that care may be given in this very urgent situation.

Do not put liquid into the mouth of an unconscious individual, as it may be aspirated into the lungs. The use of "Instant Glucose," a prepared jelly, or a sugar cube under the tongue or in the mouth of the unconscious patient has been recommended. These substances may be used when no other treatment is at hand and transportation will be prolonged. In general, however, this practice is probably not wise. Recent studies indicate that very little sugar so administered is absorbed, and the risk of an unconscious patient aspirating a pellet of sugar probably outweighs the benefits. Prompt transportation to an emergency department is the appropriate step.

The Asthmatic Athlete

44

Asthma is a Greek work describing shortness of breath. The asthmatic patient has difficulty in breathing because his normal airways have narrowed as a result of hypersecretion of mucus, bronchospasm or mucosal edema.

The narrowed airway disrupts conduction of air to the alveoli and ventilation and perfusion are mismatched. This can result in abnormal gas exchange. Narrowing of the airways with bronchospasm increases resistance to airflow and, thus, increases the work of breathing. This pathologic state may be detected during bronchospasm by the forced vital capacity maneuver described in Chapter 25. Flow rates may be reduced at any given lung volume, resulting in a reduced forced expiratory volume (FEV_1), maximum peak expiratory flow (V max) and forced expiratory flow (FEF_{25-75}). Between episodes or after the use of bronchodilators, results of this maneuver may be completely normal.

Clinically, asthma is recognized by dry, squeaky noises called wheezes, both during inspiration and expiration, that can often be heard without a stethoscope. Chest tightness is mainly bothersome during expiration. Expiration is markedly prolonged and inspiration normal. The effort to breathe out is often tiring and frightening. In contrast, with partial obstruction at a higher level in the respiratory tract, such as laryngitis or a throat infection (pharyngitis), breathing is difficult during inspiration. Sudden hyperventilation commonly occurring without obvious cause is also characterized by a feeling of not being able to get a deep enough breath and difficult inspiration but normal expiration. Dry, repetitive coughing usually accompanies wheezing and prolonged expiration. Occasionally, coughing is the only sign of asthma, which poses a more difficult diagnostic problem.

Asthma can be divided into three groups, extrinsic, intrinsic, and a combination of the two. Extrinsic, or allergic, asthma is caused by a known allergen. The patient has a history of hay fever, eczema or dermatitis as well as asthma when exposed to specific allergens such as animal dander, dust, foods and pollen. Intrinsic, or idiopathic, asthma has less clearly defined precipitating factors. Cold, exercise, or emotions may trigger an asthmatic attack. This is therefore a concern to the asthmatic athlete eager to participate in sports.

Previously, it was believed that the type of exercise performed determined the asthmatic episodes. It is now clear that bronchospasm is triggered by cooling of the respiratory mucosa due to increased ventilation during exercise. The temperature and humidity of the inspired air are important in this mechanism because the normal humidification and warming of the air by the release of moisture and heat from the respiratory mucosa cool the surrounding structures. It had long been observed that persons with exercise-induced asthma (EIA) had fewer problems when swimming than running, probably because the air inspired while swimming has a higher moisture content and is less likely to cool the respiratory mucosa. On the other hand, cool, dry air worsens bronchospasm. The intensity of exercise is also important in precipitating asthma attacks, probably because increased alveolar ventilation during vigorous exercise moves more air through the airways, further cooling the mucosa. An ideal sport for patients who suffer from exercise-induced asthma (EIA) is swimming.

Since the EIA response is also related to work intensity and duration of exercise, encourage those affected to participate in activities involving brief periods of intense work rather than those requiring sustained exercise. A pre-exercise warming may help inhibit EIA. Increased aerobic fitness eventually increases tolerance to exercise in asthmatics.

Several medications, such as inhaled metaproterenol sulfate, are highly effective in controlling EIA if used before exercising. Corticosteroids have little effect, but theophylline appears effective. Orally administered and aerosol beta-adrenergic stimulants can also reverse EIA if it occurs. Inhaled cromolyn sodium and beta-adrenergic agonists are preferred agents for blocking or reversing EIA.

While the role of exercise as the triggering medium in EIA is unclear, the reaction is identical to anaphylaxis triggered by an immunologic stimuli. Susceptible persons have a background of atopic or allergic reactions, varying in intensity, duration and frequency, and either isolated or recurrent. The combination of facial edema and syncope is usually diagnostic and should not be confused with the common faint. The mainstay of treatment is epinephrine.

EIA and asthma-induced anaphylaxis are similar in that both cause a brief attack that can be prevented or reversed by sympathomimetic agents such as cromolyn. Hypothermia and hyperthermia should also be included in the differential diagnosis.

The Physically Impaired Athlete

45

The physically impaired person has a multitude of limitations. Despite a desire to participate in sport of any kind, the barriers often seem insurmountable. They are created not only by physical and mental limitations, but also by environmental and social factors.

Physically, limitations may be due to central nervous system (CNS) dysfunction, the absence of a limb, paralysis or paresis, or orthopedic conditions. In most cases balance, equilibrium and coordinated patterns of movement and posture are disturbed.

To date, more and more medical facilities, recreation areas and schools are becoming aware of these special needs and are making facilities and programs available to the handicapped. This trend will undoubtedly continue.

When developing a sporting/recreational program for the physically handicapped, several criteria form an important foundation for a safe and enjoyable program. These include proper assessment of the handicapping condition, realistic goal setting, physical conditioning, special instructor training and, last but not least, the willingness to adapt and improvise to meet the person's special needs.

To provide an overview of the person's physical abilities assess:

1. Range of motion and flexibility of the extremities and trunk
2. Strength
3. Balance and equilibrium skills
4. Postural discrepancies
5. Associated reactions produced by increased activity (of particular importance with CNS involvement)
6. Sensory discrimination and circulation problems
7. Rhythmic and coordination skills
8. Leg length and other discrepancies of bone growth or size
9. Visual and/or auditory accuracy
10. Orthopedic or other special appliances worn

Accurate assessment of these factors is valuable in establishing realistic goals for each individual as well as the exercise or adaptations that may be necessary for specific sporting activities.

The initial assessment should include identification of any areas of concern or contraindications to participation in a particular sport. Areas of concern include:

1. Seizure activity (especially if not totally controlled)
2. Osteoporosis
3. Cardiac and respiratory conditions
4. Unstable orthopedic conditions (such as dislocated hips, instability of major weight bearing joints, scoliosis)
5. Recent trauma and surgery
6. Bleeding diatheses

Adults certainly are capable of understanding the risks involved and can usually make a judgment on the activity for themselves. Children, on the other hand, often do not realize the full implications of their conditions and proper guidance from medical personnel is valuable and necessary. Children also present another special problem. The handicaps of many conditions, although stable in an adult, can be greatly affected during the child's growth and development. Because of this, periodic reassessment is necessary during participation.

It is important to establish realistic goals, keeping in mind that the goal must be attainable within a reasonable length of time. The primary goal should be easily obtained with minimal dependence on physical equipment, geographic location and involvement of others. Higher goals can always be established. Sporting activities should be fun and enjoyable! If goals cannot be reached, the physical limitations can become an unnecessary emotional handicap. The overall goal should be to find a lifetime activity that can be easily pursued.

Proper conditioning is essential for athletes, and the handicapped are no exception. Good strength and flexibility help to reduce the possibility of injury. Cardiovascular endurance is another concern. Using assessment data, the proper conditioning program can easily be established. Balance and coordination activities should also be considered as an integral part of the exercise program for the handicapped.

An instructor working with the handicapped often requires special training. He has great responsibility for safety and without knowledge of the handicapping condition and its implications, intervention could be detrimental. With the proper guidelines, he can provide a tremendously positive experience for the handicapped.

With all these factors in mind, the creativity of the instructor is often the key to success. The ability to adapt special equipment for an individual (either as an aid or for safety) and the ability to improvise are essential.

The social and psychological difficulties are overwhelming for the physically handicapped dealing with themselves as individuals, part of a family unit and an integral part of society. Sports and recreation can be important to a healthy adjustment.

Injury prevention is of the utmost importance for the physically impaired athlete, as it is for the able-bodied athlete. Specific physical problems of each disabled athlete must be taken into consideration when using various modalities to prevent injury. For example,

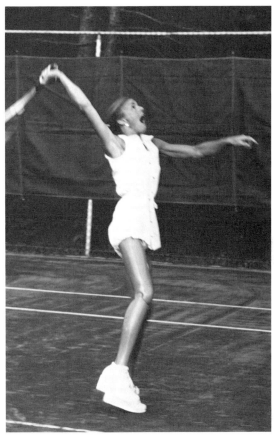

FIGURE 45:1. Athletes with prosthetic legs should be carefully watched for signs of redness on stumps.

when the amputee athlete participates in a contact sport without his prosthesis, the stump must be padded and protected. One most important aspect is physical conditioning prior to participating in a demanding sport such as alpine skiing or soccer. Strengthening the major muscle groups in conjunction with coordination should be emphasized, to the extent the physical disability allows.

In winter sports such as skiing, body temperature, a constant problem of the amputee athlete, must be maintained. Padding for warmth also assists in protecting the stump in falls. Upper extremity amputees who ski without their prostheses should also wear wool socks on the stumps to prevent frostbite. Padding either the leg or the upper extremity with

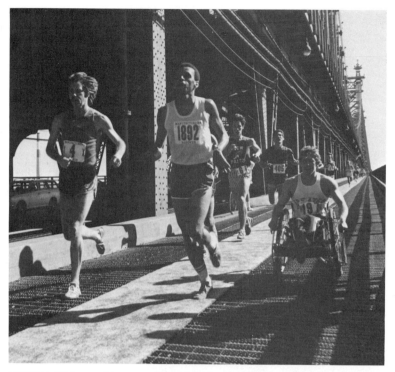

FIGURE 45:2. Athletes participating in wheel chair sports have special problems such as pressure sores below the level of protective sensation.

leather or any firm padding is not necessary since this is more cumbersome and frequently adds to the possibilities of injury.

Amputees involved in running sports need special care of their prosthetic legs as well as their stumps. They should be watched close-ly for any pressure sores or poor fitting prostheses, which contribute to problems such as blisters or eventual breakdown of their stumps. At the first sign of any redness of a lower extremity stump, direct the athlete to stop participation and seek medical attention (Fig. 45:1).

The trainer as well as the director of a sports program should have proper instruction before involving disabled athletes in any type of demanding sport. Instructors should be well qualified and specially trained to understand the problems of the disabled athlete, as well as to apply nonhandicapped modalities. Wrapping of ankles and strapping is as important for preventing injuries in the physically impaired athlete as it is in the able-bodied athlete.

Wheel chair sports have special problem areas (Fig. 45:2). In paraplegics pay special attention to preventing pressure sores below the level of protective sensation. The trainer or medical personnel should adequately evaluate the athlete prior to participation in the sport to note pressure areas over the greater trochanter or sacrum. These should be adequately padded with sponge or felt when the athlete participates in speed sports or basketball. Paraplegics have problems with heat loss in endurance events, racing and prolonged activity. The problems of one extremity conditioning are more complex than with the average athlete.

Communicable Diseases

Infection is the disease state produced in a host by the invasion of an infecting organism—virus, bacterium or parasite. Contamination is the presence of an infectious agent on body surfaces, in water or food, or on objects such as wound dressings. All surfaces, unless sterilized, should be considered contaminated. A host is the organism or person in whom an infectious agent resides. A host is infected. A carrier is a person or animal who may transmit an infectious disease while having no clinical evidence of the disease.

A reservoir is the place where the infecting organisms live and multiply. The source of infection is the thing, person or substance from which an infectious agent passes to a host. Sometimes the reservoir is also the source of the infection. The communicable period is the time during which an infectious agent may be transferred from one host to another. The incubation period is the time between infection of the host and the first appearance of signs of the disease.

A communicable disease is a contagious disease, that is, a disease that can be transmitted from one person to another person. This transmission can occur in one of three ways.

1. Directly by contact with an infected person, by ingestion of infected food or by infection of an open skin wound by an airborne organism or by contact with the contaminated person or object.
2. Indirectly by contact with contaminated objects, such as soiled dressings or clothing from an infected person. Indirect contact implies that the person being infected was not directly in contact with the host or carrier but touched some object that was contaminated.
3. Inhaling the droplets spread from an infected person who coughs or sneezes. Inhaling dust contaminated with infecting agents is also a common mode of spread.

Depending on the disease, trainers can take simple precautions to protect themselves and other personnel from contamination. Risks do exist in handling athletes with communicable disease, but proper care can minimize them. Table 46:1 reviews the types of infectious diseases and their characteristics, source, transmission, incubation, communicability and precautions.

46

TABLE 46:1. Infectious Diseases

Disease	Characteristics	Source	Mode of Transmission	Incuba-tion Period	Period of Communi-cability	Care of Personnel
AIDS*	Unexplained weight loss; fever of unknown origin; night sweats over several weeks; dry, hacking cough not associated with upper respiratory infection; persistent, unexplained diarrhea; enlarged lymph nodes in the neck, armpits and groin; small painless, purple papules or nodules on the skin or mucous membranes that gradually enlarge	Unknown	Unknown. Public Health Service recommends avoiding sexual contact with persons known or suspected of having AIDS; members of groups at increased risk for AIDS should refrain from donating plasma and blood	Unknown	Unknown	Wash hands. Use pre-cautions when disposing of needles or instruments used for AIDS patients.
Chickenpox	Acute febrile viral disease; itchy red rash that leaves scabs; more common in children	Respiratory tract secretions (scabs do not carry infection)	Direct contact; droplet contact	2–3 weeks	1 day before skin lesions appear to 6 days after skin lesions appear	Wash hands; shower; change clothing
Diphtheria	Acute bacterial infec-tion of throat, tonsils, nose and sometimes skin with local pain and swelling	Discharge from nose and throat	Direct or indirect contact	2–5 days	2–4 weeks	Immunization; wear mask if not immune
German measles (rubella)	Feverish viral illness with rash; more common in children; danger of birth defects if contracted during first 3 months of pregnancy	Discharge from nose and throat	Direct contact; indirect contact; droplet contact	14–21 days	1 week before rash appears to 4 days after rash appears	None
Gonorrhea	Bacterial venereal dis-ease characterized by thick yellow urethral discharge in males; more difficult to detect in females and may lead to chronic infec-tion	Exudate from mucous membrane	Sexual intercourse	3–4 days	Months or years unless treated	None

*Individuals at risk with suggestive symptoms should seek immediate medical evaluation. The Center for Disease Control has an AIDS task force (404) 329-3410. National Gay Task Force has current updates on AIDS (800) 221-7044 and (212) 807-6016.

TABLE 46:1.   Infectious Diseases (continued)

Disease	Characteristics	Source	Mode of Transmission	Incuba-tion Period	Period of communi-cability	Care of Personnel
Herpes I[†]	Vesiculo-ulcerative lesions of the mucous membrane of the oral cavity; irritability and local lymphadenopathy	Viral	Direct contact (saliva, stools); indirectly from utensils con-taminated with saliva of a virus carrier	3–5 days	Usually self-limiting, 1–2 weeks	Wash hands
Herpes II[‡]	Multiple vesicles surrounded by diffuse inflammation and edema; intense itching and burning along vulva, vagina and cervix or penis (often pre-ceding vesicles and associated with hemo-philus vaginitis or trichomonas vaginitis); fever, malaise and in-guinal lymphaden-opathy; with cervical or vaginal involvement, may be asymptomatic	Viral	Sexual inter-course	3–5 days; occasion-ally less than 24 hours	Recurrent, with or without sys-temic reactions, probably due to reactivation of latent viral infection	Wash hands
Herpes Zoster[§]	Inflammation of posterior nerve roots and ganglia, with crops and vesicles over skin supplied by affected sensory nerves; fever and malaise soon fol-lowed by severe pain in skin or mucosa along affected nerve route	Viral	Response of partially immune host to reactiva-tion of latent varicella virus	Unknown	To those previ-ously unexposed to varicella	Wash hands
Infectious hepatitis	Acute viral infection with fever; loss of ap-petite; jaundice; fatigue	Feces, urine, blood from infected per-son; dishes, clothing, or bed linen used by infected person; injuries from needles used by or for infected person	Fecal-oral con-tamination through handling clothes and linen; con-taminated water, food, syringes; transfusion from infected person	15–30 days	Unknown	Wash hands, use pre-cautions when dispos-ing of needles or instruments used for these patients

[†]Treatment is symptomatic. Protect patient from sources of infection at the lesion site.
[‡]Diagnosis easily made from cultures of suspected lesions. Serologic tests are also available. Symptomatic treatment with topical acyclovir ointment in initial management; topical anesthetic agents as well as drying, antipruritic agents.
[§]With severe symptoms, massive IV doses of Cytarabine inhibits further dissemination of lesions. Other IV drugs have had varying success. Topical anes-thetic and drying antipruritic agents are helpful in mild cases. Protect patient from irritation and infection.

TABLE 46:1.   Infectious Diseases (continued)

Disease	Characteristics	Source	Mode of Transmission	Incubation Period	Period of Communicability	Care of Personnel
Measles	Acute viral disease; fever; bronchitis; red blotchy rash; common in childhood	Nose and throat secretions	Direct contact; indirect contact; droplet contact	10 days	4 days before rash appears to 5 days after	None
Meningitis	Acute bacterial disease with fever; severe headache; nausea; vomiting; coma	Nose and throat secretions	Direct contact; droplet contact	2–10 days	Varies	If close contact has occurred, see physician
Mono-nucleosis	Acute viral disease with fever; sore throat, lymph node swelling	Respiratory tract secretions	Unknown; possibly person-to-person oral route	2–6 weeks	Unknown	None
Mumps	Acute viral disease with fever; swelling and tenderness of the salivary glands	Saliva of infected person	Direct contact; indirect contact; droplet contact	12–26 days	7 days before swelling appears to 9 days after	None
Pneumonia	Acute viral or bacterial disease; fever; chills; cough; chest pain	Respiratory tract secretions	Direct contact; indirect contact; droplet contact	Varies	Varies	None
Poliomyelitis	Acute viral disease with fever; headache; gastro-intestinal symptoms; stiff neck; paralysis	Nose and throat secretions; feces	Direct contact	7–12 days	6 weeks	None
Rocky Mountain spotted fever	Acute bacterial disease with fever; headache; rash over the body including palms and soles	Infected tick; reservoirs are rodents and dogs	Tick bite	3–10 days	Tick's life span	Remove ticks without crushing, protecting hands with gloves if possible

TABLE 46:1.   Infectious Diseases (continued)

Disease	Characteristics	Source	Mode of Transmission	Incubation Period	Period of Communicability	Care of Personnel
Smallpox	Acute viral disease with fever; headache; abdominal pain; rash with scabbing and eruptions	Respiratory discharge; scabs	Direct contact; indirect contact; droplet contact	7–16 days	From first symptoms to disappearance of symptoms	Revaccination
Scarlet fever	Acute bacterial disease with headache; fever, nausea; vomiting; sore throat	Respiratory discharge	Direct contact; indirect contact; droplet contact; carriers exist	2–5 days	Unknown	Wear mask; change; shower; boil clothes
Syphilis	Acute bacterial venereal disease; primary lesion seen at 3 weeks as a hard sore that erodes; secondary skin eruptions appear during next 4–6 weeks; late disabling complications of heart and brain	Saliva; semen; blood; vaginal discharge during the infectious period	Direct contact through mucosal surface or open wounds; sexual intercourse	10 days– 10 weeks	Variable	If scratched or bitten, contact physician
Tuberculosis	Chronic bacterial disease; cough; fatigue; weight loss; chest pain; coughing up of blood	Respiratory secretions; occasionally milk	Direct contact; indirect contact; droplet contact; carriers exist	4–6 weeks	As long as live tubercle bacilli are excreted	Wear mask; chest x-ray yearly; skin test periodically
Typhoid fever	Fever; loss of appetite; diarrhea	Feces and urine	Direct contact; indirect contact; raw fruits; vegetables; milk; carriers exist	2 weeks	As long as typhoid bacilli are excreted	Wash hands
Whooping cough	Acute bacterial disease with violent attacks of coughing; a high-pitched whooping; common among children	Respiratory discharge	Direct contact; indirect contact; droplet contact	7 days–3 weeks	7 days–3 weeks	Change; shower; boil clothes

Common Dermatological Problems

47

Common dermatological problems are related to the athlete's skin type as well as to environmental influences such as heat, humidity, gear and sporting activity. Therapeutic problems include acne vulgaris, fungal infections, viral infections, bacterial infections, miliaria, contact dermatitis and infestations.

ACNE VULGARIS

Acne vulgaris is most commonly a hereditary disorder of the oil glands and hair follicles that is influenced by the bacterial flora in these structures (Figs. 47:1, 2). Clinically, the disease presents as multiple blackheads, inflammatory papules, pustules or cysts. Acne lesions appear on the face, chest, shoulders, back, arms and, in severe cases, on the lower extremities. Seborrheic dermatitis (dandruff) is frequently associated with acne vulgaris and can be seen on the face as well as the scalp. Acne flares during athletic seasonal activities, probably due to increased heat, perspiration and, ultimately, oil production.

The treatment of acne consists of topical drying agents and topical antimicrobial agents as well as oral antibiotics. The common topical drying and antimicrobial agent used is benzoyl peroxide, which comes in 5% to 10% dilution. This agent reduces the number of bacteria responsible for the acneiform lesions. This is helpful since the bacteria produce an enzyme that breaks down into a highly irritating fatty acid, oil, that inflames the skin.

Benzoyl peroxide increases tissue oxygenation as well as healing. Drying or oil-removing agents such as astringent lotions and soap and water can aid healing. Mechanical and surgical removal of blackheads, while useful, must be done by a dermatologist or a trained nurse. Topical abrasive pads can be used for blackhead acne, but with the more inflammatory acnes it can exaggerate or worsen the condition. Antibiotic therapy, both topical and oral, is highly effective in treating all forms of acne. The basic antibiotic used is tetracycline, in doses between 250 and 1,000 mg daily for control of bacteria, oil production and inflammation. The worse the acne, the higher the dose of tetracycline. The newer topical tetracycline and erythromycin lotions seem effective when applied once or twice a day to areas of skin involvement and appear to equal approximately 500 mg of oral tetracycline. Topical antibiotics can be used when oral antibiotics are contraindicated or a patient is at high risk, such as a preadolescent athlete or a pregnant woman. In the preadolescent, oral tetracycline may cause pigmentation of the permanent teeth. For this reason, oral tetracyclines are avoided in this age group.

Another therapeutic modality for blackhead acne includes topical vitamin A acid, which can be obtained in various concentrations and in cream, lotion, gel or alcohol vehicles. Applying this treatment daily for at least six weeks reduces keratinization of the hair follicle, thereby reducing blackhead formation.

Low dose systemic corticosteroids, estrogens and tranquilizers, as prescribed by a physician, are adjunctive therapies used in severe resistant acne and cystic acne.

FUNGUS INFECTIONS

Ringworm

Ringworm infections are caused by a variety of different fungi—essentially microscopic plants that grow on humans. On examination, this skin disease may resemble a well-defined, slightly reddened patch(es) with some fine scaling at its periphery. Occasionally, if the patient is allergic to the fungus, blisters may be observed. When the fungal infection involves the feet, the sole of the foot may look like dry skin or may again have some redness, swelling and even blisters. Microscopic examination of the scale or the blister top reveals vegetating parts of the fungus. Bacterial and fungal cultures and Wood's light examination are diagnostic.

Ringworm infections are treated with antifungal agents such as Tinactin cream or solution, Micatin 2%, Lotrimin cream 2%, Lotrimin cream or solution, and Mycelex cream. Apply antifungal therapies twice a day for at least two to four weeks. In addition, keep the areas dry and clean. If large areas of the skin are affected or the fungus infection is blistered, oral antifungal agents are often used to reduce the infection. Treatment consists of Fulvicin, 500 mg to 1 gm a day for at least one month. Inflammatory conditions of the groin may be due to fungus, bacterial infection, contact allergy or irritant reactions. Since all of these conditions may resemble each other, if a condition fails to respond to the antifungal treatment, dermatologic consult is indicated.

Tinea Versicolor

Tinea versicolor is a ringworm infection of the skin caused by Pityrosporon orbicular, a yeast fungus (Fig. 47:6). This yeast infection is found in the keratin of the horny layer of the skin as well as in the horny layers of the hair follicle. It may appear as a salmon-pink, finely scaling patch that fails to pigment when exposed to the sun, leaving a white patch. This cutaneous fungus infection is noncontagious, but is highly visible because of its brown or white patches, usually on the trunk. Tinea versicolor is treated with antidandruff shampoo at least once a week for two weeks, repeated as necessary.

VIRAL INFECTIONS

Herpes

The most common viral infection is a herpes infection or cold sore. These infections can occur in the mouth, lips, face, trunk or the genital area. The disorder is highly contagious. It presents as a blister on a reddened base and is associated with pain locally. Frequently groups of blisters on a reddened base ulcerate and become infected with bacterial organisms. Herpes simplex can be diagnosed on inspection, but microscopic examination of the blister base confirms the diagnosis. The disorder is treated by destruction of the blisters by mechanical excoriation or the use of topical drying agents, including some of the acne medications such as the benzoyl peroxide agents. Anti-inflammatory agents with hydrocortisone may be used and appear to reduce the skin inflammation and increase comfort. The usual duration of the herpes infection is two weeks. Treatment is directed at reducing the skin pain and discomfort and decreasing the healing time. There is no specific effective antiviral therapy. During active blistering and ulceration, this disease is highly contagious and should be considered a disqualifying contagious disorder in contact sports.

Molluscum Contagiosum

Molluscum contagiosum is another viral disorder characterized by flesh-colored pink papules with a central dimpling (Fig. 47:10). The skin surrounding these papules is not inflamed. Papules may occur anywhere on the body but especially on the trunk, axilla, face, perineum and thigh, appearing singly or in multiple groups. This disorder is also contagious and is frequently passed from one athlete to another in frictional contact sports such as wrestling. Careful examination of the skin lesions by an experienced physician confirms the diagnosis. A physician should treat this disorder using destructive agents such as cryotherapy, electrodessication and a variety of topically applied acids, such as trichloroacetic acid.

Warts

Warts, also a viral infection of the skin, are caused by a papillomavirus, found within the skin of the body as well as mucous membranes (Fig. 47:11). Normal incubation time for a wart virus from contact to the formation of a lesion is approximately six months. The lesions are discrete, raised, flesh-colored to pink papules with a rough surface. On the feet they tend to grow inward, causing pain similar to a corn on walking. The treatment of warts, especially on pressure points during the athletic season, should be only palliative with paring of the keratotic lesion for comfort. The use of 40% salicyclic acid plasters applied daily reduces the raised keratotic lesion. If the lesion does not disappear, it can be treated later with 40% salicyclic acid pads with a locally destructive procedure such as cryotherapy and electrodessication. Surgical excision and superficial x-ray are contraindicated as treatment. Warts on pressure points and on areas of movement should not be treated during the athletic season, since treatment produces inflammation and a wound that heals slowly.

BACTERIAL INFECTIONS

Impetigo

Impetigo is one of the most common contagious disorders in the athlete. It is caused by two organisms: streptococcus and staphylococcus. In the younger child or adolescent, impetigo frequently presents as a blister, but in older individuals the characteristic appearance is a superficial ulcer with a yellow crust, similar to that seen in older herpes lesions. Visual inspection and bacterial culture can identify this disorder. Treatment consists of local cleansing with soap and water, or astringents or alcohol solutions. Topical antimicrobial agents can be used, but oral antibiotics are preferred. The preferred antibiotic is erythromycin, 250 mg four times a day for two weeks.

Staphylococcal folliculitis, a form of impetigo, is also a common infection in bearded men, especially black men. The curly facial or scalp hair reenters the skin, causing a small, inflammatory lesion that ultimately becomes a pustule. This condition can be treated with astringent lotions or drying agents such as those used in acne vulgaris. Broad spectrum antibiotics given for seven to ten days are helpful in controlling the folliculitis. An abrasive facial pad may prevent reentry of the facial or scalp hair.

Other Bacterial Infections

A furuncle, caused predominantly by a staphylococcal organism, is a tender inflammation around the hair follicle that becomes a fluctuant mass. It is treated by topical application of warm to hot packs and topical benzoyl peroxide in 10% dilution. Other therapy includes oral penicillin antibiotics for 7 to 14 days. Incision and drainage are usually not necessary if treatment is initiated early. An athlete with an active abscess or furuncle should be disqualified from participation until the lesion has cleared because the condition is highly contagious.

Other superficial bacterial infections or fungal infections may develop in skin abrasions, such as seen in mat burns, Astroturf burns and cinder burns. Treatment is routine first aid, cleansing with soap and water, topical drying agents or topical antibiotic ointments. Systemic antibiotic medication is rarely indicated.

CONTACT ALLERGY AND IRRITANT DERMATITIS

Substances to which an athlete is allergic or those that irritate the skin can cause inflammatory skin disorders (Fig. 47:13). Contact irritant dermatitis is a nonallergic reaction of the

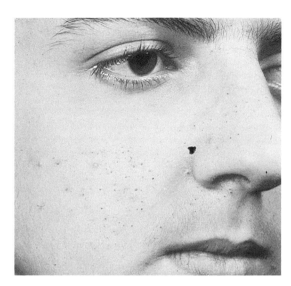

FIGURE 47:1. Acne vulgaris on the cheek and nose. This is a comedone type, presenting as multiple blackheads and papules.

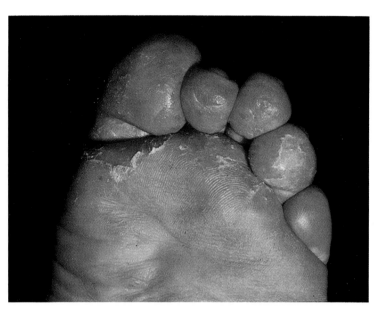

FIGURE 47:3. Tinea pedis, a fungus disease of the foot commonly known as athlete's foot

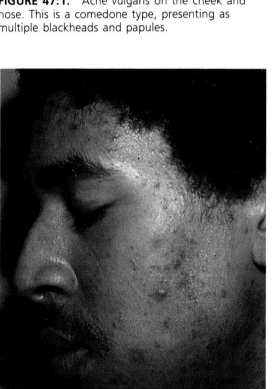

FIGURE 47:2. Severe acne vulgaris of the face and neck with multiple blackheads, inflammatory papules, pustules and cysts

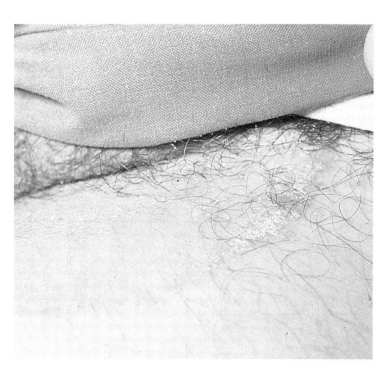

FIGURE 47:4. Tinea cruris, a fungus disease of surfaces of contact in the scrotal, crural and genital areas

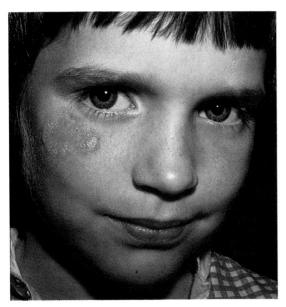

FIGURE 47:5. Tinea faciale, a fungal infection of the face

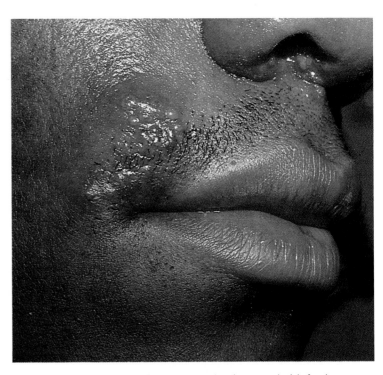

FIGURE 47:7. Post-wrestling Herpes simplex I, a viral infection perpetuated and spread by contact with the wrestling mat

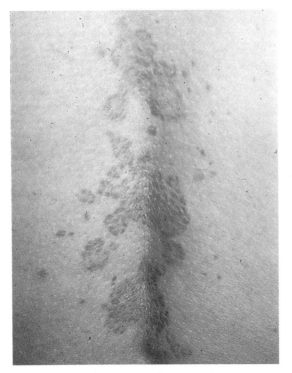

FIGURE 47:6. Tinea versicolor appearing as salmon-pink, finely scaling patches on this athlete's back

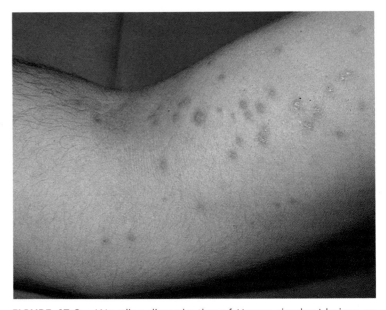

FIGURE 47:8. Wrestling dissemination of Herpes simplex I lesions on the antecubital region is frequently seen.

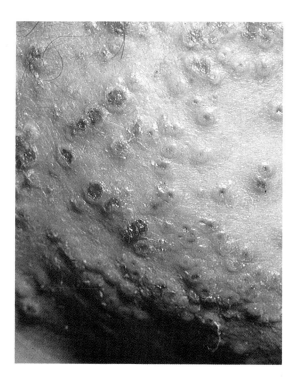

FIGURE 47:9. Wrestling dissemination of Herpes simplex I lesions on the face

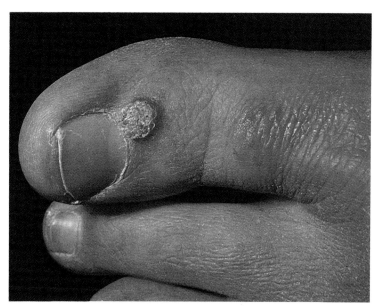

FIGURE 47:11. The wart seen on the anteromedial aspect of this great toe is erythematous at its base, secondary to irritation from this patient's shoe.

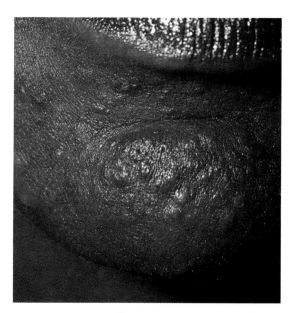

FIGURE 47:10. Molluscum contagiosum on this patient's chin shows the central dimpling of the flesh-colored papules characteristic of this disorder.

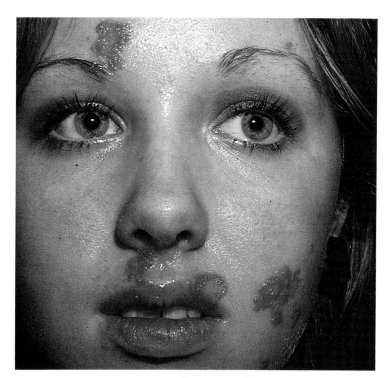

FIGURE 47:12. Impetigo, an inflammatory skin infection marked by isolated pustules occurring principally around the mouth and nose. These often become crusted and rupture.

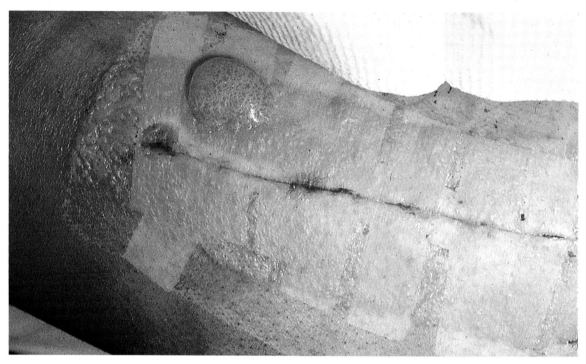

FIGURE 47:13. Contact dermatitis in a patient found to be sensitive to Benzoin used in combination with Steri-strips for skin closure

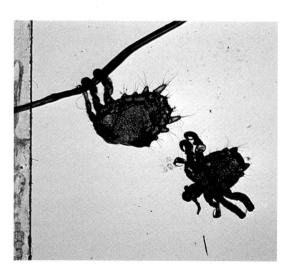

FIGURE 47:14. Pediculosis pubae, commonly known as crab lice, seen under the dissecting microscope

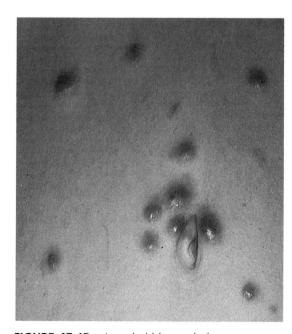

FIGURE 47:15. Lymphoid hyperplasia

skin to exposure to irritating or caustic substances or to a physical agent that damages the skin, producing pain and ulceration. Contact allergy is an allergic response of the skin, producing inflammation in those who have an allergy to an external agent.

In athletes irritant skin reactions are usually secondary to physical and mechanical agents such as:

1. Dry ice burns
2. Abrasions from Astroturf
3. Poorly fitting gear including football helmets
4. Callus formation in gymnasts and bicyclists
5. Striae in weight lifters
6. Increased sweating in hockey players
7. Loss of skin secondary to the application of caustic agents such as adhesive tape and direct contact injuries

The contact allergy skin reactions appear to be due to given contactants, for example:

1. Rhus (poison ivy, oak and sumac)
2. Paraphenylenediamine (blue and black dyes)
3. Nickel compounds (jewelry, metal protective gear)
4. Rubber compounds and chromates (tanned leather and metal parts)

The use of topical medications, however, is limited in treatment of skin disorders because of their increased allergy-inducing capabilities. These topical medications include benzocaine, topical antihistamine preparations, ammoniated mercury, neomycin, penicillin and sulfonamides. In the athlete, tincture of benzoin and paraminobenzoic acid are potent skin sensitizers. Allergic skin dermatitis may present as an acute, blistering rash on a red, swollen base or as chronically dry, thickened skin. Itching or pain is common to all contact skin rashes whether due to irritant or allergic agents.

Contact dermatitis of both irritant and allergic origin is best dealt with by avoiding the contactant responsible for the skin reaction. In addition, it is helpful to recognize early potential contact irritants or allergy.

Treat the acute skin reaction with cool compresses or soaks and topical corticosteroid preparations in vehicles that promote drying, such as aerosol sprays, gels, lotions, solutions or creams. Systemic antihistamines reduce itching but have an undesirable sedative effect. Aspirin is effective in reducing itching and pain and may be given in doses of 300 to 600 mg every four hours while the athlete is symptomatic. Short courses of corticosteroids, prednisone, 30 mg a day for 7 to 14 days with rapid reduction, is helpful but should be prescribed by a physician. Disqualification from participation totally depends on the degree of skin involvement, the site of involvement, the severity of the symptoms and the specific sport.

The chronic form of contact dermatitis can also be managed by avoiding the contactant or establishing a barrier. For example, contact dermatitis secondary to rubber materials in foot gear can be treated by applying topical corticosteroid cream to the foot and then powdering it with talcum powder and wearing a heavy white sock. Then change the sock frequently during the day, because a damp sock allows the rubber material to leach from the shoe onto the foot.

Topical corticosteroids are helpful in treating chronic contact dermatitis. Corticosteroids should be in cream or ointment so that the cortisone not only reduces the inflammation but the cream or ointment lubricates the skin. Secondary bacterial infections should be treated with parenteral antibiotics and skin cleansing techniques.

INFESTATIONS

The most common infestations observed in athletes are crab lice and scabies.

Pediculosis Pubis (Crab Louse)

Pediculosis pubis is contracted through intimate contact with affected individuals. For athletes, direct contact in the sporting event

TABLE 47:1.   Treatment Summaries for Dermatological Conditions

Condition	Treatments
Acne vulgaris	Astringent lotion, liquid cleansing agents; benzoyl peroxide 5% or 10% once or twice a day; topical vitamin A acid every other day (at night); tetracycline, 500 mg a day for six weeks gradually reduced to maintenance dose of 250 mg a day; topical antibiotics twice a day
Ringworm	Soap and water cleansing twice a day; topical antifungal agents twice a day for one month (Tinactin powder, solution, cream, Micatin cream, Lotrimin cream, solution, Mycelex cream); griseofulvin, oral fungistatic and fungicidal antibiotic, 1 gm daily for three to four weeks
Tinea versicolor	Soap and water cleansing; six to eight hour application of antidandruff shampoo, repeat weekly as necessary, or Tinver solution applied daily for three to four weeks, or other antifungal agents (Lotrimin, Micatin, Mycelex cream or solution) twice a day for one month
Herpes	Soap and water cleansing; topical drying agents three times a day (benzoyl peroxide 5% or 10%, tincture of benzoin, Camphophenique, Blistex); oral salicylates, aspirin, every three to four hours for pain
Warts and molluscum contagiosum	Salicyclic acid plaster 40% applied daily for four months; topical caustic agents (25% podophyllin in compound tincture of benzoin, applied weekly, Duofilm applied daily for two to four months); physician therapy (cryotherapy, electrodessication or topical compounded acids)
Impetigo	Cleansing of skin; topical antibiotics; oral erythromycin 250 mg four times a day for 14 days
Contact dermatitis	Avoidance of cause; acute: wet dressings twice or three times a day, topical corticosteroids, lotions, gel or cream; chronic: topical corticosteroid cream or ointment, aspirin 300–600 mg every four hours for itching
Infestations	Wash skin and clothing (set aside clothing for 7 to 14 days); gamma benzene hexachloride (Kwell) lotion or cream for 6 to 24 hour application, repeat as necessary; other therapies with lesser cure rates: Eurax cream twice a day for 48 hours, 6% precipitated sulfur in Vaseline, twice a day for three days

as well as in the dressing rooms through showers, towels and clothing may allow passage from one individual to another. Crab louse is observed in the genital area, trunk and, occasionally, the underarms and eyelashes. The lice cause extreme itching of the involved sites and, on occasion, red spots. Diagnosis is made by visually identifying the louse or its eggs. The eggs, attached to the hair shafts, appear as clear, translucent, small masses. Treatment consists of gamma benzene hexachloride (Kwell) lotion or shampoo applied after bathing to the affected areas for 6 to 24 hours. Repeat this treatment in one week if viable lice are still identified. Occasionally the hairy areas must be shaved or combed to remove the eggs. Use a fine tooth comb after rinsing it with white vinegar in a dilution of 1:4. The clothing of an affected individual should be washed, disinfected and hung away for seven days. All suspected contacts should be examined and treated. On occasion, this may include a whole team.

Scabies

Scabies is caused by a mite, Sarcoptes scabiei. This mite infestation is characterized by itching and elevated burrows on the skin surface. Commonly observed on the hands, in the athlete they are equally common on the trunk and genital area. The female mite makes these burrows in which she lays her eggs. Long-standing infestation may present as an acute dermatitis with severe itching. Diagnosis is made by scraping the burrow, examining the scraping under a microscope and then visualizing the mite.

The treatment of choice is the application of gamma benzene hexachloride, lotion or shampoo to the whole body for 6 to 24 hours. Repeat the treatment if viable mites are seen at a later date. Clothing and bed linen should be changed, washed and put aside for 14 days. Treat team members and other contacts prophylactically. Gamma benzene hexachloride is a known neurotoxin and should not be misused or overused.

Table 47:1 summarizes allergy and contact dermatitis conditions discussed in this chapter and their treatments.

Nutrition

48

Many factors affect nutrient needs and nutrient availability, including the athlete's physical condition, nutritional status, age and genetic background. In addition, the presence and concentration of other substances as well as the chemical form of the nutrient itself and the environment play a role. Finally, the body has a remarkable ability to adapt to changing conditions in order to survive.

This adaptability and the many influences on nutritional needs and physical performance combine to make it difficult to measure whether a change in dietary intake actually causes a change in performance. This lack of knowledge, coupled with the desire for a magic formula that guarantees success, leads to a great many nutritional myths and fads among athletes.

Diets do not create strong bodies or increase speed. Strength, power and endurance come only through training. The diet merely provides the necessary raw material that allows the training to build and run the human machine.

Diets must be individualized. Athletes come from many different backgrounds with widely varying beliefs regarding diet. The age, size, physical condition and metabolic rate of each player must be considered. The adolescent athlete has increased needs to support growth, while the mature athlete may remain on a constant plane or be recovering from an injury.

The scientific rationale for good nutritional practices as well as practical information on the nutritional concerns of athletes are discussed here. Registered dietitians in private practice or hospitals are also good resources for information on diet.

CALORIC BALANCE AND WEIGHT CONTROL

The focus of weight control in the athlete should be on body composition rather than on weight. An assessment of body fat percentage is far more useful than a simple scale weight measurement. The percentage of body fat and its complement of lean body weight should be assessed at regular intervals throughout the season so that corrective measures, such as changes in training and diet, may be initiated if necessary.

The body fat percentage recommended for the average man is 15% and for the woman 26%. Body fat stores of most athletes are below these averages because extra pounds of fat create more work for the body without increasing its efficiency. Male gymnasts and runners have reported body fats as low as 5% to 8%, while women involved in the same sports have reported body fats of 10% to 12%. Table 48:1 lists levels of body fat observed in athletes in various sports.

In general, the percent body fat for male athletes should be 8% to 10% and 12% to 14% for females. The optimal body fat percentage may vary according to the sport and the athlete. Many athletes perform very well at higher body fats. The goal is improved athletic performance, not a specific percentage of body fat. Women should not drop below 10% because of the possibility of cessation of menses.

The amount of body fat can be calculated either by a skinfold method or by underwater weighing. Underwater weighing, which requires calculating lung volume, is probably the most accurate, but it is not generally available. Skinfold calipers are less expensive and easily obtained. Skinfold thickness changes are a fairly sensitive indication of changes in total body fat. The method is reasonably accurate as long as the same person takes the measurements.

Caloric Requirements

Weight maintenance is accomplished by balancing caloric intake with caloric output. Calories are provided by carbohydrates, fats, protein and alcohol. The number of calories in a given food reflects its energy potential. Protein and carbohydrate are equal in calories. One gram of either yields 4 calories. One gram of fat equals 9 calories, over twice that of protein or carbohydrate. Alcohol falls in the middle, with 1 gram yielding 7 calories.

The number of calories the athlete needs (caloric output) depends upon the age, body weight, body composition, gender, basal metabolic rate and physical activity levels. The calorie per kilogram of body weight is highest in children because of the growth and development of tissues. As individuals age, the caloric need decreases.

Body weight affects total caloric requirements because it takes more calories to maintain a higher weight. Percent of body fat is also important because it takes more calories to maintain muscle tissue than to maintain fat. Therefore, even if two athletes weigh the same, the one with the lower percent body fat will have the higher caloric needs. Since men have less fat than women, men's caloric needs are greater.

Individual variations in basal metabolic rate, which range from 10% to 20%, can either increase or decrease caloric needs. Physical activity can cost an additional 1,000 to 1,500 calories. Caloric output through exercise is determined by the duration and intensity of the activity and the weight of the athlete.

All of these factors make it difficult to assess actual caloric needs from formulas and tables. The best way to determine caloric needs is, during a time of weight maintenance, to have the athlete keep track of food intake for three

TABLE 48:1. Body Composition Values for Male and Female Athletes

Sport or Position	Sex	Relative Fat %
Baseball	m	11.8–14.2
Basketball	f	20.8–26.9
	m	7.1–10.6
Football	m	
Defensive backs	m	9.6–11.5
Offensive backs	m	9.4–12.4
Linebackers	m	13.4–14.0
Offensive linemen	m	15.6–19.1
Defensive linemen	m	18.2–18.5
Quarterbacks, kickers	m	14.4
Gymnastics	m	4.6
	f	9.6–17.0
Ice hockey	m	13.0–15.1
Jockeys	m	14.1
Rowing	m	8.5–11
	f	14.0
Skiing		
Alpine	m	7.4–10.2
	f	20.6
Cross-country	m	7.9–12.5
	f	15.7–21.8
Soccer	m	9.6
Speed skating	m	11.4
Swimming	m	5.0–8.5
	f	17.1–26.3
Tennis	m	15.2–16.3
	f	20.3
Track and field	m	8.8
Distance running	m	6.3–13.6
	f	15.2–19.2
Discus	m	16.3
	f	25.0
Weight lifting	m	9.8–12.2
Power	m	15.6
Body building	m	8.3
Wrestling	m	4.0–10.7

Wilmore, J.H. "Body composition and athletic performance." In Haskell, W.; Skala, J.; Whittam, J., eds., *Nutrition and Athletic Performance.* Palo Alto, California, Bull Publishing Co., 1981.

days and then calculate the number of calories consumed. Many "calorie books" are available. Computer programs now make this calculation fairly easy. Table 48:2 lists average food intakes of university athletes.

TABLE 48:2. Caloric Intakes of University Athletes

Sport	Average	Minimum	Maximum
Men			
Basketball	4,762	1,600	9,270
Crew (no coxswain)	5,267	2,711	7,162
Football	5,557	2,516	13,517
Gymnastics	2,080	568	4,249
Lacrosse	3,926	2,467	8,147
Mountain climbing	3,829	2,441	5,959
Soccer	2,965	2,177	3,705
Wrestling	2,665	412	6,702
Women			
Basketball	2,835	500	3,879
Crew	2,339	1,262	3,577
Dancing	1,909	898	2,909
Lacrosse	2,219	1,438	3,059
Swimming	2,874	1,516	5,874
Volleyball	2,094	1,144	3,199

Adapted from Short, S., Short, W. R. "Four year study of university athletes' dietary intake." *Journal of the American Dietetic Association* 82:632, 1983.

Weight Loss

Calories consumed in excess of caloric need cause weight gain regardless of whether the calories are in the form of carbohydrate, fat, protein or alcohol. Some evidence indicates that excess fats are used more efficiently than excess proteins or carbohydrates and consequently promote greater weight gain. Alcohol intake is often under-reported and can contribute as much as 25% of the total calories. Obviously, a reduction in alcohol and fat intake can contribute substantially to weight loss without affecting the nutritional quality of the diet.

Each pound of body fat contains approximately 3,500 calories. Being 15 pounds overweight represents nearly 53,000 excess calories. If the average need for calories is about 2,000 per day, then a week of total starvation would theoretically result in only a 4 pound weight loss. The body cannot exist on calories provided by fat alone so that, in times of starvation or very low calorie intake, the body begins to break down body protein, namely muscle tissue.

Fat losses and maintenance of weight loss are best achieved by reducing daily intake by 500 to 1,000 calories, thus promoting a loss of 1 to 2 pounds per week. Rapid weight losses to make weight minimums are rarely achieved through dieting but usually through water losses. These water losses are ultimately harmful, since they make the athlete dehydrated and susceptible to muscle cramping, fatigue, weakness and loss of concentration. The use of diuretics and cathartics for weight loss should be prohibited because repeated use puts stress on the body organs.

Very low calorie diets or semistarvation techniques to cause rapid weight loss are also not recommended because a good proportion of body weight loss is from muscle protein. Repeated use of very low calorie regimens results in adaptation to lower calories, thus causing slower weight loss and faster regain.

In the first weeks of dieting, weight loss will appear more rapid because of accompanying water loss. As the diet continues, weight loss slows. Weight change is not immediately related to calorie intake. An excess intake of 1,000 calories on one day does not cause a gain of ⅓ pound on the next. Water retention, digestive processes and other factors cause fluctuations in weight. Athletes should weigh in only once a week, at the same time of day, preferably first thing in the morning in the nude.

Weight Gain

In order to gain weight in the form of muscle mass, a combination program of diet and exercise is essential. No hormone, vitamin, drug or protein supplement will increase muscle mass. Muscle tissue is approximately 70% water and 22% protein, with the rest fat and carbohydrate. A pound of muscle tissue represents about 700 to 800 calories. To provide sufficient calories for muscle synthesis, 500 to 1,000 calories per day from a balanced diet are needed for a gain of 1 to 2 pounds a week. High intakes of protein foods are not necessary, since excess protein is broken down for energy or stored as fat. A weight training program is essential in order to stimulate the growth of muscle tissue.

DIET COMPOSITION DURING TRAINING

Six classes of nutrients are necessary to build and drive the human body: carbohydrates, proteins, fats, vitamins, minerals and water. Alcohol can also be considered a nutrient since it can be used by the body for energy, but it is not essential for body functioning and can be toxic to the system.

Carbohydrates, proteins and fats are the energy-yielding nutrients, whereas vitamins, minerals and water regulate body processes. Through digestion in the stomach and intestines and metabolism in the liver, the energy nutrients are broken down or converted to their smaller, more usable compounds. They are then transported to the site in the body where they are needed for building, repair, energy or energy storage (fat or glycogen).

Carbohydrates are found in foods such as sugars, starches and fiber. The body converts sugars and starches to glucose for energy or to glycogen for energy storage in the liver and muscle tissues. When glycogen stores are filled, excess carbohydrate is converted to fat. Through a process of carbohydrate loading, glycogen stores may be increased in specific muscle tissue.

Fiber is not absorbed but is essential for gastrointestinal functioning. Low fiber diets have also been associated with several diseases, including diverticulosis, constipation, heart disease, cancer of the colon and diabetes. Consequently, a high-fiber diet is recommended. Fiber is found in fruits, vegetables, whole-grain breads and cereals.

While a high carbohydrate diet is essential to good health in all individuals, it is especially important to the athlete in training who works out for three to six hours a day—50% to 60% of calorie intake should be from carbohydrates in order to keep the glycogen stores filled. Carbohydrate loading, used to generate extra glycogen, requires a carbohydrate intake of 70% to 80%. (See Eating Before and During Event.)

Proteins are long chains of nitrogen containing compounds called amino acids. The 22 amino acids are synthesized into structural components, enzymes and hormones as needed, or are converted to fatty acids or glucose for energy or energy storage. The body cannot store nonfunctioning protein, so extra protein is used for energy or converted to fat.

Protein intake should be approximately 10% to 12% of the calories, or .8 gm/kg of body weight in the adult and 1.0 to 1.5 gm/kg in the adolescent. Even during intense training and build-up, protein intakes above these levels are unnecessary. Protein sources are meats, fish, poultry, eggs, dried beans and nuts and dairy products. Animal protein sources are usually high in fat, so a high protein diet means a high fat diet, which necessarily means a low carbohydrate diet.

Fats present in the diet synthesized by the body are triglycerides, fatty acids, phospholipids and sterols. The predominate sterol is cholesterol. Cholesterol and phospholipids function as integral parts of cell membranes.

There are two types of cholesterol. LDL-cholesterol is found in foods and is produced by the body. LDLs contribute to high circulating levels of blood cholesterol. HDL-cholesterol is produced only by the body. High blood levels of HDL-cholesterol are thought to play a preventive role in heart disease.

There is still controversy over the degree of reduction of the intake of cholesterol and saturated fats required to reduce cholesterol levels in the general population. Since exercise increases HDL-cholesterol, a protective lipid, severe reduction of cholesterol-containing foods may not be necessary unless the athlete has a family history of heart disease.

Triglycerides, the major storage form of fats, consist of a glycerol and three fatty acids. Fatty acids are the body's alternative energy source to glucose. Fatty acids may be saturated or unsaturated, and either contributes the same amount of calories.

High fat intakes are associated with heart disease, cancer of the colon, breast cancer and endometrial cancer in women. In addition, calories consumed as fat means fewer calories from carbohydrates. Therefore, 30% to 35% of calorie intake should come from fat. Meats, eggs, milk and cheese all contain fat. Other sources are fried foods, butter, margarine, salad dressings, oils and mayonnaise. Because of the large numbers of calories needed by athletes, fried foods and high fat foods may be consumed, but only in moderation.

Table 48:3 gives a recommended number of daily servings from seven food groups. These seven include the basic four plus an additional three to make up the high caloric needs of the athlete.

Observe athletes during training meals to identify those with unusual or inadequate nutritional habits. A calorie counter and nutrient composition manual are helpful references. Fortunately, almost every hospital and school system has a registered dietitian. Do not hesitate to seek consultation, support and guidance from a specialist. Regrettably, sports nutrition is just becoming recognized as needing greater attention. The trainer may need to communicate knowledge of sports energy requirements and athletes' eating habits to the dietitian. With this information and the nutritionist's knowledge, individualized programs may be worked out.

WATER AND ELECTROLYTE REPLACEMENT

Water

Water is the most critical element in the diet. Most of the other nutrients essential for life can function only in the presence of water. Under optimal conditions, the body can survive 60 days without food but only 10 to 18 days without water.

Under moderate environmental conditions and activity levels, the body needs approximately 2,000 ml (slightly more than 2 quarts) of water per day. Water is provided by fluids, foods (up to 90% of fruits and vegetables is water) and metabolic water. Metabolic water is produced when protein, carbohydrate and fat are broken down for energy. For every gram of glycogen stored, 3 gm of water are stored. This water is released into the body when the glycogen is broken down.

A loss of body water equaling 2% to 3% of body weight will begin to adversely affect performance. Loss of 4% to 5% of body weight results in reduced carrying capacity of the blood for nutrients as well as reduced ability to remove heat from the body. Unless lost water is replaced, body temperature will rise, leading to heat exhaustion, heat stroke and even death.

Continuous sweating during prolonged exercise can reach a rate of 800 to 1,000 ml per

TABLE 48:3. Daily Servings from Food Groups

Food Group	Calorie Intake		
	2,800	4,300	5,500
Meats, fish, poultry and eggs	8–10 oz	10–12 oz	16–18 oz
Lowfat milk	2 or more cups	2 or more cups	2 or more cups
Vegetables	2–4 servings*	2–4 servings	2–4 servings
Fruits and juices	4 or more servings	6 or more servings	8 or more servings
Breads, cereals, starches	10–12 servings	14–16 servings	16–18 servings
Desserts and sweets†	1–2 servings	2–3 servings	3–4 servings
Sweetened beverages	1 12 oz	4–5 12 oz	5–6 12 oz
Fats and oils	3–4 tbls	6–8 tbls	8–10 tbls

*One serving is approximately ½ cup unless specified.
†Sample dessert servings: 1/8 of pie, a piece of cake 3″×3″, 1 cup of ice cream, 5–10 cookies

hour. Under hot environmental conditions, sweating may be as great as 2,000 ml per hour. Since 1 pint of water equals 1 pound of body weight, only an athlete over 200 pounds can tolerate a continuous workout in a moderate to cold environment for 2 hours without fluid replacement. Under heated conditions, a loss of 4,000 ml is a 5% loss in a 160 pound athlete and a 4% loss in a 200 pound athlete. Both are performance- and life-threatening percentages. Football players and runners can lose 8 to 10 pounds during a two hour workout.

Sweating to make a weigh-in and then attempting to replace all water loss immediately prior to competition results in loss of strength and endurance, and is potentially dangerous if restoration is not complete (see Chapter 50).

Electrolytes

The major electrolytes lost in sweat are sodium, chloride, potassium, calcium and magnesium. Small amounts of iron and copper as well as of nitrogen and some water-soluble vitamins are also lost. Sodium and chloride account for the greatest percentage of nutrients lost through sweat. Decreased losses through the urine partially compensate for this loss. Research shows that an adequate diet prior to and during training with salt allowed as desired provides adequate electrolytes. Encourage intake of citrus juices, fruits and vegetables for potassium.

For athletes with hypertension or the strong potential for hypertension, monitor blood pressures. A mild sodium restriction (4 gm) may be indicated. Treatment should be individualized, based on blood pressures, eating habits and sweat losses.

Electrolyte replacement during exercise is of little or no value. Electrolyte concentrations in the body actually increase due to the loss of body water. Even during prolonged, strenuous exercise such as marathon running, water in combination with a balanced diet maintains electrolyte balance. Electrolyte imbalances can occur after four to seven days of hard training with inadequate food intake.

SUGAR

Small amounts of glucose taken during prolonged exercise help spare glycogen and thus can increase the amount of energy available. However, high concentrations of glucose adversely affect water absorption by slowing the gastric emptying rate. High glucose concentration formulas (10% or higher) are only recommended when exercising in a cold environment where sweat losses are not great. When exercising in a hot environment, fluid replacement takes precedence over glucose. Glucose content of formulas should not exceed 2% to 3%. In any case, the large volumes of dilute glucose solutions will result in increased consumption of glucose. Glucose polymers may be used at percentages up to 5% without delaying emptying.

The following guidelines insure adequate fluid replacement and thus lead to optimal performance.

1. Drink small volumes of water frequently rather than large volumes infrequently, e.g., 6 to 8 ounces every 15 minutes.
2. Drink cold beverages (refrigerator temperature) to reduce core temperature.
3. Have fluids accessible, since the thirst mechanism does not function adequately when large volumes of water are lost. Athletes will not seek out water if it is far away. In many cases, they need to be reminded to drink.
4. After workout, replenish fluids at the rate of 1 pint for every pound lost. Weight should be back to normal prior to the next workout. Minimal body fat is lost during a workout, so weight after an event compared to weight immediately prior to an event is a good indication of total body water lost.
5. Water is the ideal fluid replacement, although commercially prepared glucose, electrolyte solutions, juices and other beverages may be used. Consider taste preferences of athletes, since whether they like a substance will govern how much they drink. The following are recommended.

   a. Glucose content of less than 2.5 gm/100 ml of water, or 25 gm/quart. This is equal to 1½ rounded tablespoons of sugar per quart.

   b. Few or no electrolytes. If included, they should be limited to a maximum of .2 gm of sodium chloride and .2 gm of potassium per quart.

   c. Juices diluted with five parts water, and colas and sweetened sodas with three parts water to reduce the glucose concentration to 2.5%. These could be adjusted to taste.

   d. Read labels of glucose and electrolyte solutions and dilute as needed. Most need some dilution.

6. The American College of Sports Medicine recommends hyperhydration prior to prolonged exercise in a hot environment. Intake should be approximately 16 ounces of cold beverage, 15 to 30 minutes prior to workout. With experience, larger amounts (up to 2 pints) may be tolerated.

VITAMINS AND MINERALS

The Food and Nutrition Board of the National Research Council states that, even though athletic activity increases energy expenditure, the larger quantities of food consumed, if chosen wisely, meet increased needs for any essential nutrients. Athletes always have and always will believe supplements are the key to improved performance. Currently, there is little scientific basis for any vitamin or mineral supplement above and beyond normal needs. Simply the belief that a supplement will improve performance can give the athlete increased confidence, thereby a mental edge. While not encouraging the use of supplements, and in fact discouraging their use, do not take them away unless the dosage level is potentially harmful. Point out the facts to the athlete, as well as the costs and potential dangers of megadoses. The athlete should begin to realize that correct selection of food can more directly affect performance than taking supplements.

TABLE 48:4. Nutrient Allowances per 1,000 kcal Derived from the 1980 Recommended Dietary Allowances

Age and Sex Group	Energy	Protein	Fat-soluble Vitamins			Water-soluble Vitamins			
			Vitamin A	Vitamin D	Vitamin E	Ascorbic Acid	Thiamin	Ribo-flavin	Niacin
	kcal	gm	μgRE	μg	mgαTE		mg		mgNE
Children									
1–3 yr	1,300	18	303	8	4	35	0.5	0.6	7
4–6 yr	1,700	18	294	6	4	27	0.5	0.6	7
7–10 yr	2,400	14	292	4	3	19	0.5	0.6	7
Males									
11–14 yr	2,700	17	370	4	3	19	0.5	0.6	7
15–18 yr	2,800	20	357	4	4	21	0.5	0.6	6
19–22 yr	2,900	19	345	3	3	21	0.5	0.6	7
23–50 yr	2,700	21	370	2	4	22	0.5	0.6	7
51+ yr	2,400	23	417	2	4	25	0.5	0.6	7
Females									
11–14 yr	2,200	21	364	5	4	23	0.5	0.6	7
15–18 yr	2,100	22	381	5	4	29	0.5	0.6	7
19–22 yr	2,100	21	381	4	4	29	0.5	0.6	7
23–50 yr	2,000	22	400	3	4	30	0.5	0.6	7
51+ yr	1,800	24	444	3	4	33	0.5	0.7	7

Vitamins

The standard charts used for the recommended dietary allowances are difficult to use with the athlete whose weight and intake may be 50% higher than that of the reference person. Table 48:4 gives the nutrient allowances per 1,000 calories derived from the recommendations of the Food and Nutrition Council of the National Research Council.

Table 48:5 lists the vitamins and their functions, sources and toxicity. There are two types of vitamins, water soluble and fat soluble. The water-soluble vitamins include all of the B complex vitamins as well as vitamin C. These vitamins are not stored in large amounts in the body. Therefore, megadoses do not increase body stores. Many of the B vitamins are used in energy metabolism, so that need is increased as more calories are burned. As long as appropriate foods are chosen, B vitamin intake is increased in proportion to need. In a recent study of food intakes of university athletes participating on various sports teams, B

vitamin intakes were found to be adequate without supplementation.

Megadoses of B complex vitamins do not appear to be toxic except for niacin. High doses of niacin cause decreased use of free fatty acids and therefore increase fatigue. In addition, niacin supplements in the form of nicotinic acid cause tingling sensations, flushed skin and liver damage. Megadoses of B vitamins have not been shown to improve performance. B12 shots have no effect on performance and are essentially harmless.

There is still controversy surrounding vitamin C. The increased stress caused by exercise indicates an increased need for vitamin C. Some respected investigators in the field of physical performance have recommended intakes of 200 to 300 mg, levels easily achieved through appropriate food selection.

While megadoses of vitamin C are not harmful, the body does adapt to high levels. As the level of vitamin C supplement increases, the percentage absorbed decreases. If

TABLE 48:4. Nutrient Allowances per 1,000 kcal Derived from the 1980 Recommended Dietary Allowances (continued)

Water-soluble Vitamins			Minerals						
Vitamin B6	Folacin	Vitamin B12	Calcium	Phosphorus	Magnesium	Iron	Zinc	Iodine
mg	μg				mg				μg
0.7	77	1.5	615	615	115	11.5	7	54
0.8	118	1.5	471	471	118	5.9	6	53
0.7	125	1.3	333	333	104	4.2	4	50
0.7	148	1.1	444	444	130	6.7	6	56
0.7	143	1.1	429	429	143	6.4	5	54
0.8	138	1.0	276	276	121	3.5	5	52
0.8	148	1.1	296	296	130	3.7	6	56
0.9	167	1.3	333	333	146	4.2	6	63
0.8	182	1.4	546	546	136	8.2	7	68
1.0	191	1.4	571	571	143	8.6	7	71
1.0	191	1.4	381	381	143	8.6	7	71
1.0	200	1.5	400	400	150	9.0	8	75
1.1	222	1.7	444	444	167	5.5	8	83

Hansen, R.G.; Wyse, B.W. "Expression of nutrient allowances per 1000 kilocalories." *Journal of the American Dietetic Association* 76:223, 1980.

TABLE 48:5.   Vitamin Sources and Functions

Fat-soluble Vitamins		
Nomenclature	Important Sources	Physiology and Functions

Vitamin A
  Retinol
  Retinal
  Retinyl ester
  Retinoic acid
  Provitamin A
    Alpha-, beta-, gamma-
    carotene, cryptoxanthin
	Animal
	  Fish-liver oils
	  Liver
	  Butter, cream
	  Whole milk
	  Whole-milk cheeses
	  Egg yolk
	Plant
	  Dark-green leafy vegetables
	  Yellow vegetables
	  Yellow fruits
	  Fortified margarines
		Bile necessary for absorption
		Stored in liver
		Maintains integrity of mucosal epithelium, maintains visual acuity in dim light
		Large amounts are toxic

Vitamin D
  Vitamin D2
    Ergocalciferol
  Vitamin D3
    Cholecalciferol
  Antirachitic factor
	Fish-liver oils
	Fortified milk
	Activated sterols
	Exposure to sunlight
	Very small amounts in butter, liver, egg yolk, salmon, sardines
		Synthesized in skin by activity of ultraviolet light
		Liver synthesizes $25(OH)D_3$
		Kidney synthesizes $1,25(OH)_2D_3$
		Functions as steroid hormone to regulate calcium and phosphorus absorption, mobilization and mineralization of bone
		Large amounts are toxic

Vitamin E
  Alpha-, beta-, gamma-
  tocopherol
  Antisterility vitamin
	Plant tissues—vegetable oils; wheat germ, rice germ; green leafy vegetables; nuts; legumes
	Animal foods are poor sources
		Not stored in body to any extent
		Related to action of selenium
		Humans: reduces oxidation of vitamin A, carotenes, and polyunsaturated fatty acids
		Animals: normal reproduction; utilization of sex hormones, cholesterol

Vitamin K
  Phylloquinone (K1)
  Menaquinone
  Menadione
	Green leaves such as alfalfa, spinach, cabbage
	Liver
	Synthesis in intestine
		Bile necessary for absorption
		Formation of prothrombin and other clotting proteins
		Sulfa drugs and antibiotics interfere with absorption
		Large amounts are toxic

Water-soluble Vitamins		
Ascorbic acid Vitamin C	Citrus fruits; tomatoes; melons; cabbage; broccoli; strawberries; fresh potatoes; green leafy vegetables	Very little storage in body Formation of intercellular cement substance; synthesis of collagen Absorption and use of iron Prevents oxidation of folacin

TABLE 48:5.   Vitamin Sources and Functions (continued)

Water-soluble Vitamins (continued)		
Nomenclature	Important Sources	Physiology and Function
Thiamin Vitamin B1	Whole-grain and enriched breads, cereals, flours; organ meats, pork; other meats, poultry, fish; legumes, nuts; milk; green vegetables	Limited body storage Chiefly involved in carbohydrate metabolism
Riboflavin Vitamin B2	Milk; organ meats; eggs; green leafy vegetables	Limited body stores, but reserves retained carefully; involved in energy metabolism

Niacin
  Nicotinic acid
  Nicotinamide
	Meat, poultry, fish; whole-grain and enriched breads, flours, cereals; nuts, legumes
	Tryptophan as a precursor
		Coenzyme for glycolysis, fat synthesis, tissue respiration

Vitamin B6
  Three active forms
    pyridoxine, pyridoxal, pyridoxamine
	Meat, poultry, fish; potatoes, sweet potatoes, vegetables	Involved in protein metabolism; conversion of tryptophan to niacin; conversion of glycogen to glucose; requirement related to protein intake

Pantothenic acid	Meat, poultry, fish; whole-grain cereals; legumes Smaller amounts in fruits, vegetables, milk	Involved in energy metabolism
Biotin	Organ meats, egg yolk, nuts, legumes	Avidin, a protein in raw egg white, blocks absorption; large amounts must be eaten; involved in energy metabolism

Vitamin B12
  Cyanocobalamin
  Hydroxycobalamin
	In animal foods only: organ meats, muscle meats, fish, poultry; eggs; milk	Requires intrinsic factor for absorption; involved in energy and cell synthesis; synthesis of DNA and RNA; formation of mature red blood cells

Folacin
  Folic acid
  Tetrahydrofolic acid
	Organ meats, deep green leafy vegetables; muscle meats, poultry, fish, eggs; whole-grain cereals	Active form is folinic acid; requires ascorbic acid for conversion; synthesis of nucleoproteins, maturation of red blood cells; interrelated with vitamin B12

Choline	Egg yolk, meat, poultry, fish, milk, whole grains	Probably not a true vitamin; involved in cell synthesis

Lipoic acid
  Thioetic acid
  Protogen
		Probably not a true vitamin; involved in energy metabolism

Robinson, C., Lawler, M. *Normal and Therapeutic Nutrition*. New York, MacMillan Publishing Co.

the athlete stops the supplement suddenly, a deficiency can occur. Discourage megadoses of 500 mg but wean athletes off high doses slowly.

The fat-soluble vitamins, A, D, E and K, are stored in the body, especially in the liver. Excessive intakes through megadoses over long periods of time lead to toxic symptoms and, in the case of vitamin A, death. Megadoses of vitamin E appear to be nontoxic but are not recommended.

Athletes often take vitamin E supplements. Through its role as an antioxidant, vitamin E could potentially increase oxygen and fatty acid supply and thus increase endurance. However, studies have not shown improved performance with vitamin E.

Nonvitamins

Periodically, new "vitamins" are promoted to athletes. These claims are erroneous by definition as a vitamin. A vitamin is an organic compound essential to life and is involved in many specific interactions in the body. In order for a compound to be essential to life, it must be in the normal food supply of the population. Otherwise, the population would have ceased to exist or would have adapted to life without the "vitamin," in which case it would no longer be essential.

Pangamic acid is erroneously labeled B15. In fact, there is no chemical structure assigned to pangamic acid and, therefore, it can have no specific functions. In addition, when B15 supplements were analyzed, a compound was found that is mutagenic and may cause cancer.

Minerals

Minerals are also grouped into two classes. The major minerals are those needed in amounts greater than 100 mg per day. Trace minerals are those needed in very small amounts. Table 48:6 lists minerals, their sources, functions and toxicity.

Increased intakes of any minerals cannot be justified as long as diets are balanced. The only possible exception is iron. Excessive intakes of major minerals are generally nontoxic but are not recommended. One potential problem can result if the diet is low in calcium (milk and dairy products) and high in phosphorus (meat and soft drinks). The normal ratio of calcium to phosphorus is 1:1, but with a low calcium and high phosphorus, calcium may be lost from the bones.

The need for sodium and potassium was discussed under water replacement. Salt tablets are not recommended because processed foods and the salt shaker provide more than an adequate amount of sodium. Since potassium depletion has serious complications, high potassium foods should be included daily, especially in those with large sweat losses.

Iron deficiency is one of the few mineral deficiencies found, mostly in women and teenagers. Iron deficiency may seriously limit athletic performance. An intake of over 2,500 calories is needed to insure adequate iron intake. The consumption of meat enhances the absorption of the iron found in grains and vegetables. Vitamin C enhances the absorption of iron in all foods. Athletes with low calorie intakes may require iron supplements. Ferrous gluconate is usually best tolerated, but the prescription and dosage should be done in consultation with a physician, since iron can be highly toxic in excess.

Not much is known about many of the other trace minerals, and they are therefore subject to erroneous claims. Megadoses are not recommended because of the interactions between minerals and the potential of toxicity. Zinc and copper must be in a ratio much the same as calcium and phosphorus. While there is no indication that minerals are toxic at normal intake levels, there is no research to say what happens when megadoses are consumed.

The compounds the body actually requires are few. These include some eight to ten of the 22 amino acids; glucose; one fatty acid, linoleic acid; approximately 20 minerals; 16 vitamins; and water. Theoretically a body could thrive on only this handful of essential ingredients. However, the balance of chemical reac-

TABLE 48:6.   Minerals: Sources and Functions

Nomenclature	Physiology and Functions	Important Sources
Calcium	Hardness of bones, teeth Transmission of nerve impulse Muscle contraction Normal heart rhythm Activate enzymes Increase cell permeability Catalyze thrombin formation	Milk, hard cheese Ice cream, cottage cheese Greens: turnip, collards, kale, mustard, broccoli Oysters, shrimp, salmon, clams
Chlorine	Chief anion of extracellular fluid Constituent of gastric juice Acid-base balance; chloride-bicarbonate shift in red cells	Table salt
Chromium	Efficient use of insulin in glucose uptake; glucose oxidation, protein synthesis, stimulation of fat, and cholesterol synthesis Activation of enzymes	Liver, meat Cheese Whole-grain cereals
Copper	Aid absorption and use of iron in synthesis of hemoglobin Electron transport Melanin formation Myelin sheath of nerves Purine metabolism	Liver, shellfish Meats Nuts, legumes Whole-grain cereals Typical diet provides 1 to 5 mg
Fluorine	Increases resistance of teeth to decay; most effective in young children Moderate levels in bone may reduce osteoporosis	Fluoridated water: 1 ppm
Iodine	Constituent of diiodotyrosine, triidothyronine, thyroxine; regulate rate of energy metabolism	Iodized salt is most reliable source Seafood Foods grown in nongoitrous coastal areas
Iron	Constituent of hemoglobin, myoglobin and oxidative enzymes: catalase, cytochrome, xanthine oxidase	Liver, organ meats Meat, poultry Egg yolk Enriched and whole-grain breads, cereals Dark-green vegetables Legumes Molasses, dark Peaches, apricots, prunes, raisins Diets supply about 6 mg per 1,000 kcal
Magnesium	Constituents of bones, teeth Activates enzymes in carbohydrate metabolism Muscle and nerve irritability	Whole-grain cereals Nuts; legumes Meat Milk Green leafy vegetables

TABLE 48:6. Minerals: Sources and Functions (continued)

Nomenclature	Physiology and Functions	Important Sources
Manganese	Activation of many enzymes; oxidation of carbohydrates, urea formation, protein hydrolysis Bone formation	Legumes, nuts Whole-grain cereals
Molybdenum	Cofactor for flavorprotein enzymes; present in xanthine oxidase	Organ meats Legumes Whole-grain cereals
Phosphorus	Structure of bones, teeth Cell permeability Metabolism of fats and carbohydrates; storage and release of ATP Sugar-phosphate linkage in DNA and RNA Phospholipids in transport of fats Buffer salts in acid-base balance	Milk; cheese Eggs, meat, fish, poultry Legumes, nuts Whole-grain cereals
Potassium	Principal cation of intracellular fluid Osmotic pressure; water balance; acid-base balance Nerve irritability and muscle contraction, regular heart rhythm Synthesis of protein	Widely distributed in foods Meat, fish, fowl Cereals Fruits, vegetables
Selenium	Antioxidant Constitute of glutathione oxidase	Meat and seafoods Cereal foods
Sodium	Principal cation of extracellular fluid Osmotic pressure; water balance Acid-base balance Regulate nerve irritability and muscle contraction "Pump" for active transport such as for glucose	Table salt Processed foods Milk Meat, fish, poultry
Sulfur	Constituent of proteins, especially cartilage, hair, nails Constituent of melanin, glutathione, thiamin, biotin, coenzyme A, insulin High-energy sulfur bonds Detoxication reactions	Protein foods rich in sulfur-amino acids Eggs Meat, fish, poultry Milk, cheese Nuts
Zinc	Constituent of enzymes: carbonic anhydrase, carboxypeptidase, lactic dehydrogenase	Seafoods Liver and other organ meats Meat, fish Wheat germ Yeast Plant foods are generally low Usual diet supplies 10 to 15 mg

Robinson, C., Lawler, M. *Normal and Therapeutic Nutrition*. New York, MacMillan Publishing Co.

tions is such that, if the correct amount and proportions are not available when needed, a deficiency or inefficiency can occur.

For this reason, it is far more practical and logical to maintain health through a balanced diet than to try to outwit nature by depending on essential elements alone. In addition, since the nutrients are interdependent and the sources varied, there is obviously no advantage to any trick diet that is unbalanced.

EATING BEFORE AND DURING EVENTS

Carbohydrate Loading

In endurance competitions requiring high levels of energy over a prolonged time, maximizing the storage of glycogen in the muscle can improve performance. Carbohydrate loading in combination with depletion exercise can increase these stores. Most likely to benefit from a carbohydrate loading program are long-distance runners, swimmers, bicyclists and cross-country skiers. It may also benefit athletes involved in sports that require prolonged movement of varying intensities such as soccer, lacrosse and ice hockey, as well as tournament sports such as tennis and handball.

One day prior to going on a carbohydrate loading diet, the athlete exercises to exhaustion to deplete glycogen stores. The workout must be identical to the competitive event in order for the appropriate muscles and muscle fibers to become depleted. If the athlete is bicycling, he should bicycle to exhaustion. If he is involved in soccer or lacrosse, he should do interval training, alternating between high- and low-intensity running.

The two methods of carbohydrate loading (Table 48:7) have both been used successfully. The athlete's schedule and tolerances should determine which is used. During carbohydrate loading, the athlete's weight should increase 1 to 3 pounds, since water is stored with glycogen.

During the three days prior to the event, 70% to 80% of the calories should be from

TABLE 48:7. Carbohydrate Loading Methods

Method A	
1st day	Depletion exercise
2nd day	High carbohydrate diet; little or no exercise
3rd day	High carbohydrate diet; little or no exercise
4th day	High carbohydrate diet; little or no exercise
5th day	Competition

Method B	
1st day	Depletion exercise
2nd day	High carbohydrate diet; regular exercise
3rd day	High carbohydrate diet; regular exercise
4th day	High carbohydrate diet; regular exercise
5th day	High carbohydrate diet; little or no exercise
6th day	High carbohydrate diet; little or no exercise
7th day	High carbohydrate diet; little or no exercise
8th day	Competition

Williams, M. *Nutrition for Fitness and Sport.* Dubuque, IA, Wm. C. Brown Co., p. 35.

carbohydrate, 10% to 15% from fat and 10% to 15% from protein. Table 48:8 lists the number of servings.

Since the diet is necessarily low in fat, avoid high fat meats and most visible fats. High fat breads and desserts such as pastries, doughnuts and pies should be avoided. The athlete has the choice of having some butter, margarine and gravy, or higher fat meats like steak, and eggs. Table 48:9 gives sample menus.

The original carbohydrate loading program had a carbohydrate-deficient diet sandwiched between the exercise and the carbohydrate loading. Research showed that very low carbohydrate intake was not necessary. Equal benefits were derived from just high carbohydrate as from low carbohydrate, followed by high carbohydrate.

Pre-event Meal

The food eaten on the day of an athletic event does not benefit performance. High intakes of protein foods such as steak and eggs do not give the athlete extra energy, nor do they protect him from muscle injury. In fact,

TABLE 48:8.   Carbohydrate Loading: Intake Three Days Prior to Competition

Food Groups	2,800 kcal	4,300 kcal	5,500 kcal
*Low fat meats, fish, poultry; occasional eggs	6 oz 330 kcal	8 oz 440 kcal	12 oz 660 kcal
Milk, skim or low fat	2 cups 220 kcal	2 cups 220 kcal	2 cups 220 kcal
Breads and cereals	10–14 servings 980 kcal	14–18 servings 1,260 kcal	18–22 servings 1,540 kcal
Vegetables	2–4 servings 100 kcal	2–4 servings 100 kcal	4–6 servings 100 kcal
Fruits and fruit juices	3–4 servings 240 kcal	5–6 servings 360 kcal	7–8 servings 480 kcal
Fats and oils	1–2 tbls 135 kcal	1–2 tbls 135 kcal	2–4 tbls 270 kcal
Desserts and sweets	1–2 servings 470 kcal[†]	3–5 servings 1,200 kcal	4–6 servings 1,500 kcal
Beverages, sweetened	2–12 oz 320 kcal	4–12 oz 640 kcal	6–12 oz 960 kcal

*Chuck roasts, round steak, ground round, any cut of veal. If higher fat meats are desired (sirloin, rib eye, etc.), omit added gravies, fats and oils.
[†]For 3,000 calories and less, avoid high fat desserts such as pies, pastries and doughnuts.

high protein, high fat foods cause increased stress on the kidneys and take a long time to digest. General guidelines for eating prior to a competitive event follow.

1. The meal should be high carbohydrate, low fat and protein (Table 48:10), either solid food or a liquid formula.
2. Take solid food three to four hours prior to an event.
3. Take liquid meals two to three hours prior to an event. They should be low in fat and high in carbohydrate, with some vitamins and minerals added. Some examples are Nutrament, Sustacal and Instant Breakfast.
4. Foods should be easily digestable. Avoid fried foods and foods known to cause flatulence, which varies with the individual.
5. Do not ingest foods and beverages high in sugar within one hour of the start of competition. Sugars taken at the start of a game stimulate insulin production and therefore

actually cause an accelerated use of glycogen supplies.
6. Take adequate fluids to insure hydration. Unsweetened beverages may be taken within 15 to 30 minutes of competition. Hyperhydrate in hot environments (see Water and Electrolyte Replacement).

Eating During an Event

The primary concern during an event is to replenish lost fluids. Glucose feedings during athletic events of long duration at moderate to high intensity may help prevent hypoglycemia and spare glycogen stores. Marathon running, cross-country skiing, soccer and lacrosse are some examples of activities in which performance might benefit. In general, a glucose solution of 2% to 3% is recommended. (For more specific recommendations see discussion of fluid replacement.)

FOOD AND DRUG INTERACTIONS

Impact of Food on Drugs

Drug absorption is affected by gastrointestinal function, the relative lipophilic/hydrophilic character of the drug, gastrointestinal pH and the drug product dissolution rate. In general, drugs are absorbed more slowly when taken with a meal because food delays gastric emptying.

Food intake does not reduce the quantity of the drug absorbed, in most cases. It does affect the length of time it takes for the drug to reach peak levels. This is not clinically significant if the drug is used on a continual basis. However, the delay is undesirable when:

1. A rapid effect is needed to relieve acute symptoms
2. It precludes the achievement of effective plasma and tissue concentrations of drugs rapidly metabolized and excreted
3. Drugs are inactivated in the stomach

Some drugs are recommended to be taken with food because they irritate the gastrointestinal tract. Most of the anti-inflammatory drugs fall into this category, as do many of the analgesic anti-inflammatories (Table 48:11).

When food is ingested, the pH of the stomach decreases. This increased acidity may increase the destruction of antibiotics and therefore decrease the amount of active drug. Therefore, drugs like ampicillin, erythromycin and penicillin should be taken one hour before meals or two hours after meals (Table 48:12). Because of the affect of acidity on these drugs, they should not be taken with citric juices.

Tetracycline is affected by iron and calcium. These minerals bind with tetracycline to form a nonabsorbable complex. Therefore, tetracycline should be taken before meals and not at the same time as an iron or calcium supplement or milk and milk products.

Products that irritate the stomach are sometimes coated with an acid-resistant, base-susceptible "enteric coating" developed to pass through the stomach and dissolve in the intestine. Foods that increase the pH of the stomach, such as milk, may dissolve the coating while the drugs are still in the stomach. Aspirin and erythromycin are sometimes coated and should never be taken with milk.

Medication should always be taken with a glass of water and not immediately before bed

TABLE 48:9. Carbohydrate Loading Menus

2,800 kcal	5,500 kcal
1 cup orange juice 2 cups cereal 2 slices toast 2 tsp jelly 1 cup milk, low fat	2 cups orange juice 8 large pancakes with syrup 1 cup milk, low fat
Turkey hoagie Large peach 2 cupcakes Iced tea	2 turkey sandwiches with lettuce and tomato 2 large apples Large slice of cake 12 oz soda
2 cups spaghetti with 1 cup meat sauce 1½ cups green beans 1 tsp margarine ½ cup applesauce	6 oz roast beef Large baked potato 4 slices bread 1½ cup broccoli 1 cup fruit cocktail 2 tsp margarine 3 tsp jelly Large slice of pie
20 cookies 1 cup milk	1 tuna sandwich 20 cookies 1 cup milk
2 12 oz sodas during day	6 12 oz sodas during day

TABLE 48:10. Sample Pre-event Menus

Orange juice Cereal with low fat milk Toast with butter and jelly Beverage of choice	Orange juice Pancakes with syrup Toast with margarine and jelly Beverage of choice
Grapefruit juice Spaghetti with meat sauce Tossed salad with dressing Italian bread with margarine Fruit cup Beverage of choice	Fruit cup Beef chow mein Shrimp fried rice Stir fried vegetables Sherbet Beverage of choice

TABLE 48:11.   Drugs with Meals

Indomethacin (Indocin)	Oxyphenbutazone (Oxalid)
Ibuprofen (Motrin)	Naproxen (Naprosyn)
Fenoprofen calcium (Nafron)	Zomepirac sodium (Zomax)
Phenylbutazone (Butazolidin, Azolid)	Aspirin

TABLE 48:12.   Drugs One Hour Before or Two Hours After Meals

Ampicillin	Lincomycin
Erythromycin	Cephalosporins
Penicillin	Tetracycline
Enteric coated medications	

rest to avoid possible irritation or ulceration of the esophagus. This is particularly important with those known ulcerogenic drugs such as analgesics, tetracycline and nonsteroidal anti-inflammatory drugs.

Impact of Drugs on Nutrients

Overt nutritional deficiencies are unlikely to develop with drug use unless the athlete's nutritional status is borderline. The absorption of nutrients can be decreased by altering the physiochemical nature of the gastrointestinal tract, by binding nutrients, by direct toxic effects or by inhibition of mucosal cell enzyme systems. Of the drugs most commonly used by athletes, only two are likely to cause nutritional deficiencies.

Many women athletes use oral contraceptives. With long-term use oral contraceptives can cause nutritional deficiencies of B6, B12, folic acid and vitamin C. A varied diet high in fruits, vegetables and grains gives sufficient quantities of these nutrients. If caloric intake is restricted, then a vitamin supplement of 100% of the recommended daily allowances (RDA) is indicated.

Prolonged use of corticosteroids also causes nutritional problems. Corticosteroids increase protein catabolism, increase sodium retention, decrease calcium and phosphorus absorption and increase urinary loss of zinc, calcium, potassium and nitrogen. With the use of these drugs, a diet high in protein, low in sodium (2 to 4 gm), restricted in simple sugars and high in vitamins and minerals is necessary. A supplement to meet the RDA is also recommended if the corticosteroids are continued for a long period of time.

Caffeine

Caffeine stimulates the central nervous system as well as the heart. Intakes of 50 to 200 mg will cause alertness, while excessive intakes of 300 to 500 mg can cause nervousness, muscular tremors and heart palpitations. With habitual intake, the body adapts to higher levels of caffeine.

Caffeine also stimulates the release of adrenalin and causes a rise in the amount of free fatty acids in the blood. Because of this increased availability of free fatty acids, caffeine may affect performance. Most research shows that caffeine has no effect on performance in events lasting under one hour. However, for events lasting over two hours, caffeine may increase energy available from fats and thus spare glycogen. Some studies show conflicting findings. Caffeine may be beneficial only in some people. More research is needed.

The amount of caffeine needed to produce the rise in free fatty acids is low, 200 to 300 mg, equivalent to two cups of brewed coffee (Table 48:13). If the athlete feels that caffeine improves his performance, it can be allowed and should be taken one hour prior to exercise. Note that caffeine has been classified as a drug by the International Olympic Committee.

Aside from acting as a stimulant, caffeine acts as a diuretic. It may decrease body water prior to an event and thus adversely affect performance capacity. This adverse effect should be weighed against potential benefits.

Alcohol

Although consumed as a food, alcohol is classified as a drug. Alcohol is rapidly absorbed from the stomach and small intestine, particularly if little food is present in the gastrointestinal tract. The presence of sugar enhances the absorption of alcohol. Alcohol is metabolized at a relatively constant rate, approximately ¾ of an ounce an hour.

Alcohol causes diuresis in excess of fluid volume ingested and consequently should not be used for fluid replacement. Dehydration causes some of the ill effects of a hangover.

Beer and wine contain very small amounts of thiamine, niacin, riboflavin, calcium and potassium. The amounts are so low that their contribution to nutritional intake is minimal. In fact, chronic usage of alcohol in excess of 20% of caloric intake can decrease the absorption of folic acid, thiamine, B12, B6, magnesium, zinc and other trace minerals. An intake of foods high in vitamins and minerals is therefore recommended.

The combination of alcohol with drugs is potentially dangerous, especially with drugs that act on the central nervous system, including muscle relaxants and antidepressants. In addition, some drugs have a coating soluble in alcohol, so the drug may be released more quickly than desired. Antihistamines and slow-release medications should never be taken with alcohol because of this fast release.

THE DIABETIC ATHLETE

Exercise helps control diabetes by reducing the need for insulin. Therefore, upon initiation of a regular exercise program, the insulin dose will probably need to be decreased or food intake increased. Because of the pro-insulin effects of exercise, take the following precautions to avoid exercise-induced hypoglycemia.

1. Exercise should be consistent, at the same time every day and of approximately the same intensity and duration. Avoid exercising during the time of peak insulin

TABLE 48:13. Caffeine Content of Beverages

Beverage	Caffeine (mg/100 ml)	mg/8 oz
Carbonated		
Coca Cola*	18	45
Dr. Pepper*	17	43
Mountain Dew*	15	38
Diet Dr. Pepper*	15	38
Tab	13	33
Pepsi-Cola*	12	30
RC Cola*	9	23
Diet RC*	9	23
Diet Rite*	9	23
Fanta Root Beer†	0	0
Coffee		
Instant*	44	110
Percolated*	73	183
Dripolated*	97	243
Coffee: decaffeinated		
Infused‡	1–3	8–24
Instant‡	0.50–1.50	4–12
Decaf†	0.90	7.2
Nescafe†	3–6	36–47
Sanka	2	15
Tea, bagged		
Black, 5 min brew*	33	83
Black, 1 min brew*	20	50
Tea, loose		
Black, 5 min brew*	29	73
Green, 5 min brew*	25	63
Green, Japan, 5 min brew*	15	38
Cocoa; chocolate*	6	15
Ovaltine‡	0	

*Bunker, M.L., McWilliams, M. "Caffeine content of common beverages." *Journal of the American Dietetic Association* 74: 28, 1979.
†Nutritional analysis data supplied by the manufacturer.
‡Nagy, M. "Caffeine content of beverages and chocolate." *JAMA* 229: 337, 1974.
Adapted from "Caffeine Content of Beverages." *Handbook of Clinical Dietetics*, American Dietetic Association. New Haven, Yale University, p. 149.

activity. If this is unavoidable, then the athlete should eat a high carbohydrate snack (juice and crackers, milk and cookies, soda and crackers, etc.) one half hour prior to exercise.

2. For insulin doses given prior to exercise, use nonexercised injection sites such as the abdominal wall. Exercise enhances the delivery of insulin from the injection site.
3. During prolonged activity of moderate intensity or greater, approximately 10 gm of carbohydrate (4 ounces of juice or soda or a piece of fruit) should be taken for every 30 minutes of activity.
4. Stop activities at initial warnings of hypoglycemia, and give a high carbohydrate beverage. Because of rapid onset of symptoms, the diabetic should never exercise alone. Those around him should be knowledgeable about the symptoms of hypoglycemia and corrective action.
5. As with all athletes, adequate fluid replacement is essential.

ANOREXIA AND BULIMIA

Nutritional abuse is being recognized and acknowledged with increasing frequency. Anorexia nervosa and bulimia are two nutritional disorders of which the athletic trainer should be aware.

Anorexia nervosa is a disorder of severe weight loss associated with a variety of psychological and physical conditions. A person with this disorder begins dieting but then loses sight of a realistic goal for his weight. To be as thin as possible becomes an obsession, and the person loses all concept of a normal body image. Calorie input and output become a preoccupation. The fear of gaining weight is such a concern that these people often exercise constantly in an effort to "burn up" any calories consumed that day. While anorexia is primarily found in adolescent women, it is increasingly being found in men. Those athletes most susceptible are those involved in activities in which low body weight and small size are advantageous—gymnasts, dancers, wrestlers, jockeys, long-distance runners, divers, and lightweights and coxswains in crew.

Bulimia is a disorder involving a more normal weight, but the person uses vomiting, diuretics or laxatives to prevent weight gain. The person may eat an inordinate amount of food in a binge once or twice a week or as frequently as 20 times a day. The simple maneuver of vomiting often becomes addictive and uncontrollable.

Most bulimics are perfectionists and overachievers. The athlete who is or who becomes bulimic often displays this behavior in workouts or competition. Where the anorexic may become withdrawn, the bulimic has an intense desire to please everyone. Therefore, the coach and athletic trainer may be extremely influential in working with the bulimic athlete.

Unfortunately, both eating disorders create serious medical concerns. Both anorexia and bulimia share severe depression as a side effect. The anorexic has amenorrhea, while the bulimic may have irregular menses. Without medical intervention, the anorexic dies of starvation.

Hypokalemia is a concern for bulimic individuals because this potassium deficiency results from chronic vomiting or laxative/diuretic abuse. Potassium is necessary for adequate muscle functioning, and a deficiency is often marked by muscle fatigue, weakness, erratic heart beat and kidney damage. Potassium loss aggravates dehydration and electrolyte imbalances.

The stomach normally secretes acid in response to food as it initiates digestion. Chronic vomiting causes this acid to irritate the esophagus, teeth and mouth, resulting in ulcers, esophageal varices, destruction of tooth enamel and sores in the mucous membranes of the mouth. Other concerns include hiatal hernias and rupture of the esophagus.

Medical treatment is imperative for both the bulimic and anorexic. The trainer can help by insuring that the coach is not making unrealistic weight goals for his athletes and by helping the athlete determine an ideal body weight and fat content. The trainer may also help diagnose nutritional problems and encourage the athlete to seek help. These individuals must work with psychologists, psychiatrists or nutritionists experienced in working with eating disorders.

Signs of Anorexia Nervosa*

1. Feeling of obesity, even as weight loss increases
2. Altered body image
3. More than 25% weight loss
4. No desire to keep body weight over the minimum for age and height
5. No physical disorder to cause such weight loss

Signs of Bulimia

1. Binge eating repeatedly
2. Eating inconspicuously during a binge
3. Ending a binge with abdominal pain, sleep, self-induced vomiting or laxatives
4. Attempting severely restrictive diets to lose weight
5. Weight variations of more than 10 pounds due to binges and fasts
6. Realizing that the eating pattern is abnormal and not being able to stop voluntarily
7. Depression after eating binges
8. No physical disorder
9. Behavior is not anorexic

Organizations†

The following regional associations may offer more specific guidance for organizations and professionals.

*Journal of the National Athletic Trainers Association, Vol. 18, 1983, p. 138.

†Boskind, M., White, W. *Bulimarexia.* New York, W.W. Norton & Co., 1983.

West:
Anorexia Nervosa & Related Eating Disorders, Inc. (ANRED)
Post Office Box 5102
Eugene, OR 97405

Midwest:
Anorexia Nervosa & Associated Disorders, Inc. (ANAD)
Post Office Box 271
Highland Park, IL 60035

National Anorexic Aid Society, Inc. (NAAS)
Post Office Box 29461
Columbus, OH 43229

East and New England:
American Anorexia Nervosa Association, Inc. (AANA)
133 Cedar Lane
Teaneck, NJ 07666

The Anorexia Nervosa Aid Society of Massachusetts, Inc. (ANAS)
Post Office Box 213
Lincoln Center, MA 01773

South:
Maryland Association for Anorexia Nervosa and Bulimia, Inc. (MAANA)
222 Gateswood Road
Lutherville, MD 21093

Alcohol and Drugs

49

Athletes subject to the stresses and strains of athletic competition and the trauma of contact sports have special medical needs in addition to medical problems common to any group of young, active individuals. Drugs and medications and treatments for the special needs of the athlete should be available. The training room should not be a pharmacy, but should contain common medications used by the physician or by the trainer under the direction of the physician. On a road trip sufficient medical supplies to meet emergencies should travel with the team.

The needs of high school athletes differ from those of a professional team. Medications and treatments appropriate for one group of athletes may not be totally appropriate for another. A general description of the types of drugs available and their potential uses follows. The philosophy of their use and the types of treatments employed must of necessity vary from physician to physician, from sport to sport and from age group to age group.

ANTI-INFLAMMATORY MEDICATION

Systemic

Anti-inflammatory drugs are widely used for common musculoskeletal stresses, strains and trauma. Many such drugs are now available, some of which are new and relatively untried. Every drug can cause harmful side effects and should be prescribed only by a physician.

The commonest and safest drug is aspirin. Aspirin occasionally causes gastrointestinal difficulties but a buffered aspirin preparation can usually be substituted successfully. Indomethacin (Indocin), a drug useful in arthritis, also effectively reduces inflammatory conditions not only in joints but also in juxta-articular structures and tendons. Contraindications are rare in young athletes, although it may occasionally cause intestinal disturbances and dizziness. Phenylbutazone is perhaps the most effective anti-inflammatory drug in common use for musculotendinous and articular inflammations. Side effects can be more severe. They include gastritis, intestinal irritation and fluid retention. These are not uncommon in older people, but seldom occur in the young, active athlete. Very rarely, the drug may significantly depress the white blood cell count. If doses of 300 to 400 mg per day are limited to one week periods in the athlete, this complication is very rare. If phenylbutazone is used for longer than 7 to 10 days, especially in an older population, blood count to determine leukopenia must be obtained. Newer systemic anti-inflammatory agents are also used to treat musculoskeletal inflammatory conditions of the athlete.

Systemic cortical steroids, effective in generalized inflammatory conditions, are rarely indicated in the athlete. When these drugs are needed, athletic participation should be limited or terminated.

Local

Local steroids, such as cortisone or cortisone-like derivatives, may occasionally be indicated. Yet, their use in athletics is an area of continuing controversy. Undoubtedly, they can markedly decrease intra-articular inflam-

516

matory conditions, but they can also inhibit normal cartilage metabolism. Therefore, use them sparingly, if at all, in the young athlete. Local steroids can also relieve periarticular or peritendinous inflammatory conditions, but, as repeatedly demonstrated, injections into collagenous tissues, such as tendons or ligaments, cause microscopic disorganization and weakening. Repetition of injections often leads to pathologic rupture. Therefore, steroids should be injected carefully adjacent to tendons or ligaments, but not into them. If local steroid injection therapy is used to treat tendonitis, particularly in the lower extremity, the body part must be rested for 7 to 12 days following injection to minimize the risk of rupture. Many synthetic, cortisone-like derivatives are marketed, each with particular reported advantage.

Dimethyl sulfoxide (DMSO), a solvent derived from wood, aroused great interest because of claims of significant anti-inflammatory action. Its use remains restricted by the Federal Drug Administration to treatment of interstitial cystitis. No studies to date have documented the efficacy of DMSO in managing inflammatory conditions related to athletics. Also, side effects from possible impurities in preparations available commercially and the fact that high doses have induced cataracts in experimental animals have caused concern. DMSO also causes bad breath and has the potential to carry bacteria into joints.

ANALGESICS AND ANESTHETICS

While narcotics are rarely needed in athletics, meperidine (Demerol) is perhaps the most widely used. It should be employed only in serious and painful trauma as a temporary emergency measure and under physician control. Traumatic conditions are rarely so painful that propoxyphene plus aspirin (Darvon compound) or combinations of codeine and aspirin, or codeine and acetaminophen (Tylenol), cannot control them.

Local anesthetic agents should be part of every training room. Three types should be available: lidocaine 1% (Xylocaine 1%) for common use, lidocaine 2% (Xylocaine) with epinephrine for longer action, and bupivacaine 0.5% (Marcaine 0.5%) for occasional use when prolonged action is needed. Not only are these agents useful in minor surgery (e.g., wound suturing), but they also can be used as local anesthetics when, on a rare occasion, a fracture or dislocation requires reduction. Injection of local anesthesia into joints can often provide effective though temporary pain relief. The use of local anesthetics for pain relief should not be abused in an attempt to return an athlete to competition prematurely and must be under the direct control of a physician.

MUSCLE RELAXANTS

A variety of effective muscle relaxants are available. In general, for athletes use one with minimal sedative side effects to avoid depression of the central nervous system. Carisoprodol (Soma) in dosages of 350 mg is one example. It is well tolerated and has minimal central nervous system side effects. Diazepam (Valium) and chlordiazepoxide (Librium), drugs commonly used in clinical practice, should generally be avoided in athletes because of their secondary depression of the central nervous system. They may be used rarely as an injectable preparation in treating severe heat cramps. Quinine sulfate, in 5 grain capsules, is useful for treating muscle cramps that occur at night. It has few, if any, side effects and can be used with impunity in players of any age.

If a player has difficulty sleeping due to unusual circumstances, such as following a major injury or during particular physical or emotional stress, flurazepam hydrochloride (Dalmane) is preferred over barbiturates.

ANTIBIOTICS

In addition to local antibiotics described under the section on skin, eyes and ears, athletes may occasionally require systemic antibiotics. Oral tetracycline, usually coupled with an expectorant, can often help treat athletes susceptible to chronic bronchitis. A chest film can confirm the absence of alveolar disease. Tetracycline, or its relative minocycline, is also used to treat acne in small doses of 250 mg per day, a common problem among teenage athletes. Infected skin lesions (postoperative wounds, blisters and abrasions) although treated with local antibiotic preparations following sterile cleansing, occasionally require systemic antibiotics. A common causative agent in infected skin wounds is penicillinase-resistant Staphylococcus aureus. This bacterium is susceptible to many of the cephalosporins as well as dicloxacillin. Therapy with one of these can begin while awaiting results of the culture and sensitivity study.

"Strep" throat is occasionally seen in athletes, especially when resistance is decreased by long, strenuous workouts and little sleep. Athletes whose throats appear infected should have a culture, especially if exudate is present. If the culture is positive for beta hemolytic streptococci, oral penicillin is the treatment of choice.

ELECTROLYTE SOLUTIONS

Fluid replacement in athletes is crucial. Although several years ago special electrolyte drinks for athletes gained popularity, plain, free water available at all times during practice and games is all that is needed. Athletes with intact renal function adequately equilibrate their electrolytes.

IRON SUPPLEMENTS

Iron supplementation is needed when iron deficiency is documented, most commonly among menstruating women. Hemoglobin and hematocrit values document anemia, but do not detect low levels of iron deficiency that may affect oxygen-carrying capacity. When the athlete needs maximal oxygen-carrying capacity for peak performance, serum analysis for protoporphyrin to heme ratios more

precisely evaluates iron deficiency. Proper iron supplementation can then be instituted in deficient athletes. Because laboratory analysis for protoporphyrin to heme ratios may not be financially feasible, supplementing the diet of menstruating women with 320 mg of iron daily may be advisable.

ALLERGY MEDICATIONS

Antihistamines are effective in treating allergic rhinitis, conjunctivitis and hives. They will also control pruritus in contact dermatitis. However, their potential side effects of drowsiness and slow reaction time may be unacceptable to the competing athlete. In allergic rhinitis, decongestants may be as effective in alleviating upper airway obstruction and offer symptomatic relief without drowsiness.

Asthmatic athletes find their symptoms are decreased if they remain well hydrated. Cromolyn sodium (Intal), theophylline and beta-adrenergics (epinephrine, isoproterenol, metaproterenol sulfate, and terbutaline sulfate) can also be used to control bronchospasms in the asthmatic. Beclomethasone depropionate (Vanceril), a synthetic steroid, is available as an inhalant to treat allergic patients. Though effective, many physicians feel steroids (oral or inhalant) do not have a place in the daily management of the asthmatic athlete and should be employed only briefly to manage a severe allergic reaction. Exercise-induced asthma (EIA) is bronchospasm precipitated by exercise. It frequently occurs in previously nonallergic persons. Similar to treating the asthmatic athlete, treating EIA centers around hydration and the use of bronchodilators prior to exercise.

Exercise-induced anaphylaxis is a medical emergency. Like any anaphylactic reaction, the symptoms are diaphoresis, hypertension, hyperpyrexia and the feeling of "impending doom." Immediate treatment with fluids, subcutaneous epinephrine and intravenous benadryl (25 to 50 mg) is needed as the athlete is transported to the nearest emergency department. The etiology of exercise-induced anaphylaxis is not known, but is probably multifactorial. Like exercise-induced bronchospasm, the athlete may have no allergic history. One episode of exercise-induced anaphylaxis does not necessarily predispose the athlete to future attacks.

GASTROINTESTINAL DRUGS

Occasionally the nervous or agitated athlete will have gastric upsets and problems of hyperacidity for which magnesium and aluminum hydroxide preparations (Maalox, Amphojel, Gelusil, etc.) are useful. An effective drug for nausea is prochlorperazine (Compazine) or promethazine hydrochloride (Phenergan) in oral doses of 5 to 15 mg. When vomiting is severe, both can be used in a suppository or injectable form. Diarrhea, either functional or organic, may be a problem on road trips, particularly with indiscriminate or irregular eating. In most conditions, Lomotil has replaced other antidiarrheal agents because of its convenience, low toxicity, and effectiveness. It is given in doses of one to two tablets, four to six hours apart.

RESPIRATORY DRUGS

The symptoms of the common cold are difficult to treat, at best. With the athlete's high level exertion and fatigue, they can be particularly troublesome. Decongestants open up nasal passages and because of their drying effect can secondarily reduce cough. Combinations of decongestants and antihistamines are even more effective in relieving congestion. As in the treatment of allergic rhinitis, the secondary effects of decreased reaction time and drowsiness of the antihistamines must be balanced against their increased effectiveness over decongestants alone. Timing may be an important factor in choosing a medication. Prescribing decongestants during the day and an antihistamine at night (when drowsiness may be a benefit and not a detriment) is often a good treatment plan.

MEDICATIONS FOR EYES AND EARS

External otitis and inflammatory conditions about the external auditory canal can be treated easily with cortisone plus neomycin or lidocaine plus neosporin.

Eye trauma is not infrequently encountered in sports. Foreign bodies can often be removed by thoroughly washing the eye with sterile saline or using copious amounts of a commercially available irrigating solution such as Dacriose. Pain can often be relieved with proparacine ointment 0.5% instilled locally into the eye by eyedropper. A patch is useful in traumatic eye conditions, either a proprietary device or a gauze dressing. Patching the eye prevents repeated irritation of the cornea by the lid. The eye is subject to inflammatory conditions as well as trauma. Cortisporin Otic solution is effective in relieving noninfectious inflammation, but steroid solutions such as this should be avoided in cases of infectious conjunctivitis, either bacterial or viral. Bacterial conjunctivitis can be effectively treated with Neosporin ophthalmic solution (or ointment) or sodium sulfacetamide ointment 10% instilled locally into the eye.

In addition to purely medical supplies, the training room and the physician's traveling bag should include blood pressure cuffs, stethoscope, small flashlight, thermometer and heavy bandage scissors. A small mirror for use in replacing lenses and a patch for corneal irritations and abrasions should be included, as well as sterilized suture kits with needle holder and prepackaged sutures.

DRUG ABUSE

Although drugs are an indispensable therapeutic aid, they should not be used as artificial adjuncts to the athlete's desire to improve performance. Drug abuse in sports has been referred to as ''doping.'' Specifically, doping is defined by the International Olympic Committee as ''the administration of, or the use by a competing athlete, of any substance foreign to the body, or of any physiological substance taken in abnormal quantity by an abnormal route of entry into the body, with the sole intention of increasing in an artificial and unfair manner his performance in competition.'' Multiple tests can now detect these drugs in the blood or urine of competing athletes. Not surprisingly, many of these drugs have greater potential for physiological harm than for giving a ''competitive edge.''

A partial list of substances presently banned by the medical commission of the International Olympic Committee and the International Amateur Athletic Federation follows.

Stimulants

Psychomotor stimulants: amphetamines, benzphetamine, cocaine, diethylpropion, methylphenidate, ephedrine, pemoline, phendimetrazine, phenmetrazine, phentermine

Sympathomimetic amines: Ephedrine, methylephedrine

Miscellaneous central nervous system stimulants: nikethamide, strychnine

Depressants

Narcotic analgesics: morphine, heroin, methadone

Muscle relaxants: ethanol

Tranquilizers: phenothiazine, butyrophenones, meprobamate, chlordiazepoxide, barbiturates

Anabolic steroids

A more complete list is available by writing to Colonel F. Don Miller, Olympic House, 1750 East Boulder Street, Colorado Springs, CO 80909.

PSYCHOMOTOR DRUGS

Stimulants

The primary effect of psychomotor stimulants is on the brain and central nervous system. They increase motor activity and delay the onset of the subjective feeling of fatigue. Because they cause excessive energy expenditure, they probably do not improve muscular performance. Depending on the dosage, individual sensitivity and other factors, they may be toxic, and often create psychological dependence.

Caffeine, considered one of the least dangerous of the psychomotor stimulants, is one of the most common, and is found in tea, coffee, cocoa and colas. It is not only a psychomotor stimulant, but also stimulates cardiac muscle. Recently it was shown that 330 mg of caffeine (equivalent to about 2½ cups of coffee) increases plasma fatty acids by enhancing lipolysis. This spares glycogen depletion and, hence, aids performance in endurance exercise. Yet, caffeine still remains an ''acceptable stimulant'' and is not barred by athletic committees.

Depressants

These drugs include narcotic analgesics, sedatives, antidepressants, hypnotics and alcohol. They decrease activity of the central nervous system and have been used to increase physical and psychological tolerance of pain in an attempt to improve athletic performance. Because many psychomotor depressants are used legitimately to lessen pain or relieve muscle spasms following an injury, they highlight the major problem that drug regulation committees for organized sports must face: where does therapy end and ''doping'' begin?

Alcohol is the most widely (used) abused drug among both teenagers and adults. Its abuse in sports stems from a misguided belief that it will decrease nervous tremors and, therefore, increase precision in marksmanship sports—riflery, archery, etc. Others wrongly believe alcohol decreases anxiety and, therefore, improves concentration as well as serves as a readily available source of carbohydrates for endurance events. Actually, its benefit in a carbohydrate loading diet is far below that of other high carbohydrate sources such as pastas and sweetened juices. Moreover, it provokes dehydration by blocking antidiuretic hormones (ADH) produced by the pituitary to prevent water loss from the kidneys. Alcohol decreases alertness, slows reaction time and impairs coordination and judgment. It causes fat to accumulate in the liver and can lead to fatty degeneration of this organ.

ANABOLIC STEROIDS

Anabolic steroids are synthetic modifications of testosterone developed to increase the anabolic action of this compound relative to its androgenic effects. Athletes combine anabolic steroids with an intense progressive resistance exercise program and a high protein diet during their training periods in an attempt to increase body weight and muscle mass. Although there is general agreement that anabolic steroids increase muscle mass if taken in combination with adequate weight training programs and protein rich diets, this increase in muscle bulk does not appear to provide any increase in strength or endurance. The risks of taking anabolic steroids are significant, including sterilization in women, premature epiphyseal closure in the adolescent, salt and water retention, testicular atrophy, oligospermia, prostatic hypertrophy, hypercalcemia, choleostatic jaundice and hepatocellular carcinoma.

BIRTH CONTROL PILLS

Although presently not listed as a prescribed drug by any organized athletic committee, birth control pills should not be used to alter normal monthly hormonal cycling. No data indicate that the female athlete's performance is influenced by progesterone or estrogen peaks. A survey of Olympic champions in the 1972 Olympics found gold medalists in all phases of the menstrual cycle. Recent work demonstrates augmented responses to decreased O_2 and increased CO_2 resulting in an increase in ventilation at submaximal levels of exercise during the luteal (high progesterone)

phase of the menstrual cycle. This increase in ventilation (respiratory rate) did not, however, appear to affect the performance of trained athletes adversely. Further research is needed in this area.

MEGADOSE VITAMINS

Vitamins are organic compounds essential in minute amounts to maintain normal anabolic function. Since vitamins are not synthesized, or not synthesized in adequate amounts, within the body, small amounts are a dietary necessity. The athlete's need for vitamins may be slightly greater than that of the normal population due to his high anabolic turnover. However, if the athlete maintains an increased caloric intake with well-balanced meals, he will, on the basis of diet alone, increase his intake of vitamins in sufficient amounts to supply his daily needs.

The ingestion of large quantities of vitamin preparations is currently popular among athletes. These megadose vitamins have not been determined to be beneficial, and overdoses of vitamins, especially the fat-soluble vitamins (A, D, E and K), can lead to toxicity. Excessive doses of vitamin D can cause hypercalcemia, with side effects as mild as gastrointestinal irritability or as serious as renal cardiac failure. Vitamin E toxicity can result in headaches, nausea, fatigue, dizziness and blurred vision. Vitamin A is a neurotoxin and results in malaise, lethargy, insomnia and restlessness, as well as increased intracranial pressure.

Of all the vitamins, vitamin C has perhaps received the most publicity. It is well established that 45 mg of vitamin C—the Federal Drug Administration minimal daily requirement—is sufficient for this vitamin's role in maintaining normal blood clotting mechanisms, collagen repair (healing) and in enhancing absorption. Claims that large ingestions of vitamin C in the range of 1,500 to 5,000 mg per day can prevent the common cold, cure herpes virus infections, prevent cancer and retard the onset of arteriosclerotic heart disease have not been substantiated. Since this vitamin is water soluble, most ingested vitamin C in excess of the daily minimal requirement is excreted by the kidneys. However, nausea and diarrhea are reported complications from excessive doses of this vitamin.

Pangamic acid, an apricot pit derivative, is supposedly a mixture of sodium and calcium glucamate and deisoporpylkmine dichloroacetate. Some claim it is an essential nutrient and should be considered a vitamin, terming pangamic acid vitamin B-15. Authorities such as Goodhart, the author of many nutritional texts, maintain that pangamic acid is not an essential nutrient and, therefore, should not be considered a vitamin. The Federal Drug Administration agrees with this last point of view.

"BLOOD DOPING"

"Blood doping" refers to withdrawing a unit of blood from the athlete and storing it for several weeks prior to competition. Normal homeostatic mechanisms then begin synthesizing red cells to return the red cell count to the "predraw" level. Prior to the event, the athlete is transfused his previously drawn unit of blood. These added cells raise the red blood cell count to greater than normal levels, in the hope that additional red cells will increase oxygen-carrying capacity and, hence, improve aerobic endurance. Data substantiating this conclusion are controversial. Sludging of red cells secondary to sudden increase in number in an athlete whose total fluid level may be somewhat depleted is a risk of this procedure. It is not advised.

EMERGENCY TREATMENT OF DRUG ABUSE

When faced with drug abuse, an overall assessment of the patient is necessary, as in any illness or injury, and treatment priorities must sometimes be established. In general, airway maintenance is the first priority. Preventing self-injury, maintaining level of consciousness and observing for other injuries are the other crucial parts of the initial assessment.

Most patients who have abused drugs have an altered sense of consciousness, often depressed. Do not induce vomiting in any patient who is not fully conscious and fully alert due to the danger of aspiration of the vomited material into the tracheobronchial tree.

Convulsions, often major seizures, are frequently seen in drug abuse patients from a number of different causes. Protect the patient from falls or biting the tongue by the usual techniques for managing patients with convulsions.

Maintain the level of consciousness by constant stimulation, either by gentle shaking, conversation or light pinching. Once the patient is unconscious, severe respiratory depression may follow rapidly. It is sometimes necessary to insert an airway and ventilate these patients if respirations are severely depressed.

Approach patients under the influence of hallucinogenic or stimulant drugs in a calm, professional, sympathetic manner. Often it is possible to "talk the patient down," that is, to calm the patient. Gain the patient's confidence, and avoid the use of restraints if possible.

Patients in severely depressed states often injure themselves and may not be aware that they have done so. Quickly check the patient for suspected fractures or other injuries. Sometimes the patient has a head injury as well as a drug overdose and it is difficult, if not impossible, to separate the effects of the two. These patients should be promptly taken to the hospital and treated as though they had sustained a serious head injury.

Patients who abuse injectable drugs may have fever from deep infections of the brain, heart or other organs resulting from the use of contaminated equipment and unsterile drugs. The source of these infections may not be apparent. The incidence of hepatitis is particularly high in these patients, and they may be jaundiced. Jaundice can be detected by observing the yellow coloring of the sclera (white portion of the eye) or the skin. Always remember that hepatitis is extremely contagious and handle these patients carefully to avoid infection.

Patients who fall asleep or into a coma from drug overdose may lie with their arms and legs twisted in contorted positions for several hours, impairing the blood supply to extremities, which may be cold, swollen, paralyzed, cyanotic or numb and often permanently injured. These injuries should be noted, the extremity splinted and the patient promptly transported to the hospital.

Superficial infections of the hands and forearms are common in patients who abuse injectable drugs. The extremity will be hot, swollen, red and obviously inflamed. Treat the extremity as though injured, with a bulky, soft dressing and a splint.

Stimulants

Frequently abused stimulant drugs include amphetamines ("speed," "bennies") and cocaine ("coke," "snow"). Caffeine, found in coffee and cola drinks, is a mild stimulant, as are certain antiasthmatic drugs such as adrenalin and aminophylline. Certain drugs commonly used as nasal decongestants, such as ephedrine and isoproterenol, are also mild stimulants. These drugs are taken by mouth with the exception of cocaine, which is frequently sniffed.

The sale of certain equipment, particularly that used to prepare cocaine, is legal in many states. Look around the patient and his environment for spoons, lamps, pipes and other evidence of cocaine paraphernalia.

All of these stimulants can cause a profound reactive depression when they are stopped or if they are suddenly taken in large amounts. However, the usual manifestation of overdose of a stimulant drug is an obviously excited, agitated patient with rapid pulse and respirations, and even convulsions.

These patients require emotional support. They occasionally ask to be taken to a hospital and should be carried without restraint if at all possible. Never leave this patient alone, but treat him like any other emotionally ill patient.

If the patient has depressed respirations, maintain the airway and provide assisted ventilation, if necessary, during transport to the hospital.

Depressants

Physical findings that suggest addiction to depressants include small, nonreactive pupils and needle marks on the skin of the forearms and hands, left by multiple intravenous injections. An overdose patient is seriously ill and should have an adequate airway established and maintained and be promptly transported to the emergency department.

Hallucinogens

A patient who has taken a hallucinogenic drug such as LSD or marijuana usually is in an altered state of awareness. These patients rarely take a large enough overdose to cause coma or unconsciousness, but occasionally the hallucinatory effect may be extremely unpleasant and result in a panic state—the "bad trip." The emergency care of these patients is the same as for any other emotionally ill patient: emotional support; a calm, professional, straightforward manner; and prompt transportation to the hospital. Do not restrain these patients unless they are physically dangerous, and do not leave them alone.

Allergic Reactions

Any drug can cause allergic reactions. Penicillin is the most common widely used drug that causes an allergic reaction. The most serious allergic reactions are sudden cardiovascular collapse (anaphylactic shock), wheezing respirations, itching, rashes and urticaria (hives) on the skin, vomiting and fever. Many persons who know they have an allergy wear identifying bracelets or tags. Always search for this on a patient with a suspected allergic reaction. Allergic reactions may be fatal. Give these patients basic life support and transport them immediately to the emergency department.

Virtually any drug taken in improper amounts may result in undesirable reactions (see Chapter 41 for further information).

Multiple Drug Abuse

Persons who abuse drugs often take more than one drug at a time, creating combined drug reactions. Try to find out as much as possible about what drug or drugs the patient has been taking. Look for empty bottles, needles, syringes and paper wrappers that may contain powdered drugs, bottles, spoons, alcohol lamps or other evidence of drug paraphernalia. Send all these to the hospital with the patient. These patients are seriously ill. Drug combinations result in effects far greater than those of individual drugs taken separately. The patient or an acquaintance may be able to tell you exactly what drug or drugs have been taken.

Drug Withdrawal

Patients who are addicted to drugs, that is, who are physically dependent upon a constant supply of a drug, may experience a severe reaction when the drug is withdrawn. These reactions may be in the form of anxiety, nausea and vomiting, convulsions, delirium, profuse sweating, severe abdominal cramps and, ultimately, death.

Alcohol Abuse

Alcohol is a powerful central nervous system depressant. It is the most commonly abused drug in modern American society. Alcoholics can be young, middle-aged, elderly, men, women, executives, businessmen or blue-collar factory workers as well as "bums." More than 50% of all traffic fatalities or injuries involve at least one drunken driver. Chronic alcoholics are often suicidal. Alcohol, like all other drugs, builds up a certain tolerance. Patients addicted to alcohol require larger amounts to get the same effect.

As a depressant alcohol dulls the sense of awareness, slows reflexes and decreases reac-

tion time. Patients under the influence of alcohol may show the same signs as patients with physical illnesses or injuries, specifically head injuries, toxic reactions or uncontrolled diabetes. Always bear in mind that a patient suffering from the effects of alcohol could have a physical illness as well. If there is the slightest question a person may have some illness other than alcoholic overdose, bring the patient to the hospital. Often the family or acquaintances can provide a good history of the patient's drinking pattern.

Drunken patients may show aggressive, inappropriate behavior, fall easily and be combative. Take steps to protect them from self-injury. Occasionally, a patient consumes so much alcohol that signs of central nervous system depression appear and respiratory support may be necessary. Take these patients promptly to the hospital.

Alcohol Withdrawal

When a person used to a constant supply of alcohol withdraws from it, he develops a very specific syndrome. Perhaps the person can no longer buy alcohol, is ill or, for some other reason, is cut off from the source. The alcoholic withdrawal syndrome may manifest itself in two ways—alcoholic hallucinations and delirium tremens. In alcoholic hallucinations the patient perceives figures, often walking on the wall, sometimes seeming to attack the patient. These hallucinations are frightening but are temporary.

Alcoholic hallucinations usually lead to delirium tremens, a much more severe complication. Delirium tremens may occur from one to seven days after the withdrawal and are characterized by restlessness followed by fever, sweating, confusion and disorientation, agitation, delusions and hallucinations. A history of chronic alcohol ingestion, with one or more days of withdrawal, can usually be obtained from the patient's family or an acquaintance. The mortality rate in delirium tremens is high. These patients are extremely ill and need to be hospitalized. During transportation, protect the patient from further self-injury and watch for the development of convulsions. Should convulsions occur, treat them appropriately. These patients may also suffer from hypovolemic shock due to sweating and fluid loss. Should signs of vascular collapse (low blood pressure, rapid pulse) appear, transport the patient with the feet slightly elevated and the head turned to one side to avoid aspiration if vomiting occurs. These patients are usually irrational and respond inappropriately to suggestions or conversation. Nonetheless, try to approach the patient calmly, with reassurance and emotional support.

Alcohol in large amounts is a gastric irritant. Persons who have consumed large amounts of alcohol may vomit forcefully. Sometimes they will vomit up blood, either from laceration of the lower portion of the esophagus caused by repeated vomiting, irritation of the stomach wall, or the rupture of lower esophageal veins enlarged because of underlying liver disease (esophageal varices). Bring anyone who vomits blood to the hospital immediately since blood loss can produce shock.

Long-term, chronic abuse of alcohol produces muscular incoordination, memory loss, apathy and lack of interest, and other obvious evidences of chronic brain deterioration. Always search for fractures and other injuries in the alcoholic who is so prone to falling and self-injury.

Environmental Problems

50

HEAT DISORDERS

The main center for thermal regulation in the body is in the hypothalamus, where thermal receptors sense the local temperature of the heated or cooled blood to this area. Autonomic impulses to increase body sweating and peripheral vasodilatation result from hypothalamic temperature elevations.

Normal body temperature is maintained by precise balance between heat production and heat loss. Body heat is produced by basic metabolic processes, by food intake (specific dynamic action) and by muscular activity. Heat loss occurs in five ways.

1. *Conduction:* When the body comes in contact with a cooler object, for example, a cold wet shirt, heat is directly transferred from the warmer body to the cooler object.
2. *Convection:* When cool air moves across the body surface, heat is transferred to the cooler air, warming it and cooling the body.
3. *Evaporation:* When water on the body surface is transformed from a liquid to a vapor, the body loses heat. Vaporization of approximately 1 gm of water removes about .6 kcal of heat by perspiration.
4. *Respiration:* When inspired, cooler air is raised to the body temperature in the lung and heat is lost through respiration.
5. *Radiation:* Heat can be radiated by the body to the environment.

Most of these mechanisms depend upon the fact that the environmental temperature is lower than the body temperature. If the external temperature is higher than the body temperature, the primary source of heat loss is vaporization of sweat, assuming the humidity is low enough to accept the vaporization.

When the body is challenged by an elevated environmental temperature, mechanisms to increase heat loss are activated that include cutaneous vasodilatation, sweating and increased respiratory rate.

Extreme heat produces both an immediate and delayed effect on the body physiology. The immediate response is vasodilatation of the vessels in the skin with increased blood flow to the skin and increased sweat production, maximizing losses through radiation and convection. With moderate heat exposure, the increased blood flow to the skin is achieved at the expense of flow to other organs. Greater heat stress increases the pulse rate to maintain cardiac output. Respiratory rate also increases to assist in cooling when the air temperature is less than body temperature.

There are approximately 2 million eccrine, or sweat, glands in the body. Sweat production increases sharply with increasing temperature and may result in the loss of 2 to 8 liters of water per 24 hours. The average person loses about 2 gm of sodium chloride in each liter of sweat at the beginning of warm weather. With acclimatization, the body conserves sodium chloride. Sweating is an efficient means of cooling when the humidity is low, with up to 600 kcal dissipated for each liter of sweat that evaporates. When the humidity rises, evaporation of sweat decreases. No heat loss results from sweat that drips off or remains in clothing. When the environmental temperature is less than skin temperature, 30.6 C (87 F), heat is transferred out of the body. At rest with the temperature below 30.6 C (87 F), about two thirds of the body's normal heat loss occurs due to radiation and convection of heat. The rest of the heat is lost through evaporation from the skin and the lungs, and a small amount is lost through the urine and feces. As the ambient temperature approaches skin temperature and exceeds 30.6 C (87 F), loss of body heat through radiation and convection is sharply curtailed. As heat transfer is reversed, heat loss is mostly achieved by evaporation.

There are five principal mechanisms of human thermal regulation:

1. Excitation of sweating by the central heat receptors
2. Vasodilatation elicited by central heat receptors
3. Inhibition of sweating by cold receptors of the skin
4. Excitation of metabolic heat production by cold receptors of the skin
5. Inhibition of thermal regulatory heat centers

The rate of water loss can be substantially increased by sweating. Evaporation over most of the body surface directly cools the blood that runs through the capillary skin. The rate of cooling by evaporation depends on the amount of body surface exposed, the condition and nature of the covering material, the degree of humidity in the air in contact with the skin and the rate of air circulation over the surface.

Salt in Warm Weather

For years controversy has existed as to whether or not athletes who perspire heavily consume more salt in the summer than they do in the winter, or more than the average population. An adequate consumption of salt is rarely a problem in the typical American diet. In fact typical Americans consume an excessive amount of sodium, i.e., 5 to 10 gm of sodium per day, although we probably require only 1 to 3 gm. Sodium is widely used as a flavoring agent, a preservative in packaged foods, and most Americans use table salt on food. One ''Big Mac'' supplies the sodium needs for one day.

Several key electrolytes are lost in sweat, namely, sodium, chloride, potassium and magnesium. The quantity of electrolytes varies from day to day and from individual to individual, depending in part on the person's degree of conditioning or acclimatization. The well conditioned athlete loses fewer electrolytes than his poorly conditioned counterpart. The electrolyte concentrations in sweat vary greatly: .3 to 2.7 gm of sodium, .3 to 2.8 gm of chloride, and .2 to 1.2 gm of potassium per liter. Since a typical mixed diet furnishes 3 to 10 gm of sodium, 2.5 to 8 gm of chloride and 2 to 6 gm of potassium, net deficiencies of these electrolytes are highly unlikely even with profuse sweating.

Most electrolyte losses can be made up at meals following athletic events. Rarely, an athlete may lose 5 to 6 liters of sweat per athletic event, manifested by weight loss of 2 to 10 pounds, and probably require electrolyte replacement. Water is most important to replace electrolytes during and immediately after the event. Then a diet including potassium-rich foods such as potatoes, tomatoes, tomato juice, citrus fruits, vegetables, meat, peas, fish and beans is recommended. Whenever athletes add extra sodium to their diets, they should drink liberal amounts of water simultaneously. Otherwise, excessive sodium can draw water out of the body cells, accentuating the dehydration.

Water loss in a sweating athlete exceeds sodium loss and is generally of greater concern. Adequate fluid intake is essential to maintain the hydrated state and prevent an abnormal rise in body temperature. An average adult exercising in a neutral environment requires approximately 2.5 liters of water a day. This water comes from all fluids consumed as well as from food. The average runner requires an additional 1.5 to 2 liters of water per hour of active sweating and 2 to 4 liters of water per hour when competing in endurance events.

An athlete should conscientiously consume fluids before, during and after an event to insure hydration. Thirst alone is not an adequate indicator of fluid needs. The athlete should be weighed before and after the event to determine the amount of fluid that needs to be replaced. Advise those players losing over 3% of the body weight in a vigorous practice to take water frequently during practice, and to adequately rehydrate prior to the next practice.

While maintaining hydration, the athlete should avoid excessive protein, caffeine, alcoholic beverages and foods that increase urine production, which might result in dehydration. Most authorities agree plain water is the best replacement. Salt-containing hypertonic beverages probably should be avoided as a salt replacement because their sodium content aggravates dehydration. Salt tablets are not recommended for sodium replacement because they cause gastric fullness and distress.

Heat Exposure Syndromes

Aside from skin disorders such as prickly heat and sunburn, basically three types of syndromes result from exposure to heat.

Heat Cramps

Normal muscle contractions or relaxations require a strict balance of salt and water within the muscle. With excessive perspiration, both water and salt are lost. Some physicians believe cramps are due to excessive fluid loss in the muscles; others believe electrolyte imbalance causes the muscle spasm. Blood volume is usually well preserved and the individual is alert. Heat cramps occur in persons who sweat profusely and, like all disorders due to heat, usually take place at the beginning of the warm weather season before acclimatization. These persons usually are otherwise in good condition. These cramps may involve the legs, abdominal muscles or arms. They are different from cramps from overexertion, and there is no history of injury, such as a pulled muscle. The diagnosis is largely by exclusion to rule out an acute muscle injury. These persons may have a history of heat cramps.

Once the cramps have developed, treatment is rest from the exertional stress and passive stretching. Ingestion of water or a hypotonic saline solution (made by mixing 1 teaspoon of table salt to 1 quart of water) may help reverse the cramps. Prevention involves insuring adequate fluid and a normal salt diet during times of excessive sweating. Conditioning and acclimatization also help reduce the incidence of cramps.

Heat Exhaustion

This is a more severe heat syndrome caused by inadequate cardiovascular responsiveness to circulatory stresses induced by heat. Vasoconstriction in other parts of the body or volume expansion normally compensates for initial diversion of blood flow to the skin. Otherwise fit individuals involved in extreme physical exertion in a hot environment can develop heat exhaustion. Under these conditions the muscle mass of the body and the brain require increased blood flow. At the same time the skin needs an increased blood flow to radiate heat from the skin in the form of sweat. Because the vascular system is inadequate to meet the simultaneous demands placed upon it by the skin, muscle and viscera, heat exhaustion results. It is an insidious, slowly progressive, peripheral vascular collapse, or "shock" syndrome.

Heat exhaustion, also called heat prostration, then, is characterized principally by the signs of peripheral vascular collapse or shock—weakness, faintness, dizziness, headache, loss of appetite, nausea, pallor, diffuse sweating, vomiting, an urge to defecate and postural syncopy.

Heat exhaustion is known to be of two types. One occurs with excessive salt loss and the other with excessive water loss, which is more common in athletes. In the water depletion type, more water than salt has been lost.

The symptoms develop due to reduced blood volume from fluid loss. The patient may appear ashen and gray. In salt depletion heat exhaustion, the skin is cold and clammy. With water depletion heat exhaustion, the skin is hot and dry. Vital signs, however, are normal and body temperature may even be below normal. A hypertonic state is caused by a relative increase in electrolytes. These persons may become unconscious if not treated. This type of "too much salt" heat exhaustion is also seen in people who take excessive salt tablets as well as with water depletion.

In addition to replenishing electrolytes and fluids, treat the patient's mild state of hypovolemic shock by having him lie down in a cool room. He may or may not need intravenous fluids. Rest diminishes the demands on his circulatory system. Heat exhaustion is common and is ordinarily promptly reversed. Pre-existing conditions such as cardiovascular disease, vomiting and diarrhea, however, can aggravate it. Monitor the athlete closely during activity. Be alert for poorly conditioned athletes who are more susceptible to these conditions. Prevent physical activity in the athlete who suffers heat exhaustion until he has returned to the predehydrated state.

Heat Stroke

Heat stroke is the third and most serious syndrome. In heat stroke all of the mechanisms for body cooling have failed to the extent that severe hyperpyrexia ensues. It may develop suddenly or progress from water depletion heat exhaustion. Heat stroke is a true emergency with a very high mortality rate. Untreated victims of heat stroke die because of damage to the cells of the central nervous system. Since some survivors may have permanent nerve damage because of hyperpyrexia, rapid and vigorous treatment is essential for full recovery. Heat stroke in the athlete is almost always precipitated by prolonged, strenuous physical exercise, either when the athlete is poorly acclimatized or in situations that do not allow evaporation of sweat. Strenuous muscular work contributes to the development of heat stroke by increasing the production of body heat.

Pathophysiology of Heat Stroke. Under conditions of maximum heat stress when the ambient temperature approaches the skin temperature and the humidity increases, evaporation of sweat efficiently removes heat from the body. Under conditions of maximum heat stress, however, the initially high rates of sweat production cannot be maintained indefinitely. When the rate of sweat production falls, the body temperature rises abruptly. This failure of perspiration is known as "sweat fatigue" or anhidrosis. The maximum amount of sweat that can be produced upon exposure to heat is related to the humidity. The absence of sweating and presence of moderate dehydration in the exercising athlete intensifies hyperpyrexia. For every rise of one degree Fahrenheit in core temperature, metabolism increases 7%, creating a vicious circle. Heat stroke usually occurs when the ambient temperature is over 35 C (95 F) for a day or two and the relative humidity is in the range of 50% to 75%, as heat illness is cumulative.

Although heat stroke is the least common of the heat disorders, it is often a problem for distance runners in hot environments. In football, it is second only to head injury as the most frequent cause of fatalities. Wrestlers dehydrated through weight loss are also particularly susceptible to heat stroke.

With fluid loss from exercise, the heat regulatory mechanism fails and the central sweating mechanism shuts off to avoid further dehydration. As the heat generated by metabolic activity builds up, body temperature rises yet the skin is dry. The rising temperature increases cell metabolism, especially in the central nervous system where damage occurs.

Premonitory symptoms are irritability, aggressiveness, emotional instability and hysteria, progressing to apathy, failure to respond to questions and disorientation. The patient may have an unsteady gait and glassy stare. Hot and dry skin accompanies the final signs of collapse and unconsciousness. Early in the course of the disease, the pulse is rapid and full. As the changes of heat stroke become established and tissue is damaged by body heat, vasomotor collapse occurs, blood pressure falls and the pulses become rapid and weak.

Treatment must begin as soon as heat stroke is diagnosed. Emergency care is designed to rid the body of excessive heat as rapidly as possible, reducing temperature below 38 C (100 F). Immerse the patient in a bathtub in water cooled with ice if available or use wet sheets or compresses and fans while transporting the patient to the hospital. Begin any form of cooling immediately. Treatment for shock may require intravenous fluids, but cooling is the priority and must be continued during transportation to the hospital. Medication may be required to prevent shivering during body cooling.

Air conditioned room cooling is effective only for minor hyperpyrexia. Antipyretic drugs, such as aspirin, do not help because they require an intact heat-losing mechanism. Although external cooling should be carried out until the patient's temperature falls to 38 C (100 F), the patient should be observed for secondary rises in temperature.

Preventing Heat Stress Syndromes

Heat stress syndromes are obviously related to climate, determined by temperature and humidity. Since climate and humidity cannot be controlled, other factors must be, especially the athlete's condition and acclimatization. Coaching techniques, color and type of uniforms, the time of day and the intensity of training all contribute to heat injuries. Table 50:1 lists the causes, clinical signs and symptoms and treatments for the heat stress syndromes.

TABLE 50:1.   Heat Stress Syndromes

Disorder	Cause	Clinical Signs and Symptoms	Treatment
Heat cramps	Excessive fluid loss in muscles Electrolyte imbalance Athlete is not acclimated to local climate	Profuse sweating Cramps involving abdominal muscles, or extremities	Rest in cool environment Passive stretching Ingestion of H_2O or hypotonic solution
Heat exhaustion (excessive salt loss)	Profuse sweating; with inadequate replacement of body salts; vomiting or diarrhea	Weakness, faintness, dizziness, headache, loss of appetite, nausea, pallor, profuse sweating, urge to defecate Skin is gray and ashen, cold and clammy	Rest in a cool room in recumbent position Fluids or IV if unconscious, increase fluid and salt intake in normal diet Discontinue activity until well under control
Heat exhaustion (excessive H_2O loss)	Profuse sweating with inadequate replacement of body fluids, vomiting or diarrhea	Skin is hot and dry, small urine volume, excessive thirst, weakness, headache, unconsciousness	Rest in cool room in recumbent position Sponge with cool H_2O Increase intake of fluids Keep record of body weight Discontinue activity until well under control
Heat stroke	Progress from H_2O depletion Failure of all mechanisms for body cooling This is a true medical emergency	Irritability, aggressiveness, emotional instability, hysteria, progression to apathy, disorientation, unsteady gait, glassy stare Skin is hot and dry, pulse is rapid and full, blood pressure falls	Immerse patient in bathtub cooled with ice or wet compresses with fan blowing Transport to hospital immediately, treat for shock Cooling is top priority

Acclimatization

Acclimatization is the body's adaptation to heat stress and increases capacity to work at high environmental temperatures. It was first studied when military personnel were exposed to tropical climates. Unable to work for the first few days, they gradually became able to tolerate high temperatures without becoming exhausted. Acclimatization involves modification in neural, hormonal and cardiovascular physiology. The changes in cardiovascular physiology are very similar to those observed during general physical training. After acclimatization, there is less subjective discomfort during heat exposure, with less increase in pulse and respiratory rate under the same conditions of heat and stress. Cardiovascular stability with postural changes and activity is also greater. Skin and rectal temperatures remain close to normal and sweat production increases after acclimatization. Sweating begins sooner after exposure to heat and work, or at a lower environmental temperature, than before acclimatization.

There is a diversity of opinion as to how long full acclimatization takes. Many say that in four to seven days and as little as 90 minutes of exposure to heat per day, the body can fully adapt to the stress of heat, whereas others say that full acclimatization may take two months. Previous physical conditioning and exercise enhances the ability to adapt to heat. Once achieved, acclimatization is maintained for several weeks with short periods of re-exposure. After six weeks of heat exposure, the body may be able to produce 2½ times the person's normal volume of sweat.

Preseason Conditioning

The body's heat regulating mechanism becomes accustomed to the elevation of internal temperature that accompanies vigorous exercise, often as high as 39.4 C (103 F) in the trained athlete. When tested under conditions of high heat and high humidity, the physically fit require much less acclimatization to heat than those out of condition. Because the long-distance runner characteristically can produce elevated internal temperatures, running is a good preseason conditioning exercise. At least four weeks of long-distance running should be carried out in the preseason.

Environment

Test the air a short time prior to any practice or game using a wet bulb, globe, temperature index (WBGT index), which is based upon the combined effects of air temperature, relative humidity, radiant heat and air movement. The military has established standards for when training is allowed to continue. A sling psychrometer can be used to correlate the dry ball temperature with relative humidity. Again, existing standards should be followed on when to allow, modify or prohibit training when the humidity is high (Fig. 50:1). In the event of severe thunderstorms with lightning, all outdoor athletic activities, practices and games should be suspended.

Coaching Techniques

Equipment and Uniforms. These should be light weight, porous and light in color. Sleeves should be short and socks should be low. The

Temp. (°F.)	Humidity	Procedure
80°–90°	Under 70%	Watch those athletes who tend toward obesity.
80°–90° 90°–100°	Over 70% Under 70%	Athletes should take a 10-minute rest every hour and tee shirts should be changed when wet. All athletes should be under constant and careful supervision.
90°–100° Over 100°	Over 70%	Under these conditions it would be well to suspend practice. A shortened program conducted in shorts and tee shirts could be established.

FIGURE 50:1.

athlete should have the opportunity to change perspiration-soaked uniforms during the practice session. Expose as much skin as possible to the air.

Schedules. Practices during hot, humid weather should be early in the morning or late in the afternoon to avoid the worst heat. Early in the season, schedule night games. However, if games must be played during the late mornings or early afternoons in hot, humid climates, the players must be acclimatized to those conditions. Practice sessions during high temperature-high humidity conditions to acclimatize athletes should be shorter and less intense, with less clothing or uniforms and more frequent rest and water breaks than a normal practice session held during the cool part of the day. Allow frequent rest breaks during the practice, i.e., ten minutes every half hour. Consider canceling practice in extreme temperature and humidity.

Free Fluid Quantity. Encourage free intake of fluid during games and practice sessions, but avoid large amounts at any one time. The rate of water replacement should be about 1 pint for each pound lost, or 10 ounces every half hour. In ideal situations, control the rate of dehydration by weighing the athlete and rehydrating him between practice sessions. Weight should be checked daily and recorded. It has been proven that a well hydrated athlete achieves good physical conditioning faster than a poorly hydrated athlete.

Salt Tablets. Most trainers and physicians feel that adequate table salt with meals is all that is necessary to replace electrolytes lost in practice and games. However, hypotonic electrolyte solutions with .10 solution of salt may be helpful in very warm areas where perspiration results in considerable salt and fluid loss.

COLD INJURIES

The human body is a heat-generating mechanism. Its temperature must remain within a very narrow range simply for survival, i.e.,

23.9 C to 44.4 C (75 F to 112 F). For proper bodily function the range is even narrower: 37 C (98.6 F) ± a few degrees. In addition to the warmth and heat the body produces, it also gains heat from external sources such as sun, fire and ingestion of warm foods.

For the purpose of heat regulation, the body consists of a "core," i.e., the brain, heart, lungs and major abdominal organs, and a "shell," i.e., the skin, muscles and extremities. When exposed to cold, the body attempts to increase internal heat production by increasing muscular activity, such as shivering, and by increasing the basal metabolic rate at which food stored within the body is burned. Heat loss is decreased by reducing the circulation of blood in the shell.

Cold injury occurs in two ways. In the first, the core temperature is maintained but the shell temperature falls, resulting in local injuries that include frostnip, superficial frost bite, deep frost bite, chilblains, trench foot or immersion foot. In the other, both the core and the shell temperatures fall, systemic hypothermia occurs, all body processes slow down, and the patient may die if not treated.

Body parts freeze when not enough heat is available to counteract external cold resulting in local injury. Predisposing factors include:

1. Inadequate insulation from cold and wind
2. Restricted circulation because of arterial disease or tight clothing, especially footwear
3. Fatigue
4. Poor nutrition
5. The use of alcohol
6. The body's normal effort to maintain its core temperature by shunting blood flow away from the shell

Most commonly affected are hands, feet, ears and exposed parts of the face. All of these areas are located far from the heart and normally subjected to rapid heat loss because of a large surface area to volume ratio.

Freezing temperatures affect the cells in the body in a predictable fashion. A cell is mostly water, which becomes cool and eventually freezes, no longer able to function. The resulting ice crystals destroy the cell. Local cold injuries are the result of injuries of the capillary blood vessels and other tissue components of the skin and the subcutaneous cells. Cell injuries are all essentially the same, varying only in degree and depth. Duration of the exposure, the temperature to which the skin has been exposed and the wind velocity are the three most important factors in determining the severity of a local injury.

Frostnip, or Incipient Frostbite

Frostnip usually affects the tips of the ears, nose, cheeks, chin, tips of the fingers and toes, usually in conditions of high wind, extreme cold or both. It is manifested as a sudden blanching or whiteness of the skin. Frostnip comes on slowly and painlessly. The afflicted person often does not notice it, and frequently a companion first perceives it. There may be no permanent tissue damage, and it can be treated effectively by the firm, steady pressure of a warm hand, blowing hot breath or by holding the nipped fingers motionless in the arm pit. Do not rub the skin with snow. As warmth and color return, tingling may occur. After thawing, the skin may turn red and may flake for several days.

Superficial Frostbite

Superficial frostbite usually involves the skin and the underlying superficial tissue. The skin appears white and waxy and is firm to the touch, but the tissue beneath it is soft and resilient. The person should be taken indoors, protected from the cold and subjected to the same, steady, careful rewarming as for frostnip. Again, do not rub with snow or the hand. When the injured area thaws, it is first numb, then mottled blue or purple. Capillary damage and plasma leaks into the tissue cause swelling. If the frostbite is severe, the tissue beneath the outer layers of skin is involved and blisters may form. Throbbing, aching and burning may last for weeks. The skin may remain per-

manently red and tender and sensitive to re-exposure to cold so that these susceptible areas should receive extra protection.

Deep Frostbite

Deep frostbite is extremely serious and usually involves the hands and feet. The tissues are cold, pale and solid. The tissues deep to the skin and subcutaneous layers are usually injured and may be completely destroyed. Render emergency treatment as quickly as possible keeping the patient dry and providing external warming. The injured area turns purplish blue and becomes extremely painful after thawing. Large blisters or gangrene may develop in the first day or two. Permanent tissue damage depends on the temperature and the duration of freezing.

The treatment of the above three conditions calls for early and rapid rewarming by whatever means possible, including warm water baths. If a prolonged delay is anticipated before reaching a medical facility, rapid rewarming with warm water should be instituted. Keep the temperature of the water between 38 C to 40.6 C (100 F to 105 F) with thermometer control, making sure it does not become too hot, yet maintaining a temperature 6 F or 7 F warmer than normal body temperature. Check the warmth continually because immersing the cold extremity causes loss of heat. The container should be large enough so that neither the extremity nor the patient touches the sides. Continue rewarming until the frozen area is deep red or bluish in color. Maintain the patient's body temperature with warm drinks. Analgesic medication may be needed. Always guard against infection. Apply bandages loosely under sterile conditions, do not rupture blisters and insert pads between the toes.

Chilblains

Chilblains result from repeated exposure of bare skin to temperatures in the low teens Centigrade (or 60s F) for prolonged periods. The injury results in red, swollen, hot, tender, itching areas, usually on the fingers or toes, and the lesions tend to recur in the same areas during cold weather each season. There may be permanent skin changes between the periods of recurrence. This injury represents a chronic injury of the skin and the peripheral capillary circulation. There is no treatment for chilblains once the skin injury has been established except to prevent recurrence and to protect the area from further exposure to cold.

Trench or Immersion Foot

Trench or immersion foot results from the wet cooling of an extremity over hours or days at temperatures slightly above freezing. It is frequently seen in military personnel and shipwrecked seamen. The lesion represents primary damage to the capillary circulation of the skin, which may progress to necrosis or gangrene of the skin, muscle and nerves. The involved extremity is cold, swollen, waxy, mottled and numb. After it is warmed, it becomes red, swollen and hot, and blisters may develop as well as gangrene. The treatment is to remove the wet, cold foot gear and gently rewarm the extremity, maintaining good local hygiene and applying warm, dry covering.

General Treatment for Local Injuries

Only frostnip and superficial frostbite should be treated in the field, with direct application of body heat. The remaining patients should be taken to a hospital as soon as possible. Enroute, protect the damaged area from further injury, especially from rubbing, chafing and contusion. If absolutely necessary, a patient may be allowed to walk on a frostbitten extremity providing that no thawing has occurred. Walking even a long distance on a frostbitten limb does not lessen the chance of successful treatment if the limb has not thawed. However, once the frozen limb has thawed, the patient becomes a stretcher case. Walking on a thawed limb with the resulting chance of refreezing is extremely painful and dangerous. Blisters are usually a good prognostic sign, indicating that only a partial thickness of skin has been damaged.

Systemic Hypothermia

General, severe body cooling can occur at temperatures well above freezing. It is usually caused by exposure to low or rapidly dropping temperatures, cold moisture, snow or ice. It is aggravated by hunger, fatigue and exertion and may be associated with other local cold injuries. Documentation of the extent of hypothermia requires a clinical thermometer that can reach a low temperature.

Generalized body cooling has five states.

1. Shivering, an attempt by the body to generate heat
2. Apathy, sleeplessness, listlessness and indifference, which may accompany rapid cooling of the body
3. Unconsciousness with a glassy stare, a very slow pulse rate and slow respiratory rate
4. Freezing of the extremities
5. Death

Shivering usually begins at a rectal temperature of 35 C (95 F) and, as the cooling proceeds, clumsiness, fumbling, stumbling, falling, slow reactions, mental confusion and difficulty in speaking follow. Death may occur within two hours of the onset of the first symptoms.

Systemic hypothermia is an acute first priority medical emergency and requires the rapid transfer of the patient to emergency facilities. The basic principles of emergency care are:

1. Prevent further heat loss
2. Rewarm the patient as rapidly and safely as possible
3. Be alert for complications

Mild to moderate hypothermia (rectal temperature of 27.2 C to 38 C [81 to 95 F] with the patient conscious) is treated by preventing further heat loss by removing the patient from the wind, replacing wet clothing, adding appropriate insulating material and providing external heat in any way possible, e.g., hot water bottles, electric blankets, camp fires, or body heat from rescuers. If the patient is conscious, hot liquids may be given. An effective way of rewarming a patient with systemic hypothermia is to immerse him in a tub of warm water kept between 40.6 C to 43.3 C (105 F to 110 F).

Severe hypothermia (rectal temperature below 27.2 C [81 F] with unconsciousness) carries serious dangers from cardiac arrhythmias and rewarming shock. While the above procedures are carried out, facilities to diagnose and treat cardiac arrhythmias, especially ventricular fibrillation, should be available. Rewarming shock occurs as the circulatory system of the body warms and veins dilate before the heart becomes able to support the expanded circulation within a dilated system. Evacuate this patient to a medical facility; do not warm him in the field. Start intravenous fluid and monitor vital signs. These patients may appear dead yet may still be revived.

Contributing Factors in Cold Injuries

Local injuries obviously occur in colder climates when the ambient temperature is closer to freezing and the skin is exposed (Table 50:2).

Systemic hypothermia, however, occurs in all months of the year, depending upon the activities and the altitude—temperatures of 50 F with a mild wind. Hunters, hikers, skiers and climbers exposed to unusually severe weather for which they have not prepared are in danger of hypothermia. The alcoholic or other ill person whose normal defenses from cold are insufficient can also experience hypothermia in mild conditions.

Athletes cannot acclimatize to cold as they can to heat. Rather they must prepare for cold by anticipating weather changes, by having the right clothing available in layers when possible, by having dry clothing available and, above all, recognizing the ever present possibility of hypothermia regardless of the season. Yet, the athlete should avoid overdressing, especially with synthetic materials that promote sweating and prevent evaporation.

All people subjected to a cold environment are susceptible to these injuries. They should be fully aware of the effect not only of cold but of windchill and understand the value of insulating materials and the layering principle in clothing.

TABLE 50:2. Wind-chill Factor

Wind Speed (miles per hour)	Equivalent Temperature (°F)													
Calm*	35	30	25	20	15	10	5	0	−5	−10	−15	−20	−25	−30
		COLD												
5	32	27	22	16	11	6	0	−5	−10	−15	−21	−26	−31	−36
			VERY COLD											
10	22	16	10	3	−3	−9	−15	−22	−27	−34	−40	−46	−52	−58
				BITTER COLD										
15	16	9	2	−5	−11	−18	−25	−31	−38	−45	−51	−58	−65	−72
20	12	4	−3	−10	−17	−24	−31	−39	−46	−53	−60	−67	−74	−81
25	8	1	−7	−15	−22	−29	−36	−44	−51	−59	−66	−74	−81	−88
						EXTREME COLD								
30	6	−2	−10	−18	−25	−33	−41	−49	−56	−64	−71	−79	−86	−93
35	4	−4	−12	−20	−27	−35	−43	−52	−58	−67	−74	−82	−89	−97
40	3	−5	−13	−21	−29	−37	−45	−53	−60	−69	−76	−84	−92	−100

*"Calm-air" as used in wind-chill determinations actually refers to the conditions created by a person walking briskly (at 4 miles-per-hour) under calm wind conditions.

National Oceanic and Atmospheric Administration

ALTITUDE DISORDERS

Altitude sickness is a maladjustment of the individual to the hypoxia of a high altitude and is generally divided into three syndromes.

1. *Acute mountain sickness* (AMS)
2. *High altitude pulmonary edema* (HAPE)
3. *High altitude cerebral edema* (HACE)

These three forms may appear separately or simultaneously. They are not clear-cut entities and probably represent a common, underlying physiologic response to hypoxia. Almost everyone gets acute mountain sickness when exposed to high altitudes, but few develop the advanced stages. HAPE and HACE are serious and potentially fatal.

The basic cause of mountain sickness is not proven. The severity of symptoms and rapidity of onset vary from patient to patient. Some people are inherently more susceptible than others, especially young people who have made a rapid ascent. The symptoms are directly proportional to the rapidity of the ascent, the duration and degree of exertion, and are inversely proportional to acclimatization and physical conditioning. The initial signs and symptoms of altitude sickness are from oxygen lack or hypoxia. They are thought to be secondary changes since there may be a lag period before symptoms develop.

Altitude sickness is becoming more common as more people are trekking, skiing and taking part in recreational activities at higher altitudes than ever before. Inadequate time on weekend trips to acclimatize to high altitudes is definitely a factor in this disease. Symptoms may appear at 7,500 to 8,000 feet, and death has occurred at altitudes of 8,000 or 9,000 feet. In addition to the problems of hypoxia, people at higher altitudes face insidious temperature changes and increases in ultraviolet and radiation exposure.

Acute Mountain Sickness

Acute mountain sickness is the mildest form of altitude sickness, and most people will experience it. There is no direct relationship between the altitude and the severity of the illness. Mild to moderate cases occur at all altitudes. There is a time lag of 6 to 96 hours between arrival and the onset of symptoms, which include headache, difficulty sleeping, early morning arousal, dyspnea on exertion, loss of appetite, light headedness, fatigue, confusion, weakness, tachycardia or bradycardia and edema.

High Altitude Pulmonary Edema

High altitude pulmonary edema is a more dramatic form of altitude illness, and is an unusual form of noncardiac pulmonary edema. It may develop on the first exposure to high altitude, but frequently is seen after descent and re-ascent. Symptoms vary in severity. After the symptoms of acute mountain sickness subside, shortness of breath, increased rate of respiration and an irritating cough that progresses to hemoptysis and substernal chest pain may develop. The cough produces bloody, frothy sputum.

The diagnosis is suspected when rales are heard in the chest. It is imperative that these people return to a lower altitude quickly and that they be given oxygen when possible. They must be thoroughly re-evaluated before allowing re-ascent.

High Altitude Cerebral Edema

High altitude cerebral edema is a less common but very dangerous form of altitude sickness. Death has occurred as low as 8,000 feet but is rare below 12,000 feet. Its relationship to high altitude pulmonary edema is unclear. The symptoms are initially those of acute mountain sickness but with increasingly severe headaches followed by mental confusion, forgetfulness and emotional instability, hallucinations and, finally, localized motor weakness and reflex changes. The condition may progress to coma and death. Bradycardia is an initial finding and may be related to increased cerebral pressure. Judgment and coordination are impaired due to direct local swelling of the brain, especially the cerebellum. Occular signs and symptoms such as blurring of vision, papilledema, retinal and vitreous hemorrhage may develop.

Preventing Altitude Illness

Preparation for high altitude activities should include months of cardiovascular training, strength training and aerobic conditioning (running 12 to 15 miles a day). A person who is aerobically fit has a higher altitude threshold than an unfit person.

The symptoms of altitude illness are proportional to altitude and duration and degree of exertion divided by acclimatization and physical conditioning. Acclimatization involves a long, slow ascent, going up higher during the day and coming down lower to sleep and rest. Persons with coronary vascular disease or chronic obstructive pulmonary disease should avoid areas of low oxygen tension.

Acute mountain sickness is usually self-limited, lasting two to five days. Headaches usually respond to aspirin. Reduce activities during the early days in high altitudes, since most people adapt to higher altitudes in a few days. Avoiding fatty foods and encouraging a high carbohydrate diet helps control nausea.

High altitude pulmonary edema and cerebral edema are emergencies and when suspected, persons should descend. Oxygen should be used when available, and the patient should be carried down since exercise aggravates HAPE and HACE. Corticosteroids, such as dexamethasone or betamethasone, may be used to treat HACE, but all of these measures are secondary to descent. A diuretic such as acetazolamide may stabilize breathing.

DEPTH DISORDERS

The effect of barometric pressure on gas exchange causes three types of depth problems: descent, bottom and ascent.

Descent Problems

Descent causes compression problems commonly called ''squeeze'' injuries. Areas in the body normally hollow and containing air at atmospheric pressure are subjected to a ''squeeze'' from increasing external pressure as the diver descends. If the passage connecting the area to the throat or mouth is blocked, pressure within the cavity then cannot equalize readily. Such areas include the middle ear, the sinus cavities, the lung and the facial areas, especially the area around the eyes and nose. Equalization occurs if the diver pauses at intervals during descent to breathe compressed air at about the same pressure as the surrounding water. Swelling from an upper respiratory infection or an allergy can block the eustachian tubes connecting the middle ear to the outside. Individuals with these conditions are more susceptible to ''ear squeeze'' and should avoid diving until the condition clears. Ordinarily, pain prevents further descent and in effect limits damage.

Uncomplicated squeeze injuries of these areas are not medical emergencies and frequently do not need medical treatment. Sinus squeezes and mask area squeezes can be treated by cold packs. Ear squeeze can be complicated by rupture of the ear drum and immediate treatment is indicated to minimize the chances of middle ear infection, with subsequent hearing loss and balance disturbances. Transport people with a suspected ruptured eardrum to an emergency department immediately. A diver who sustains a perforated eardrum must avoid diving until the injury heals, usually a matter of several weeks.

If cold water enters the middle ear, the diver may suddenly lose his balance, panic and rapidly sprint to the surface with lungs full of air under excess pressure and develop air embolism, discussed later with problems of ascent. Of course, loss of balance can cause mental confusion and lead to drowning.

An exceedingly rare descent condition is lung compression or thoracic squeeze, which occurs when the diver descends deeply and rapidly while holding his breath. Emergency treatment consists of resuscitation and life support during transportation to a medical facility.

Bottom Problems

Bottom problems are related to the duration and depth of a given dive, especially in dives using rebreathing or deep-sea diving equipment. Five specific conditions all can lead to unconsciousness under water and drowning. Treatment includes prompt rescue and basic life support.

Nitrogen Narcosis

If a diver descends too deeply, increasing pressure of nitrogen in his body affects the brain as alcoholic intoxication does—nitrogen narcosis or "rapture of the deep." Divers at or below 100 feet have impaired judgment even though they do not think so. It is immediately corrected by rising to shallower water. The diver who fails to ascend may become so narcotized that he disregards his own safety and removes his breathing equipment while in water. Most sports diving instructors limit dives to 130 feet because of the insidious danger of nitrogen narcosis.

Oxygen Toxicity

Oxygen toxicity occurs when pure or enriched oxygen mixtures are used instead of air. The symptoms may begin with convulsions or dizziness, numbness and muscle twitching. Immediate correction follows ascent and switching to breathing plain air instead of a mixture of enriched oxygen. Self-contained under water breathing apparatus (SCUBA) should never deliver pure oxygen to the swimmer under water.

Carbon Dioxide (CO_2) Toxicity

Carbon dioxide toxicity occurs when special rebreathing equipment is defective and carbon dioxide is not reabsorbed adequately. CO_2 accumulates in the diver, causing shortness of breath, headache and panic. Ascent to uncontaminated surface air is necessary to correct the condition.

Hypoxia

Exhaustion of the oxygen in the air supply from faulty breathing equipment diminishes the oxygen level in the blood and produces unconsciousness and death unless rescue and resuscitation are prompt.

Carbon Monoxide Poisoning

Carbon monoxide poisoning results from filling tanks with air contaminated with carbon monoxide. The symptoms are similar to those seen on the surface, i.e., headaches, shortness of breath and, ultimately, unconsciousness as carbon monoxide combines with hemoglobin, thus decreasing the oxygen going to the brain. Carbon monoxide poisoning is treated by the immediate breathing of oxygen, which forces the carbon monoxide from the hemoglobin molecule. It can be prevented by careful inspection of all facilities selling compressed air to divers.

Ascent Problems

The two major ascent problems, air embolism and decompression sickness, are both caused by rapid ascents allowing expanding gas bubbles to enter the blood stream. Treatment is the same for both these ascent problems, i.e., recompression.

Air Embolism

Air embolism is the most dangerous, most common and least recognized hazard in sports diving. It can occur in dives as shallow as 6 feet if the diver holds his breath during a rapid ascent. When water pressure on the chest is rapidly reduced, air within the lungs expands. Rapid expansion of air can rupture alveoli within the lung and damage the adjacent blood vessels. The air can then be forced from the lungs into the blood vessels to travel as emboli in the vascular system to any part of the body. Air bubbles act as plugs preventing body tissue from receiving its normal supply of blood and oxygen. Brain damage is obviously the most serious result of air embolisms. Additionally, air can be forced from the lungs into the pleural space or into the mediastinum to create a pneumothorax or a pneumomediastinum.

Signs and symptoms of air embolus are:

1. Mottling or blotching of the skin
2. Frothy or bloody fluid at the nose and mouth
3. Pain in muscles, joints, tendons or abdomen
4. Difficult breathing with chest pain
5. Dizziness and vomiting
6. Difficulty in speaking and seeing
7. Paralysis and coma

Immediate treatment is to rescue the patient from the water, keep him calm and quiet and transport him to an emergency department while giving basic life support, including oxygen inhalation. Keep the patient on his left side with the head and chest lower than the feet, to reduce the chance of air embolization to the brain. The patient may require immediate recompression in a pressure chamber.

Decompression Sickness

Decompression sickness, also known as the bends or caisson's disease, is primarily caused by bubbles of nitrogen gas plugging small vessels within the body. Decompression sickness is related to the depth and duration of the dive in contradistinction to air embolism. It is seen following long, deep dives and is not frequent in sports scuba divers, who usually exhaust their air supply before their body tissues have absorbed sufficient nitrogen to make them subject to decompression sickness when they ascend.

When a diver breathes air under pressure, he absorbs much more than the usual amount of air into his tissues. Inspired air is about four fifths nitrogen and one fifth oxygen and carbon dioxide. The oxygen and carbon dioxide diffuse rapidly throughout the body and present no problems in blood or tissues, but nitrogen, which is absorbed into fat, is released slowly and carried as small bubbles in the blood. As long as the pressure of the dive is maintained, nitrogen is released very slowly and bubbbles remain very small. If pressure is released quickly, as when a diver ascends rapidly without pause, nitrogen is released

rapidly, and the bubbles become much larger and actually obstruct the vessels in which they lie. This results in decompression sickness or the ''bends.'' The term ''bends'' has been used because of the bent over position these people assume from their severe joint pains. The symptoms are directly referable to the obstructed arteries, which may be muscular, cerebral, skin or visceral.

If a diver ascends at a rate not exceeding 25 feet per minute and pauses for 10 minutes at specific levels, depending upon the depth and duration of his dive, his body can be depleted of nitrogen gradually and he avoids the bends. Specific dive tables are available that give the rate of ascent and the number and length of pauses necessary for a dive of a given duration at a given depth.

The proper treatment for decompression sickness is obviously recompression. The patient is placed in a pressure chamber and subjected to high pressure once again. The nitrogen that was released into the blood is forced back into the tissues, the bubbles are reduced in size, and the symptoms subside. The patient is then gradually decompressed to allow him to release excess nitrogen slowly and steadily.

Damage from the bends may be transient. However, if a major cerebral or spinal vessel is blocked, tissue damage may produce permanent effects, including paralysis.

Oxygen should be administered while en route to a recompression chamber to try to minimize brain damage. Remember that symptoms of decompression disease may not occur until some hours after a dive is concluded, while the symptoms of air embolism are usually immediate.

To prevent these potentially serious injuries, the diver must understand the physiology of gas exchange and the need to use proper breathing techniques while ascending and descending. He must plan the duration and depth of his dives based on the available charts and tables and his level of experience. Finally, his equipment must be checked regularly to assure proper function.

Poisons, Stings and Bites

51

Each year approximately 1 million children and thousands of adults accidentally swallow poisons. From 5,000 to 10,000 in the United States die annually from accidental or intentional poisoning. Of all poisonings 80% occur in children under the age of 6. Approximately 15% of all poisonings require some sort of emergency treatment.

The several hundred poison control centers throughout the United States are usually located in emergency departments of large hospitals. The telephone numbers of these poison control centers are readily available. Medical personnel who staff the poison control centers have access to information on virtually all of the commonly used drugs, chemicals, and substances that could possibly be poisons. Each of these substances is listed on a card, as is the specific antidote, if any, and any specific emergency treatment for that poison. The poison control centers are usually staffed 24 hours a day, and they should be contacted for help whenever there is a poisoning problem.

POISONINGS

A poison is any substance that can produce a harmful effect on the body processes. Poisons may act by modifying normal metabolism of cells or by actually destroying the cells. Poisoning can result from ingestion, inhalation, injection, surface contact or absorption through the skin and mucous membranes of substances in toxic amounts.

The first decision to make when faced with a possible poisoning victim is whether a poisoning has actually occurred. Some substances are harmless and require no treatment.

Others require nothing more than drinking a glass of milk or water to offset an upset stomach. However, if there is the slightest doubt, contact the poison control center and begin emergency treatment.

Some of the more common symptoms of poisoning are nausea, vomiting, abdominal pain, diarrhea, dilation or constriction of the pupils, excessive salivation or sweating, difficulty in breathing, unconsciousness or even convulsions. If respiration is inadequate, cyanosis occurs. Chemical burns or surface irritants cause inflammation of the skin or mucous membranes with blisters or even full-thickness burns.

Attempt to determine the nature of the poison. Look for objects at the scene, such as overturned bottles, pills lying around or toxic fumes from spilled chemicals or gases. The remains of any food or drink at the scene may also be important. Collect all suspicious material, put it into a plastic bag and take it to the hospital. If the patient vomits, attempt to collect some or all of the vomitus in a plastic bag and bring that to the hospital for chemical analysis. The most important thing, in addition to resuscitating the patient, is to identify and bring along any suspicious medicines, drugs or substances that may have caused the poisoning, or the bottle or can that contained the material. The ingredients of many substances are often listed on the label, which can be of great help to the poison control center. In addition, knowing how much material is left in the container can give the physician some idea of how much has been ingested. If the brand name of the material is known, sometimes the manufacturer can be contacted for a specific description of the material in the container. By bringing the container with the patient, proper treatment may be hastened and a life saved.

Treatment

Most poisons do not have a specific antidote or remedy. Supportive care is the first rule of emergency management of a poison victim. In general, the most important treatment for ingested poison is to dilute the poison in the stomach and then induce its removal by vomiting, provided that the patient is alert and conscious. Contact the poison control center first. Under their direction, dilute the poison by having the patient drink one or two glasses of milk or water. If the patient is alert and the poison control center says to do it, the next step is to induce vomiting.

Do not induce vomiting under the following circumstances.

1. If the patient is unconscious or semi-conscious, or is having a convulsion
2. If the swallowed poison is strongly corrosive, such as a strong acid, lye or drain cleaner, or has caused obvious burns on the lips or throat
3. If the poison contains any petroleum product, such as kerosene, gasoline, lighter fluid or clear furniture polish. These agents may cause chemical pneumonia if aspirated into the lungs

Vomiting is most easily induced by administering syrup of ipecac, 1 tablespoon followed by a glass of water. Transport the patient to the hospital promptly after the dose of ipecac, anticipating that most patients will vomit within 15 to 20 minutes, frequently inside the transport vehicle. Do not forget to collect the vomitus. If vomiting has not occurred after 20 minutes, repeat the dose once only.

When the patient does vomit, make sure the airway remains clear. If the patient is lying down, turn his head to one side. The standing patient should lean over a basin or sink.

Some substances are best managed by immobilization in the stomach with activated charcoal, 1 tablespoonful well mixed in a glass of water. This should be done under the direction of the poison control center. Activated charcoal inhibits the action of ipecac and should not be given right after a dose of ipecac. Many children do not want to swallow this dirty, inky, messy substance (charcoal), and may require some coaxing. Never force it into someone's mouth.

Soothing agents such as milk or milk of magnesia may be used when the poison is a gastric irritant. Again, follow the directions of the poison control center.

Inhaled Poisons

For inhaled poisons, such as natural gas or carbon monoxide, move the patient into fresh air. This protects the patient as well as those assisting him. Give supplementary oxygen and begin basic life support if necessary.

Injected Poisons

Poisoning by injection is almost always the result of self-administered drug overdose. Other sources of injected poisons are the bites and stings of insects or animals. If swelling from an injection is apparent in an extremity, remove all rings, watches and bracelets. Apply a constricting band above and below the site of the injection just tightly enough to occlude the venous flow so the patient's pulse is still palpable distal to the constricting bands. Application of an ice pack decreases the local pain and swelling.

Surface (Contact) Poisons

Many corrosive substances, such as acids, alkalis and some petroleum or benzine products, damage the skin, mucous membranes or eyes by direct contact. Contact with these agents causes inflammation or chemical burns in the affected areas.

Remove the irritating or corrosive poison as rapidly as possible by first dusting off any dry materials and then washing the affected area with soap and water, or flooding it under a shower if a large amount of material has spilled on the patient. Direct a stream of water on the patient's clothes as they are being removed. Treat chemical poison in the eyes by immediately irrigating the eye for several minutes. Do not waste time attempting to neutralize the substance on the patient, but rather immediately wash it off with water.

Plant Poisons

Ingestion of small amounts of some plants can produce severe gastrointestinal disturbances similar to those caused by other toxic substances: vomiting, diarrhea and cramps. Symptoms can occur within 20 to 30 minutes after ingestion. If the patient vomits, bring the vomitus to the hospital. Give the patient supportive care, allow vomiting as needed, and take the patient to the hospital promptly with a sample of the plant ingested if possible.

Poisonous plants sometimes affect the central nervous system, causing depression, hyperactivity, excitement, stupor, mental confusion or even coma.

Treatment for this kind of poisoning is also directed toward basic life support. Do not induce vomiting if these patients show any signs at all of stupor or coma. Bring the patient promptly to the hospital, again with a sample of the plant.

Skin Irritants

Skin irritation is the most common form of plant poisoning, producing symptoms of itching, burning and blister formation. These plants rarely produce systemic symptoms. Emergency treatment is thorough cleansing with soap and water. These patients occasionally need medical attention for prolonged symptoms.

The Dieffenbachia, a common house plant, is a special case. A leaf of this plant accidentally placed in the mouth produces irritation of the mucous membranes of the upper airway severe enough to cause difficulty in swallowing, breathing and speaking. The airway can be partially or even completely obstructed.

Emergency treatment involves maintaining an open airway, giving oxygen and transporting the patient immediately to the hospital.

INSECT STINGS AND BITES

Many kinds of insects can inflict painful stings or bites. However, only a very few are potentially dangerous. Bees, wasps, ants, scorpions and spiders are considered under this category.

Bees, Wasps and Ants

Stings and bites from bees, wasps and ants are among the most common insect injuries. Most of these insects sting with a small, hollow spine that projects from the abdomen and injects venom (animal poison) directly into the skin. The honeybee's stinger is attached to its intestines, part of which it leaves behind with the stinger. The insect invariably dies after it stings. Wasps, hornets and ants, however, can sting or bite repeatedly. Identification of the stinging insect is often impossible, because the insect tends to fly away immediately after stinging.

These stings or bites produce either local or systemic symptoms. Local symptoms are the most common: sudden pain, swelling, heat and redness about the affected area. Sometimes a white, firm elevation (wheal) with itching occurs in the skin. While there is no specific treatment for these injuries, applying ice may ease the pain. Swelling may be considerable, and sometimes these patients are extremely frightened. However, the local manifestations of these stings are not serious.

Attempt to remove the stinger and the portion of the abdomen with it by gently scraping it off the skin. Do not use tweezers or forceps, as squeezing the stinger only injects more venom into the patient.

Approximately 5% of the population is allergic to the venom of the bee, wasp or ant. This allergy accounts for approximately 200 deaths per year. The honeybee venom is most commonly associated with allergy. Insect stings in an allergic person produce a hypersensitive reaction, manifested by generalized itching, skin wheals, weakness, headache, dyspnea, anxiety and abdominal cramps. This reaction may even proceed to anaphylactic shock and death. The rapid development of wheals and wheezing respirations means hypersensitivity reaction. Administer basic life support at once, and transport the patient immediately to the hospital. Give oxygen, and be prepared to maintain the airway and cardiac function. Place a venous tourniquet on the extremity above and below the site of the sting. To minimize the absorption of toxin, attempt to remove the stinger from the wound by gentle scraping. Place an ice bag over the injury site to help slow the absorption rate of the toxin.

Patients with a history of severe allergic reactions to bee stings may have commercially manufactured ''bee sting kits'' prescribed specifically for them by a physician. These kits usually contain epinephrine prepared in the syringe ready for injection and, sometimes, antihistamine pills. Where local laws permit, assist the patient in administering the medication, as it may save the life of someone with a severe anaphylactic reaction. Follow the specific instructions for epinephrine injections outlined in the package insert. Following administration, epinephrine produces tachycardia and, on occasion, increased anxiety or nervousness in the patient. Complete other emergency care as outlined earlier, and promptly transport the patient to the hospital.

Scorpions

Scorpions are rare and found primarily in deserts. Scorpion stings, except for that of a specific scorpion in the Arizona desert, are painful but not dangerous, causing localized swelling, pain and discoloration. The sting from the Arizona scorpion may produce a severe systemic reaction resulting in circulatory collapse, severe muscle contractions, excessive salivation, hypertension, convulsions and cardiac failure. Emergency treatment for

this insect sting is basic life support. Antivenin (antitoxin to a venom) is available and should be administered by a physician. Notify the hospital as soon as possible that a patient with a suspected Arizona scorpion sting is on the way. Remember, however, that only the scorpion found in Arizona causes this serious problem.

Spiders

Two spiders commonly found in the United States have bites that can be serious, even life-threatening—the black widow spider and the brown recluse spider. Many other spiders will bite, but do not produce serious complications. The black widow spider measures approximately 1 inch in length with its legs extended. It is glossy black in color and has a distinctive yellow-orange hourglass-shape marking on its belly. On its back, however, there is no marking. The danger of the black widow spider bite lies in its systemic manifestations. The venom attacks the nervous system, resulting in severe muscle cramps with boardlike rigidity of the abdominal muscles, tightness in the chest, and difficulty in breathing accompanied by sweating, nausea and vomiting.

Emergency treatment for the black widow spider bite is basic life support. Sometimes the individual is not even aware of having been bitten, or where. Apply cold to the site of the bite if identified. A physician must administer the specific antivenin for this spider bite. It is particularly important to identify the spider and bring it to the hospital whenever possible.

The brown recluse spider is a little smaller than the black widow spider and dull brown in color. It has a violin-shaped mark on its back, which can be seen from above. The spider gets its name because it tends to live in dark areas, corners and in old unused buildings. The bite from this spider produces local rather than systemic manifestations. Its venom causes severe local tissue damage and can lead to an ulcer and gangrene. The bitten area becomes red, swollen and tender within a few hours. A small blister forms and, several days later, may become a large scab, covering a deep ulcer. Death is rare but these bites need local surgical treatment, and these patients should be brought to the hospital. Again, if possible, identify the spider.

SNAKEBITES

Snakebites are fairly common throughout the United States. Some 45,000 to 50,000 snakebites are reported annually, approximately 7,000 of which are caused by poisonous snakes. However, fatalities from snakebites are extremely rare, about 15 a year for the entire country.

Of the approximately 150 different species of snakes in the United States, about 20 are poisonous. Snakes are generally timid and bite only when provoked, angered or accidentally injured, as when stepped on. In general, four different species of poisonous snakes are seen in the United States: several species of rattlesnake, the copperhead, the cottonmouth (water moccasin) and the coral snake. Rattlesnakes can usually be identified by the rattle on their tails. A small nubbin on the end of the tail prevents the skin from being completely shed. Succeeding layers of skin leave dried remnants that form the characteristic rattle.

In handling snakebites, it is extremely important to identify whether envenomation (deposit of venom into the wound) has occurred. Approximately one third of all poisonous snakebites do not result in envenomation because the snake has either recently struck another animal or, for some other reason, no venom gets into the wound.

With the exception of the coral snake, the poisonous snakes in the United States all have hollow fangs in the roofs of their mouths that literally inject the poison from two sacs in the back of the head. The characteristic appearance of a poisonous snakebite, therefore, is two small holes, usually about a half inch apart, with surrounding discoloration, swelling and pain. The bites of nonpoisonous snakes leave tooth marks rather than fang holes. Yet, some poisonous snakes have teeth as well as fangs.

The mere presence of tooth marks does not necessarily mean that the snake was not poisonous.

Pit Vipers

Rattlesnakes, copperheads and cottonmouth water moccasins are all pit vipers. The head of a pit viper is triangular with a small pit located just behind the nostril and in front of the eye. The pupil of the eye is vertical and slitlike. The pit is a heat-sensing organ that allows the snake to strike accurately at any warm target, even in the dark. The fangs of the pit viper normally lie flat against the roof of its mouth. When the snake is attacking, the mouth opens wide and the fangs drop down, so that if the mouth strikes an object, the fangs penetrate it.

The cardinal signs of envenomation by a pit viper are severe, burning pain at the site of the injury, followed by swelling and discoloration. This begins within 5 to 10 minutes and spreads slowly over the next 8 to 36 hours. Bleeding under the skin may result in ecchymotic discoloration. Systemic signs, which may or may not occur, include weakness, sweating, faintness and the signs of shock. Often a patient bitten by a snake will faint from anxiety. This is a temporary state and should not be confused with shock.

The venom of the pit viper destroys all tissues locally and causes internal bleeding systemically. If there are no local signs of envenomation (swelling, discoloration and severe local pain) by one hour after the bite, no venom has entered the wound.

The emergency treatment of pit viper bites is directed at the systemic and local effects.

1. Calm and reassure the patient. Have him lie down and keep quiet to decrease the spread of any venom through the system. Patients will often vomit, from anxiety as well as from systemic effects of the poison. Never give the patient alcohol.
2. Locate the bite area.
3. Wrap soft rubber tubes around the extremity above and below the fang marks, and

tighten them just enough to occlude the venous circulation. The pulse in the distal extremity should not disappear. This maneuver limits the spread of the venom.

4. Clean the bite gently with soap and water or a mild antiseptic.
5. Immobilize the extremity with a splint to minimize movement and spread of the venom.
6. Monitor vital signs: blood pressure, pulse and respiration.
7. If there are any signs of shock, place the patient in the shock position and administer oxygen.
8. Promptly transport the patient to the hospital. Notify the hospital that a snakebite victim will arrive and, if possible, describe the snake.
9. If the snake has been killed, as it often has, bring it to the hospital. Identification of the offending snake is extremely important in administering the correct antivenin.

If the patient shows no signs of envenomation, or can reach a hospital in under four to five hours, then the only treatment necessary is basic life support, a clean dressing over the suspected bite area, and venous constricting bands above and below the bite.

If the patient shows signs of envenomation and more than four to five hours will pass before a hospital is reached, further local wound treatment may be necessary. It should be carried out upon the specific instructions of a physician. After the bite, the poison remains locally in the tissues for about 30 minutes, and some can be mechanically removed by making a small, half inch long incision through the skin in the long axis of the extremity over each fang mark. The incision should be just deep enough to go through the skin to expose the subcutaneous fat. Do not go deeper than a quarter inch to avoid injuring important tendons, nerves and blood vessels. Then use the suction cup from a snakebite kit to mechanically suck out some of the poison.

This technique, incision and suction, should be used only on a bite of an extremity, not on the head or trunk, only under the direction of a physician in a patient showing definite signs of envenomation, and less than 30 minutes after the bite occurs. Bring all suspected snakebite victims to a hospital, whether they show immediate signs of envenomation or not.

In areas where poisonous snakes are found, always keep a snakebite kit in the trainer's kit. Know the address of the nearest facility where antivenin is available—a nearby zoo or the local or state public health department.

Coral Snake

The coral snake is a small, very colorful snake with a series of bright red, yellow and black bands completely encircling its body. The red bands are next to the yellow bands. This is an important point because many harmless snakes are colored similarly to the coral snake, but none have the red and yellow bands next to each other, completely encircling the animal's body. A rhyme for remembering this is ''Red on yellow will kill a fellow. Red on black, venom will lack.''

The coral snake is rare, living primarily in Florida and the desert Southwest. It is not found in the northern part of the United States. Like the pit vipers, it is shy and bites only when provoked. The coral snake, a relative of the cobra, has tiny fangs and injects venom with its teeth as well as its fangs. Therefore, the coral snake must use a chewing motion to inject its poison. Because of its small mouth and teeth and limited jaw expansion, the coral snake usually bites its victim on a small part of the body, i.e., a hand, foot or, especially, a finger. The bite of a coral snake leaves one or more tiny punctures or scratch-like wounds.

The danger of this particular snake is that its venom is toxic to the brain, causing paralysis of the nervous system. There are minimal local manifestations of the coral snakebite, but paralysis of respiration, movement of the eyes and eyelids, as well as bizarre behavior, occur as a result of the toxic effects on the central nervous system.

Treatment depends upon positive identification of the snake. Antivenin is available, but most hospitals or physicians will have to order it from a central supply area, often in another city. Therefore, the need for it should be made known as soon as possible.

The steps of emergency care in the event of a coral snake bite are listed below.

1. Immediately quiet and reassure the patient. Do not give alcohol.
2. Lightly apply soft rubber tubes around the extremity above and below the bite.
3. Flush the area of the bite with 1 to 2 quarts of water to wash away any poison left on the surface of the skin.
4. Splint the extremity to minimize movement and the spread of the venom to the central nervous system.
5. Check and monitor the patient's vital signs.
6. Keep the patient warm and elevate the lower extremities to help to prevent shock.
7. Give artificial ventilation with oxygen if needed.
8. Apply an ice bag or coolant bag to the bite area if the physician so recommends. Under no circumstances should the extremity be packed in ice.
9. Promptly transport to the Emergency Department, giving advance notice that the patient has been bitten by a coral snake.

Incision and suction should not be done in the case of a coral snake bite, as there is little local effect from this bite. The danger is to the central nervous system.

DOG BITES AND RABIES

The exact incidence of dog bites is unknown. Most people bitten by dogs do not report the bite, but dog bites are potentially serious injuries. The animal's mouth is heavily contaminated with virulent bacteria and, particularly if the bite is on the hand or the face, serious infection may result. Therefore, consider all dog bites infected wounds and treat them with dry, sterile dressings.

Often, the person is extremely apprehensive, upset and frightened; therefore, calm reassurance is extremely important. Most dog bites are not serious but should be treated by a physician. Usually antibiotics are given while the wound may or may not need suturing.

The greatest concern about dog bites, or any animal bite, is the spread of rabies. Although rabies is extremely rare today due to widespread inoculation of pets, it still exists. Uninoculated stray dogs could be rabies carriers. Certain other animals, including squirrels, bats, foxes, skunks and raccoons, may also carry rabies.

Rabies is a fatal disease. Antibiotics are of no use. Once the disease develops in an animal or a person, there is no treatment. A rabid animal may act perfectly normal, or it may appear vicious, salivate or act in any other abnormal way. Behavior alone does not indicate rabies with certainty.

If the animal has been inoculated against rabies, it may have a tag so stating on its collar. Be sure to check for this. In most cases the animal will be a pet. If it does not have a rabies tag, it should be captured (not killed) and turned over to the Health Department for observation. If the animal is then suspected of having rabies, it is killed and the brain studied. If the animal cannot be identified or found, the patient usually must undergo a series of rabies inoculations which, if begun early enough, prevent rabies from developing. They are painful, with some side effects, and are administered over a two-week period.

In 1980 a new rabies vaccine was developed from material grown in human tissue. It is much simpler to use and has fewer side effects. It is expensive and difficult to produce, and may be in short supply. Know the location of the local rabies control center and the institution that has the human rabies vaccine.

MARINE ANIMAL INJURIES

Despite much publicity about shark bites, they are extremely rare. Emergency treatment of a large marine animal bite is the same as for any other major open wound. After removing the patient from the water, control hemorrhage, apply dressings and splints, treat for shock and promptly transport the patient to the hospital.

With the exception of the shark and barracuda, most marine animals are nonaggressive and will not deliberately attack. Injuries from these animals occur when they are accidentally stepped on or are otherwise provoked.

Injuries from marine animals occur most often from swimming into the tentacles of a jellyfish, stepping on the back of a stingray or falling onto a sea urchin. Be familiar with the marine animals in your locality. Stings from the tentacles of a jellyfish, Portuguese man-of-war, various anemones, corals or hydras can be treated by removing the patient from the water and sprinkling the affected area with alcohol. Then, sprinkle meat tenderizer over the area, followed by talcum powder. This inactivates the poison deposited on the skin and is usually the only treatment necessary. On rare occasions, a person will have a systemic allergy to the sting of one of these animals, which is managed by anaphylactic shock treatment, administering basic life support and transporting promptly to the hospital.

Punctures from the spines of sea urchins, stingrays or certain spiny fish such as catfish are best treated by immobilizing the area and soaking it in water as hot as the patient can stand without risking a burn for 30 minutes. The toxin from these fish is heat sensitive, and simply applying hot water can dramatically relieve local pain. Again, some persons may have allergic reactions. As with any other wound, tetanus and other infections are possible.

Some water animals may bite, such as the nonpoisonous water snake or the cottonmouth water moccasin. In contrast to most other snakes, the cottonmouth water moccasin can be aggressive and may attack deliberately. The treatment of the cottonmouth bite is the same as that of any other pit viper.

Many fish are poisonous if eaten. Emergency treatment for such poisoning is the same as for any other poisoning. Give basic life support, prevent injury from convulsions and promptly transport the victim to the hospital.

Other rare conditions include shocks from electric fish or skin rashes from certain marine parasites. These injuries are usually mild, although a person may panic from contact with an electric eel.

Glossary

A band: one of the transverse bands making up the repeating striated pattern of skeletal and cardiac muscle; located in the middle of a sarcomere; corresponds to the length of the thick filaments.

abdomen: more inferior of the two major body cavities, lying between the thorax and the pelvis.

abdominal catastrophe: most severe form of acute abdomen.

abdominal cavity: cavity between the diaphragm and the pelvis that contains all the abdominal organs.

abdominal quadrants: four equal parts into which the abdomen is divided, separated by two lines intersecting at right angles at the umbilicus—right upper, right lower, left upper and left lower quadrants.

abdominal thrust: series of manual thrusts to the upper abdomen to relieve upper airway obstruction.

abduction: motion of a limb away from the midline.

abrasion: rubbing off or scraping off of the skin or a mucous membrane.

abscess: localized collection of pus (white blood cells) into a cavity formed by the disintegration of tissues.

acceleration: rate of increase in speed of a moving body.

acetabulum: the socket of the hip joint into which the femoral head fits.

acetone: colorless liquid found in small quantities in normal urine and in larger amounts in diabetic urine; a metabolic end product of the use of fat for routine energy needs.

acetylcholine: substance found in many parts of the body having important physiologic functions such as being involved in transmitting an impulse from one nerve fiber to another.

Achilles tendon: tendon joining the gastrocnemius and soleus muscles in the calf of the leg to the bone of the heel.

acidosis: condition caused by accumulation of acid or loss of base in the body.

acromioclavicular joint: joint at the top of the shoulder, formed by bony articulations of the scapula and clavicle.

acromion process: lateral extension of the spine of the scapula; the highest point of the shoulder.

actin: one of the proteins in muscle fiber; the other is myosin.

acute: having a short and relatively severe course.

acute abdomen: abdominal condition causing acute irritation or inflammation of the peritoneum, which in turn causes severe pain.

acute myocardial infarction: death of heart muscle; ''heart attack,'' caused by lack of oxygen to the muscle.

addiction: physical or emotional dependence on a specific drug.

adduction: motion of a limb toward the midline.

adenosine diphosphate (ADP): adenosine compound containing two phosphoric acid groups. This enzyme is produced during muscle contraction.

adenosine triphosphate (ATP): adenosine compound containing three phosphoric acids found in all cells representing energy storage.

adrenal glands: flattened bodies located in the retroperitoneal tissues above the kidneys;

549

produces steroid hormones and epinephrine (adrenaline).

agonist: the muscle directly engaged in contraction as distinguished from those that relax in a given movement.

air embolism: bubbles of air released into the blood from rupture of lung alveoli during ascent from the water or while flying too high in an unpressurized plane.

air exchange: exchange of air between the organism and the environment in respiration.

air hunger: distressing dyspnea occurring in paroxysms; found in diabetic coma.

air pressure splint: double-walled plastic tube that immobilizes a limb when the space between the walls is inflated. When sufficiently inflated, it forms a secure splint. Inflation should always be by mouth.

airway: route for passage of air in and out of the lungs. **upper airway:** portion of the airway that includes the mouth, pharynx and throat.

alkalosis: pathologic condition resulting from accumulation of base or loss of acid in the body.

allergic: suffering from allergy.

allergy: altered reaction of body tissue to a specific substance that nonsensitive persons would not have.

alveoli: air sacs of the lungs.

amino acids: building blocks for protein construction; end product of protein digestion and hydrolysis. There are 20 or more amino acids; ten are essential for life.

aminophylline: antiasthmatic drug; a stimulant.

amnesia: loss of memory.

amphetamines: group of stimulant drugs.

amputation: removal of a body part.

anabolic steroid: testosterone, or a steroid hormone resembling testosterone, that stimulates anabolism in the body as a whole.

anabolism: process by which living cells convert simple substances into more complex compounds.

anal canal: lower end of the alimentary canal.

anal fissure: ulcer at the margin of the anus.

anaphylactic shock: shock caused by an allergic reaction.

androgenic steroid: substance producing or stimulating male characteristics, as in male sex hormones.

anemia: condition in which there is a reduction in the number of circulating red blood cells, hemoglobin or volume of red cells.

aneurysm: weakened, bulging area of a blood vessel.

angina pectoris: attacks of chest pain with squeezing or tightness in the chest and difficulty breathing; caused by lack of oxygen for the heart.

angle of Louis: bony prominence on the breastbone, just inferior to the junction of the clavicle and sternum and just opposite the second intercostal space.

angulation: departure from a straight line, as in a broken bone.

anisocoria: unequal size of the pupils of the eyes.

ankle: joint between the foot and the leg (tibia and talus).

ankle hitch: part of a traction splint that applies traction to the foot.

antagonist: that which counteracts the action of a muscle or drug.

antecubital fossa: depression in the anterior region of the elbow.

anterior: term indicating the front part of the body or any structure.

anterior chamber of eye: front part of the space containing aqueous humor, behind the cornea and in front of the iris.

anterior drawer: manual stress test to determine the amount of anterior displacement of the tibia on the femur when the knee is flexed.

anterior superior iliac spine: blunt bony projection on the anterior border of the ilium, forming the anterior end of the iliac crest.

anterior surface: surface at the front of the body, facing the examiner.

antibiotic: chemical substance produced by a

microorganism that has the capacity to kill other microorganisms.

antibodies: protein substances developed by the body, usually in response to the presence of an antigen found in the body.

anticonvulsant: drug used to prevent seizures.

antigen: substance that triggers a specific immune response against itself when formed within or introduced into the body, i.e., causes the formation of antibodies.

antihistamine: drug that counteracts the effects of histamine and relieves the symptoms of an allergic reaction.

anus: distal or terminal ending of the alimentary canal.

aorta: major artery leaving the left side of the heart that carries freshly oxygenated blood to the body.

aortic valve: valve that guards the aortic opening in the left ventricle of the heart and prevents backflow.

apex: top of a body organ or part, tip of a pointed structure.

apneic: having no spontaneous breathing.

aponeurosis: broad fibrous sheet attaching a muscle to another muscle.

appendicitis: inflammation of the appendix.

appendix: small, closed end tube that opens into the cecum in the lower right quadrant of the abdomen.

aqueous humor: fluid in front of the lens of the eye.

arachnoid: the middle of the three layers of tissue that envelop the brain and spinal cord; lies between the dura mater and the pia mater.

arm: part of the upper extremity extending from the shoulder to the elbow.

arrhythmia: any disturbance in the rhythm of the heartbeat.

arterial pressure points (pulse points): points where arteries pass over bony prominences or lie close to the skin; here an artery can be palpated and the arterial pulse taken.

arteries: tubular vessels that carry oxygenated blood from the heart to the body tissues.

arterioles: small arterial branches.

arteriosclerosis: group of diseases characterized by thickening and loss of elasticity of the arterial walls.

articular: pertaining to a joint.

articular cartilage: thin layer of cartilage covering the ends of bones to form the joint surfaces.

articular surface: surface relating to a joint.

articulation: joint, juncture.

artificial circulation: means of starting the patient's circulation by external chest compression.

artificial respiration: see artificial ventilation.

artificial ventilation: opening the airway and restoring breathing by mouth-to-mouth, mouth-to-nose or mouth-to-stoma ventilation, or by the use of mechanical devices.

ascending colon: part of the colon that lies in the vertical position on the right side of the abdomen, extending up to the lower border of the liver from the cecum.

ascent injuries: injuries in ascent from a dive, especially air embolism and decompression sickness.

aspiration: taking foreign matter into the respiratory tract during inhalation.

assisted ventilation: see artificial ventilation.

asthma: condition marked by labored breathing and wheezing due to contraction of the bronchi.

asystole: lack of a heartbeat.

ataxia: muscular incoordination manifested when voluntary movements are attempted.

atelectasis: areas of lung collapse.

atherosclerosis: form of arteriosclerosis in which yellowish plaques containing cholesterol and other fatty substances are deposited beneath the inner layer of the arteries.

atmospheric pressure: unit of pressure equal to the pressure of the air at sea level, approximately 14.7 pounds per square inch.

atrial fibrillation: atrial arrhythmia caused by rapid, random contractions of the atrial heart muscle. Ventricular heart rate is irregular, often rapid.

atrium: either of the two upper chambers of the heart.

auditory nerves: nerves transmitting hearing sensations to the brain.

auscultation: listening to sounds within the organs to aid diagnosis and treatment.

automatic: involuntary.

autonomic nervous system: portion of the nervous system regulating involuntary functions, such as digestion or sweating.

avulsion: injury in which a whole piece of skin, with varying portions of subcutaneous tissue or muscle, is torn loose completely or partially.

axilla: armpit.

bacilli: members of a specific group of microorganisms, including the tubercle (tuberculosis) and typhoid bacillus.

bacterium: microorganism that causes infections and is not a virus or a parasite.

ball-and-socket joint: joint that allows internal and external rotation as well as bending.

basal skull fracture: fracture of the base of the skull; cerebrospinal fluid may leak from the ear, nose or a scalp laceration, or there may be hemorrhage from the ear without apparent cause.

basic life support: emergency lifesaving procedure of recognizing and correcting respiratory or cardiovascular system failure.

basket litter: see Stokes' basket.

basophils: cells or cell parts readily stained by methylene blue. An increased number is found during the healing phase of inflammation or chronic inflammation.

Bennett's fracture: fracture dislocation of the base of the first metacarpal.

bilateral: on both sides.

bile: fluid secreted by the liver and transmitted to the large intestine through the bile ducts; required for normal fat digestion.

bile ducts: ducts conveying bile from the liver to the intestines.

biliary system: ductal system consisting of the gallbladder and the bile ducts connecting the liver to the intestine.

bite block: block to put in the patient's mouth to prevent biting of the tongue.

bladder, urinary: musculomembranous sac where urine is collected and stored.

blood: red, sticky fluid composed of plasma, red blood cells, white blood cells and platelets; means by which oxygen and nutrients are transported to the tissues to sustain life, and carbon dioxide and various metabolic products are removed to cleanse the body.

blood pressure: pressure of the blood against the walls of the arteries as it passes through.

blood volume: total quantity of blood in the body.

blunt abdominal wound: injury to the abdomen caused by a blunt object such as a football helmet or shoulder pad (see closed abdominal injury).

body of a vertebra: front part; a round, solid block of bone.

bone: hard form of connective tissue that makes up the skeleton.

bone necrosis: death of bone structure.

boutonnière deformity: deformity of the finger characterized by flexion of the proximal IP joint and hyperextension of the distal joint.

bowel: see intestine.

brachial artery: artery on the inside of the arm between the elbow and the shoulder; used in taking blood pressure and for checking pulse in infants.

brachial plexus: network of nerves originating from branches of the spinal nerves; located in the neck and axilla.

bradycardia: slow heart action; a sinus rhythm with a rate below 60 in an adult, or below 70 in a child.

brain: controlling organ of the body; center of consciousness; functions include perception, control of reactions to the environment, emotional responses and judgment.

brain stem: area of the brain between the spinal cord and cerebrum, surrounded by the cerebellum; controls functions necessary for life, such as respiration.

breath-holding blackout: blackout under water because of hypoxia; swimmer does not realize the need to take a breath; usually occurs after forced hyperventilation that reduces arterial pCO_2 and obliterates the normal respiratory drive.

bronchi: two main branches of the trachea that lead into the right and left lungs.

bronchial asthma: common form of asthma.

bronchiole: fine subdivision of the bronchi, less than 1 mm in diameter, having no cartilage but abundant smooth muscle and elastic fibers in its wall.

bronchitis: inflammation of the mucous membrane of the bronchi.

bulb syringe: rubber or plastic device of defined capacity (60 cc) used for gentle suction and irrigation in neonates and small infants.

bulky hand dressing: dressing and splint for hand and wrist injuries; the hand is formed into the "position of function," a rolled soft roller bandage is placed in the palm, the hand is completely wrapped with soft roller dressing, a padded board splint is applied to the palmar side and secured with a soft roller bandage.

bunion: inflammation and thickening of the bursa of the joint of the great toe usually associated with marked joint enlargement and toe displacement laterally.

burn: lesion caused by heat exposure or exposure to chemicals or electricity.

calcaneus: heelbone.

calcium: bivalent metallic ion found in nearly all organized tissues, especially bone.

capillary: minute vessel that connects the arterioles and venules. The wall functions as a membrane for the interchange of various substances between the blood and tissue fluid.

capillary adhesion: adhesion between two moist surfaces effected by the water molecules of each surface; the normal mechanism by which the lung expands, following the motions of the chest wall.

capillary filling: filling of the capillary bed (best seen in the finger or toe under the nail) with blood, causing a normal pink color.

capillary perfusion: passing of blood through the appropriate capillary bed to nourish tissues.

capsule: fibrous tissues enclosing a joint.

carbohydrate: compound derived from alcohols, e.g., starches, sugars, celluloses and gums.

carbon dioxide (CO_2): waste product formed in body tissues by the metabolism of sugars.

carbon dioxide drive: stimulus to breathe caused by the carbon dioxide level in arterial blood.

carbon dioxide exchange: process by which carbon dioxide leaves the blood and oxygen enters it.

carbon dioxide narcosis: condition in which the carbon dioxide in the blood rises to high levels and the respiratory center becomes narcotized, or depressed.

carbon monoxide (CO): colorless, odorless, poisonous gas formed by the incomplete combustion of carbone; when inhaled, it blocks oxygen transport and use.

carcinoma: cancerous growth made up of epithelial cells.

cardiac arrest: sudden ceasing of heart function.

cardiac arrhythmia: see arrhythmia.

cardiac compression: external heart massage to restore circulation and the pumping action of the heart.

cardiac failure: condition in which damage of the heart muscle interferes with its function, characterized by disturbances in cardiac output and increased venous pressure.

cardiac muscle: specialized form of striated muscle that makes up the walls of the heart.

cardiac output: effective volume of blood expelled by either ventricle per unit of time.

cardiac pacemaker: device that imposes a regular rhythm on the heart by delivering an electrical impulse through wires sewn into the heart muscle.

cardiac standstill: absence of contraction or electrical activity of the heart.

cardiogenic shock: shock resulting from inadequate functioning of the heart.

cardiopulmonary: of the heart and lungs.

cardiopulmonary resuscitation: artificial establishment of circulation of the blood and movement of air into and out of the lungs in a pulseless, nonbreathing patient.

cardiorespiratory arrest: see cardiac arrest; respiratory arrest.

cardiovascular collapse: see cardiac arrest.

cardiovascular system: heart and blood vessels.

cardioversion: restoration of heart sinus rhythm by electrical shock.

carotid arteries: principal arteries of the neck running upward in the neck and dividing into the external and internal carotid arteries to supply the face and head and brain, respectively; can be palpated on either side of the neck.

carotid pulse (carotid artery pulse): pulse felt in the upper portion of the neck.

carpal bones: bones of the wrist.

carpal tunnel syndrome: pressure on the median nerve where it passes through the carpal tunnel of the wrist causing soreness, tenderness, numbness and weakness of the thumb muscles.

carpometacarpal joint: joint between the wrist and the metacarpal bones.

carrier: person or animal who transmits an infectious disease while not being affected.

cartilage: connective tissue containing a tough, elastic substance; found in joints, at the developing ends of bones and in specific areas such as the nose and ear.

cartilaginous: composed of cartilage.

cataract: opacity of the lens of the eye impairing vision.

cauda equina: spinal nerves descending from the lower part of the spinal cord, separately within the spinal canal, lying below the second lumbar vertebra. The horse's tail appearance gives it its name.

cecum: first part of the large bowel into which the ileum opens.

cell: small mass of protoplasm (living matter) bounded by a membrane; the smallest unit of living matter that can function independently.

cellular component: part of a cell.

center of mass: point where the weight of a vehicle is concentrated.

central nervous system: brain and spinal cord.

cephalad: toward the head.

cerebellum: part of the brain that occupies the posterior cranial fossa behind the brain stem; involved in synergic control of skeletal muscles; plays important role in coordination of voluntary muscle movements.

cerebral: pertaining to the brain, specifically the cerebral cortex.

cerebral arteries: arteries supplying the brain.

cerebral concussion: see concussion.

cerebral embolus: see embolus.

cerebrospinal fluid: fluid contained in the four ventricles of the brain and in the subarachnoid space about the brain and spinal cord.

cerebrovascular accident: see stroke.

cerebrum: main brain area with two hemispheres controlling movement, hearing, balance, speech and visual perception.

cervical collar: neck brace that partially stabilizes the neck following injury.

cervical fracture: fracture of the cervical spine.

cervical spine: upper seven bones of the back, found in the neck.

cervix: the lower and narrow end of the uterus.

chambers: cavities.

chemical burns: burns caused by exposure to chemicals.

chemical pneumonia: inflammation of pulmonary parenchyma and bronchial tissue caused by direct chemical irritation as in the aspiration of acid gastric juice.

chest thrust: series of manual thrusts to the chest to relieve upper airway obstruction.

chicken pox: acute viral disease with fever and itchy red rash (varicella); more common in children.

chin-lift maneuver: see head tilt-chin lift.

cholecystitis: inflammation of the gallbladder.

choline: amine essential in fat and carbohydrate metabolism; prevents fat from being deposited in the liver.

choroid: layer of blood vessels between the retina and the sclera that nourishes the eye and especially the retina.

chronic bronchitis: long-standing form of bronchitis, with attacks of coughing and changes in the lung tissue.

chronic congestive heart failure: condition due to heart disease and characterized by breathlessness and edema, both in the lungs and generalized in the body.

chronic obstructive lung disease: slow process of disruption of the airways, alveoli and pulmonary blood vessels caused by chronic bronchial obstruction.

circulate: to follow a course that returns to the starting point, as blood circulates through the body.

circulatory collapse: failure of the circulation, either cardiac or peripheral (shock).

circulatory system: channels through which the nutrient fluids of the body circulate; often used to mean only the channels conveying blood.

circumoral: around the mouth.

circumorbital: around the orbit.

cirrhosis: loss of normal liver cell structure with fibrosis (formation of fibrous tissue—scarring).

clammy: cold, damp skin.

clavicle: collarbone.

clinical: pertaining to or founded on actual observation and treatment of patients.

clinical syndrome: set of clinical signs or symptoms occurring together.

closed abdominal injury: abdomen is damaged by a severe blow but the skin remains intact (see blunt abdominal wound).

closed chest compression: method of manual compression of the heart to aid or replace its own beat in which the chest is not opened and the heart is compressed between the sternum and spine; used to restore circulation in an acute situation when heart action has ceased.

closed chest injuries: skin is not broken.

closed fracture: skin has not been penetrated by the bone ends and no wound exists near the fracture site; the fracture has not been exposed to air or contaminated.

closed wound: soft tissue damage occurs beneath the skin but there is no break in the surface of the skin.

coccygeal spine: coccyx, or tailbone; last four vertebrae.

coffee ground vomitus: vomitus consisting of dark-colored matter, usually digested blood, with the appearance of coffee grounds.

colic: painful intestinal cramp caused by strong or interrupted peristaltic waves.

colitis: inflammation of the colon.

collateral circulation: circulation carried on through secondary channels after the principal vessel is obstructed.

collecting system of kidney: little tubes in the kidney that collect the end products of body metabolism, which the kidney will excrete as urine.

Colles' fracture: fracture of the distal radius, with dorsal displacement of the fragments, producing the ''silver fork deformity'' in which the injured wrist assumes a curvature similar to the side view of a dinner fork.

colon: part of the large intestine that extends from the ileocecal valve to the rectum.

coma: state of unconsciousness from which the patient cannot be aroused.

comatose: in a coma.

comminuted fracture: bone is broken into more than two fragments.

common bile duct: bile duct that empties into the duodenum, along with the pancreatic duct.

communicable disease: see contagious disease.

communicable period: time during which an infectious agent may be transferred from one host to another.

complex partial seizure: consciousness is clouded and the patient displays automatic behavior.

compound fracture: open fracture; exposed to air and contamination.

compression dressing: dressing that applies pressure to slow down or decrease edema or hemorrhage.

concussion: jarring injury of the brain resulting in disturbance of brain function.

conduction: loss of heat from a body by direct contact with a cold object.

condyle: rounded protuberance at the end of a bone forming an articulation with another bone.

confusion: mental state marked by the mingling of ideas with disturbance of understanding.

congenital: existing at birth.

congested: excessively full, for example, blood vessels.

congestive heart failure: heart disease characterized by breathlessness and sodium and water retention. There may be fluid in the lungs as well as generalized fluid swelling in the body.

conjunctiva: delicate membrane that lines the eyelids and covers the exposed surface of the eye.

consciousness: state of being conscious; responsiveness of the mind to the impressions made by the senses.

consistency: degree of firmness of substance.

constricted: becoming narrow by drawing together or squeezing.

contact lens: shell of plastic applied directly over the globe or cornea to correct refractive errors of the eye.

contagious disease: disease that can be transmitted from one person to another; a disease that is ''catching.''

contamination: soiling, staining or infection by contact with bacteria or other infectious agents.

contraindicated: a treatment or medication should not be given.

contusion: bruising; reaction of soft tissue to a direct blow.

convection: loss of heat from a body by a moving current of air.

convulsion: violent involuntary contraction or series of contractions of the skeletal muscles.

core: central portion of the body: trunk, thoracic and abdominal viscera, head and brain. The core temperature is the temperature of this body portion.

cornea: transparent tissue layer in front of the pupil and the iris of the eye.

coronary arteries: arteries of the heart.

coronary arteriosclerosis: arteriosclerosis of the coronary artery.

cortex (compacta): outer layer of an organ, as of the brain—cerebral cortex.

cortisone: hormone from the adrenal cortex used as a medication.

costal arch: fused costal cartilages of the seventh to tenth ribs forming the upper limit of the abdomen.

costal cartilage: bar of cartilage attaching a rib to the sternum or to adjacent ribs.

costochondral separation: separation of a rib and its cartilage.

counteragent: a drug or agent that opposes the effects of another drug or agent.

counterpressure: pressure countering already existing pressure.

countertraction: traction applied against other traction as in reduction of a dislocation.

CPR: cardiopulmonary resuscitation.

cramp: painful spasm, usually of a muscle; a gripping pain in the abdominal area; colic.

cranium: area of the head above the ears and eyes; the bones forming the vault that lodges the brain.

cravat: bandage made by folding a triangular piece of cloth from its apex toward the base.

crepitus: grating or grinding sensation when two irritated surfaces rub together, i.e., fractured bone ends, patellofemoral chondromalacia.

cricoid cartilage: lowermost cartilage of the larynx.

cricothyroid membrane: substantial sheet of fascia connecting the thyroid and cricoid cartilages.

critical burns: burns complicated by respiratory tract injury; third-degree burns involving critical areas or more than 10% of body surface; second-degree burns involving more than 20% to 25% of body surface.

cross-finger technique: method of opening the patient's mouth with the trainer's crossed fingers to probe the mouth for foreign bodies.

croup: acute obstruction of the larynx, with barking cough and hoarseness and a harsh, high-pitched breathing sound.

crural: pertaining to the leg or thigh; femoral.

crushed chest: see flail chest.

CVA: cardiovascular accident; see stroke.

cyanosis: blue color around the lips, fingernails or fingertips, resulting from poor oxygenation of the circulating blood; the blood is very dark.

cystitis: inflammation of the bladder.

decerebrate response: characteristic stiffening of the extremities in response to pain indicating loss of cerebral control.

decompression sickness: the "bends"; bubbles of nitrogen are released in the bloodstream during rapid ascent from deep water causing arterial block.

decongestants: drugs that reduce congestion or swelling (usually of the nasal passages).

decontamination: ridding a person or object of some contaminating substance.

deep frostbite: cold injury through the skin and subcutaneous tissue to the muscle and bone; usually involves the hands and feet.

defecate: move the bowels.

defibrillation: termination of atrial or ventricular fibrillation, usually by electroshock.

deformity: distortion (twisting out of the natural shape) of a body part; general disfigurement of the body.

dehydration: loss of body water.

delirium: mental disturbance marked by hallucinations, cerebral excitement and physical restlessness, usually lasting only a short time.

delirium tremens: serious manifestation of the alcohol withdrawal syndrome, with restlessness, fever, confusion, disorientation and hallucinations.

delusional: having false beliefs or ideas.

dementia: severe emotionally disturbed state, in which the patient acts irrationally due to his own distortion of his environment.

Demerol: meperidine hydrochloride; a narcotic, analgesic, sedative and antispasmodic; may produce physiological and psychological dependence.

denervated: condition in which nerve supply is cut off or blocked.

depressants: drugs that decrease awareness and mental capacity to function, slow reflexes; may decrease respiratory and heart rates.

depressed fracture (of the skull): a fragment or fragments of bone are pushed inward against the brain.

derangement: mental disorder; disarrangement of a part or organ.

dermis: the inner layer of the skin, containing hair follicles, sweat glands, sebaceous glands, nerve endings and blood vessels.

descending colon: part of the colon that lies on the left side of the abdomen, extending from a point below the stomach to the level of the iliac crest.

descent injury: compression problems caused by outside pressure on the diver's body.

detoxification: treatment designed to free an addict from a drug habit.

diabetes mellitus: disease in which the body is unable to use sugar normally because of a deficiency of insulin.

diabetic: one who has diabetes; pertaining to diabetes.

diabetic coma: state of unconsciousness caused by loss of fluid and increased acidity in diabetes mellitus.

diabetic ketoacidosis: condition caused by excessive fluid and sugar loss in the kidneys and an excessive build-up in the bloodstream of acid metabolic products (ketones) caused by the body's use of substances other than sugar for energy.

diagnosis: identifying a disease or injury from its signs and symptoms.

diameter: length of a straight line through the center of a circle or an object.

diaphragm: flat, circular sheet of muscle separating the thoracic and abdominal cavities.

diaphysis: shaft or middle part of a long cylindrical bone.

diarrhea: an abnormally large number of liquid bowel movements.

diastole: relaxation of the heart while the ventricles fill with blood.

diastolic blood pressure: lower blood pressure noted during ventricular relaxation as the heart fills with blood.

differential diagnosis: distinguishing among various diseases to determine the one from which the patient suffers.

diffuse: not definitely limited or localized; widely spread.

digestion: process of breaking food down to its basic chemical components that can be absorbed by the intestine.

digestive system: gastrointestinal tract (stomach and intestines), mouth, salivary glands, pharynx, esophagus, liver, gallbladder, pancreas, rectum and anus.

Dilantin: anticonvulsant drug.

dilate: swell, become wide, enlarge.

Dilaudid: trade name for a narcotic drug, a depressant.

diphtheria: acute bacterial infection of throat, tonsils, nose and sometimes skin with local pain and swelling.

dislocation: displacement of the ends of two bones at their joint so that the joint surfaces are no longer in proper contact.

disoriented: having lost the sense of familiarity with one's surroundings; not knowing one's position in space or time.

displaced fracture: deformity of the limb; fragments are not aligned.

distal: location in an extremity nearer the free end; location on the trunk farther from the midline or from the point of reference.

distensibility: ability to distend, or swell, from inner pressure.

diverticulitis: inflammation of congenitally abnormal pouches along the distal colon.

dorsal: posterior.

dorsal spine: portion of the spine that attaches to the 12 ribs—the thoracic spine.

dorsalis pedis artery: artery on the anterior surface of the foot; can be palpated when present.

dorsiflexion: motion of a joint towards the dorsal surface.

double vision: perception of two images of a single object.

dressing: wound covering, usually gauze.

droplet: small drop, such as expelled from the mouth in coughing, sneezing or speaking, which may carry infection through the air.

drowning: suffocation in or under water.

drug: any substance that produces a physical or mental effect on the body.

drug abuse: overuse of a drug to the point of addiction.

drug withdrawal: physical reaction characterized by anxiety, nausea, vomiting, convulsions, delirium, sweating or cramps that occurs when an addict is unable to get drugs.

duodenum: first or most proximal portion of the small intestine, connecting the stomach to the jejunum.

dura mater: outermost of the three layers of tissue that envelop the brain and spinal cord.

dysfunction: impaired or abnormal functioning.

dysphagia: sensation of difficulty in swallowing.

dyspnea: difficulty or pain with breathing.

dyspneic: suffering from dyspnea.

dysuria: difficulty in urination.

eardrum: thin, tense membrane forming the greater part of the outer wall of the middle ear and separating it from the outer ear canal.

ecchymosis: bruise; a discoloration of the skin due to subcutaneous and intracutaneous bleeding. Bluish at first, it changes later to a greenish yellow because of chemical changes in the pooled blood.

edema: condition in which fluid escapes into the tissues from vascular or lymphatic spaces and causes local or generalized swelling.

edematous: swollen, with excessive fluid in the tissues.

effusion: escape of fluid into a joint.

elbow: joint between the arm and the forearm.

electrocardiographic: pertaining to an electrocardiogram, tracing of the electrical activity of the heart muscle.

embolus: clot or other plug brought by the blood from one vessel and forced into a smaller one, obstructing the circulation.

Emergency Medical Information Card or Tag: card carried or worn as a bracelet or necklace to warn of a serious medical problem the patient has.

emphysema: disease of the lung in which there is extreme dilation of pulmonary air sacs and poor exchange of oxygen and carbon dioxide. It causes rapid, shallow breathing and frequently results in secondary impairment of heart action.

enchondral ossification: process whereby a cartilage anlage (model) is replaced by bone.

endomysium: thin sheath of connective tissue consisting principally of reticular fibers that invests each striated muscle fiber and binds the fibers together within a fasciculus.

endothelium: layer of epithelial cells that lines the cavities of the heart and blood vessels.

energy: capacity to work; power to produce motion.

enteritis: inflammation of the intestine, especially the small intestine.

enzyme: protein capable of producing or accelerating some change in a given substance.

eosinophil: white blood cell characterized by red granules in the cytoplasm when stained.

ephedrine: nasal decongestant and mild stimulant.

epicondyles, medial and lateral: eminences on either side of a bone above the condyles.

epidemiology: study of the frequency and distribution of diseases in a community.

epidermis: the outermost layer of the skin, varying in thickness from 1/200 to 1/20 inch, and containing keratinized, or horny, external protecting cells constantly being rubbed away.

epidural: outside the dura mater and under the skull.

epidural hematoma: hematoma outside the dura mater and under the skull.

epigastric: related to the epigastrium.

epigastrium: upper middle region of the abdomen.

epiglottis: lidlike cartilaginous structure overhanging the superior entrance to the larynx and serving to prevent food from entering the larynx and trachea while swallowing.

epilepsy: condition manifested by seizures caused by an abnormal focus of activity within the brain that produces severe motor responses or changes in consciousness.

epimysium: fibrous sheath about a muscle fiber.

epinephrine: hormone that stimulates the heart and the sympathetic nervous system.

epiphyseal fracture: injury to the growth plate of a long bone in children; may lead to arrested bone growth.

epiphyseal plate: transverse cartilage plate near the end of a child's bone responsible for growth in length of the bone.

epiphysis: end of a long bone.

epistaxis: nosebleed.

epithelium: covering of internal and external surfaces of the body; consists of cells joined by cementing substances.

erythema: reddening.

erythrocytes: red blood cells.

esophageal varices: huge collateral veins in the esophagus that develop when cirrhosis of the liver is established and blood flow from the gastrointestinal tract is shunted around the liver.

esophagus: passage leading from the pharynx to the stomach; a muscular tube lined with squamous, or skinlike, epithelium.

estradiol: most potent, naturally occurring estrogen in humans; considered a true ovarian hormone.

estrogen: female sex hormones responsible for secondary sexual characteristics and cyclic changes in the vagina.

estrone: an estrogic hormone less active than estradiol; also called follicular hormone.

etiological: pertaining to the cause of a disease.

evaporation: loss of heat from the body by conversion of moisture or perspiration on the body's surface to a vapor.

eversion: turning outward.

eversion (of eyelid): pulling the lid away from the eyeball, forward and upward.

evisceration: protruding of internal organs through a wound.

excitable focus: area of the brain responsible for causing epileptic seizures.

excretion: eliminating material from the body.

expiration: exhaling, breathing out, or expelling air from the lungs.

extend: to straighten (a joint).

extension: motion of straightening a joint or moving the joint towards the dorsal surface of the body.

external: outer; outside the body.

external bleeding: hemorrhage that can be seen coming from a wound.

external chest compression: see cardiac compression.

external genitalia: genitalia outside the body.

extracellular: outside the cell.

extrasystoles: irregular, extra heartbeats.

extremities: arms and legs.

face: front part of the head, including eyes, nose, cheeks, mouth and forehead; made up of bones fused together to protect important structures.

face mask: mask fitted to the face through which gas is delivered to the patient.

faint: psychogenic shock; a temporary loss of consciousness, usually of brief duration and not serious.

false motion: motion at a point in a limb where it usually does not occur; positive indication of bone fracture.

fascia: sheet or band of tough fibrous connective tissue; it lies deep under the skin and forms an outer layer for the muscles and various organs of the body.

fat: adipose tissue; white or yellowish tissue that forms soft pads in the body and supplies reserve energy.

fatigue fracture: see stress fracture.

fatty acid: hydrocarbon that has a hydrogen atom replaced by a carboxyl group. There are saturated and unsaturated fatty acids.

febrile: elevations of body temperature above normal range—36–37.5 C (96.8–99.5 F).

fecal: pertaining to feces.

feces: excrement discharged from the intestines.

felon: purulent infection of the pulp of the distal phalanx of the finger.

femoral artery: principal artery of the thigh, a continuation of the external iliac artery. It supplies blood to the lower abdominal wall, external genitalia and leg.

femoral condyles: two surfaces at the distal end of the femur that articulate with the superior surfaces of the tibia.

femoral head: proximal end of the femur, articulating with the acetabulum.

femoral neck: heavy column of bone connecting the head and the shaft of the femur.

femoral nerve: major peripheral nerve, immediately lateral to the femoral artery.

femoral shaft: main part of the femur.

femoral vein: continuation of the popliteal vein that becomes the external iliac vein; the major vein draining the thigh.

femur: bone that extends from the pelvis to the knee, the longest and largest bone in the body; the "thigh bone."

fibrillation: uncontrolled and ineffective beating of the heart occurring when individual muscle fibers take up independent, irregular activity; it causes loss of effective cardiac function.

fibula: outer and smaller of the two bones of the leg, extending from just below the knee to form the lateral portion of the ankle joint.

finger probe: technique for probing the patient's mouth for foreign bodies.

first-degree burn: burn limited to the most superficial layer of the epidermis and resulting only in reddening of the skin.

flail chest: condition of the chest wall characterized by a free segment that moves paradoxically (opposite to normal motion) when the patient breathes; caused by fractures of several ribs in two or more places each.

flail segment: segment of the chest wall in a flail chest injury that lies between the rib fractures and moves paradoxically as the patient breathes.

flexion: bending of a joint; in contrast to extension.

floating ribs: 11th and 12th ribs, which do not connect to the sternum.

flotation device: device that keeps one from sinking in water, such as a life jacket.

fluid therapy: treatment with intravenous fluids to correct the patient's condition.

follicle: small secretory sac or cavity.

follicle stimulating hormone (FSH): gonadotropic hormone released by the pituitary gland. In the female it induces ovarian follicular growth; in the male, proliferation of the seminiferous tubules.

foot drop: paralysis of the dorsiflexor muscles of the foot and ankle, so that the foot falls and the toes drag on the ground in walking.

four-person logroll: method of placing a person on a carrying device, usually a long spine board or a flat litter, by rolling the patient on one side and then back onto a litter.

fracture: any break in the continuity of a bone.

fracture-dislocation: combined injury in which the joint is dislocated and a part of the bone near the joint is fractured.

frostbite: localized cold injury to body part that is partially or completely frozen.

frostnip: incipient frostbite, with superficial local tissue destruction.

full-thickness burn: see third-degree burn.

gallbladder: pear-shaped, membranous sac on the undersurface of the liver; collects bile from the liver and discharges it into the duodenum through the common bile duct.

gamekeeper's thumb: tear of the ulnar collateral ligament of metacarpophalangeal joint of thumb (also skier's thumb).

gangrene: death of tissues, usually the result of a loss of blood supply.

gastric juice: digestive fluid secreted by the glands of the stomach; it contains mainly hydrochloric acid, pepsin and mucus.

gastritis: inflammation of the lining of the stomach.

gastroenteritis: inflammation of the lining of the stomach and intestines.

generalized seizure: seizure in which most of the brain is involved; manifested by motor activity of all parts of the body.

genitalia: male and female reproductive systems and the male urethra.

genitourinary system: organs of reproduction together with the organs concerned in the production and excretion of urine.

genu: knee.

germinal layer: layer of skin cells that constantly reproduce to replace outer cells that are being shed or rubbed off.

glenohumeral joint: true shoulder joint.

glenoid fossa: recess in the scapula for the articulation of the humeral head laterally forming the glenohumeral joint.

glucose: sugar occurring in certain foods, especially fruits, and in normal blood; in diabetes mellitus it is present in the urine.

gonorrhea: common venereal disease; a contagious infection of the genital mucous membrane.

Good Samaritan laws: laws providing that a person who voluntarily undertakes to help an injured or ill person at the scene is not liable with any fault or responsibility at law for errors or omissions in the care rendered.

gout: hereditary form of arthritis, with excessive uric acid in the blood and recurrent painful attacks of arthritis in joints.

granulocyte: any cell containing granules, especially a leukocyte.

great vessels: large vessels entering or leaving the heart, including aorta, pulmonary arteries and veins, and venae cavae.

greater trochanter: broad, flat process at the upper end of the lateral surface of the femur to which several muscles are attached.

greenstick fracture: an incomplete fracture that passes only part way through the shaft of a bone; occurs only in children.

guarding: refusal to use an injured part because motion causes pain; involuntary or voluntary abdominal muscular contraction reflecting inflammation and pain within the peritoneal cavity.

gums: dense fibrous tissue, covered by mucous membrane, that envelops the alveolar process of the upper and lower jaws and surrounds the necks of the teeth.

hair follicles: small organs that produce hair; there is one for each hair connected with a sebaceous gland and a tiny muscle.

hallucination: sense perception not founded on objective reality.

hammer toe: toe with dorsal flexion of the first phalanx and plantar flexion of the second and third phalanges.

hamstring: large muscle groups at the back of the thigh that flex the knee.

hard palate: bony plate; the anterior part of the roof of the mouth.

haversian system (osteon): architectural unit of bone consisting of a central tube with alternate layers of intercellular material.

head of a bone: rounded end, allowing joint rotation.

head tilt-chin lift: opening the airway by tilting the patient's head backward and lifting the chin.

head-tilt maneuver: opening the airway by tilting the patient's head backward as far as possible.

head tilt-neck lift: opening the airway by tilting the patient's head backward and lifting the neck upward.

heart: hollow muscular organ that receives the blood from the veins and propels it into the arteries.

heart attack: see myocardial infarction.

heart failure: see cardiac failure.

heat cramps: painful muscle spasms of arms or legs caused by excessive body heat and depletion of fluids and electrolytes.

heat exhaustion (prostration, collapse): mild form of shock caused by loss of fluid and electrolytes from the circulation because of excessive sweating when exposed to heat.

heat exposure: dose of excessive energy received by the body, either locally or over its entire surface, for which normal protective mechanisms are insufficient.

heat stroke: condition of rapidly rising internal body temperature that overwhelms the body's mechanisms for release of heat.

hematemesis: vomiting of blood.

hematochezia: passage of bloody stools.

hematoma: a pool of blood collecting within the damaged tissue.

hematuria: blood in the urine.

hemiplegia: paralysis of one side of the body.

hemithorax: one side (one half) of the chest.

hemolysis: destruction of red blood cells.

hemophilia: hereditary bleeding disorder due to deficiency of coagulation factor VIII.

hemoptysis: coughing up of bright red blood.

hemorrhage: bleeding; blood escaping from arteries or veins.

hemorrhagic shock: shock resulting from blood loss.

hemorrhoid: varicose dilation of a vein near the rectum.

hemostasis: arrest of bleeding or circulation.

hemostat: any agent that arrests, chemically or mechanically, the flow of blood from an open vessel; an instrument for arresting hemorrhage by compression of the bleeding vessel.

hemothorax: presence of blood in the chest cavity within the pleural space outside the lung.

hepatitis: see infectious hepatitis.

hernia: protrusion of a loop of an organ or tissue through an abnormal opening.

hinge joints: joints that can bend and straighten but cannot rotate.

hives: urticaria; allergic skin disorder marked by patches of swelling and intense itching; caused by contact with something to which the person is allergic.

hollow organs: tubes through which materials pass, such as the stomach, intestines, ureters and bladder.

hormones: chemical substances produced in the body by a gland or cells of a gland that have special regulatory effects on the activity of another distant organ.

host: organism or person in or on whom an infectious agent resides.

humerus: bone of the arm articulating with the scapula to form the shoulder joint and with the ulna and radius distally at the elbow.

humidified: with moisture added to (as of room air).

hyaline articular cartilage: true cartilage; smooth and pearly, it covers the articular surfaces of bones.

hydrochloric acid: normal component of gastric juice.

hydroxyapatite: inorganic compound that gives rigidity to bones and teeth.

hyperextension: extreme extension, straightening, of a limb or body part.

hyperflexion: extreme bending.

hyperglycemia: abnormally increased content of sugar in the blood.

hypersensitive: allergic.

hypersensitive reaction: severe allergic reaction with wheezing, cardiovascular collapse and skin wheals (hives).

hypertension: abnormally and persistently high blood pressure.

hyperventilation (primary): dyspnea without lung abnormalities; overbreathing to the extent that arterial carbon dioxide is abnormally lowered.

hyphema: bleeding into the anterior chamber of the eye, obscuring the iris.

hypoglycemia: abnormally low sugar content in the blood.

hypotension: abnormally low blood pressure.

hypothalamus: part of the brain stem that activates, controls, and integrates peripheral autonomic mechanisms, endocrine gland activity, water balance in the body and automatic functions such as sleep.

hypothermia: systemic lowering of the body temperature below 33.3 C (95 F).

hypovolemia: decrease in the volume of the circulating blood.

hypovolemic shock: hemorrhagic shock; shock caused by insufficient blood within the body.

hypoxia: deficiency of oxygen reaching the tissues of the body.

hysteria: neurotic disturbance marked by excitement and self-consciousness, anxiety, symptoms of imaginary illness, and lack of emotional control.

iatrogenic illness: an undesired physical or mental condition resulting from medical intervention.

idiopathic illness: conditions without clear origin; of unknown cause.

ileocecal valve: protrusion of the terminal ileum into the large intestine at the junction of the ileum and colon; protects the terminal ileum from feces forced back into the cecum.

ileum: more distal portion of the small intestine, between the jejunum and the colon.

ileus: obstruction of the bowel.

iliac crests: thickened, expanded upper borders of the ilium.

iliac spines: blunt, bony projections on the borders of the ilium.

ilium: expansive superior portion of the hip bone; a separate bone in early childhood.

immersion foot: see trench foot.

immunization: process by which resistance to an infectious disease is produced.

impaled foreign object: object such as a knife, splinter of wood or piece of glass in a puncture wound.

implied consent: consent implied by the fact that the person voluntarily entered a situation.

incontinence: inability to control the bowels or bladder.

incubation period: time between exposure and the first appearance of signs of an infectious disease in a host.

indirect contact: transmission of a communicable disease by contaminated object.

inelastic: unable to expand.

infarct: area of a tissue that is damaged or dies as a result of insufficient blood supply; see myocardial infarction.

infecting organism: see infectious agent.

infection: disease state produced in a host by the invasion of an infecting organism (virus, bacterium).

infectious agent: cause of an infectious disease, such as a virus or bacterium.

infectious hepatitis: acute viral infection of the liver causing fever, loss of appetite, jaundice and fatigue.

inferior: lying lower in the body.

inferior vena cava: see vena cava.

infestation: disease state produced by parasites.

informed consent: consent given by a person who understands the nature and extent of any procedure to which he or she is agreeing and has sufficient mental and physical capacity to make such a judgment.

infusion: introduction of a fluid (other than blood or blood products) into a vein.

inguinal ligament: fibrous band running from the anterior superior spine of the ilium to the tubercle of the pubis.

injection: forcing a fluid into, as for medical purposes.

innoculation: introduction of an attenuated disease agent into a healthy person to produce a mild form of the disease followed by immunity.

innominate bone: bone forming one half of the pelvic girdle and arising from a fusion of the ilium, ischium and pubis.

insertion: site of attachment of a muscle.

inspiration: inhaling; breathing in, drawing air, into the lungs.

insulin: hormone produced by the pancreas that enables glucose to be converted to glycogen and stored till needed; used in treatment and control of diabetes mellitus.

insulin shock: shock caused by an overdose of insulin or failure to eat enough food to balance the insulin, resulting in a sudden drop in the blood sugar level; chief symptoms are sweating, tremor, anxiety, vertigo and double vision, followed by delirium, convulsions and collapse.

intercellular: between cells.

intercostal: between the ribs.

intermittent positive pressure breathing: active inflation of the lungs during inspiration under positive pressure from a cycling valve.

internal jugular vein: major vein draining the brain.

internal temperature: body temperature.

internuncial neurons: neurons interconnecting the sensory nerves with the motor nerves.

intertrochanteric: between the two trochanters of the femur.

intervertebral disc: cartilaginous cushion between two vertebral bodies.

intestine: part of the alimentary canal extending from the pyloric opening of the stomach to the anus.

intra-abdominal: within the abdomen.

intracellular: within cells.

intracerebral bleeding: bleeding within the brain.

intracerebral hematoma: hematoma within the brain.

intracranial: within the skull.

intracranial hematoma: hematoma, or collection of blood, inside the skull.

intramembranous ossification: formation of bone within a membrane.

intramuscular: within a muscle.

intrapericardial: within the pericardium.

intraperitoneal: within the peritoneal cavity.

intrathoracic: within the chest.

intravascular: within a vessel.

intravenous: within a vein.

intravenous fluid: fluid given by way of a vein.

intravenous line: polyethylene catheter through which fluids are given directly into a vein.

inversion: turning inward toward the body.

involuntary muscle: muscle that continues to contract rhythmically regardless of conscious control.

involuntary nervous system: see autonomic nervous system.

iris: muscle behind the cornea that dilates and constricts the pupil regulating the amount of light that enters the eye.

irrigation: washing by a stream of water or other fluid.

ischemia: lacking blood; local or temporary anemia due to obstruction of circulation to a body part.

ischial tuberosities: bony prominences felt in the middle of each buttock.

ischium: inferior dorsal part of the innominate bone; a separate bone in early childhood.

isometric exercise: contraction of muscles without motion of the part.

isotonic exercise: contraction of muscles against resistance with movement of the part.

jaundice: yellow tissue seen in liver disease caused by bilirubin deposited in the skin.

jaw-thrust: opening the airway by bringing the patient's jaw forward, tilting the head backward and pulling the lower lip down.

jejunum: portion of the small intestine that extends from the duodenum to the ileum.

jersey finger: rupture of the insertion of the flexor digitorum longus tendon by forced extension of the flexed finger.

joint: articulation, place of union or junction between two or more bones of the skeleton.

joint capsule: fibrous sac with synovial lining that encloses a joint.

ketoacidosis: acidosis seen in diabetic patients and associated with an enhanced production of ketone bodies from incomplete metabolism of fats.

ketone: metabolic end products of the use of fat for routine energy needs.

kidneys: two retroperitoneal organs that filter the blood, excreting the end products of metabolism as urine, and regulating salt and water content in the body. They lie in the same plane as the pancreas, behind the abdominal cavity.

knee joint: articulation between the distal femur and the tibia.

"knocked-down" shoulder: a dislocation of the acromioclavicular joint.

laceration: cut that may leave a smooth or jagged wound through the skin, subcutaneous tissues, muscles and associated nerves and blood vessels.

Lachman test: test for instability of anterior cruciate ligament of the knee. Originally described by Lanbrinudi, an anterior drawer test performed with the knee flexed 20°.

lacrimal system: system pertaining to the tear, consisting of lacrimal (tear) glands and ducts.

lamellar bone: thin leaf or plate of bone.

large intestine: portion of the digestive tube extending from the ileocecal valve to the anus, made up of the cecum, colon and rectum.

larynx: voice box; a musculocartilaginous structure lined with mucous membrane, above the trachea and below the base of the tongue, guarding the entrance to the trachea and functioning secondarily as the organ of the voice.

laser: a beam of nonspreading, monochromatic, visible light; high energies are concentrated into a narrow beam.

lateral: lying away from the midline.

lens: transparent body of the eye, through which images are focused on the retina.

leukocytes: white blood cells.

Leydig's cells: furnish the internal secretions of the testes.

licensure: formal permission to perform certain acts.

ligament: band of fibrous tissue that connects bone to bone or bone to cartilage and supports and strengthens joints.

light rescue: movement of injured patients from uncomplicated car crashes and from buildings.

linear fracture (of the skull): thin line crack in the skull.

liver: large, solid organ situated in the upper right abdomen; produces bile, stores sugar for immediate use by the body and chemically treats all products of absorption in the gastrointestinal tract.

localized abdominal tenderness: tenderness in a specific part of the abdomen.

"locked" joint: joint in which there is a marked loss of normal motion.

lower urinary tract: bladder and urethra.

lucid interval: time in which the patient seems normal between periods of unconsciousness.

lumbar spine: lower part of the back formed by the lowest five nonfused vertebrae.

lumbar vertebra: vertebra of the lumbar spine.

lumbosacral plexus: network of nerves serving the lower extremity.

lumen: cavity of a tube-shaped organ such as a blood vessel.

lungs: organs that aerate the blood, occupying the lateral cavities of the chest and separated from each other by the heart and mediastinal structures.

lymphatic system: system of vessels that convey lymph from the tissues to the blood.

lymphocyte: type of leukocyte; mainly responsible for the specific defenses of the body against foreign invaders.

malleolus: rounded projection on either side of the ankle joint.

mallet finger: avulsion of the insertion of the tendon of the exterior digitorum communis into the distal phalanx of the finger caused by forced flexion of the extended joint.

mandible: bone of the lower jaw.

manipulation: moving with the hands.

manually controlled resuscitators: resuscitators with manual control, used in ambulances.

manubrium: the upper bone of the sternum articulating with the clavicle and first pair of costal cartilages.

mastoid process: prominent, hard, bony mass at the base of the skull behind the ear.

maxilla: irregularly shaped bone, formed by the fusion of several smaller bones, that helps to form the upper jaw on either side of the face; it contains the upper teeth and the orbit of the eye, the nasal cavity and the palate.

mechanism of injury: factors involved in producing the injury.

medial: lying toward the midline.

median nerve: nerve that controls sensation of the central palm, the thumb and the first three fingers, as well as the ability to oppose the thumb to the little finger.

mediastinum: median or middle area in the thorax, between the lungs, in which lie the heart, great vessels, esophagus and trachea.

Medic-Alert: bracelet, necklace or card stating the patient's medical problems.

medicolegal: relating to both medicine and law.

medulla oblongata: cone of nerve tissue continuous with the pons above and the spinal cord below; controls vital functions such as respiration, circulation and the five senses.

melena: passage of dark black stools with the consistency of tar.

meninges: three membranes that envelop the brain and spinal cord: the dura mater, pia mater and arachnoid.

meningitis: inflammation of the meninges.

meniscus: cushion of cartilage that fills up a space between bones and aids in the gliding motion and stability of the joint.

menstrual cycle: period of the regularly recurring changes in the endometrium, ending in its shedding (menstruation).

menstruation: periodic bleeding from the vagina at approximately four week intervals in which the lining of the uterus is shed.

mesentery: delicate tissue formed by peritoneum that suspends the organs within the abdomen from the body walls and carries blood vessels and nerves to all these organs.

metabolic: pertaining to metabolism.

metabolic shock: shock caused by loss of body fluid.

metabolism: series of chemical processes that extract the energy needed for life from food.

metacarpal bones: five bones of the hand extending from the wrist to the fingers.

metaphysis: portion of long bone in the wide part at the extremity containing the growth zone in children.

metatarsal bones: five long bones of the foot between the instep and the toes.

middle ear: tympanic cavity with its ossicles.

midline: imaginary straight vertical line drawn from midforehead through the nose and the umbilicus to the floor.

milliliter: one-thousandth of a liter.

millimeters of mercury (mm Hg): unit of pressure used in measuring blood pressure. The amount of pressure needed to raise 1 mm of mercury 1 ml.

minerals: nonorganic substances usually occurring in the earth's crust.

minor's consent: consent to treatment given by a minor.

monitoring: checking constantly on physiological signs (cardiac, respiratory).

monocyte: phagocytic leukocyte found in small numbers in normal blood.

mononucleosis: acute viral disease with fever, sore throat and lymph node swelling.

morbidity: state of being diseased.

morphine: narcotic drug, a derivative of opium.

mortality: death rate.

Morton's neuroma: pain in the metatarsal region due to abnormality or osteochondrosis of the heads of the metatarsals.

Morton's toe: abnormally long second metatarsal.

motor nerves: nerves that transmit impulses to muscles, causing them to move.

mouth: lips, cheeks, gums, teeth and tongue.

mouth-to-mask ventilation: system of artificial ventilation in which the trainer ventilates the patient with supplemental oxygen through a mask while supplying air from his or her own lungs at the same time.

mouth-to-mouth ventilation: artificial ventilation performed by the resuscitator's mouth making a seal around the patient's mouth as he exhales into the patient's mouth.

mouth-to-nose ventilation: artificial ventilation in which the resuscitator's lips make a seal around the patient's nose.

mouth-to-stoma ventilation: artificial ventilation for patients with a tracheal stoma, in which the resuscitator blows into the tube or stoma.

mucous membrane: lining of body cavities and passages that communicate directly or indirectly with environment outside body.

mucus: opaque, sticky secretion of the mucous membranes, consisting of mucin, epithelial cells, leukocytes and water, in which various inorganic salts are dissolved.

multipennate: term used for muscles with more than two muscle bellies, i.e., pectoralis major.

musculoskeletal system: all the bones, joints, muscles and tendons of the body, collectively.

mutation: alterations in the genes, causing altered heredity of offspring.

myocardial: of the heart muscle.

myocardial contusion: bruise of the heart muscle.

myocardial infarction: heart attack; damaging or death of an area of the heart muscle.

myocardium: heart muscle.

myofibrils: small fibrils found in muscle tissue running parallel to the cellular long axis.

myosin: protein present in muscle fibrils and comprising about 65% of total muscle protein.

nasal cannula: tube for insertion into the nose; oxygen can be administered with it through two small tubular prongs that fit into the nostrils.

nasal septum: partition separating the two nostrils; composed of membrane, cartilage and bone.

nasopharyngeal airway: artificial airway positioned in the nasal cavity; the curvature of the airway follows the nasal floor.

nasopharynx: part of the pharynx that lies above the level of the soft palate.

neck of a bone: region below the head of the bone.

necrosis: destruction and death of tissues.

negligence: instance where the actions or behavior of an individual who had a duty to act did not conform to the required standard of care and injury resulted.

nerve root: proximal (nearest) end of a spinal nerve.

nerves: branches from the spinal cord and brain; either sensory, motor or a combination of both.

nervous system: brain, spinal cord and nerves.

neurology: the branch of medical science concerned with the nervous system and its disorders.

neuron: nerve cell; the fundamental functional unit of nervous tissue.

neurosurgery: surgery of the nervous system.

neutralize: to render neutral; specifically, the chemical combination of hydrogen and hydroxyl ions to form water, thus rendering each ion harmless.

nitrogen (N): colorless, gaseous element; when released as bubbles of gas in the bloodstream under conditions of reduced atmospheric pressure, it can cause arterial embolization.

nitrogen narcosis: state of euphoria caused by increased blood nitrogen during a deep dive.

nitroglycerine: medicine used in treating angina pectoris; it relaxes vascular smooth muscle and increases blood flow and oxygen supply to the heart muscle.

NOCSAE: National Operating Committee on Standards for Athletic Equipment.

nocturia: necessary passage of urine at night.

nonconductive: inability to transmit an electrical current or any other source of energy.

nondisplaced fracture: no deformity of the bone.

nontraumatic: injury not due to trauma.

nose: facial organ of smell and part of the respiratory system.

nostril: one of the nose's external openings.

nutrients: substances that nourish the body.

obesity: excessive body weight; an excessive amount of body fat.

occiput: back part of the head.

occlusive dressing: dressing or bandage that closes a wound and protects it from the air.

olecranon process: most posterior portion of the elbow at its apex.

open abdominal injuries: injuries, e.g., stab or gunshot wounds, in which the abdominal cavity has been penetrated.

open chest injuries: injuries in which the chest wall has been penetrated.

open fracture: fracture in which the bone is exposed to air and contaminated.

open wound: break in the surface of the skin or in the mucous membrane that lines the mouth, nose, anus or vagina.

opium: highly addictive narcotic drug.

optic nerves: nerves transmitting visual sensations to the brain.

orbit: eye socket.

organism: individual living thing, plant or animal.

oriented: knowing one's position in person, space or time.

origin: more fixed end or attachment of a muscle.

oropharynx: division of the pharynx between soft palate and upper edge of the epiglottis.

osteoblast: cell associated with production of osteoid.

osteoclast: large multinuclear bone associated with absorption and removal of bone.

osteocyte: osteoblast imbedded within bone.

osteoid: protein substance secreted by the osteoblast in which the calcium salts are precipitated giving rigidity to the bone.

osteomalacia: condition produced by a loss of calcium from bones.

osteon: see haversian system.

osteoporosis: abnormal brittleness of the bones caused by loss of protein matrix.

ovaries: female glands that produce sex hormones and ova.

oxygen exchange: the process by which oxygen is provided to the blood and carbon dioxide is taken from the blood to be expelled in exhalation.

oxygenated: supplied with oxygen.

pacemaker, cardiac: a device that stimulates the contraction of the heart muscle at a certain rate by electrical impulses; imposes a regular rhythm and rate on the heart.

palate: the roof of the mouth.

pallor: paleness, absence of skin color.

palmar: pertaining to the palm of the hand.

palpable: able to be touched or felt.

palpate: to examine by touch.

pancreas: large, elongated gland situated transversely behind the stomach, between the spleen and the duodenum; major source of digestive enzymes and produces the hormone, insulin, that regulates the metabolism of sugar.

pancreatic juice: juice secreted by the pancreas that contains many enzymes acting in the digestion of fat, starch and protein; flows directly into the duodenum through the pancreatic ducts.

pancreatitis: inflammation of the pancreas.

papilledema: edema of the optic papilla of the eye.

paradoxical motion: motion of the injured segment of a flail chest, opposite to the normal motion of the chest wall.

paralysis: complete or partial loss of the ability to move.

paralytic ileus: cessation of bowel mobility.

parasite: organism that lives within or on another living organism.

parasympathetic nervous system: craniosacral part of the autonomic nervous system; causes dilation of blood vessels, increases tone and contractility of smooth muscle and induces secretion.

parietal peritoneum: lining of the abdominal and pelvic walls and the undersurface of the diaphragm.

parietal pleura: portion of the pleura lining the inside of the chest cavity.

parietal regions: more lateral portions of the cranium.

paronychia: inflammation of folds of tissue surrounding the fingernail.

parotid gland: largest of the three chief, paired salivary glands.

paroxysm: a sudden recurrence or intensification of symptoms: a spasm or seizure.

partial seizure: seizure involving less extensive areas of the brain than a generalized seizure.

patella: kneecap.

patella alta: high positioned patella.

patella baja: low positioned patella.

pathologic fracture: occurs through weak or diseased bone and can be produced by minimal force.

pediatric: study and treatment of children in health and disease.

pelvic cavity: space within the walls of the pelvis.

pelvic floor: coccygeus and levator ani muscles and the perineal fascia, closing the pelvic outlet.

pelvic inflammatory disease: venereal infection usually involving the fallopian tubes and surrounding tissue; commonly gonorrheal.

pelvis: bony ring connecting the trunk to the lower extremities.

penetrating abdominal wound: wound caused by the penetration of the abdomen by an instrument or missile, such as a knife or bullet.

penetrating chest injuries: injuries in which an object has penetrated the chest.

penicillin: antibiotic extracted from cultures of certain molds.

penis: male organ of urinary excretion and copulation.

pepsin: only digestive enzyme produced in the stomach; initiates the digestion of protein.

peptic ulcer: ulcers in the stomach or duodenum caused by the action of pepsin.

perforating wounds: wounds that transverse a limb or body to exit on the opposite side; through-and-through wounds.

perforation: hole made through a part of substance.

perfusion: process of blood entering an organ or a tissue through its arteries and leaving through the veins, providing tissue nourishment.

pericardial sac: sac that surrounds the heart and the roots of the great vessels.

pericardial tamponade: condition in which blood or other fluid is present in the pericardial sac outside the heart exerting an unusual pressure on the heart.

perineum: pelvic floor and associated structures occupying the pelvic outlet.

periosteum: specialized connective tissue covering all bones of the body.

peripheral nervous system: portion of the nervous system that consists of the nerves and ganglia outside the brain and spinal cord.

peristalsis: wormlike movement by which the alimentary canal and other tubular organs move their contents.

peritoneal fluid: fluid in the abdominal cavity bathing the organs.

peritoneum: membrane lining the abdominopelvic walls (parietal peritoneum) and reflected inward over the viscera (visceral peritoneum).

peritonitis: inflammation of the lining of the abdomen.

perspiration: sweat.

pH: scale representing acidity and alkalinity; pH of 7 is neutral, less than 7 shows increasing acidity and greater than 7 shows increasing alkalinity (alkalosis).

phalanges: 14 bones making up the skeleton of the fingers or toes.

pharyngeal: relating to the pharynx.

pharynx: cavity at the back of nose and mouth; the throat.

physical dependence: addiction.

physiologic: characteristic of the state or functioning of the body or of a tissue or organ.

physiology: branch of biology that deals with the functions and actions of living matter and the physical and chemical factors involved.

physis: segment of tubular bone concerned with growth in bone length.

pia mater: innermost of the three layers of tissue that envelop the brain and spinal cord.

pinna: external ear.

pituitary: endocrine gland secreting hormones essential for regulating growth and water excretion, as well as hormones that regulate other endocrine glands.

plasma: liquid portion of whole blood within which the red and white cells lie; carries the blood cells and transports nutrients to all tissues.

platelets: disc-shaped elements of the blood,

smaller than red blood cells; essential in the formation of blood clots.

plethoric: having dark reddish-purple skin color; all visible blood vessels are full.

pleura: membrane lining the thoracic cavity and surrounding the lungs.

pleural space: potential space between the pleural surfaces.

pneumomediastinum: presence of air or gas in the mediastinum.

pneumonia: inflammation of the lungs.

pneumothorax: presence of air within the chest cavity in the pleural space but outside the lung.

poison: substance producing a harmful effect on body processes.

poison control center: center that gives advice and help by telephone in poisoning emergencies.

poliomyelitis: acute viral disease with fever, headache, gastrointestinal symptoms, stiff neck and paralysis.

polydipsia: excessive thirst for long periods of time, as in diabetes.

polymorphonuclear leukocytes: granular leukocyte; a white blood cell with a nucleus composed of two or more lobes or parts.

polyuria: passage of a large volume of urine in a given period, as in diabetes.

popliteal artery: continuation of the superficial femoral artery in the popliteal space (posterior surface of the knee).

posterior: behind; back.

posterior surface: surface at the back of the body.

posterior tibial artery: artery just posterior to the medial malleolus; easily palpable.

precordial: pertaining to the precordium, lying anterior to the heart.

precordium: chest wall over the heart.

pressure point: point where a blood vessel runs near a bone; pressure can be applied to these points to stop or slow bleeding.

professional standards: published recommendations of organizations and societies.

prominence: projection, protrusion.

pronation: assuming a prone position; turning the palm of the hand backward.

prostate gland: small gland that surrounds the male urethra where it emerges from the urinary bladder; it secretes a fluid that is part of the ejaculatory fluid.

prosthesis: artificial substitute for a missing body part.

protein: one of a group of complex organic compounds; essential combinations of amino acids; principal constituent of the animal cell.

protons: particles of an atom with a positive electrical charge.

proximal: location on an extremity nearer the trunk; location on the trunk nearer the midline or to the point of reference.

psychiatry: branch of medicine dealing with the study, treatment and prevention of mental illness.

psychogenic shock: common faint.

psychosis: severely disturbed state of mind; mental disorder characterized by defective or lost contact with reality.

ptyalin: digestive enzyme in saliva that converts starch to simple sugar.

puberty: period in growth when secondary sex characteristics appear and reproduction becomes possible.

pubis: anteriormost of the three bones (pubis, ilium and ischium) that fuse to make up the innominate bone.

pulmonary: of the lung.

pulmonary artery: major arterial vessel leading from the right ventricle to the lungs.

pulmonary contusion: bruise of the lung.

pulmonary edema: abnormal accumulation of fluid in the pulmonary tissues and air spaces.

pulmonary embolus: see embolus.

pulmonary oxygen toxicity: damage to the lungs caused by high oxygen concentration.

pulmonary veins: four veins that return blood from the lungs to the left atrium of the heart.

pulse: regular throbbing in the arteries caused by the contraction of the left ventricle of the heart.

pulse rate: rate of the pulse; reflects the rapidity of heart contractions.

pupil: circular opening in the middle of the iris of the eye.

pupillary reaction: contraction of the pupil in reaction to a bright light.

pus: liquid inflammation product made up of white cells and a thin fluid called liquor puris.

pyelonephritis: inflammation of the kidney and renal pelvis due to bacterial infection.

pylorus: distal or duodenal aperture of the stomach.

Q angle: the angle made by the rectus femoris and patellar tendon as it attaches to the tibial tuberosity.

quadriceps: great extensor muscle of the front of the thigh, divided into four parts.

rabid: having rabies.

rabies: acute virus disease of the nervous system spread by the saliva of a rabid animal.

radial artery: artery palpated at the base of the thumb.

radial nerve: nerve carrying sensation to the greater portion of the back of the hand; controls extension of the hand at the wrist.

radial nerve palsy: injury to the radial nerve in which the patient is unable to extend the wrist or fingers; produces wrist drop.

radial pulse: pulse of the radial artery.

radial styloid process: bony process felt on the lateral (thumb) side of the wrist.

radiant energy: any energy radiated from any source: electromagnetic waves, radio waves, visible light, x-rays or nuclear radiation.

radiation: sending forth of radiant energy.

radioactivity: nuclear emission of mass or energy.

radium: radioactive element used in clinical therapy.

radius: bone on the thumb side of the forearm.

rales: sound of air bubbling through liquid in the alveoli and bronchi, much like sand falling on an empty tin can.

''rapture of the deep'': nitrogen narcosis.

reactive depression: depression caused by some external situation and relieved when the situation is removed.

recessed: below the surface in a cavity.

recompression: restoration of normal pressure after the patient has been in conditions of greatly lowered atmospheric pressure.

recompression chamber: pressure chamber constructed to give air under greater than atmospheric pressure to a patient with the ''bends'' or to one who needs oxygen under pressure.

rectosigmoid colon: part of the large intestine that courses downward below the iliac crest, describing an S-shaped curve; the lower part of the curve joins the rectum.

recurvatum: deformity in which a joint is bent backwards, i.e., beyond normal extension.

red blood cells: erythrocytes.

referred pain: pain felt on a body surface other than the location of the pathological lesion.

reflex: motor response to a sensory stimulus not involving a conscious action.

reflex arc: neutral arc used in a reflex action, such as pulling the hand away from a hot stove; it involves sensory, short-circuiting internuncial and motor nerves.

regurgitation: casting up of incompletely digested food because the stomach is too full or overdistended with air and fluid.

rehabilitation: restoration of the patient to self-sufficiency.

renal: pertaining to the kidney.

renal colic: colicky pain caused by obstruction of the ureter by a stone, as the ureter tries to overcome the obstruction by peristalsis.

renal pelvis: cone-shaped collecting area that connects the ureter and the kidney.

resistance: ability of an organism to remain unaffected by infectious agents.

respiration: breathing.

respiratory: pertaining to breathing.

respiratory center: area in the brain that senses the level of carbon dioxide and controls respiration.

respiratory distress: difficulty in breathing.

respiratory shock: shock resulting from inadequate oxygen supply.

respiratory tract: organs and structures of respiration, chiefly the nose, larynx, trachea, bronchi, bronchioles and lungs.

resuscitation: restoring to life or consciousness using assisted breathing to restore ventilation and cardiac massage to restore circulation.

retina: light-sensitive area of the eye where images are projected; a layer of cells at the back of the eye that change the light image into electrical impulses that are carried by the optic nerve to the brain.

retrograde amnesia: loss of memory for the events preceding the injury.

retroperitoneal: behind the peritoneum.

retroperitoneal space: the space between the posterior parietal peritoneum and the posterior abdominal wall containing the kidneys, adrenal glands, ureters, duodenum, ascending and descending colon, pancreas and large vessels and nerves.

rewarming shock: shock in patients with severe hypothermia when the circulatory system dilates and the blood is shunted from the heart and lungs as the patient is warmed.

rhonchi: whistling, snoring sounds in breathing.

ribs: the paired arches of bone, 12 on either side, that extend from the thoracic vertebrae toward the anterior midline of the trunk.

roentgen: the amount of radiation that produces one unit of ionization in 1 cc of dry air under standard temperature and pressure conditions.

rotation: a turning around on an axis. **external rotation:** to the outside. **internal rotation:** to the inside.

rubella: German measles.

rubeola: measles.

rule of nines: rule dividing the body into sections, each of which constitutes approximately 9% of the total body surface area; used to estimate the amount of body surface burned.

sacral spine: see sacrum.

sacroiliac joint: joint or articulation between the sacrum and ilium.

sacrum: triangular bone just below the lumbar vertebrae formed by five fused sacral vertebrae.

saliva: secretion of water, protein and salts, secreted into the mouth by salivary glands; makes food easier to chew and begins breaking starch down for digestion.

salivary ducts: ducts (tubes or passages) through which the saliva passes.

salivary glands: glands that produce saliva to keep the mouth and pharynx moist.

sarcolemma: delicate plasma membrane in every striated muscle fiber.

sarcomere: unit of length of a myofibril.

scalp: that part of the skin of the head normally covered with hair.

scapula: shoulder blade.

scarlet fever: acute bacterial disease with headache, fever, nausea and vomiting, sore throat and rash.

sciatic nerve: nerve that carries major motor and sensory innervation to the foot and leg.

sclera: white portion of the eye; the tough outer coat of the eye that protects the delicate, light-sensitive inner layer.

scrotum: pouch of thickened skin hanging at the base of the penis containing the testicles and their accessory ducts and vessels.

scuba: self-contained underwater breathing apparatus.

sebaceous glands: glands producing an oily substance called sebum, discharged along the shafts of the hairs on the head and body.

second-degree burn: damage into, but not through, the dermis and resulting in blisters on the skin.

seizure: attack of epilepsy.

semiconscious: partly conscious.

seminal vesicles: storage sacs for sperm and seminal fluid that empty into the urethra at the prostate.

sensitivity: allergy.

sensory nerves: nerves that carry sensations of touch, taste, heat, cold, pain or other modalities.

sepsis: presence in the blood or other tissues of harmful microorganisms or their poisons.

septic shock: shock resulting from severe infection.

septum: dividing wall or membrane between body spaces or masses of soft tissue.

sera: blood serum from animals inoculated with bacteria or toxins; produces passive immunization in the body because of the antibodies it contains.

serosa: peritoneum that covers organs.

serous: relating to or resembling serum, that is, thin and watery.

serum: clear liquid that separates from the clot and the corpuscles in the clotting of blood.

shaft of a bone: long, straight, cylindrical mid-portion.

shell: appendages of the body: arms and legs, hands and feet. The temperature of these parts is called shell temperature.

shin splints: slang term meaning pain in the lower legs.

shivering: trembling of the body caused by contraction of the muscles; automatic attempt of the body to generate more heat through muscular action.

shock: state of collapse of the cardiovascular system; discrepancy between the cardiovascular system and its contents.

shock position: supine with legs elevated and knees straight so that blood drains from the enlarged vessels in the legs and returns to the heart for active circulation.

shoulder girdle: proximal portion of the upper extremity, made up of the clavicle and the scapula.

shoulder separation: dislocation of the acromioclavicular joint.

side effect: effect of a drug other than the one for which it is given.

signs: readily apparent manifestations of changes in body functions.

simple fracture: closed fracture.

simple partial seizure: one in which seizure activity is limited to one or more extremities or one side of the body.

sinus: general term for spaces, such as the channels for venous blood in the cranium or the air cavities within the cranial bones.

sinusitis: inflammation of a sinus.

skeletal muscles: striated (marked by streaks) muscles that are attached to bones and usually cross at least one joint.

skeleton: supporting framework of the human body, composed of 206 bones.

skier's thumb: see gamekeeper's thumb.

skin: outer covering of the body, consisting of the dermis and the epidermis and resting on subcutaneous tissue; the largest organ of the body; isolates the body from its environment, protects it from bacterial invasion, controls temperature, retains fluids and furnishes information about the external environment to the brain through its nerve endings.

skull: bones of the head, collectively.

small bowel juice: juice secreted by the small intestine, containing mucus and potent enzymes.

small intestine: portion of the digestive tube between the stomach and the cecum, consisting of the duodenum, jejunum and ileum.

smallpox (variola): acute viral disease with fever, headache, abdominal pain, rash with scabbing eruptions and pneumonia.

smooth muscles: nonstriated, involuntary muscles; smooth muscles constitute the bulk of the gastrointestinal tract and are present in nearly every organ to regulate automatic activity.

snow blindness: blindness caused by the glare of the sun upon snow.

soft palate: fold of mucous membrane and

muscle extending posteriorly into the pharynx from the hard palate.

solid organs: organs without a central lumen or cavity.

somatic nervous system: portion of the nervous system that regulates voluntarily controlled functions.

somnolent: sleepy.

Spanish windlass: tourniquet consisting of a handkerchief tied around a body part and twisted by a stick passed under it.

spasm: sudden, violent, involuntary contraction of a group of muscles.

sphincters: circular muscles that encircle a duct or opening in such a way that their contraction constricts the opening.

sphygmomanometer: instrument for measuring blood pressure in the arteries; a rubber cuff attached by a rubber tube to a compressible bulb and by another tube to a column of mercury marked off in millimeters.

spinal canal: tunnel created by a series of arches formed by the back part of each vertebra that runs the length of the spine and encloses and protects the spinal cord.

spinal column: central supporting bony structure of the body; vertebral column.

spinal cord: extension of the brain, composed of virtually all the nerves carrying messages between the brain and the rest of the body; is contained within the spinal canal and thus protected by the vertebrae of the spinal column.

spinal discs: see intervertebral disc.

spinal nerves: 31 pairs of nerves that arise from the spinal cord and pass out between the vertebrae.

spine: column of 33 vertebrae extending from the base of the skull to the tip of the coccyx.

spine board: wooden board primarily used for extrication and transportation of patients with actual or suspected spinal injuries; also serves as a litter; can be used to raise or lower patients or to provide rigid support during cardiac compression. The long spine board is 6 feet and the short board 32 to 34 inches.

spleen: large, solid organ situated in the left upper quadrant of the abdomen; major function is the normal production and destruction of blood cells.

splinting: immobilizing an injured part by means of a device applying pull or applying a rigid support to that part.

"splinting" (by patient): any clinical situation in which the contraction of the patient's own muscles immobilizes an injured or diseased area.

spontaneous pneumothorax: pneumothorax caused by the rupture of a congenitally weak area of the surface of the lungs.

sprain: injury in which a joint is partially, temporarily dislocated at the moment of injury and supporting ligaments are stretched or torn.

stabilizing dressing: dressing used to keep bandages in place during transport—soft roller bandages, rolls of gauze, triangular bandages or adhesive tape.

standard of care: manner in which the individual must act or behave when giving care.

starch: compound present in various plant tissues, composed of many linked molecules of glucose or simple sugar.

state of consciousness: degrees of consciousness or unconsciousness of the patient.

status epilepticus: condition in which one major attack of epilepsy succeeds another with little or no intermission.

statutes: laws.

sterile pressure dressing: sterile bandage made up of gauze pads, with a universal dressing applied over them at the point where pressure is needed.

sterilize: to make sterile—free from bacterial contamination.

sternoclavicular joint: articulation between the sternum and the clavicle.

sternocleidomastoid muscle: cervical muscle that produces rotation of the head.

sternum: breastbone.

steroids: compounds composed of fatty molecules called sterols.

stethoscope: instrument used to determine blood pressure and to detect heart, breath and bowel sounds.

stimulants: drugs that excite the mind and cause rapid heart rate, increased blood pressure, rapid breathing and a sense of euphoria or well-being.

stimulus: something that rouses or attempts to rouse the patient to activity.

sting: injury caused by venom of a plant or animal.

Stokes' basket: basket stretcher shaped like an oblong plastic shell, used to remove patients from heights or to move them over difficult terrain or debris.

stoma: opening or mouth.

stomach: expansion of the alimentary canal between the esophagus and the duodenum, which receives food, stores it, and moves it into the small bowel.

stool: fecal discharge from the bowels.

straddle slide: method for placing a patient on the long spineboard by straddling both board and patient and sliding the patient onto the board.

strain: stretching or tearing of a muscle.

stress fracture: occurs when the bone is subjected to frequent, repeated stresses, such as in running or marching long distances.

stretcher: two-person carrying device to transport supine patients to, from and in an ambulance.

striated muscle: muscle with characteristic stripes, or striations, under the microscope; voluntary, skeletal muscle.

stroke: sudden lessening or loss of consciousness, sensation and voluntary movement caused by rupture or obstruction of an artery in the brain.

styloid process: pointed projection of a bone.

subatomic particle: particle smaller than an atom.

subcutaneous: under the skin.

subcutaneous emphysema: presence of air in soft tissues, giving a very characteristic crackling sensation on palpation.

subcutaneous tissue: tissue, largely fat, that lies directly under the dermis and insulates the body.

subdural: beneath the dura mater and outside the brain.

subdural hematoma: hematoma beneath the dura mater and outside the brain.

substernal: under the breastbone.

subungual hematoma: hematoma beneath a finger or toe nail.

sucking chest wounds: open wounds of the chest wall which let air pass into and out of the pleural space with each respiration.

suctioning: aspirating material by mechanical means.

suffocate: stop breathing; blocking a person's breath; suffer from lack of oxygen.

sunstroke: see heatstroke.

superficial frostbite: cold injury involving the skin and the superficial tissue.

superficial temporal arteries: arteries supplying the scalp palpable just anterior to the ears at the temporomandibular joints.

superior: toward the head; lying higher in the body.

superior vena cava: see vena cava.

supination: state of being supine; turning the palm of the hand forward.

supine: lying on the back or with the face upward.

supraclavicular: above the collarbone.

supracondylar fracture: fracture of the distal end of the humerus or femur in which the fracture line extends across the bone just above the condyles.

suprasternal: above the sternum.

swallow: to take a substance through the mouth, pharynx and esophagus into the stomach.

swathe: bandage that passes around the chest to secure an injured arm to the chest.

sweat: liquid secreted by the sweat glands.

sweat glands: glands that secrete sweat are of two types: the ordinary sweat glands are distributed all over the body and promote cooling by evaporation; specialized, or apocrine, sweat glands are found only in certain areas of the body, such as the armpit.

swelling: transient abnormal enlargement, often due to pooling of blood at site of injury.

swimmer's ear: inflammation in the outer ear canal.

sympathetic nervous system: portion of the autonomic nervous system that lies outside the spinal canal; controls many automatic functions such as constriction of blood vessels and increases in heart rate.

symphysis: line of fusion between the bones that are separate in early childhood.

symphysis pubis: firm fibrocartilaginous joint between the two pubic bones.

symptoms: evidence of changes in body functions apparent to the patient and expressed to the examiner on questioning.

synchondrosis: temporary cartilaginous joint.

syncope: fainting.

syndesmosis: fibrous joint where connective tissue forms an interosseus membrane or ligament.

synostosis: union between bones formed by an osseus bridge.

synovial joint: articulation permitting more or less free movement; the opposing surfaces are composed of hyaline cartilage; a synovial membrane is present.

synovial membrane: see synovium.

synovium: inner surface of the joint capsule.

syringe: instrument for injecting liquids into or withdrawing them from any vessel or cavity.

systemic reaction: affecting the body generally.

systole: contraction of the heart muscle.

systolic blood pressure: higher blood pressure noted at the moment of ventricular contraction of the heart.

tachycardia: abnormally fast heart rate; high pulse rate.

tailbone: the coccyx.

Tailor's bunion: enlargement of the lateral aspect of the fifth metatarsal.

talus: anklebone.

tamponade (cardiac): compression of the heart by pericardial fluid.

tarsal bones: bones of the instep of the foot.

tarsal plate: firm framework of connective tissue that gives shape to the upper eyelid.

tears: fluid that lubricates the eye and flushes foreign material from it.

teeth: small, hard structures in the jaw, used for chewing food.

temples: lateral and most anterior portions of the cranium.

temporomandibular joint: mandible and cranium joint, just in front of the ear.

tendons: tough, ropelike cords of fibrous tissue attaching skeletal muscles to bones.

tenesmus: straining of the anal sphincter with an urge to defecate that cannot be satisfied.

tension pneumothorax: condition in which air continuously leaks out of the lung into the pleural space, increasing pressure within the space at every breath.

terminal: at the end; near death.

terminal ileum: end of the ileum.

testicles (singular, testis): male genital glands containing specialized cells that produce hormones and sperm.

testosterone: hormone responsible for the appearance and development of male secondary sex organs.

tetanus: infectious disease in which muscle spasm causes "lockjaw," arching of the back and seizures.

thalamus: part of the brain stem; the site of certain involuntary nervous controls.

thermal burn: burn caused by heat.

thigh: upper portion of the lower extremity from the hip joint to the knee.

third-degree burn: skin is destroyed down to the subcutaneous fat; the skin may appear pale, dry and white or brown or charred.

thoracic cage: bony chest.

thoracic spine: portion of the spine to which ribs attach.

thoracic squeeze: compression of the chest.

thorax: upper part of the trunk between the neck and abdomen; the chest.

throat: pharynx.

thrombosis: formation or presence of a blood clot within a blood vessel.

thrombus: clot within a vessel.

thyroid cartilage: largest cartilage of the larynx.

thyroid gland: ductless gland lying on the upper part of the trachea; it produces thyroid hormone.

tibia: shinbone.

tibial tuberosity: prominence on the tibia for the insertion of the quadriceps tendon.

tidal volume: amount of air breathed in and out during one respiratory cycle.

tolerance: reaction to a drug by a chronic user; more and more of the drug is needed to obtain the same effect.

tongue: movable muscular organ on the floor of the mouth, used in taste, chewing, swallowing and speech.

tongue-jaw lift: method of opening the patient's mouth by grasping the tongue and lower jaw between the thumb and fingers and lifting forward to probe for foreign bodies.

tonic-clonic seizure: see generalized seizure.

topographic anatomy: superficial landmarks of the body.

torso: human trunk.

tourniquet: device, such as a bandage, twisted tightly around an extremity with a stick; used to stop bleeding that cannot be controlled by any other means.

toxic: poisonous.

toxins: poisons.

trachea: windpipe; main trunk for air passing to and from the lungs.

traction: action of drawing or pulling on an object.

traction splint: holds a lower-extremity fracture or dislocation immobile; allows steady longitudinal pull on the extremity.

tragus: small, rounded, fleshy protuberance immediately at the front of the ear canal.

tranquilizers: drugs that calm and quiet the patient without affecting the state of consciousness.

transverse colon: part of the colon that runs transversely across the upper part of the abdomen.

trauma: wound or injury, either physical or psychological.

trench foot: form of cold exposure to the feet in which they are immersed in cold, but not freezing, water or moisture for long periods of time.

triage: sorting or selection of patients to determine priority of care.

triangular bandage: piece of cloth cut in the shape of a right-angled triangle; used as a sling for the arm and for other purposes.

trochanters: prominences on a bone where tendons insert; specifically, two protuberances, greater and lesser, on the femur.

tuberosities: prominences on bones where tendons insert.

tympanic membrane: eardrum.

type I (red) muscle fiber: fiber containing large amounts of myoglobin and that is slow twitch, resistant to fatigue.

type II (white) muscle fiber: fiber containing small amounts of myoglobin and that is fast twitch and fatiguable.

ulcer: lesion on the skin or mucous surface caused by the superficial loss of tissue, usually with inflammation.

ulcerative colitis: chronic ulceration in the colon.

ulna: inner and larger bone of the forearm, on the side opposite the thumb.

ulnar artery: artery palpated at the base of the little finger.

ulnar nerve: controls sensation over the fifth and fourth fingers; controls most of the muscular function of the hand.

ulnar styloid process: bony prominence felt on the medial side of the wrist.

ultraviolet light: invisible rays of the spectrum beyond the violet rays.

unconscious: having lost consciousness.

unilateral: on one side.

universal dressing: dressing made of thick, absorbent material, measuring 9 × 36 inches and packed folded into a compact size.

upper urinary tract: kidney and ureter.

uremia: toxic condition caused by waste products of metabolism accumulating in the blood as a result of a failure of kidney function.

ureteral colic: colicky pains due to obstruction of the ureter.

ureters: fibromuscular tubes that convey urine from the kidney to the bladder.

urethra: membranous canal conveying urine from the bladder to outside the body.

uric acid: end product of metabolism of nucleic acids.

urinary bladder: see bladder.

urinary system: organs for production and excretion of urine.

urinate: excrete urine.

urine: fluid waste product of the body; excreted by the kidneys, passed through the ureters, stored in the bladder and discharged through the urethra.

urticaria: hives; allergic reaction characterized by bumps on the skin.

uterus: muscular organ that holds and nourishes the fetus; opens into the vagina through the cervix.

vaccine: preparation of killed microorganisms or living organisms administered to produce or increase immunity to a disease.

vagina: muscular, distensible tube connecting the uterus with the external female genitalia; receives the penis during intercourse.

vagus nerve: tenth cranial nerve; serves the larynx, lungs, heart, esophagus, stomach and most of the abdominal viscera.

valgus: angulation outward and away from the midline of the body.

Valium: drug used as a tranquilizer and muscle relaxant.

varus: angulation inward and toward the midline of the body.

vasa deferentia (singular: vas deferens): spermatic ducts of testicles.

vascular: relating to or containing blood vessels.

veins: tubular vessels that carry blood from the capillaries toward the heart.

vena cava: one of the two large veins conducting blood to the right upper chamber of the heart. **inferior vena cava:** venous trunk returning blood from the lower extremities and the pelvic and abdominal viscera. **superior vena cava:** venous trunk returning blood from the upper extremities and the head, neck and chest.

venereal disease: disease transmitted by sexual contact.

venom: poison secreted by animals and deposited in bite wounds.

venous pressure: pressure of the blood in the veins.

ventilation: exchange of air between the lungs and the air of the environment; breathing.

ventilator: device to aid breathing.

ventricle: either of the two lower chambers of the heart.

ventricular extrasystoles: extra heartbeats in the ventricle.

ventricular fibrillation: see fibrillation.

ventricular premature contractions: extra heartbeats arising in a damaged ventricle; can produce ventricular tachycardia.

ventricular tachycardia: see tachycardia.

venturi mask: breathing unit that provides a specific concentration of oxygen through a delivery tube connected to a standard face mask.

venules: small veins into which blood passes from the capillaries.

vertebrae: 33 bones of the spinal column; 7 cervical, 12 thoracic, 5 lumbar, 5 sacral and 4 coccygeal vertebrae.

virus: specific agent of an infectious disease; specifically, a group of microbes that can pass through fine filters that bacteria cannot pass through. An incomplete organism, it cannot sustain life alone but is an obligate intracellular parasite and lives with the cells of the host or organism attached.

viscera: internal organs of the body.

visceral peritoneum: continuation of the parietal peritoneum that covers the stomach, spleen, liver, intestines, bladder and female reproductive organs.

visceral pleura: part of the pleura that surrounds the lungs and separates their lobes.

vital signs: pulse rate, respiratory rate, body temperature and blood pressure.

vital statistics: age, sex and kin of the patient.

vitamins: organic substances that occur in many foods and are necessary for normal metabolism in the body.

vitreous humor: fluid behind the lens of the eye.

void: see urinate.

volar: located on the same side as the palm of the hand.

Volkmann's contracture: irreversible contracture of muscles produced by fibrosis of dead muscle cells killed by ischemia.

voluntary muscle: muscle under direct voluntary control of the brain, which can be contracted or relaxed at will; skeletal muscle.

voluntary nervous system: see somatic nervous system.

vomiting: disgorging the stomach contents through the mouth.

vomitus: vomited material.

vulva: external female genitalia.

wheal: raised area on the skin resulting from an allergic reaction.

wheezes: whistling sounds made in breathing.

white cells: leukocytes.

whooping cough: acute bacterial disease with violent attacks of coughing and high-pitched whooping.

windpipe: trachea.

withdrawal: physical or physiological removal of oneself from a situation.

woven bone: bony tissue in the embryo and young children; also in pathologic conditions in adults.

wrist: joint between the forearm and the hand.

wrist joint: a modified ball-and-socket articulation formed by the radius, ulna and carpal bones.

xiphoid process: the pointed process of cartilage supported by a core of bone connected with the lower end of the body of the sternum.

x-rays: electromagnetic waves that penetrate various substances and can also affect a photographic plate; used in diagnosis and therapy.

zygoma: the quadrangular bone of the cheek, articulating with the frontal bone, the maxilla, the zygomatic process of the temporal bone and the great wing of the sphenoid bone.

Index

Page numbers in italics refer to figures;
page numbers followed by t refer to tables.

A

Abdomen
  acute, 425–428t, *426t, 427t*
  anatomy of, *28–30, 29, 417–420,*
    418, 419
  diseases of, 427, 428t
  injuries of, 419, 429–431, 430t
Abdominal cavity, *28–30, 29, 417–420,*
    418, 419
Abdominal thrusts, *382–383*
Abrasion, defined, *151,* 152
Achilles tendon, 165, 326, 327,
    rupture, 311
    taping, *74–75*
Achilles tendonitis, 79, 310–311
Acne vulgaris, 486, *489,* 494t
Acute cervical intervertebral disc
    herniation, 405
Acute mountain sickness (AMS), 536
Acute myocardial infarction (AMI),
    447, 448–451, 450t
Acute pulmonary edema, *453,* 454
Acute tears, 282
Adhesive capsulitis, 202–203
Adhesive taping, *47–48*
  of the lower extremities, 66–80
  of the upper extremities, 51–65
Aerobic capacity, 122, 123–124
  of women vs. men, 466
Aerobic system, 116
Air embolism, 538–539
Airway obstruction, *376–377*
  as cause of dyspnea, 453, 454–455
  recognizing, 381–382
  relieving, *382–384, 383*
Alcohol, 499, 513
  abuse, 520–521, 524
  withdrawal, 524–525
Allergic reactions, 453–454, 455,
    523–524
Allergy
  contact, 488–493, *492*
  medications, 518–519

Altitude disorders, 536–537
  acute mountain sickness, 536
  high altitude cerebral edema,
    536–537
  high altitude pulmonary edema,
    536
  preventing, 537
Alveoli, 331, *332*
Amenorrhea, 470
  secondary, 470–471
American College of Sports Medicine,
    5
American Medical Association, 5
American Orthopaedic Society for
    Sports Medicine, 5
AMI. *See* Acute myocardial infarction.
Anabolic steroids, 521
Anaerobic systems, 115–116
Analgesics, 517
Anaphylactic shock, 368, 373, 543
Anaphylaxis, 477
  exercise-induced, 518–519
Anatomy. *See also* individual body
    structures.
  of arterial pulse points, *35*
  of a bone, 156–157
  general and topographic, 23–35
  language of, 23–24
  of the respiratory system, *331–333,*
    332
Anemia, 351
Anesthetics, 517
Aneurysm, 458
Angina pectoris, 447, 448
Angle of Louis, 28
Ankle
  anatomy, 314–316, *315*
  hitches, 175, 176
  injuries, clinical evaluation of,
    316–317, *318*
  injuries, management procedures
    for, 319, *320*
  injuries, mechanisms of, 316

injuries, rehabilitation following, 320
injuries, types of, 316
joint, *165*
taping, *71–74, 72, 73*
Anorexia nervosa, 471, 514–515
Ant bites, 542–543
Anterior compartment syndrome, 308–309
Anterior dislocation, 199–201, *200*
Anterior drawer test, *182–183, 250, 251,* 317, *318*
Anterior surface, defined, 23
Anterolateral/posterolateral rotatory instability, 262–263
Anterolateral rotary instability, 257–261, *258, 259, 260*
Anteromedial/anterolateral instability, 262
Anteromedial/posteromedial rotatory, instability, 263
Anteromedial rotary instability, *254–257, 255, 256*
Antibiotics, 517–518
Anti-inflammatory drugs, 516–517
  local steroids, 516–517
  systemic cortical steroids, 516
Antivenin, 543, 545
Anus, *420,* 423
Apley's compression test, 246–247
Aponeurosis, 150
Appendicitis, 423, 426, 430
Appendix, *419, 420,* 423
Arches, foot, 321–322
Arm, upper, 209–217
  anatomy, *162–163,* 209–210, *212*
  injuries, *211–213*
  ligaments, 210, *211*
  muscles, 210–211
  nerves, vessels and bursae, 211, *212*
Arrhythmia, 448
Arterial pulse points, *35*
Arteries, pulmonary, 332, *333*
Arteriosclerosis, 456, 457t, 458
Arthritis, joint, 270
Artificial circulation, *384–387, 385, 386*
  using external chest compression, *385–387, 388*
Artificial ventilation, 376–381
  gastric distention during, 381
  mouth-to-mouth, *379–380*
  mouth-to-nose, *380–*381
  mouth-to-stoma, 381
  using head-tilt maneuver, *377*
  using head tilt-neck lift, *377–378*
Ascent problems (of divers) 538–539
  air embolism, 538–539
  decompression sickness, 539

Assumption-of-risk doctrine, 17
Asthma
  and allergic reactions, 453–454, 455
  bronchial, 453–454
  exercise-induced, 337, 454, 476–477, 518
  extrinsic (allergic), 476
  intrinsic (idiopathic), 476
Astroturf burns, 488
Atherosclerosis, 447
Athletes
  asthmatic, 476–477
  diabetic, 473–475, 513–514
  legal responsibilities of, 17–19
  physically impaired, 478–480, *479*
  psychological considerations in working with, 111–114
  role of, on sports medicine team, 11
  women, *465–472, 467, 469*
Athletic director, role of, 10
Athletic injury data sources, list of, 6
Athletic trainer
  personal liability of, 17
  role of, in evaluating injuries and illness, 13–14
  role of, on sports medicine team, 10–11
Athletic trainers associations, list of, 6
ATP (adenosine triphosphate), 149
Automobile racing
  and frequency of distal femur fractures, 293–294
Autonomic nervous system, 404–405
Avulsion, defined, *151,* 152

B

Back blows, 382
  plus manual thrusts, 383–384
Baker's cyst, 288–289
Bandages
  pressure, 152, *153,* 155
  soft roller, 155
  for soft tissue injuries, 154–155
  triangular, 155
Bandaging. *See also* Strapping; Taping.
  adhesive taping, 47–48
  with cotton wraps, 49–50
  elastic, 48–49, 81–92
  elastic, for soft tissue support, 48–49
  introduction to, 47–50
  lower extremity, 60–80
  upper extremity, 51–65
Bankart lesion, 199, *200*

Baseball
  and epicondylitis, 215–216
  exercises for pitchers and throwers,
    209
  finger, *221*
  protective devices for, 95, 100, 101,
    103, 436
  shoulder injuries, 194
Basic life support. *See* CPR.
Basketball
  and Achilles tendonitis, 310–311
  and fracture-dislocations of the
    ankle, 319
  protective devices for, 101
  and stress fractures, 312–313
Bee stings, 542–543
Bile ducts, 417, *418*, 422
Biliary system, *419*, 422
Biomechanics
  of foot, *323, 324*
  laws and definitions of, 178–188
  of the patella, *271–272, 273*
Birth control pills, 521
Bites
  ant, 542–543
  dog, 546
  human, 227
  scorpion, 543
  snake, 544–546
  spider, 543–544
Black eye, 412
Bladder, urinary, 417, *418, 433*
Bleeding
  control of, 152–153, *361–364, 363*
  external, 361–362
Blisters, foot, 328
Blood
  cells, function of, 350
  circulation, 357–*358*
  "doping," 522
  loss, controlling, *361–364, 363*
  parameters, 351–352t
  plasma, 351
  plasma alterations, 352
  pressure, 37–39, 355, 357
Blowout fracture, 24
Body fat percentage, 496–497t
Bone
  anatomy, 155–*157, 156, 158*
  composition and remodeling,
    157–158
  fracture, *166, 185–186*
  strength and stiffness, 180–182
Bottom problems (of divers), 538
  carbon dioxide toxicity, 538
  carbon monoxide poisoning, 538
  hypoxia, 538

  nitrogen narcosis, 538
  oxygen toxicity, 538
Boutonnière deformity, 222, *223*
Bowling, tennis elbow and, 215
Boxing, protective gloves for, *98,* 101
Braces (protective device), 96, 99, *100*
Brain
  anatomy, 394–*395*
  and cerebral spinal fluid, *395–397*
  circulation, *396*
  cranial nerves of, *397*
  injuries to, 397–*399*, 398t
  lobes of, *396–397*
Bras, sports, 471–472
Breast support, myths concerning,
    472
Bronchi, *331,* 332
Bronchiole, terminal, 331, *332*
Bronchitis
  chronic obstructive, *337*
  viral, 338–339
Bruise. *See* Contusions.
Bucket handle derangement, 186, *187*
Bucket handle tear, 283, *284, 285*
Budding taping, 63, *65*
Bulimia, 514–515
Bunions, 470
"Burner" injury, *406*
Bursitis of the elbow, *214*
Bursitis of the foot, 326
Bursitis of the hip, 230, *231*
Bursitis of the knee, 286–289
  anserine, 288
  and Baker's cyst, 288–289
  bicipital, 288
  deep infrapatellar, 287–288
  and iliotibial band-friction
    syndrome, 288
  prepatellar, *287*
  superficial infrapatellar, 288
Bursitis of the shoulder joint, 199

C

Cable tension dynamometer, 127, *129*
Caffeine, 512, 513t, 520
Calcaneus (heelbone), *165*
Callosity, 326
Caloric requirements, 497, 498t
Carbohydrate loading, 509–510t
  menus, 511t
  methods, 509t
Carbohydrate, 496, 499
Carbon dioxide toxicity, 538
Carbon monoxide poisoning, 538
Cardiac cycle, *353–354, 355, 356*
Cardiac function, *447–448*

Cardiogenic shock, 367, 372
Cardiopulmonary resuscitation. *See* CPR.
Cardiovascular endurance, 122–124, 123t, 360
Cardiovascular system, 353–360
    cardiac cycle of, *353–354, 355, 356*
    cardiac output of, 354–*357*
    cardiovascular endurance of, 360
    circulation of blood in, 232, *233,* 357–*358*
    effects of exercise on, 358–359
    and shock, 365–373, *371*
Carpals, *163, 164*
Carpal tunnel syndrome, 219
Cartilage, articular, 158–159, 160
Cartilaginous cushions, 159
Caudad end, defined, 23
Cauliflower ear, 414
Cavus foot, *324*
CBC (complete blood cell) count, 352
Central nervous system, 393
Cephalad end, defined, 23
Cerebral spinal fluid, *395–397*
Cerebrovascular accident (CVA), 458–459
Cervical spine fractures, 406–408, *407*
Chest
    colds, 338–339
    flail, 342–*344*
    injuries, 340–349
    pain, acute, 447–451
    thrusts, *383*
Chilblains, 533–534
Choking. *See* Airway obstruction.
Cholesterol, 499
Chronic tears, 282–283
Cilia, 332
Cinder burns, 488
Circular finger strapping, 63
Circulation, artificial, 384–*387, 385, 386*
    in the abdomen, 417, 418, 420
    in the arm, 211, *212, 218*
    in the brain, *396*
    in the hand, 219–*220*
    in the knee, 239
    in the shoulder region, 192, *193*
    in the thigh, 233, 235
Clavicle, *162*
Clawing of the toes, *324,* 325
Coach
    role of, in evaluating injury and illness, 13–14
    role of, on sports medicine team, 10
Cocaine, 523
Coccyx, 160, 161, 404
Codman pendulum exercise, 204–215, 207–208

Cold injury, 532–535t
Cold packs
    chemical, 136, 176
    flexible gel, 136
Colic, 424, 425, 441
    renal, 442
College sports medicine organizations, list of, 6
Coma
    diabetic, 474
    as diagnostic sign, 40
Comaneci, Nadia, *466*
Common cold, 519
Communicable diseases, 481–485, 482t
Compression wrap. *See* Elastic bandaging.
Concussion, cerebral, 397–398t
    first-degree, 397–398
    second-degree, 398
    third-degree, 398
Conditioning (of women vs. men), 467–468
Congestive heart failure, 448, 449
Conjunctivitis, 519
Consciousness, state of
    as diagnostic sign, 40, *41*
    during airway obstruction, 381–382
Consent for treatment, 18, 19
Consultants, general (on sports medicine team), 8
Contraceptive devices, 471
Contrast therapy, 136
Contributory negligence, 17
Contusions
    cerebral, 398
    definition of, 151
    elbow, 213–214
    facial, 413
    fingertip, 220
    forearm, 218–219
    hand, 224
    male and female genitalia, 436–437
    myocardial, 348
    pulmonary, 348
    thenar and hypothenar, 224
    thigh, 233
    upper arm, 211–213
    upper back muscle, 408–409
Coral snake bites, 545–546
Corticosteroids, 212
Costal arch, 161, *162*
Cotton wraps, 49–*50*
Counseling athletes, 112
CPR (cardiopulmonary resuscitation), 374–389
    by artificial circulation, 384–*387, 385, 386*

by artificial ventilation, 376–381, *377, 378, 379, 380*
for children, 389
effectiveness of, 388
following acute myocardial infarction, 448
following electric shock, 460
interruption, 389
positioning patient for, *375–376*
relieving airway obstruction before, *382–384*
training coaches in, 10
using external chest compression, *385–387, 386*
when to use, 374–375
Crab louse, 493–495
Cramps
  heat, 528, 530t
  muscle, 148–149, 308
Cranium, 160
Cryokinetics, 133, 136–137
Cryotherapy, 133, 134t–137
  modalities, 135–137
CVA (cerebrovascular accident), 458–459
Cyanosis, 39, 341
Cycling
  carbohydrate loading before, 509t, 511t
  protective devices for, 101

D

Daily medical report form, *16*
Decompression sickness, 539
Deformities, foot, *324–325*
Delirium tremens, 524–525
Depressants, 520–521
Depression, 113
Depth disorders, 537–539
  ascent problems, 538–539
  bottom problems, 538
  descent problems, 537
Dermatitis, contact irritant, 488–493, 494t
Dermatological problems, 486–495
  acne vulgaris, 486, *489*, 494t
  bacterial infections, 488, 494t
  contact allergy and irritant dermatitis, 488–493, *492*, 494t
  fungus infections, 487, *490*, 494t
  infestations, 493–495, 494t
  viral infections, 487–488, *491*, 494t
Descent problems (of divers), 537
Diabetes, 473–475
  as cause of unconsciousness, 456, 457t

and how to distinguish diabetic coma from insulin shock, 474–475
  and the insulin-dependent athlete, 473–474
Diabetic coma, 474–475
Diabetic ketoacidosis, 474–475
Diagnostic signs, 36–41
Diaphragm, 150, 332, *334*
Diarrhea, 440
Diastolic blood pressure, 38
Diathermy, 138–*139*
Diet
  composition during training, 116, 499–500t
  role of, 496
  sugar in, 501–502
  vitamins and minerals in, 502t–509, 504t, 507t
  water in, 500–501
Diffusion (of air in lungs), 335–337, *336*
Digestive system, *420–424*
Disc, herniated, *409*
Disclosure of information, 18
Disease
  abdominal, 427, 428t
  as cause of unconsciousness, 456–459, 457t
  communicable, 481–485, 482t
  Osgood-Schlatter, *289*–290
Dislocations
  ankle, 319
  anterior, 199–201, *200*
  causes of, 166–168
  definition of, *166*
  elbow, *216*
  finger, 222
  foot, 327
  fracture, 166, *167*
  hip, 232
  knee, 270–271
  of MCP joints, 224
  patellar, 276
  posterior, *201–202*
  recurrent anterior, 208
  shoulder, *195–196*, 199–201, *200*
  signs of, 170–171
  splinting, 172–174
  sternoclavicular, *195–196*
Distal, defined, 23
Diving
  disorders, 537–539
  injuries, splinting, 411
Dog bites, 546
''Doping,'' 519
Dressings
  occlusive, 155
  pressure, 155

for soft tissue injuries, 154–155
stabilizing, 155
to stop bleeding, 362
universal, 154–155
Drug abuse, 519–520
depressants and, 520
emergency treatment of, 522–524
multiple, 524
stimulants and, 520
Drugs. *See also* Alcohol; Caffeine.
abuse of, 519–520, 522–524
allergy medications, 518–519
anabolic steroids, 521
analgesics and anesthetics, 517
antibiotics, 517–518
anti-inflammatory, 516–517
birth control pills, 521
''blood doping'' and, 522
electrolyte solutions, 518
gastrointestinal, 519
impact of, on nutrients, 512
impact of food on, 511–512t
influence of, on cardiovascular
  system, 358
interaction of, with food, 511–513
iron supplements as, 518
as medications for eyes and ears,
  519
megadose vitamins as, 521–522
muscle relaxants as, 517
psychomotor, 520–521
responsibilities of team physician in
  prescribing, 19
withdrawal from, 524
Dysmenorrhea, 471
Dysphagia, 438
Dyspnea, 340–341, 349, 452–455
and pulmonary physiology,
  452–453
in sports, 453–454t
treatment of, 454–455
without lung abnormalities, 454
Dysuria, 441

E

Ear
injuries, 414
medications, 519
Edema
high altitude cerebral, 536–537
high altitude pulmonary, 536
Elastic bandaging
application/removal guidelines for,
  48, *81–83*, *82*
common application methods for,
  83–92, *84*, *85*, *86*, *87*, *88*, *89*, *90*,
  91

procedures, 81–92
purpose of, 48
for soft tissue support, 48–49
Elbow, 209–217
anatomy, 209–*210*, *212*
hyperextension taping, *55–56*
injuries, 213–217, *214*, *216*
ligaments, 210, *211*
muscles, 210–211
nerves, vessels and bursae, 211, *212*
Electrical muscle stimulation, 140–*141*
Electric shock, 460
Electrolyte replacement, 502, 527
Electrolyte solutions, 518
Embolism, 459
Emotions (causing fainting), 460
Emphysema, 337, 349
subcutaneous, 348
Enchondral ossification, 158
Environmental problems, 526–539
altitude disorders, 536–537
cold injuries, 532–*535*
depth disorders, 537–539
heat disorders, 526–532, 530t, *531*
Environmental testing, 13
Epicondylitis, 215–216
Epilepsy, 460
Equipment, protective
evaluating, 13
principles of, 95–96
selection and fitting of, 101–106
special, 106, 107
for upper and lower extremities,
  97–101
Esophagus, *420*, *421*
Evisceration, 430
Examination
of athletes by team physician, 18–19
of injury site, 43–44
of knee injury, 243–247, *244*, *246*
of lower leg injury, 307–308
of musculoskeletal injuries, 171
of shoulder injuries, 203–204
Exercise. *See also* Training.
active assistive, 125
aerobic, 360
anaerobic, 360, 454
flexibility, *121–122*
and the heart, 358–359
isokinetic, 129–*130*, *131*
isometric, 127, *129*, 301–302
isotonic, 127–128, *129*
muscle training, 117–119t, 127
passive, 125–126
for pitchers and throwers, 209
program of, 130–131
resistive, 127–*130*, 128t, *129*, *131*
shoulder, 204–205

shoulder, after surgery, 207–209
shoulder flexibility, *205–206*
after shoulder joint sprains, 209
for strength training, 206–207
underwater, 125, 130–131, 303
variable resistance, 128–129
Exercise order, defined, 117
Extensor mechanism deficiencies, 273–274
External chest compression, *385–387, 386*
External rotation recurvatum test, *261–262*
Eye
  black, 412
  injuries, *412–413*
  medications, 519
  removing foreign body from, *412*

F

Fabrication (of protective equipment), 104–106, *105*
Face, 160, 394
Face mask, 101
Facial injuries
  to the ear, 414
  to the eye, *412–413*
  fractures, *413*
  to the mouth, 414
  nasal fractures, 413
  to the teeth, 414
Family physician, role of, 9
Faradic muscle stimulators, 140–141
Fatigue curve, *185*
Fatigue fracture, *185–186*
Fats, 499–500
Federation of Sports Medicine, 5
Felon, 221
Female athletes. *See* Women athletes.
Femur, 164, *165,* 232
Fencing, protective devices for, 101
Fibula, 164–*165,* 306
Field hockey, protective devices for, 95, 98, 100
Figure-of-eight wrap, *83–85, 84, 86*
Figure-of-eight wrist hyperextension taping, 59
Figure-of-eight wrist hyperflexion taping, 58
Finger joint hyperextension/flexion stop strapping, 63
Finger taping, *63–65*
Flail chest, 342–343, *344*
''Flak jackets,'' 98
Flat feet, 324–*325*
Flexion rotation drawer test, 259–*260, 261*

Fluids replacement, 501–502, 527–528, 532
Fontanelles, 158
Food. *See also* Nutrition.
  before and after events, 509–510
  and drug interactions, 511–513
  groups, daily servings from, 500t
  impact of, on drugs, 511–512t
Foot
  anatomy, *321–323, 322*
  biomechanics of, *323–324*
  cavus, *324*
  deformities, 324–325
  flat (pronated), 324–*325*
  injuries, mechanics of and types of, 325–328
  injuries, rehabilitation following, 328
  Morton's, 325
Foot/ankle pressure wrap, 89, *91–92*
Football
  coaches, responsibilities of, 10
  and gamekeeper's thumb, *223*
  and heat stroke, 529
  knee, 270
  lower leg contusions, frequency of, 306–307
  protective devices for, 95, 97, 98, 99, *100,* 101, *102, 103*
  shoulder injuries, frequency of, *194*
  ''stinger'' or ''burner,'' *406*
  upper arm injuries, frequency of, 211–212
Footwear, design of, 95, 96
Force, effects of, 178–179
Forearm
  anatomy, *209–210*
  injuries, *218–219*
  ligaments, 210, *211*
  muscles, 210–211
  nerves, vessels and bursae, 211, *212, 218*
4 S wrap, *88–89*
Fracture, dislocation, 166, *167,* 170–171
Fractures, 165–177.
  bone, under repetitive loading, *185–186*
  causes of, 166–168
  classifying, 168
  definition of, *166*
  fatigue, *185–186*
  signs and symptoms of, 168–170
  splinting, 172–174
  stress, in women vs. men, 469
  types of, 168, *169, 170*
Fractures, ankle, 317, 319–320
  fracture-dislocations, 319, *320*

Fractures, cervical spine, 406–408
  of the atlantoaxial joint, 407
  hangman's fracture, *407–408*
  Jefferson fracture, *407*
  of the odontoid process, 407
Fractures, elbow, *217*
  avulsion, of the medial epicondyle, 217
  in children's elbows, 217
  of the olecranon, 217
  supracondylar, of the humerus, *217*
  undisplaced, of the radial head, 217
  Volkmann's contracture, *217*, 218
Fractures, facial bone, 413
  compression, of the zygomatic arch, *413*
  nasal, 413
  orbital, 412–413
Fractures, finger, hand and wrist, 223–225
  base of second and third metacarpals, 225
  carpal scaphoid, 225
  finger, 223
  first metacarpal, 224–225
  Hamate hook, 225, *226*
  metacarpal, 224
Fractures, foot, 327
  fatigue, 327
  stress, 327
Fractures, forearm, 218–219
  Galeazzi, 218
  Monteggia, 218
Fractures, hip, 232
Fractures, knee, 293–297
  about the knee, 293–297
  chondral and osteochondral, 290, *292–293*
  distal femur, 293–*294*
  femoral condyle, 294–295
  of the growth plate, 296, *297*
  intercondylar femur, 294, *295*
  patellar, 296–297
  proximal tibia, 295–*296*
  supracondylar, 294
  tibial spine, 296
Fractures, lower leg, 312–313
  fibula, 313
  stress, 312–313
  tibia, 313
Fractures, pelvic, 229
Fractures, rib, 342, *343*
  immobilizing, *341*, 342
Fractures, shoulder
  clavicle, *196*
  proximal humerus, 202
  scapular, 199, 346
Fractures, skull, 394, *395*

Fractures, spinal, 161, 172
Fractures, thigh
  femoral shaft, 235
  stress, of the femur, 235
Fractures, upper arm, *213*
  humeral shaft, *213*
Fractures, upper back and thoracic spine, 408–409
  dorsal spine, 408
  posterior rib, 408
  spinal, 408
Free weight exercise program, 118, 119t, 206–*207*, *208*
Freiberg's disease, 328
Frequency (voiding episodes), 442
Frostbite, 533, 534
Frostnip, 533, 534
Frozen shoulder (adhesive capsulitis), 202–203
Fungo routine (for pitchers), 209
Funnelization, 158
Furuncle, 488

G

Gallbladder, 417, *418*, *419*, *420*, 422
Galvanic muscle stimulators, 140, 141
Gamekeeper's thumb, 223–224, 228
Gastric distention, 381
Gastroenteritis, 438
Gastrointestinal complaints, 438–441
  colic, 441
  diarrhea, 440
  dysphagia, 438
  hematemesis, 439–440
  hematochezia, 440–441
  jaundice, 441
  melena, 440
  vomiting, 438–439
Gastrointestinal drugs, 519
Gastrointestinal system, 438–441
Genitalia
  anatomy, *433*
  female, injury to, 436–437
  male, injury to, 436
  protective devices for, 99
Genital system, *433*
  injuries, 436–437
Genitourinary complaints, 441–443
  dysuria, 441
  frequency, 442
  hematuria, 441–442
  incontinence, 442
  renal colic, 442–443
  urethra discharge, 442
Genitourinary system, 432–437
  female reproductive system, 434

common complaints about, 441–443
genital system, *433*
injuries, 434–435
male reproductive system, 433–434
urinary system, *432–433*
Genu recurvatum, *254*
Glass (inury), 153–154
Golf, tennis elbow and, 215
Gravity external rotation test, 262, *263*
Great toe taping, *76–78, 77*
Growth plate, injuries to, 296
Gymnast hand taping, *61–62*

H

Hallucinogens, 523
Hallux valgus, 325
Hammer toe, 325
Hamstring strains, 234–235
Hand
    anatomy, *163, 164, 219*
    injuries, 220–225, *221, 223, 226–227*
    injuries, rehabilitation following,
        227–228
Hand strapping, *61–63, 62*
Head
    anatomy, 24–*25*, 393–*397, 394, 395,
        396*
    injury, initial assessment of,
        399–400, *401*
    injury to the brain, 397–*399*, 398t
    injury to the skull, *394, 395*
    protective devices for, 101
Head tilt-chin lift, *378*
Head-tilt maneuver, *377*
Head tilt-neck lift, 377–*378*
Heart. *See also* Cardiovascular system.
    as a cardiac special muscle, 150–151
    circulation, 232, *233*, 357–*358*
    damage from chest injuries, 340,
        348–349
    disease, coronary, 447–448, *449*
    exercise and the, 358–359
    locating the, in CPR, *385*
Heat cramps, 528, 530t
Heat disorders, 526–532
    heat exposure syndromes, 528–532,
        530t, *531*
    heat loss, 526–527
    salt in warm weather, 527–528
Heat exhaustion, 528–529, 530t
    from salt depletion, 529, 530t
    from water depletion, 528–529, 530t
Heat exposure syndromes, 528–532
    heat cramps, 528
    heat exhaustion, 528–529
    heat stroke, 529–530t

Heat loss, 526–528
Heat regulation, 526–527, 532
Heat stroke, 529–530t
    as cause of high body temperature,
        39
    pathophysiology of, 529–530
Heel spur, 327
Helmets, 95, 101, *102, 103*
    maintenance of, 104
Hematemesis, 439–440
Hematochezia, 440–441
Hematologic system, 350–352
Hematoma
    acute anterior, 307
    cerebral, 398–399
    definition of, 151
Hematuria, 441–442
Hemiplegia, 40
Hemoglobin content (of blood), 351
Hemoptysis, 341
Hemorrhage, controlling, *361–364,
        363*
Hemorrhagic shock, 366, 370–372
Hemothorax, *343*, 347
Hepatitis, 522–523
Hernia, 436
Herpes, 487, 494t
High altitude cerebral edema
    (HACE), 536–537
High altitude pulmonary edema
    (HAPE), 536
High school sports medicine organi-
    zations, list of, 6
Hill-Sach lesion, 199, *200*
    reverse, 201
Hip, 230–232
    anatomy, *230, 231*
    dislocation, 232
    fractures, 232
    and groin sprain, 231–232
    injuries and pelvis injuries, 232
    joint sprain, 231
    overuse injuries to, 230
    protective devices for, 98, *99*
    synovitis, 230–231
Hormones, influence of, on cardio-
    vascular system, 358
Hughston jerk test, 259, *260*, 261
Humerus, *162, 163*
Hydrocollator packs, 137–*138*
Hyperpyrexia, 529, 530
Hyperventilation, 454, 455
Hyphema, 412
Hypoglycemia, 473, 474–475,
        513–514
Hypothermia, systemic, 534–535
Hypovolemic shock, 528–529
Hypoxia, 538, 536–537

I

Ice hockey, protective devices for, 95, 97, 98, 100, 101, 103, 436
Ice packs, 136
ICE (ice, compression, elevation) treatment, 134, 143, 300
Illness
    prevention of, 12–13
    prompt evaluation and initial treatment of, 13–16
Immersion, cold water, 136
Immobilization-of-one-digit finger taping, 63–64, 65
Immobilization-of-multiple digits finger taping, 64
Impaled foreign objects, 153–154
Impetigo, 488, 494t
Incontinence, 442
Inertia, moment of, defined, 178
Infections
    bacterial, 488
    furuncle, 488
    impetigo, 488
Infections, fungus, 487
    ringworm, 487
    tinea versicolor, 487, 490
Infections, secondary, 153
Infections, upper and lower respiratory, 338–339
    about the tonsils, 338
    bronchitis, 338–339
    ear, 338
    infectious mononucleosis, 338
    influenza, 339
    pneumonia, 339
    sinus, 338
    streptococcal bacterial, 338
    viral throat, 338
Infections, viral, 487–488
    herpes, 487
        molluscum, 487–488, 491
        warts, 488, 491
Infectious diseases, 482t
Inferior end, defined, 23
Infestations, 493–495, 494t
    pediculosis pubis (crab louse), 493–495
    scabies, 495
Influenza, 339
Informed consent, defined, 18
Infrared lamps, 138
Injuries
    from athletes' perspective, 112–113
    as cause of unconsciousness, 457t, 459–460
    examination for, 24–35
    keeping records of, 14

ligament, 183–184
marine animal, 546–547
to the musculoskeletal system, 147–177
prompt evaluation and initial treatment of, 13–16
referral of extensive, 14
rehabilitation after, 14
soft tissue, 151–154
Injuries, abdominal, 419, 429–431
    blunt abdominal wounds, 430t
    evaluating, 429–431
    penetrating, 430t, 431
Injuries, ankle
    clinical evaluation of, 316–317, 318
    fractures, 317
    management procedures for, 319, 320
    rehabilitation following, 320
    types of, 316
Injuries, brain, 397–399
    cerebral contusion, 398
    cerebral hematoma, 398–399
    concussion, 397–398t
Injuries, chest
    to the back of the chest, 345–346
    care of, 341–342
    classification of, 340
    compression, 345
    dyspnea, 349
    flail chest, 342–344
    hemothorax, 343, 347
    myocardial contusion, 348
    penetrating, 344–345
    pericardial tamponade, 348–349
    pneumothorax, 343, 346
    pulmonary contusion, 348
    results of, 346–349
    rib fractures, 342, 343
    spontaneous pneumothorax, 346
    subcutaneous emphysema, 348
    sucking chest wounds, 345, 347–348
    tension pneumothorax, 346–347
    types of and emergency care of, 342–349, 343, 344, 345, 347
Injuries, cold, 532–535
    chilblains, 533–534
    contributing factors in, 535t
    deep frostbite, 533
    frostnip, 533
    superficial frostbite, 533
    systemic hypothermia, 534–535
    trench or immersion foot, 534
Injuries, elbow, 213–217
    bursitis, 214
    contusions, 213–214
    dislocation, 216

epicondylitis, 215–216
fractures, *217*
sprains, 216
strains, 214–215
Injuries, facial, 412–414
Injuries, finger, hand and wrist, 220–227
    base of second and third meta-carpals fractures, 225
    boutonnière deformity, 222, *223*
    carpal scaphoid fracture, 225
    collateral ligament tears, 222
    dislocation of MCP joints, 224, 225
    dislocations, 222, 224
    finger fractures, 223
    fingertip, 220–*221*
    first metacarpal fracture, 224–225
    Hamate hook fracture, 225, *226*
    hand abrasions, 226
    human bites, 227
    hyperextension, 222
    metacarpal fracture, 224
    nerve, vessel and tendon, 226–227
    palm and dorsum, 224–*225*
    proximal finger joint, 222, *223*
    puncture, 227
    radiocarpal joint, 225–*226*
    rotary dislocation of the radioulnar joint, 225
    rupture of the transverse meta-carpal ligament, 224
    simple contusions of the hand, 224
    superficial lacerations, 226
    thenar and hypothenar eminence contusions, 224
    thumb, 223–224,
    wrist, 225–*226*
Injuries, foot
    fractures, 327
    mechanics of and types of, 325–328
    rehabilitation following, 328
    soft tissue, 326–327
Injuries, forearm, 218–219
    contusions, 218–219
    fractures, *218*
    nerve entrapment, 219
    tenosynovitis, 219
Injuries, genitourinary
    to the female genitalia, 434–435
    of the kidney, 434–435
    to the male genitalia, 434
    of the urinary bladder, *435*–436
Injuries, head. *See also* Injuries, brain
    initial assessment of, 339t–400, *401*
Injuries, hip
    fractures, 232
    groin sprain, 231–232
    hip dislocation, 232

hip joint sprain, 231
    overuse, 230
    pelvis and hip, 232
    synovitis, 230–231
Injuries, knee
    bursitis, *286–289, 287*
    chondral and osteochondral frac-tures, *292–293*
    evaluation of, 242–263
    fractures about the knee, 293–297, *294, 295, 296*
    ligament, 263–271, 265t, 266t, 267t, 268t
    management of, 298–300
    meniscus disorders, *279–286, 281, 282, 283, 284*
    Osgood-Schlatter disease, *289*–290
    patellofemoral disorders, *271–279, 272, 273, 277*
    rehabilitation following, 300–305, 301t, 302t, 304t
Injuries, lower leg
    fractures, 313
    overuse syndromes, 308–313
    soft tissue, 306–308
Injuries, lumbar spine
    fractures, 410
    pars interarticularis defects, 409–*410*
    symptomatic lumbar disc, *409*
Injuries, musculoskeletal, 165–*166*
    causes of, 166–167
    dislocation, 170–171
    examination of, 171–172
    fractures, 168–*170, 169*
    sprains, 171
    and transporting, 176
    treatment of, 172–176, *173, 174, 177*
Injuries, neck
    acute cervical intervertebral disc herniation, 405
    cervical sprain, 405
    cervical strain, 405
    forced lateral deviation of the neck, 405–*406*
    treating severe head injuries as, 410–411
Injuries, pelvic, 229
Injuries, shoulder
    acromioclavicular joint, 196–*197*
    acute trauma, 193–*194*
    acute traumatic tears, 198
    adhesive capsulitis, 202–203
    bicipital tendonitis, 198–199
    brachial plexus traction, 203
    bursitis of the shoulder joint, 199
    chronic repetitive movements, 194
    chronic rotator cuff tears, 198

clavicle fractures, *196*
fractures of the proximal humerus, 202
initial examination of and first aid for, 203–204
pathology and treatment of, *195–203, 196, 197, 200, 201*
recurrent anterior subluxation, 202
rehabilitation after, 204–209, *205, 206, 207, 208*
rotator cuff, 197–198
scapular fractures, 199
shoulder dislocations, 199–202, *200, 201*
sternoclavicular dislocation, *195*–196
Injuries, spinal
cervical spine fractures, 406–408, *407*
to the intervertebral disc, 405
thoracic fractures, 408
Injuries, thigh
contusions, 233
fractures, 235
muscle strains, 234–235
myositis ossificans, *233–234*
soft tissue, 233
Injuries, upper arm, 211–*213*
contusions, 211–213
fractures, *213*
Injuries, upper back
fractures, 408
musculotendinous, 408–409
Injury
diagnostic signs and symptoms of, 36–44
effects of, on body tissues, 133
management of acute, 124
psychological phases of, 113–114
report form, 15
use of protective devices after, 95–96
Injury prevention
by adhesive taping, 47
for physically impaired athletes, 479–480
preseason physical examination for, 12–13
by sports medicine team, 12–13
using protective devices, 95
Insect stings and bites, 542–544
from bees, wasps and ants, 542–543
from scorpions, 543
from spiders, 543–544
Instability (knee), testing for, 249–263
anterolateral/posterolateral rotary, 262–263
anterolateral rotatory, 257–261, *258, 259, 260*

anteromedial/anterolateral, 262
anteromedial/posteromedial rotatory, 263
anteromedial rotatory, 254–257, *255, 256*
genu recurvatum, *254*
posterolateral rotatory, *261–262, 263*
posteromedial rotatory, 262
straight anterior laxity, *250–251*
straight lateral laxity, 253–254
straight medial laxity, 252–253
straight posterior laxity, *251–252*
Instant center analysis, 186, *187*
Insulin, 422
dependent diabetic athlete, 473–474
reaction, 473, 474–475
shock, 474–475
Insurance coverage (for athletes), 14
Intermittent compression, 143
Intestine
large, 417, *418, 419, 420,* 423
small, 417, *418, 419, 420,* 422–423
Intramembranous ossification, 158
Iontophoresis, 141
Iron
deficiency, 470
supplements, 518

J

Jaundice, 441, 522
Jaw-thrust maneuver, 378–*379*
''Jersey finger,'' 221
Jobst Compression Boot, 143
Jobst Cryotemp Unit, 143
Joint, 158–160, *159*
finger, 159
hip, 159, *230*
knee, 164, 236, 263–264, 264–265
shoulder, 189–190
using kinematics data to analyze motion in, 186–188, *187*
Joint flexibility, 119–122, *120, 121*
exercises, *121–122*
in reconditioning, 125–126
Joint play, defined, 142

K

Kenny Howard sling, *197*
Ketoacidosis, diabetic, 474
Kidney, 417, *418,* 432
anatomy, 432
injuries, 434–*435*
stones. *See* Renal colic.
Kinematics, 186–188, *187*
Knee
anatomy, 236–242, *237, 238, 239, 240, 241*

bursitis, *286–289*, *287*
chondral and osteochondral fractures, *292–293*
dislocation, 270–271
football, 270
fractures about the, 293–*297*, *294*, *295*
injuries, evaluation of, 242–*263*, *244*, *247*, *248*, *250*, *251*, *253*, *254*, *255*, *256*, *257*, *258*, *259*, *260*, *261*
injuries, management of, 249, 298–305, 301t, 302t, 304t
instabilities, testing for, 249–*263*, *250*, *251*, *252*, *253*, *254*, *255*, *256*, *257*, *258*, *259*, *260*, *261*
joint, 164, *236*, 263–264, 264–265
joint motion, using kinematics data to analyze, 186–188, *187*
laxity, 249–*263*, 266, 267t, 268–269, 274
ligament injuries, 263–271, *265*t, 266t, 267t, 268t
meniscus disorders, *279–286*, *281*, *282*, *283*, *284*
Osgood-Schlatter disease, *289*–290
osteochondritis dissecans, 290–292
overuse syndrome in women, frequency of, 465
patellofemoral disorders, *271–279*, *272*, *273*, *277*
protection, 99, *100*
Knee taping, 66–70
of hyperextension injury, *69–71*, *70*
of medial collateral ligament (MCL) sprain, *67–69*, *68*
''Knobby knees.'' *See* Osgood-Schlatter disease.
Kyphosis, 400–401

L

Laceration, *151*, 152
of the hand, 226
Lachman drawer test, *250–251*, 257, 261
Lacrosse, protective devices for, 95, 97, 101
Lactic acid system, 116
Language of topographic anatomy, 23–24
Laryngitis, 338
Larynx, *331*
Lateral, defined, 23
Lateral aspect of the knee, *239–240*
Lateral inversion sprains, taping of, *71–73*
Lateral patellar compression syndrome, 274–275

Lateral pivot shift test, *258–259*
Law of valgus, 272–273
Laxity, knee
amount of, with ligament injury, 266, 267t, 268–269
direction of, with ligament injury, 266, 267t
generalized joint, 274
with sprains, 266, 267
testing for, 249–*263*, *250*, *251*, *252*, *253*, *254*, *255*, *256*, *257*, *258*, *260*, *261*
Leg, lower
anatomy, 164–*165*, *306*
fractures, 313
overuse syndromes of, 308–313, *309*, *311*
soft tissue injuries to, 306–308
Legal responsibilities (of sports medicine team), 17–19
Leukocyte count, alterations in, 351–352
Liability
medical malpractice, principles of, 17–18
negligence, general principles of, 17, 19
personal, of athletic trainer, 17
Ligaments, 150, 159
injury to, 183–184
Ligaments, hip, 230
Ligaments, knee, *237–240*, *238*, *239*
and classification of ligament injury, 265–267, 266t, 267t
cruciate, *240–241*
and functional capacity of injured knee, 267–269, 268t
and functional stability of injured knee, 269–271
and ligament injuries, 263–271, *265*t, 266t, 267t, 268t
and mechanisms of ligament injury, 264–265t
Ligaments, shoulder, 189, *190*
Liver, 417, *418*, *419*, *420*, 422
Load deformation curve, *180*
Loads (on bones and joints), 178–188, *180*, *181*, *182*, *183*, *184*, *185*, *186*, *187*
Longitudinal arch, 321, *322*
taping, *75–76*, *77*
Lordosis, 400–401
Louisiana ankle wrap, *49–50*
Lower extremity
anatomy, 30–*33*, *32*, 164–*165*
definition of, 23
protective devices for, *99–100*
taping and strapping techniques, 66–80

Lungs
air flow through, *333–337, 334, 335, 336*
anatomy of, *331*, 332, *452–453*
collapsed, *343, 346–347*, 349
damage to, from chest injuries, 340–345, 346–348, 349
musculoskeletal structures surrounding, 332, *333*
perforation of, by fractured rib, 342, *343*
vital capacity of, 333–334

M

McMurry's test, 246, *247*, 284
''Mallet'' finger, *221*
Manipulative therapy, 142
Manual thrusts, *382–383*
Marine animal injuries, 546–547
Massage, 141–142
ice, 135–136
Mat burns, 488
Mechanical therapy, 133, 135, 141–143, *142*
Medial, defined, 23
Medial aspect (of knee), *237–238*
Medial collateral ligament (MCL) sprain, taping a, *67–69, 68*
Medical insurance, 10
Medical malpractice liability, 17–18
Medical specialists (for sports medicine team), 7
Megadose vitamins, 521–522
Melena, 440
Meniscectomy, 285–286
Menisci
disorders, *279–286, 281, 282, 283, 284*
description of, *279–280*
functions of, 281
gross anatomy of, *279, 280, 281*
lateral meniscus, 280
medial meniscus, 280
and meniscus tears, classification of, *281–285, 282, 283, 284*
Menstruation, 470, 471, 521
Menus (for athletes)
carbohydrate loading, 511t
sample pre-event, 511t
Metabolic shock, 368, 373
Metabolism, 147
Metacarpals, 163, *164*
Metacarpal strapping, 62–63
Metatarsals, 165
Metatarsus valgus, 325
Metatarsus varus, 325
Midline defined, 23

Minerals, 502t, 503, 506–509
sources and functions of, 507t
Modalities (in athletic training), 133–143
cryotherapy, 134, 135–137, 136t
mechanical therapy, 135, 141–143, *142*
penetrating/electrical therapy, 135, 138–*141, 142*
thermotherapy, 134–135, 137–*138*, 136t
types of, 133–135
Modules of elasticity, 182
Molluscum contagiosum, 487–488, *491*, 494t
Mononucleosis, 338
Morton's foot, 325
Morton's neuroma, 326
Motorcycle racing, protective devices for, 101
Mouth, *331*, 420–421
lacerations, 414
Mouthguards, 95, 101
Mouth-to-mouth ventilation, 379–*380*
Mouth-to-nose ventilation, *380*–381
Mouth-to-stoma ventilation, 381
Movement, degree of, as diagnostic sign, 40–41
Movement time, defined, 117
Mucus, 332, 421
Muscle
contraction, *184–185*
control, 116–117
cramps, 308
fiber types, 117
relaxants, 517
response to training, 118
rupture, plantaris, 312
skeletal, 148–*150, 149*
strains, 312
strength, power and endurance, 115–119, *116*, 117t, 119t, 120t, *126–127*
training, periodization of, 118
training, principles of, 117–119
training, in women, 119
training, in youths, 118
training prescription, 117–118, 119t, 120t
Muscles, hip, 230, *231*
Muscles, knee, *237–240, 238, 239*
Muscles, lower leg, 306, *307*
Muscles, shoulder, 189, *190–192, 191*
Muscles, special, 150–151
Muscles, thigh, 232–233
injuries to, 233–235
Muscular spasm, 133
decreasing, with cryotherapy, 134

decreasing, with thermotherapy, 135
Musculoskeletal injuries, 147–177
    causes of, 166–168
    examination of, 171–172
    treatment of, 172–*174, 173*
Myocardial infarction, 357
Myositis ossificans, 233–*234*

N

National Athletic Trainers Association, 5
Nautilus system, 118, 120t, 129, 206
Neck
    anatomy, 25–*26, 405*
    injuries, 405–406
    soft tissue structures of, *405*
Neer's classification, 294, *295*
Negligence liability
    general principles of, 17
    in prescribing drugs, 19
Nerve entrapment, 219
Nerves
    axillary, 200
    cranial, *397*
    in the forearm, *218*
    in the hand and wrist, *220,* 226–227
    in the knee, 238–239
    median, 219
    radial, 212–*213,* 218
    sciatic, 233, 238
    that supply shoulder musculature, 192
    in the thigh, 233
    ulnar, 213–214, 218
    of the upper extremity, 210, 218
Neuritis (foot), 326
    and Morton's neuroma, 326
    and tarsal tunnel syndrome, 326
Neurogenic shock, 367, 372
Neuromuscular system, 117
Neurovascular evaluation, 171–172, 175
    of musculoskeletal injuries, 165–166
Nitrogen narcosis, 538
NOCSAE certification standards (for protective devices), 96, 103–104
Nonvitamins, 506
Nose, *331*
    fractures, 413
Nutrition, 496–515
    and anorexia and bulimia, 514–515
    and caloric balance and weight control, 496–498t, 497t
    and the diabetic athlete, 513–514
    and diet composition during training, 499–500t

and eating before and after events, 509t–510t
and food and drug interactions, 511t–513t, 512t
for strength training, 116
and sugar, 501–502
and vitamins and minerals, 502t–509, 504t, 507t
and water and electrolyte replacement, 500–501

O

Obligatory exercise, 3
Obstruction, airway. *See* Airway obstruction.
One-repetition maximum (1RM), defined, 117, 118
Oral contraceptives, 471, 512
Organs, abdominal, 419
    hollow, *419*
    solid, *419*
Orthoplast, *98, 99, 104, 107*
Osgood-Schlatter disease, 288, *289*–290
Osteochondritis dissecans, 290–292
    clinical presentation of, 291
    pathology of, 291
    treatment of, 291–292
Osteoporosis of disuse, 158
Osteosynthesis, 297
Overdose (of toxic substances), 460
Overuse syndromes, 194, 308–313
    Achilles tendonitis, 310–311
    Achilles tendon rupture, 311
    anterior compartment syndrome, 308–309
    muscle cramps, 308
    muscle strains, 312
    plantaris muscle rupture, 312
    posterior tibial syndrome, *309*–310
    stress fractures, 312–313
Oxygen
    administering, to shock victims, 369
    toxicity, 538

P

Packs
    chemical cold, 136
    flexible gel cold, 136
    hydrocollator, 137–138
    ice, 136
    moist heat, 137–138
Padding, protective
    design and fabrication of, 104–*106, 105*
    maintenance of, 104

for primary contact points, 95, 96, *97–100, 98, 99*
Pain
  as diagnostic sign, 41
  symptoms in knee injuries, 247
Pain-spasm cycle, 133
  breaking, with thermotherapy, 135
  decreasing, with cryotherapy, 134
Pancake thumb strapping, 61
Pancreas, 417, *419, 420,* 421–422
Pancreatitis, 426, 428t, 430
Pangamic acid, 522
Paraffin bath, 138
Paralysis (as diagnostic sign), 40–41
Parents
  legal responsibilities of, 17
  role of, on sports medicine team, 11
Paronychia, 221
Parrot beak tear, 282
Patella, 164, *165, 236, 237,* 271–272, *273*
Patellar dislocation, 276
Patellar subluxation, 275–276
Patellar tendonitis, 275
Patellectomy, 297
Patellofemoral arthralgia, 274
Patellofemoral disorders, 271–279
  anatomy and biomechanics to understand, *271–272, 273*
  extensor mechanism deficiencies, 273–274
  lateral patellar compression syndrome, 274–275
  patellar dislocation, 276
  patellar subluxation, 275–276
  patellar tendonitis, 275
  patellofemoral malalignment, surgery for, 276–279, *277*
Patellofemoral malalignment, surgery for, 276–279
  distal realignment of the extensor mechanism, 278
  lateral retinacular release, *277*
  potential complications of, 278–279
  prognosis for, 279
  proximal realignment, 277–278
Patient assessment, 41–44
  and injury site duties, 43–44
  and primary survey, 41
  and secondary survey, 41–43
  and triage, 43
Pediatrician, role of, on sports medicine team, 9
Pediculosis pubis (crab louse), 493–495
Pelvis, 30, *31,* 163–*164*
  and hip injuries, 232
  injuries of, 229

Penetrating/electrical therapy, 133, 135, 138–*141, 139, 142*
Perfusion, 365–366
Pericardial tamponade, 348–349
Periodization of muscle training, 118
Peristalsis, 423–424
Peritoneum, 417–419, *418,* 427
Peritonitis, 419, 425, 426, 427, 429
Personal liability (of athletic trainer), 18
Phalanges, 163, *164*
Pharyngitis (tonsilitis), 338
Pharynx, *331, 420*–421
Phonophoresis, 140
Physical education, history of, 4
Physically impaired athletes, 478–*480, 479*
Physician-athlete relationship, 18
Physician organizations, list of, 5
Physician-school relationships, 18
Physician-trainer relationship, 8
Pit viper bites, 544–545
Plantar fascia, 326–327
Platelet count, 352
Playing surfaces, evaluation of, 13, 96
Plicae, knee, 241–242
Pneumatic counterpressure device, 369, 370, *371*
Pneumonia, 339
Pneumothorax, *343, 346*
  spontaneous, 346
  tension, 346–*347*
Poiseuille's law, 357–358
Poison control centers, 540, 541
Poisoning, 540–542
  identifying cause of, 540–541
  treatment of, 541–542
Poisons
  definition of, 540
  inhaled, 541
  injected, 541
  plant, 542
  surface (contact), 541–542
  symptoms of, 540
Posterior aspect (of knee), *238–239*
Posterior dislocations (shoulder), *201–202*
Posterior tibial syndrome, *309–310*
Posterolateral rotatory instability, *261–262, 263*
Posteromedial rotatory instability, 262
Prescription drugs, prescribing, 19
Preseason conditioning programs, 13
Preseason physical examination, 12–13, 18–19
Primary survey, 41, *42*
Progressive overload principle, 118
Pronator teres syndrome, 219

Protective acromioclavicular joint
  taping, *51–52*
Protective devices
  for the head and face, 101
  made of silicone rubber, *98, 99*
  other, 101–107
  purpose of, 95
  regulation of, 96, 104
  selecting and fitting, 101–106, *102,
    103*
  special, 106, 107
  for upper and lower extremities,
    97–100
Proteins, 496, 499
Proximal, defined, 23
Proximal finger joint injuries, 222
Psychiatrists, sport, 114
Psychogenic shock, 367, 372
Psychologists, sport, 114
Psychomotor drugs, 520–521
Pulmonary physiology, 452–453
Pulse
  as diagnostic sign, 36–37
  feeling for carotid, *385*
Puncture wound, *151*, 152, *153–154*,
    227
Pupils, dilated, as a diagnostic sign,
    40

Q

Q angle, *272*
Quadriceps tendon, *237*

R

Rabies, 546
Racquetball, protective devices for, 95
Radial deviation assist taping, 59
Radius, *163*
Reconditioning procedures, 124–132
  flexibility in, 125–126
  and functional activity progression,
    131
  and management of acute injury,
    124
  and muscle strength, power and
    endurance, *126–127*
  principles of, 124–125
  and program of exercise, 130–*131*
  and resistive exercises, 127–130,
    128t, *129, 130, 131*
Record keeping (by sports medicine
    team), 14–*16, 15*
Rectum, 417, *419, 420*, 423
Regulations (for protective equip-
    ment), 96, 103, 104
Rehabilitation
  from athlete's perspective, 113, 114

following ankle injuries, 320
following foot injuries, 328
following hand injuries, 227–228
following knee injuries, 300–305
following shoulder injuries,
    204–209, *205, 206, 207, 208*
  and functional activity progression,
    131–132
  plans for, as provided by sports
    medicine team, 14
Reinjury, protecting against, 47, 96
Relief time, defined, 117
Renal colic, 442–443
Repetition (reps), defined, 117
Reproductive system
  and female organs, *433, 434*
  and male organs, *433–434*
  and menstrual cycle, 434
Resistance, defined, 117
Respiration
  determining, in CPR, *379*
  as diagnostic sign, 37
Respiratory shock, 366–367, 372
Respiratory system
  anatomy of, *331–333, 332*
  function of, 331
  infections, 338–339
  pathophysiology, *337*
  physiology of, 333–337, *334, 335,
    336*
Retropatellar pain (in women vs.
    men), 468
Retroperitoneal organs, *418*
Ribs, 161–*162*, *332, 333*
Ringworm, 487, 494t
Roentgenograms (of knee), *248–249*
Rotator cuff, 189, 190, *191*, 192, *193*
  injuries, 197–198
  surgery, rehabilitation following,
    208–209
  tendonitis, 194
Rowing, tenosynovitis and, 219
Runner's knee, 274
Running
  and carbohydrate loading, 509t
  gait, biomechanics of, *323–324*
  and heat stroke, 529
  and overuse syndromes, 306,
    308–313, *309*
  and plasma alterations in runners,
    352

S

Sacrum, 160, 161, 403–404
SAID principle, 115
Salivary glands, *420, 421*

Salt
  tablets, 552
  using, in warm weather, 527–528
Salter-Harris classification, 296, *297*
Scabies, 495
Scalp, 393
Scapula, *162*
School nurse, role of, on sports
    medicine team, 11
Scoliosis, 402
Scorpion bites, 543
Screening exams, 125
Screw-home mechanism, *187, 188,*
    283
Screw home movement, 280, *281*
Secondary amenorrhea, 470–471
Secondary survey, 41–43, *42*
Seizures, 461–462
  epileptic, 460–461
  generalized, 461
  management of, 461–462
  partial, 461
Septic shock, 367, 373
Set, defined, 117
Shin splints, 308
Shock, 365–373
  anaphylactic, 368, 373, 454, 543
  cardiogenic, 367, 372, 449
  care and treatment of, 369–373, *371*
  electric, 460
  hemorrhagic, 366, 370–372
  hypovolemic, 440, 528–529
  insulin, 474–475
  metabolic, 368, 373, 439, 440
  neurogenic, 367, 372
  psychogenic, 367, 372
  respiratory, 366–367, 372
  septic, 367, 373
  with severe soft tissue injuries, 152
  signs and symptoms of, 341,
    368–369
  types and causes of, 366–368
Shortness of breath. *See* Dyspnea.
Shoulder, 189–209
  anatomy, *33, 162*–163, *189*
  biomechanics of, 192–193
  dislocations, 193–194, *195*–196,
    199–202, *200, 201*
  dislocations, taping, 53–55, *54*
  girdle, *33, 162*–163
  injuries, causes of, *193*–194
  injuries, first aid following, 203–204
  injuries, pathology and treatment
    of, *195*–203, *196, 197, 200, 201*
  injuries, rehabilitation following,
    204–209, *205, 206, 207, 208*
  injuries, shoulder point, *196*–197
  joints, 189–*190*
  motion, 191–*192*
  muscles, *190–191*
  nerves and circulation, 192–*193*
  pads, *97*–98, 104
  pain, evaluating, 204
  pain in women vs. men, 468–469
  protective devices for, *97*–98, 104
  strappings, *51*–55, *52, 54*
Skeletal system, 155–*165, 156, 157,*
    158, 159, 160, 161, 162, 163, 164
Skeleton
  knee, *236–237*
  shoulder, *189*
  upper arm and elbow, 209–*210*
Skiing
  and carbohydrate loading, 509t,
    511t
  and gamekeeper's thumb, *223*
  and tibial fractures, 167
Skin, 147–*148*
  color (as diagnostic sign), 39
  injuries, 226–*227*
  irritants, 541, 542
Skull, 158, 160, 161, 393–*394*
  fractures, 394, *395*
Sling
  Kenny Howard, *197*
  wrap, 89, *90*
Slocum anterolateral rotatory in-
    stability test, 257
Slocum external rotation test, *255*–256
Snakebites, 544–546
  from coral snakes, 545–546
  from pit vipers, 544
Soccer
  protective devices for, 100
  and soft tissue injuries (lower leg),
    306–307
  and stress fractures, 312–313
Soft tissue, 147–151, *148, 149, 150. See
    also* Soft tissue injuries.
  failure under loading, 182–*184, 183*
Soft tissue injuries, 151–154, *153*
  dressings and bandages for,
    154–155
  to the foot, 326–327
  to the lower leg, 306–308
  to the male and female genitalia,
    436–437
  to the thigh muscles, 233
Sphygmomanometer, *38*
Spica thumb taping, 59–*60*
Spica wraps, 85–*92, 87, 88, 89, 90, 91*
Spider bites, 543–544
Spinal column, 160–*161*
Spinal cord, *404*
  injury, 40–41
  lack of protective equipment for, 410

Spine, *393*
    anatomy of, 160–*161*
    cervical fractures of, 406–408, *407*
    curvature of, 400–*402*
Spiral wrap, *82, 83*
Spleen, 417, *418, 419,* 424
Splinters, 153–154
Splinting
    benefits of, 172
    diving injuries, 411
    fractures to combat shock, 369–370, *371*
    rules of, 173
    spine-injured victims, 411
Splints
    air, 152, *153,* 175
    to control hemorrhage, 362, *363*
    rigid, 174–175
    soft, 175
    Thomas, 175
    traction, 175–176
    types of, *173,* 174
Spondylolysis, 468, *469*
Sports Equipment Facilities Committee of ASTM, 96
Sports medicine
    goal of, 7
    organizations, list of 5–6
    pioneers in, 3–5
    program, organizing a, 12–19
    team, responsibilities of, 7–11
Sprains
    ankle, 316, 317, 319
    back, 409
    cervical, 405
    definition of, 150, 166, *167*
    elbow, 216
    foot, 327
    hip joint, 231
    knee, 265–266t
    lateral inversion, taping, *71–74, 72, 73*
    signs of, 171
    splinting, 172–174
''Squeeze'' injuries, 537
Stability (of knee joint), 263–264
    functional, 269–271
Stabilizing A-C joint straps, 89, *90, 91*
Standard anatomic position, 23
Status epilepticus, 461
Sternoclavicular joint, 158
    dislocations, *195–196*
Sternum, 161–*162*
Steroids, anabolic, 521
Stethoscope, *38–39*
Stimulants, 520, 523
''Stinger'' injury, *406*
Stings, 542–543

Stomach, 417, *418, 419, 420,* 421
Stone bruise, 327
Straight anterior laxity, *250–251*
Straight lateral laxity, 253–254
Straight medial laxity, *252–253*
Straight posterior laxity, 251–*252*
Strains
    cervical, 405
    definition of, 166, 181
    elbow, 214–215
    groin, 231–232
    hamstring, 234–235
    lower leg, 312
    musculotendinous, 409
Strappings. *See also* Taping.
    hand, 61–63, *62*
    shoulder, *51–55, 52, 53, 54*
Strep throat, 518
Streptococcal bacterial infection, 338
Stress, defined, 180–181
Stress fractures (in women vs. men), 469
Stress-strain curve, 180, *181–182*
Stroke, 456, 457t, 458–459
    heat, 529–530
Student trainer, role of, on sports medicine team, 11
Subcutaneous emphysema, 348
Subluxation
    patellar, 275–276
    recurrent anterior, 202
Subungual hematomas, 220
Sucking chest wounds, 344, *345,* 347–348
Sugar (in diet), 501–502
Superior end, defined, 23
Supportive pads, *79–80*
Surgery, arthroscopic, 285
Swathe wrap, 89, *90*
Sweating, 500–501, 526–528
Swelling (in knee injuries), 247–248
Swimming, carbohydrate loading and, 509t, 511t
Synovial fluid, 160
Synovitis (of the hip), 230
Systolic blood pressure, defined, 38

T

Tailor's bunion, 325
Talus, *165, 314, 321*
Taping. *See also* Strapping.
    Achilles tendon, *74–75*
    adhesive, *47–48*
    ankle, *71–74, 72, 73*
    and bandaging, introduction to, 47–50
    budding, 63–65

elbow hyperextension, *55–56*
finger, *63–65*
great toe, *76–78, 77*
knee, *66–71, 67, 68, 69, 70*
longitudinal arch, *75–76, 77*
lower extremity, 66–80
shoulder dislocation, *53–54*
and supportive pads, *79–80*
thumb, 59–61, *60*
upper extremity, 51–65
wrist, *56–59, 57, 58*
Tarsal bones, 165
Tarsal tunnel syndrome, 326
Team approach (to sports medicine),
  7–11
Team physician
  legal responsibilities of, 17–18
  role of, on sports medicine team,
    9–10
Tears, meniscus, 281–285
  acute, 282–283
  bucket handle, 283, 284, 285
  classification of, 281–285, *282, 283,
    284*
  chronic, 282
  diagnosis of, 283–285
  discoid meniscus, *283*
  horizontal, 282
  longitudinal, 281
  parrot beak, 282
  posterior horn, 284
  treatment of, 285–286
Teeth injuries, 414
Temperature (as diagnostic sign), 39
Tendonitis
  Achilles, 79, 310–311
  bicipital, 198–199
  patellar, 275
Tendons, 150
  in the hand, *219, 227*
Tennis
  "elbow," 215
  and injury to the median curve, 219
  "leg," 312
Tenosynovitis (in wrist), 219
TENS (transcutaneous electrical nerve
    stimulation), 141, *142*
Testicle, undescended, 436
Therapy
  contrast, 136
  cryotherapy, 133, 134t–137
  manipulative, 142
  mechanical, 135, 141–143, *142*
  penetrating/electrical, 133, 135,
    138–141, *139, 142*
  thermotherapy, 133, 134t–135,
    137–*138*

Thigh, 232–235, *234*
  anatomy, 232–233
  injuries, 233–235
Thompson test, *311*
Thorax, 26–28, *27*, 161–*162*
Thumb. *See also* Hand.
  checkrains, 60–61
  injuries, 223–224
  pancake strapping of, 61
  spica taping of, 59–*60*
Tibia, 164–*165*, 306
Tinea versicolor, 487, *490*, 494t
Tissue, soft. *See* Soft tissue.
Toes. *See* Foot.
Tonsilitis (pharyngitis), 338
Torque, moment of, defined, 178
Tourniquets, 362–364
Tachea, *331–332*
Traction, *142*, 143
  goals of, in the field, 173–*174*
  to reduce shoulder dislocations,
    200, 201
  splints, 175–176, *177*
Trainer
  relationship of, with athlete,
    111–114
  role of, in patient assessment,
    41–44
Training. *See also* Exercise.
  aerobic, 360
  anaerobic, 360
  athletic, modalities in, 133–143
  and conditioning, 115–132
  diet composition during, 499–500t
  during hot weather, 530–532
  muscle, periodization of, 118
  muscle, principles of, 117–119t,
    120t
  muscle, in women, 119
  muscle, in youth, 118
  muscle response to, 118
  strength, for shoulder muscles,
    206–*207, 208*
Transportation
  for head or spine injured athletes,
    410–411
  for musculoskeletal injuries, 176
Transverse arch (foot), 321, *322*
Trench (or immersion) foot, 534
Triage, 9, 43
Triceps, *160*
Turf toe, 327

U

Ulna, *163*
Ulnar deviation assist taping, 59
Ulnar nerve, 213–214

Ultrasound therapy, *139*–140
Ultraviolet lamps, 138
Unconsciousness
    causes of, 456–460, 457t, *458*
    in the diabetic, 474–475
    emergency care following, 43, 375, 382, 456
    and epilepsy, 460–462
Universal gym, 118, 119t, 206–*207*, *208*
Upper extremity, 189–228
    anatomy, *34–35, 162–163, 164, 189–191, 209–211, 210,* 219–*220*
    definition of, 23
    protective devices for, *97–98*
    taping, *51–65, 52, 53, 54, 55, 56, 57, 58, 60, 61, 62*
Ureters, *432*
Urethra, *433*
Urethral discharge, 442
Urinary bladder
    anatomy of, *433*
    injuries, 435–436
Urinary system, *432–433*

V

Vaginitis, 471
Veins, pulmonary, 332, *333*
Ventilation, artificial. *See* Artificial ventilation.
Vertebrae, 160–161, 402–404, *403*
Vertebral column, 400–405
    anatomy, 400, 402–404, *403*
    and the autonomic nervous system, 404–405
    curves of, 400–*402, 403*
    and the spinal cord, *404*
    vertebrae of, 160–161, 402–404, *403*
Vital capacity, 333–334
Vitamins, 502t–506, 504t
    megadose, 521–522
    and nonvitamins, 506
    sources and functions of, 504t
Volkmann's contracture, *217,* 218
Volleyball, fracture-dislocations of the ankle and, 319
Vomiting, 438–439

W

Warts, 488, *491,* 494t
Wasp stings, 542–543
Water
    loss, 527–528
    replacement, 500

Water on the knee, 160
Weight
    control, 496–499, 497t
    gain, 498–499
    loss, 498
Wheel chair sports, 480
Whirlpool bath, 137
Wolff's law, 158
Women athletes, 465–472
    anatomic and physiologic sex differences of, *465–467*
    common medical problems of, 470–472
    common orthopedic problems of, 468–470, *469*
    conditioning and rehabilitation of, 467–468
    muscle training for, 119
    psychological adjustment of, 467
Wounds
    blunt abdominal, 430t
    closed soft tissue, *151,* 152
    gunshot, 334–345
    open soft tissue, 152–*154, 153*
    penetrating, 344–*345,* 430t, 431
    penetrating abdominal, 429
    stab, 341, 344
    sucking chest, 344, *345,* 347–348
Wraps. *See also* Elastic bandaging.
    cotton, 49–*50*
    figure-of-eight, *83–85, 84, 86*
    foot/ankle pressure, 89, *91–92*
    4-S, 88–89, *90*
    Louisiana ankle, 49–*50*
    spica, 85–*92, 87, 88, 89, 90, 91*
    spiral, *82, 83*
Wrestling
    and gamekeeper's thumb, *223*
    and heat stroke, 529
    protective devices for, 99
Wrist
    bands, 56
    bony anatomy of, 219
    nerves, 226
    taping, 56–59, *57, 58*

X

Xiphoid process, avoiding, during CPR, *385*
X-ray, weighted shoulder, 196–197

Y

Young's modulus, 182

FIGURE CREDITS AND PERMISSIONS

Figures 17:1 (p. 180), **17:2** (p. 181), **17:3** (p. 181), **17:4** (p. 182), **17:5** (p. 182), **17:7** (p. 184), **17:8** (p. 184), **17:9** (p. 185), **17:10** (p. 185), **17:11** (p. 186), **17:12** (p. 187), **17:13** (p. 187): Frankel, V.H., Nordin, M. *Basic Biomechanics of the Skeletal System* (Philadelphia: Lea and Febiger, 1980).

Figure 17:6 (p. 183): Frankel, V.H., Nordin, M. *Basic Biomechanics of the Skeletal System* (Philadephia: Lea and Febiger, 1980), Figure 3-5 courtesy of Frank R. Noyes, M.D. and Edward S. Grood, Ph.D.

Figure 17:14 (p. 187): Frankel, V.H., Nordin, M. *Basic Biomechanics of the Skeletal System* (Philadelphia: Lea and Febiger, 1980), Figure 4-9B adapted from A. Helfet, *Disorders of the Knee* (Philadelphia: J.B. Lippincott and Co., 1974).

Figures 18:34 (p. 225) and **18:35** (p. 226): Weeks, Paul M.: Acute bone and joint injuries of the hand and wrist, St. Louis, 1981, The C. V. Mosby Co.

Figure 21:14 (p. 248): Ogden, John A.: Skeletal Injury in the Child. Lea & Febiger, Philadelphia, 1982.

Figure 21:43 (p. 292): O'Donoghue, Don H.: Treatment of acute dislocations of the patella. In American Academy of Orthopaedic Surgeons: Symposium on the athlete's knee, St. Louis, 1980, The C. V. Mosby Co.

Figure 25:6B (p. 334): Vander et al., *Human physiology: The mechanisms of body function* (New York: McGraw-Hill, 1980). Reprinted by permission.

Figure 25:8 (p. 336): Vander et al., *Human physiology: The mechanisms of body function* (New York: McGraw-Hill, 1980), fig. 12:18. Reprinted by permission.

Figure 25:9 (p. 336): Vander et al., *Human physiology: The mechanisms of body function* (New York: McGraw-Hill, 1980). Reprinted by permission.

Table 27:1 (p. 352): Price, Sylvia Anderson and Wilson, Lorraine McCarty, *Pathophysiology: Clinical Concepts of Disease Processes* (New York: McGraw-Hill, 1978). Reprinted by permission.

Figure 28:1 (p. 353): Modified from Vinsant, Marielle Ortiz, Spence, Martha I., and Hagen, Dianne Chapell: A commonsense approach to coronary care, ed. 2, St. Louis, 1975, The C. V. Mosby Co.

Figure 28:3 (p. 355): *(left)* from Jules Constant, *Learning Electrocardiography*, page 3. Copyright © 1973 by Jules Constant. Reprinted by permission of Little, Brown and Co. *(right)* reproduced, with permission, from Ganong WF: *Review of Medical Physiology*, 11th ed. Copyright 1983 by Lange Medical Publications, Los Altos, California.

Figure 28:4 (p. 356): Reproduced, with permission, from Ganong WF: *Review of Medical Physiology*, 11th ed. Copyright 1983 by Lange Medical Publications, Los Altos, California.

Figure 28:5 (p. 357): Price, Sylvia Anderson and Wilson, Lorraine McCarty, *Pathophysiology: Clinical Concepts of Disease Processes* (New York: McGraw-Hill, 1978). Reprinted by permission.

Figure 42:2 (p. 467): AP/Wide World Photos, Inc.

Figure 42:3 (p. 469): Kevin Fitzgerald, Focus on Sports, Inc.

Figure 45:1 (p. 479): C. Ursillo, Leo deWys, Inc.

Figure 45:2 (p. 480): R. Nedlin, Leo deWys, Inc.

Figure 47:1 through 47:15 (pp. 489–92), courtesy of Dr. Wilma F. Bergfeld, Department of Dermatology and Pathology, Cleveland Clinic Foundation.

Table 48:1 (p. 497): Jack H. Wilmore, "Body Composition and Athletic Performance," in *Nutrition and Athletic Performance*, edited by William Haskell, James Skala, and James Whittam (Palo Alto, Calif.: Bull Pub. Co., 1981). Reprinted by permission.

Table 48:2 (p. 498): S. H. Short and W. R. Short, "Four-year study of university athletes' dietary intake." Copyright The American Dietetic Association. Reprinted by permission from *Journal of the American Dietetic Association*, vol. 82:632, 1983.

Table 48:4 (pp. 502–3): R. G. Hansen and B. W. Wyse, "Expression of nutrient allowances per 1000 kilocalories." Copyright The American Dietetic Association. Reprinted by permission from *Journal of the American Dietetic Association*, vol. 76:223, 1980.

Table 48:5 (pp. 504–5) and **48:6** (pp. 507–8): Reprinted with permission of Macmillan Publishing Company from *Normal and Therapeutic Nutrition*, 16th ed. by Corinne H. Robinson and Marilyn R. Lawler. Copyright © 1982 by Macmillan Publishing Co., Inc.

Table 48:7 (p. 509): Adapted by special permission from Melvin Williams, *Nutrition for Fitness and Sport* (Dubuque, Iowa: Wm. C. Brown), p. 35.

Table 48:13 (p. 513): Adapted from "Caffeine Content of Beverages," *Handbook of Clinical Dietetics* by the American Dietetic Association (New Haven: Yale University Press), p. 149. Reprinted by permission.